# Most Commons in
Surgery

# Most Commons in
## Surgery

■ **Edward F. Goljan, MD**
Professor and Chairman of Pathology
Oklahoma State University
College of Osteopathic Medicine
Tulsa, Oklahoma

■ **Paul Peter Koro, DO, FACOS**
Senior Associate Dean for Academic Affairs
Oklahoma State University
College of Osteopathic Medicine
Tulsa, Oklahoma

**W.B. SAUNDERS COMPANY**
*A Harcourt Health Sciences Company*
Philadelphia ■ London ■ New York ■ St. Louis ■ Sydney ■ Toronto

**W.B. SAUNDERS COMPANY**
*A Harcourt Health Sciences Company*

The Curtis Center
Independence Square West
Philadelphia, Pennsylvania 19106

**Library of Congress Cataloging-in-Publication Data**

Goljan, Edward F.
  Most commons in surgery/Edward F. Goljan, Paul Peter Koro

p.; cm.

ISBN 0–7216–9291–5

1. Surgery.    2. Surgery, Operative.    I. Koro, Paul Peter.    II. Title.
  [DNLM: 1. Surgical Procedures, Operative.    WO 500 G626m 2001]

RD31.G64 2001      617–dc21                                    2001020285

*Acquisitions Editor:* William Schmitt
*Project Manager:* Edna Dick
*Production Manager:* Guy Barber
*Illustration Specialist:* Robert Quinn

MOST COMMONS IN SURGERY                    ISBN 0–7216–9291–5

Printed in the United States of America.

Last digit is the print number:    9   8   7   6   5   4   3   2   1

*This book is dedicated to our lovely spouses, Joyce and Margaret. When the 10th verse in Proverbs 31 poses the question "a wife of noble character who can find?" and then continues in verse 12 to state that "she brings [her husband] good, not harm, all the days of her life," we believe that these verses written by King Solomon centuries ago must have had our soulmates in mind.*

# ■ PREFACE

*Most Commons in Surgery* is the third book in the *Most Commons* series. The series thus far includes *Most Commons in Pathology and Laboratory Medicine* and *Most Commons in Medicine*.

In the authors' opinion, there are very few review books that specifically target third- and fourth-year medical students who are rotating through surgery and the surgical subspecialties. *Most Commons in Surgery* provides the student physician with an overview of the key concepts emphasized during clinical rotations in surgery and the factual information that is most often asked on in-service exams as well as on the USMLE and COMLEX Step 2 and 3 exams.

*Most Commons in Surgery* covers such topics as fluid and acid-base disorders, perioperative and postoperative care, critical care issues, surgical oncology, surgical hematology, organ-specific surgery, and selected topics in neurosurgery, orthopedics, and urology. The material is arranged in a table format, with a *Most Common. . .* column on the left and an *Answer and Explanation* column on the right. The most common causes of a condition, its signs/symptoms, and other information in the left column is followed by a concise answer and explanation in the right column. The leading cause/sign and other information is always highlighted in **bold letters**, while less common causes/signs and the like are in *italics*. When there is no clear-cut leading cause/sign, or the like, all the answers are presented in *italics*. Every aspect of a condition, disease, or topic is covered, including pathogenesis, signs/symptoms, complications, laboratory diagnosis, and management. A review question and discussion follows every table. In most cases, the question has a multiple-answer type format (e.g., SELECT 3 ANSWERS), similar to those currently used on the USMLE Step 2 and 3 exams. An extensive index cross-references items that may be present in different tables and chapters. The book is pocket-sized, which makes it useful for quick reference. Since the feedback from medical students from here and abroad has been outstanding for the previous *Most Commons* books, we believe that *Most Commons in Surgery* will enjoy the same enthusiastic reception.

*EDWARD F. GOLJAN, MD*

# NOTICE

Surgery is an ever-changing field. Standard safety precautions must be followed, but as new research and clinical experience broaden our knowledge, changes in treatment and drug therapy may become necessary or appropriate. Readers are advised to check the most current product information provided by the manufacturer of each drug to be administered to verify the recommended dose, the method and duration of administration, and the contraindications. It is the responsibility of the treating physician, relying on experience and knowledge of the patient, to determine dosages and the best treatment for each individual patient. Neither the Publisher nor the editor assume any liability for any injury and/or damage to persons or property arising from this publication.

THE PUBLISHER

# ■ CONTENTS

# CHAPTER

## 1

# PULMONARY FUNCTION, ACID-BASE, AND VOLUME AND ELECTROLYTE DISORDERS

## CONTENTS

### Table 1–1. EVALUATION OF PULMONARY FUNCTION AND PULMONARY DISEASE

| Most Common... | Answer and Explanation |
|---|---|
| method of evaluating oxygenation/ ventilation | **arterial blood gases** (ABGs) (see Table 1–2) |
| method of measuring lung volumes/ capacities | **spirometry** |
| volumes/capacities not directly measured by spirometry | • **RV**—volume remaining after maximal expiration, • **TLC**— * amount of air in a fully expanded lung, * measured with a nitrogen or helium dilution method, • **FRC**— * total amount of air in the lungs at the end of a normal expiration (end of the TV), * obtained by a helium dilution technique or body plethysmography, normal FRC is 2–3 liters |
| outpatient method of evaluating forced vital capacity (FVC) | **peak expiratory flow meter**—the FVC is the total amount of air that is expelled after a maximal inspiration: ~5 liters |
| method of measuring RV | **calculated as follows: RV = functional residual capacity (FRC) − expiratory reserve volume (ERV)**— * ERV is the amount of air that is forcibly expelled at the end of a normal expiration (end of TV), * FRC: * see above definition, * FRC = ERV + RV |

*Table continued on following page*

1

**Table 1–1. EVALUATION OF PULMONARY FUNCTION
AND PULMONARY DISEASE** *Continued*

| Most Common... | Answer and Explanation |
|---|---|
| method of measuring diffusion of oxygen through the alveolar/capillary interface | **DL$_{CO}$**—diffusion capacity (DL) using carbon monoxide (CO) |
| factors affecting the DL$_{CO}$ | • **CO must reach the alveoli**—DL$_{CO}$ is decreased if the airways are blocked (e.g., foreign body) or collapsed (e.g., atelectasis), • **CO must cross alveolar/capillary interface**—DL$_{CO}$ is decreased in the presence of pulmonary fibrosis (e.g., sarcoidosis), pulmonary edema, removal of an entire lung, • **CO must bind to Hgb in RBCs**— * binding to Hgb depends on the pulmonary capillary blood volume, * DL$_{CO}$ is decreased if there is decreased perfusion (e.g., PE), loss of the capillary bed (e.g., COPD), low Hgb (anemia) |
| causes of an increased DL$_{CO}$ | • **pulmonary congestion**—increases the pulmonary capillary blood volume (more Hgb to bind to), • **air trapping**—increases the overall cross-sectional area of the lungs (e.g., bronchial asthma) |
| effect of restrictive lung disease on compliance/elasticity | • **compliance is decreased**— * lungs cannot fully expand with air due to fibrosis, * analogous to trying to blow up a thick rubber hot water bottle with air, • **elasticity is increased**—increased lung recoil on expiration due to interstitial fibrosis [**Note:** examples of restrictive lung disease include sarcoidosis, silicosis, and mesothelioma.] |
| effect of restrictive lung disease on PFTs | • **all lung volumes and capacities are equally reduced**—due to the decrease in compliance, • **decreased FEV$_{1sec}$**— * refers to the amount of air expelled in 1 sec after maximal inspiration, * normal FEV$_{1sec}$ is 4 liters, * patients with restrictive disease have values <3 liters, • **decreased FVC**—patients with restrictive disease usually have values <4 liters, • **FEV$_{1sec}$/FVC ratio increased**— * increased lung elasticity results in similar values for FEV$_{1sec}$ and FVC, * most of the air is expelled in 1 sec, hence FEV$_{1sec}$ ≈ FVC |

### Table 1–1. EVALUATION OF PULMONARY FUNCTION AND PULMONARY DISEASE *Continued*

| Most Common... | Answer and Explanation |
| --- | --- |
| effect of obstructive lung disease on compliance/elasticity | • **compliance is increased**— * the lungs fill easily with air since elastic tissue support is destroyed, * analogous to blowing up an overstretched rubber balloon, • **elasticity is decreased**— * due to destruction of elastic tissue, * airways collapse on expiration and trap the air, * lungs are constantly hyperinflated [**Note:** examples of obstructive lung disease include emphysema, asthma.] |
| effect of obstructive lung disease on PFTs | • **RV is increased**—air is trapped in the small airways on expiration, • **TLC is increased**— * due to increased RV, * lungs are hyperinflated and increase the AP diameter and depress the diaphragms, • **other volumes/capacities are decreased**— * the increase in RV eventually reduces all the other volumes/capacities, * analogous to a garbage compactor, • **FEV$_{1sec}$, FVC, and FEV$_{1sec}$/FVC ratio are all decreased**— * the reduction in these parameters is much greater than in restrictive disease, * e.g., FEV$_{1sec}$ in restrictive disease = 3 liters (normal 4 liters) compared with 1 liter in obstructive disease |
| formula used to calculate A–a gradient | **PAO$_2$ = % O$_2$ (713) − PaCO$_2$/0.8, where PAO$_2$ is alveolar O$_2$, % O$_2$ is the % O$_2$ the patient is breathing, PaCO$_2$ is the arterial PCO$_2$, and 0.8 is the respiratory quotient** [Note: the *A*lveolar O$_2$ never equals *a*rterial PO$_2$ owing to ventilation and perfusion mismatches in the lungs (best match is in the lower lobes). The difference between the PAO$_2$ and PaO$_2$ is called the A–a gradient. Using normal values, the PAO$_2$ is calculated as follows: PAO$_2$ = 0.21 (713) − 40/0.8 = 100 mm Hg. If the patient is on a respirator, use the % oxygen the patient is breathing in the formula: e.g., **0.30** (713) − PaCO$_2$/0.8. The A–a gradient is obtained by subtracting the PaO$_2$ from the PAO$_2$. A medically significant A–a gradient is ≥ 30 mm Hg.] |

*Table continued on following page*

## Table 1–1. EVALUATION OF PULMONARY FUNCTION AND PULMONARY DISEASE *Continued*

| Most Common... | Answer and Explanation |
|---|---|
| causes of an increased A–a gradient | • **perfusion without ventilation**— * this produces intrapulmonary shunting, * e.g., postoperative atelectasis, ARDS, • *ventilation without perfusion*— * this increases dead space, * e.g., PE, • *diffusion abnormalities*— * $O_2$ exchange problems at alveolar/capillary interface, * e.g., interstitial fibrosis, pulmonary edema, • *right to left cardiac shunting*— * unoxygenated blood from the right heart enters the left heart, * e.g., tetralogy of Fallot |
| effect of breathing 100% $O_2$ on $PaO_2$ when there is perfusion without ventilation | **$PaO_2$ does not significantly increase**— * this defines the presence of intrapulmonary shunting, * collapse of the respiratory unit (respiratory bronchioles, alveolar duct, alveoli) reduces the amount of $O_2$ available for uptake by the capillaries |
| treatment modality for ventilation defects | **PEEP therapy**—positive end-expiratory pressure (PEEP) therapy provides positive pressure that keeps the airways open on expiration, which allows gas exchange |
| effect of breathing 100% $O_2$ on $PaO_2$ when there is ventilation but no perfusion | **$PaO_2$ increases**—delivery of 100% $O_2$ to areas of lung that are perfused compensates for areas of lung that are not perfused |
| causes of hypoxemia with a normal A–a gradient | • **depression of the medullary respiratory center**—e.g., * barbiturates, * CNS injury, • *chest bellows dysfunction*—e.g., * paralyzed diaphragm, * flail chest [**Note:** hypoxemia in the presence of a normal A–a gradient indicates that hypoxemia must be extrapulmonary in origin.] |

## Table 1–1. EVALUATION OF PULMONARY FUNCTION AND PULMONARY DISEASE *Continued*

| Most Common... | Answer and Explanation |
|---|---|
| uses of a chest x-ray | • **detects parenchymal, vascular, pleural space disease**—e.g., * atelectasis, * PH, * pleural effusions, • *defines rib cage/diaphragmatic abnormalities*—e.g., diaphragmatic hernia, • *evaluates cardiac size and chamber contours* |
| uses of pulmonary CT | • **detects pleural effusions/pleural thickening,** • **fine definition of pulmonary lesions**—e.g., calcification in solitary nodules, • **staging primary lung cancer**—identification of hilar/mediastinal lymph nodes [**Note:** spiral CT, though expensive, is fast becoming the diagnostic test of choice for lung disease, e.g., pulmonary embolism.] |
| uses of pulmonary cytology | • **sputum cytology is the gold standard for Dx of primary lung cancer**—most sensitive in centrally located cancers (sensitivity ~65%), • **pleural fluid cytology**—sensitivity ~60% in Dx of malignant pleural effusions |
| use of a Gram stain of sputum | **ancillary screen for pneumonia**— * in the past, the sputum Gram stain was the gold standard as the initial screen for pneumonia, * chest x-ray is now the gold standard for screening for pneumonia |
| uses of bronchoscopy | • **evaluation of airway disorders,** • **Dx/staging of cancer,** • **work-up of hemoptysis,** • **obtain material for culture/cytology**—e.g., bronchoalveolar lavage, • *remove foreign bodies* |

*Table continued on following page*

## Table 1–1. EVALUATION OF PULMONARY FUNCTION AND PULMONARY DISEASE *Continued*

**Question:** A 68-yr-old man with chronic lung disease from smoking presents with a recent history of cough, weight loss, and radiographic evidence of a centrally located mass on a chest x-ray. Which of the following laboratory test findings are expected in this patient? **SELECT 3**

(A) Decreased RV
(B) Decreased $FEV_{1sec}$/FVC ratio
(C) Normal A–a gradient
(D) Benign sputum cytology
(E) Increased FRC
(F) Hypoxemia

**Answer: (B), (E), (F):** The patient has COPD caused by smoking. He will most likely have an increased RV due to trapping of air behind collapsed airways **(choice A is incorrect).** The $FEV_{1sec}$/FVC ratio will most likely be decreased owing to a reduction in both the $FEV_{1sec}$ and FVC from decreased pulmonary elasticity **(choice B is correct).** The A–a gradient will most likely be increased owing to ventilation and perfusion defects in the lungs **(choice C is incorrect).** With the history of cough, weight loss, and a centrally located mass, the sputum cytology will most likely uncover either malignant squamous cells or the small hyperchromatic cells of a small cell carcinoma **(choice D is incorrect).** The FRC will most likely be increased owing to an increase in RV (FRC = ERV + RV, **choice E is correct).** Hypoxemia is inevitable in a patient with COPD **(choice F is correct).**

A–a = Alveolar–arterial gradient, COPD = chronic obstructive pulmonary disease, $DL_{CO}$ = diffusion capacity using carbon monoxide, Dx = diagnosis, ERV = expiratory reserve volume, $FEV_{1sec}$ = forced expiratory volume 1 second, FRC = functional residual capacity, FVC = forced vital capacity, $PaCO_2$ = arterial $PCO_2$, $PAO_2$ = alveolar $PO_2$, PE = pulmonary embolus, PFTs = pulmonary function tests, PH = pulmonary hypertension, RV = residual volume, TLC = total lung capacity, TV = tidal volume.

## Table 1–2. ACID-BASE DISORDERS

| Most Common... | Answer and Explanation |
|---|---|
| ABG components that are directly measured | • pH, • $PaCO_2$, • $PaO_2$ [Note: $SaO_2$, $O_2$ content, $HCO_3^-$, base excess/deficit are all calculated.] |

## Table 1–2. ACID-BASE DISORDERS *Continued*

| Most Common... | Answer and Explanation |
|---|---|
| disorders with a normal $PaO_2$ but low $SaO_2$ | • **carbon monoxide (CO) poisoning**— * CO attaches to heme on Hgb in RBCs, hence reducing the $SaO_2$ of the 4 heme groups in Hgb, * the $PaO_2$ is normal because CO does not inhibit normal gas exchange between the alveoli and plasma in pulmonary capillaries, * 100% $O_2$ is the Rx of choice • *methemoglobinemia*— * methemoglobin refers to heme iron in the ferric rather than ferrous condition, * iron in the ferric condition cannot bind $O_2$, hence the $SaO_2$ is decreased, * intravenous methylene blue is the Rx of choice, * ascorbic acid, a reducing agent, is an ancillary Rx |
| noninvasive method for measuring $SaO_2$ | **pulse oximeter**—dependent on: * rate of blood flow (e.g., vasoconstriction alters readings), * position of the ODC, * type of Hgb (e.g., cannot detect carboxyhemoglobin) |
| acid-base disorders | • **respiratory acidosis**—$PaCO_2 > 45$ mm Hg, • *respiratory alkalosis*—$PaCO_2 < 33$ mm Hg, • *metabolic acidosis*—$HCO_3^- < 22$ mEq/L, • *metabolic alkalosis*—$HCO_3^- > 28$ mEq/L |
| term applied when two or more primary ABG disorders occur simultaneously | **mixed ABG disorders**—the most common mixed disorder is a cardiorespiratory arrest combining respiratory acidosis (no ventilation) and metabolic acidosis (lactic acidosis from tissue hypoxia) |
| clues suggesting a mixed ABG disorder | • **Hx and physical exam**—know what ABGs to expect based on the Hx and physical exam, • *normal pH*— * a normal pH defines full compensation, which rarely occurs with a single acid-base disorder, * compensation brings pH close to but not into the normal range, • *exaggerated increase in arterial pH*— * this represents a combined respiratory and metabolic alkalosis, * e.g., patient with anxiety (respiratory alkalosis) who is vomiting (metabolic alkalosis), • *exaggerated decrease in arterial pH*— * this represents a combined metabolic and respiratory acidosis, * e.g., cardiorespiratory arrest: no ventilation (respiratory acidosis) and no perfusion (e.g., lactic acidosis), • *formulas*—see Table 6–2 in MOST COMMONS IN MEDICINE for formulas that calculate the expected value for the compensation |

*Table continued on following page*

**Table 1–2. ACID-BASE DISORDERS** *Continued*

| Most Common... | Answer and Explanation |
|---|---|
| compensation for respiratory acidosis | **metabolic alkalosis**— * retention of $HCO_3^-$ to produce a compensatory metabolic alkalosis requires renal reclamation and regeneration of $HCO_3^-$, * renal compensation may take 3–4 days to occur [**Note:** the abbreviated formula for pH is as follows: pH = $HCO_3^-/PCO_2$. Normally, the ratio of $HCO_3^-$ to $PCO_2$ must be 20/1 in order to maintain the pH at 7.40. Hence, a primary increase in $PCO_2$ (respiratory acidosis) must be accompanied by a compensatory increase in $HCO_3^-$ (metabolic alkalosis) to bring the pH back toward the normal range.] |
| compensation for respiratory alkalosis | **metabolic acidosis**—elimination of $HCO_3^-$ in the urine to produce compensatory metabolic acidosis requires at least 3–4 days [**Note:** a primary decrease in $PCO_2$ (respiratory alkalosis) must be accompanied by a corresponding compensatory decrease in $HCO_3^-$ (metabolic acidosis) in order to bring the pH back toward the normal range.] |
| compensation for metabolic alkalosis | **respiratory acidosis**—respiratory compensation for metabolic disorders usually occurs within a few hours [**Note:** a primary increase in $HCO_3^-$ (metabolic alkalosis) must be accompanied by a corresponding compensatory increase in $PCO_2$ (respiratory acidosis) to bring the pH back toward the normal range. Furthermore, an increase in $PaCO_2$ automatically decreases $PaO_2$ (hypoxemia). Alkalosis also left shifts the ODC, causing less release of $O_2$ to tissue. Hence, the tissue hypoxia caused by metabolic alkalosis gives this acid-base disorder the dubious distinction of being the most dangerous of the acid-base disorders for inducing cardiac arrhythmias.] |
| compensation for metabolic acidosis | **respiratory alkalosis** [**Note:** a primary decrease in $HCO_3^-$ (metabolic acidosis) must be accompanied by a corresponding compensatory decrease in $PCO_2$ (respiratory alkalosis) to bring the pH back toward the normal range. In contradistinction to respiratory acidosis, respiratory alkalosis causes an increase in the $PaO_2$.] |

## Table 1–2. ACID-BASE DISORDERS *Continued*

| Most Common... | Answer and Explanation |
|---|---|
| types of compensation | • **uncompensated**—the expected compensation for an acid-base disorder is in the normal range, e.g., in respiratory acidosis, the measured $HCO_3^-$ is 24 mEq/L (22–28 mEq/L) and has not increased in concentration (metabolic alkalosis) for compensation, • **partial compensation**— * expected compensation and pH are outside the normal ranges, * e.g., in respiratory acidosis, the serum $HCO_3^-$ is >28 mEq/L (metabolic alkalosis); however the pH is not in the normal range of 7.35–7.45, • **full compensation**— * measured arterial pH is brought into the normal range, * this rarely occurs with a single acid-base disorder: exception is living at very high altitude, where chronic respiratory alkalosis may occur with compensation into the normal range of pH |
| causes of acute respiratory acidosis (pH < 7.35, $PaCO_2$ > 45 mm Hg, $HCO_3^-$ ≤ 30 mEq/L) | • **depression of the medullary respiratory center**— * drug overdose, * CNS trauma, • *upper airway obstruction*— * cafe coronary: food lodged in the larynx, * laryngospasm, • *chest bellows disease*— * paralysis of the diaphragms, * flail chest, • *primary lung disease*— * ARDS, * severe lobar pneumonia |
| causes of chronic respiratory acidosis (pH < 7.35, $PaCO_2$ > 45 mm Hg, $HCO_3^-$ > 30 mEq/L) | • **primary lung disease**— * COPD, * bronchiectasis, • *kyphoscoliosis* [**Note:** a bicarbonate value beyond 30 mEq/L indicates that renal compensation is present, hence the condition is now considered chronic.] |
| S/S of respiratory acidosis | • **somnolence,** • *intracranial hypertension*—a high $PaCO_2$ vasodilates cerebral vessels causing cerebral edema, • *pseudotumor cerebri*—manifests with headache |
| Hgb alteration noted in respiratory acidosis | **secondary polycythemia**—respiratory acidosis always causes a drop in the $PaO_2$ (hypoxemia), which stimulates renal release of erythropoietin |

*Table continued on following page*

**Table 1–2. ACID-BASE DISORDERS** *Continued*

| Most Common... | Answer and Explanation |
|---|---|
| causes of acute respiratory alkalosis (pH > 7.45, $PaCO_2$ < 33 mm Hg, $HCO_3^-$ ≥ 18 mEq/L) | • **hyperventilation syndrome**— * anxiety, * tissue hypoxia (e.g., severe anemia), • *overstimulation of the medullary respiratory center*— * endotoxemia, * salicylates, * toxic metabolites in liver failure, * normal pregnancy: due to estrogen and progesterone stimulation, • *primary lung disease*— * PE, * acute bronchial asthma: respiratory acidosis in an asthmatic indicates that the patient is tiring and requires hospitalization with immediate intubation |
| causes of chronic respiratory alkalosis (pH > 7.45, $PaCO_2$ < 33 mm Hg, $HCO_3^-$ < 18 mEq/L but >12 mEq/L) | • **high altitude,** • *liver failure*—e.g., cirrhosis, • *chronic ILD*—e.g., sarcoidosis |
| S/S in respiratory alkalosis | • **lightheadedness,** • *tetany*— * alkalosis increases negative charges on albumin, hence there is greater binding of calcium to albumin at the expense of the ionized calcium level, * positive Chvostek's sign: facial twitching when facial nerve is tapped, * Trousseau's sign: thumb adducts into the palm when a blood pressure cuff is applied and the pressure is taken, * laryngeal stridor [**Note:** alkalosis lowers the threshold potential in muscle and nerves (normally −90) and brings it closer to the resting membrane potential (normally −60). Hence, muscle and nerves are partially depolarized and a smaller stimulus is required to initiate an action potential.] |
| types of metabolic acidosis | • **increased anion gap,** • *normal anion gap metabolic acidosis* |

**Table 1–2. ACID-BASE DISORDERS** *Continued*

| Most Common... | Answer and Explanation |
|---|---|
| formula used to distinguish increased from normal anion gap (AG) metabolic acidosis | **AG = serum Na$^+$ − (serum Cl$^-$ + serum HCO$_3^-$)** [**Note:** using normal values: AG = 140 − (104 + 24) = 12 mEq/L +/− 4 (8–16). The normal AG of 12 mEq/L represents normal anions that are not represented in the formula (e.g., albumin, PO$_4^{--}$, SO$_4^{--}$). Therefore, an increase in the AG indicates that other anions have been introduced into the extracellular fluid compartment. These include anions like lactate, salicylate, acetoacetate, to name a few. Serum bicarbonate is lowered since it is used up in buffering the excess H$^+$ ions of the acid (e.g., H$^+$ + HCO$_3^-$ → H$_2$CO$_3$ → H$_2$O + CO$_2$). An example of increased AG metabolic acidosis: serum Na$^+$ 140 mEq/L (136–145), serum Cl$^-$ 90 mEq/L (95–105), serum HCO$_3^-$ 15 mEq/L (22–28); therefore, 140 − (90 + 15) = 35 mEq/L. A normal AG is due to a loss of HCO$_3^-$ ions (see below) in the stool or urine. The lost HCO$_3^-$ anions are replaced mEq for mEq by Cl$^-$ ions, hence the term hyperchloremic normal AG metabolic acidosis. An example of a normal AG metabolic acidosis: serum Na$^+$ 140 mEq/L (136–145), serum Cl$^-$ 115 mEq/L (95–105), serum HCO$_3^-$ 15 mEq/L (22–28); therefore, 140 − (115 + 15) = 10 mEq/L.] |
| anions causing an increased AG metabolic acidosis in DKA | **AcAc/β-OHB anions**—the acetyl CoA produced from increased β-oxidation of fatty acids is used by the liver to synthesize ketone bodies (acetone, AcAc, β-OHB) |
| anions causing an increased AG metabolic acidosis in alcoholics | **lactate/β-OHB anions**— * the increase in NADH$^+$ derived from metabolism of alcohol results in conversion of pyruvate into lactate, * the increase in acetyl CoA in metabolism of alcohol is used by the liver to produce ketone bodies, particularly β-OHB (increase in NADH$^+$ causes AcAc to convert into β-OHB) |

*Table continued on following page*

**Table 1–2. ACID-BASE DISORDERS** *Continued*

| Most Common... | Answer and Explanation |
|---|---|
| anions causing an increased AG metabolic acidosis in starvation | **AcAc/β-OHB anions**— * in starvation, β-oxidation of fatty acids is the primary fuel for muscle, * acetyl CoA from β-oxidation of fatty acids is converted into ketone bodies in the liver, * ketone bodies (acetone, AcAc, β-OHB) are primarily used by the brain for energy in starvation |
| anions causing an increased AG metabolic acidosis in shock | **lactate anions**—lactic acid is the end-product of anaerobic glycolysis |
| anions causing increased AG metabolic acidosis in salicylate intoxication | **salicylate/lactate anions**— * salicylate is an acid, * salicylates are mitochondrial poisons (they uncouple oxidative phosphorylation), which produces tissue hypoxia and accumulation of lactate anions |
| anions causing increased AG metabolic acidosis in methyl alcohol poisoning | **formate anions**— * formate anions are derived from metabolism of methyl alcohol (windshield wiper fluid, Sterno), * optic nerve neuritis occurs, leading to blindness |
| anions causing increased AG metabolic acidosis in ethylene glycol poisoning | **oxalate anions**— * derived from metabolism of ethylene glycol (antifreeze), * calcium oxalate crystals block the renal tubules, resulting in renal failure |
| anions causing increased AG metabolic acidosis in CRF | **phosphate/sulfate anions**—these anions are the end products of metabolism of meat products |
| causes of a normal AG metabolic acidosis | • **loss of $HCO_3^-$ in the GI tract**— * diarrhea, * loss of pancreatic fluid, • *loss of $HCO_3^-$ in GU tract*— * proximal/distal RTA, * proximal RTA is due to a lowering of the renal threshold for reclaiming $HCO_3^-$ in the proximal tubule, * distal RTA is due to a dysfunctional $H^+/K^+$ pump in the collecting tubule |

## Table 1–2. ACID-BASE DISORDERS *Continued*

| Most Common... | Answer and Explanation |
|---|---|
| S/S of metabolic acidosis | • **hyperventilation**—respiratory alkalosis is compensation (called Kussmaul breathing), • *negative inotropic effect*—decreased response of cardiac muscle to catecholamines, • *osteoporosis*—bone buffers excess $H^+$ ions, • *warm shock*—acidosis vasodilates peripheral arterioles |
| electrolyte findings in metabolic acidosis | • **low serum $HCO_3^-$**—primary abnormality in metabolic acidosis, • *hyperkalemia*— * shift of $K^+$ out of cells in exchange for $H^+$ ions occurs mainly with inorganic types of increased AG metabolic acidosis (e.g., increased phosphate, sulfate), • *hypokalemia*—diarrhea and type I/II RTA have a greater loss of $K^+$ in the urine than gain by transcellular shifting of $K^+$ for $H^+$ ions, • *hyperglycemia*—acidosis inhibits glycolysis, • *hyperuricemia*—acids associated with metabolic acidosis compete with uric acid for excretion in the kidneys |
| causes of metabolic alkalosis (pH > 7.45, $HCO_3^- > 28$ mEq/L) | • **loop/thiazide diuretics**— * blockage of the $Na^+/K^+/2Cl^-$ cotransport pump in the thick ascending limb (TAL) of the medullary segment and the $Na^+/Cl^-$ pump in the TAL of the cortical segment, respectively, increases distal delivery of $Na^+$: leads to increased exchange of $Na^+$ ions for $H^+$ ions in the $Na^+/K^+/H^+$ aldosterone-mediated pump in the collecting tubules, * $H^+$ ions in urine reclaim $HCO_3^-$, leading to metabolic alkalosis, • *vomiting*— * loss of $H^+$ ions in gastric juice, * volume depletion results in increased proximal tubule reclamation of $HCO_3^-$, which maintains metabolic alkalosis, • *loss of anions in urine*—drug anions in urine (e.g., penicillin, ticarcillin) with their strong negative charges draw $H^+$ ions out of tubules with subsequent increase in reclamation of bicarbonate, • *mineralocorticoid excess*—e.g., primary aldosteronism results in increased exchange of $Na^+$ ions for $H^+$ ions, the latter leading to increased reclamation of $HCO_3^-$ |
| S/S of metabolic alkalosis | • **arrhythmias**—ventricular arrhythmias occur due to tissue hypoxia, • *tetany*—see above discussion |

*Table continued on following page*

## Table 1–2. ACID-BASE DISORDERS *Continued*

**Questions: 1–7**

|  | pH<br>(7.35–7.45) | PaCO$_2$<br>(33–45 mm Hg) | HCO$_3$$^-$<br>(22–28 mEq/L) |
|---|---|---|---|
| (A) | 7.22 | 69 | 27 |
| (B) | 7.26 | 26 | 11 |
| (C) | 7.33 | 68 | 34 |
| (D) | 7.37 | 62 | 36 |
| (E) | 7.42 | 22 | 14 |
| (F) | 7.50 | 29 | 22 |
| (G) | 7.51 | 48 | 38 |

Match the above arterial blood gases with the clinical scenarios.

1. A 48-yr-old man with COPD is on nasogastric suction for pyloric stenosis secondary to chronic duodenal ulcer disease.

2. A 62-yr-old man with urinary retention secondary to benign prostatic hyperplasia has fever, chills, warm skin, and a hyperdynamic circulation.

3. A 45-yr-old woman develops a sudden onset of tachypnea and dyspnea 3 days after removal of a gangrenous gallbladder.

4. A 48-yr-old man develops hypovolemic shock due to a splenic rupture secondary to a car accident.

5. A 55-yr-old man is taking a loop diuretic for chronic congestive heart failure. He has signs of volume depletion.

6. A semicomatose 28-yr-old woman presents to the emergency department with a history of barbiturate overdose.

7. A 58-yr-old man has a 60-pack-year history of smoking cigarettes. He is obese and cyanotic.

## Table 1–2. ACID-BASE DISORDERS *Continued*

**Answers: 1. (D), 2. (E), 3. (F), 4. (B), 5. (G), 6. (A), 7. (C):** Recall that respiratory conditions are defined on the basis of the $PaCO_2$—<33 mm Hg = respiratory alkalosis, >45 mm Hg = respiratory acidosis. Metabolic conditions are defined on the basis of the $HCO_3^-$—<22 mEq/L = metabolic acidosis, >28 mEq/L = metabolic alkalosis. The first patient has a mixed ABG disorder. Nasogastric suction leads to metabolic alkalosis ($HCO_3^-$ 36 mEq/L), and COPD is associated with chronic respiratory acidosis ($PaCO_2$ 62 mm Hg). The pH is normal (7.37), which is a clue that a mixed disorder is present consisting of a primary respiratory acidosis and primary metabolic alkalosis (**choice D is correct**). Note how the acid and alkaline pH of the two primary disorders causes the pH to be in the normal range. The second patient has endotoxic shock most likely due to *E. coli* sepsis from urinary retention. Endotoxic shock produces an increased AG metabolic acidosis due to lactic acidosis ($HCO_3^-$ 14 mEq/L) and primary respiratory alkalosis ($PaCO_2$ 22 mm Hg) due to overstimulation of the medullary respiratory center by endotoxins. The pH is normal (7.42) owing to a combined primary metabolic acidosis and primary respiratory alkalosis (**choice E is correct**). The third patient has a pulmonary embolus, which produces a primary respiratory alkalosis. Note that the $PaCO_2$ is 29 mm Hg (respiratory alkalosis), the $HCO_3^-$ is normal (22 mEq/L), and the pH is alkaline (7.50). Hence the patient has an uncompensated respiratory alkalosis (**choice F is correct**). The fourth patient has hypovolemic shock from blood loss and would be expected to have lactic acidosis (**choice B is correct**). Lactic acidosis is an example of metabolic acidosis—7.26 = acidemia, $PaCO_2$ = 26 mm Hg (respiratory alkalosis), $HCO_3^-$ = 11 mEq/L (metabolic acidosis). Note how the pH determines which of the two disorders is primary versus the compensation. Metabolic acidosis is subdivided into an increased AG (e.g., ketoacidosis) and normal AG (e.g., diarrhea) metabolic acidosis. The fifth patient is taking a loop diuretic and is volume depleted. Loop diuretics produce metabolic alkalosis (**choice G is correct**)—7.51 = alkalemia, $PaCO_2$ = 48 (respiratory acidosis, partial compensation), $HCO_3^-$ = 38 mEq/L (metabolic alkalosis). Note how the pH determines which of the two disorders is primary versus the compensation. Diuretics are the most common cause of metabolic alkalosis. The sixth patient has an acute barbiturate overdose, which causes acute respiratory acidosis (**choice A is correct**). The ABG is an example of an acute uncompensated respiratory acidosis—7.22 = acidemia, $PaCO_2$ 69 mm Hg = acidemia, $HCO_3^-$ = 27 mEq/L is normal (no compensation). The seventh patient has chronic obstructive pulmonary disease from smoking. COPD is an example of chronic respiratory acidosis (**choice C is correct**)—7.33 = acidemia, $PaCO_2$ = 68 mm Hg (respiratory acidosis), $HCO_3^-$ = 34 mEq/L (>30 mEq/L indicates a chronic rather than an acute respiratory acidosis, partial compensation).

*Table continued on following page*

### Table 1–2. ACID-BASE DISORDERS *Continued*

A–a = Alveolar–arterial gradient, ABG = arterial blood gas, AcAc = acetoacetate, AG = anion gap, ARDS = adult respiratory distress syndrome, β-OHB = beta-hydroxybutyrate, $Cl^-$ = chloride, COPD = chronic obstructive pulmonary disease, CRF = chronic renal failure, DKA = diabetic ketoacidosis, $H^+$ = hydrogen ions (protons), $HCO_3^-$ = bicarbonate, ILD = interstitial lung disease, $Na^+$ = sodium, ODC = oxygen dissociation curve, PE = pulmonary embolus, PFTs = pulmonary function tests, $PO_4^{--}$ = phosphate, RTA = renal tubular acidosis, $SaO_2$ = oxygen saturation, $SO_4^{--}$ = sulfate, S/S = signs/symptoms.

### Table 1–3. FLUID AND ELECTROLYTE DISORDERS

| Most Common... | Answer and Explanation |
|---|---|
| sites housing total body water (TBW) | • **ICF compartment**—contains ~two-thirds of the TBW, • *ECF compartment*— * contains ~one-third of TBW, * the ECF compartment is subdivided into the interstitial fluid (ISF) compartment (two-thirds of the ECF) and vascular compartment (one-third of the ECF) |
| site housing total body sodium ($TBNa^+$) | **ECF compartment**— * $Na^+$, unlike water, is not freely permeable through cell membranes, * $Na^+$ is an effective osmole (see below), * the $Na^+/K^+$ ATPase pump keeps $Na^+$ out of ICF and $K^+$ in the ICF |
| site housing $TBK^+$ and $Mg^{++}$ | **ICF compartment** |
| clinical index used to evaluate TBW status | **serum $Na^+$ concentration**— * serum $Na^+$ is most responsible for controlling water movements between ECF/ICF by osmosis: water moves from a point of low solute to high solute concentration, * serum $Na^+$ does not always directly correlate with $TBNa^+$, * serum $Na^+$ concentration $\approx TBNa^+/TBW$: since the serum $Na^+$ is really a ratio of $TBNa^+$ to TBW, it is possible to have hyponatremia in the presence of an increase in $TBNa^+$ by a greater increase in TBW |
| clinical index used to evaluate $TBNa^+$ | **physical examination** |

## Table 1–3. FLUID AND ELECTROLYTE DISORDERS
*Continued*

| Most Common... | Answer and Explanation |
|---|---|
| clinical indices of a decrease in TBNa$^+$ | **signs of volume depletion**— * *changes in ISF volume*— ♦ decreased skin turgor (tenting of skin), ♦ sunken fontanelles in infant, ♦ dry mucous membranes, ♦ dry axilla, * *changes in the vascular compartment*— ♦ orthostatic hypotension, ♦ oliguria (decreased GFR), ♦ flat neck veins, ♦ sinus tachycardia, ♦ hemoconcentration (increased Hct), ♦ prerenal azotemia, * *increased thirst*—due to increased AT II or an increase in plasma osmolality [**Note:** volume depletion is a better term than dehydration. Dehydration specifically refers to a loss of pure water without salt, which generally does not produce signs of volume depletion. Volume depletion is associated with the previous signs owing to the loss of Na$^+$.] |
| clinical indices of an increase in TBNa$^+$ | • **dependent pitting edema**—reflects increased TBNa$^+$ in the ISF compartment, • *transudates in body cavities*—e.g., ascites, • *increase in body weight* |
| clinical index of a normal TBNa$^+$ | **absence of above clinical signs** |
| lab test evaluating plasma solute concentration | **plasma osmolality (POsm)**— * osmolality is the number of osmoles of solute per kg, * osmoles may be effective or ineffective in controlling water movements (see below) |
| formula used for calculating POsm | **POsm = (2) Na$^+$ + serum glucose/18 + serum BUN/2.8 = 275–295 mOsm/kg**— * calculated POsm is normally within 10 mOsm/kg of measured POsm, * the POsm reflects the osmolality in both the ECF and ICF compartments |
| effective osmoles normally present in the ECF compartment | • **Na$^+$**, • *glucose* [**Note:** effective osmoles are unable to diffuse through cell membranes. Therefore, alterations in their concentration (particularly Na$^+$) establish osmotic gradients that allow water to move between the ECF/ICF compartments.] |

*Table continued on following page*

## Table 1–3. FLUID AND ELECTROLYTE DISORDERS
*Continued*

| Most Common... | Answer and Explanation |
| --- | --- |
| effective osmoles that are not normally present in the ECF compartment | • **mannitol**—this osmotic diuretic is commonly used in reducing intracranial/intraocular pressure, • *glycine*—this is an irrigating fluid used in prostate surgery |
| cause of a low POsm | **hyponatremia**— * water moves into the ICF compartment, * in the CNS, it produces cerebral edema and mental status abnormalities |
| ineffective osmole that is normally present in the ECF | **urea**— * ineffective osmoles freely permeate cell membranes, * urea is equally distributed between the ECF and ICF, hence no water movements occur (no osmotic gradient) |
| ineffective osmoles that are not normally present in the ECF | • **ethyl alcohol,** • *methyl alcohol*— * windshield wiper fluid, * Sterno, • *ethylene glycol*—antifreeze, • *isopropyl alcohol*—rubbing alcohol |
| effect of azotemia on water movements | **no effect**— * azotemia is an increase in serum BUN, * urea is an ineffective osmole, hence no water shifts from the ICF to the ECF in azotemia |
| formula used to evaluate ECF tonicity | **effective osmolality (EOsm) = 2 (serum Na$^+$) + glucose/18**— * note the absence of urea (ineffective osmole) in the formula and presence of the effective osmoles Na$^+$ and glucose, * EOsm is synonymous with the tonicity of the ECF compartment, * tonicity rather than osmolality is physiologically regulated (see below) |
| types of tonicity in the ECF compartment | • **hypotonicity**— * equates with hyponatremia, * water moves into the ICF compartment, • *isotonicity*— * equates with a normal serum Na$^+$, * no water movements occur because there is no gradient, • *hypertonicity*— * equates with either hypernatremia or hyperglycemia, * water moves into the ECF compartment, * hyperosmolality (increased POsm) and hypertonicity are not always synonymous (e.g., azotemia increases POsm but tonicity is normal) |

## Table 1–3. FLUID AND ELECTROLYTE DISORDERS
*Continued*

| Most Common... | Answer and Explanation |
|---|---|
| effect of hyperglycemia on the serum $Na^+$ concentration | **dilutional hyponatremia**—water movement from the ICF to the ECF compartment dilutes ECF $Na^+$ [**Note:** glucosuria is commonly present when hyperglycemia is present. Glucose in the urine is an osmotic diuretic and results in the loss of a hypotonic salt solution leading to hypovolemia.] |
| formula used to correct serum $Na^+$ for the dilutional effect of hyperglycemia | **corrected serum $Na^+$ = measured serum $Na^+$ + (glucose mg/dL/100 × 1.6)**— * correction of the serum $Na^+$ allows the clinician to see what the serum $Na^+$ concentration would be in the absence of the dilutional effect due to hyperglycemia, * e.g., serum $Na^+$ = 132 mEq/L (136–145 mEq/L), serum glucose = 1000 mg/dL (70–110 mg/dL): corrected serum $Na^+$ = 132 + (1000/100 × 1.6) = 148 mEq/L, which is increased (due to osmotic diuresis and loss of more water than $Na^+$ in the urine) |
| factors controlling plasma volume | • **kidney reabsorption of salt/water,** • *thirst*— * low POsm inhibits thirst, * high POsm stimulates thirst, * high AT II stimulates thirst, • *low/high pressure baroreceptors,* • *RAA system,* • *ADH*— * low POsm inhibits ADH release, * high POsm stimulates ADH release, * volume depletion automatically stimulates ADH release |
| factors activating the RAA system | • **increase in catecholamines**—activation of baroreceptors from decreased cardiac output, • *decrease in renal blood flow*—decrease in cardiac output [**Note:** the RAA system is usually activated when there is a decrease in cardiac output. Examples include hypovolemia, cardiogenic shock.] |
| sequence of events in activation of RAA system | • **JG apparatus releases renin (an enzyme)** → renin cleaves angiotensinogen into AT I → ACE converts AT I into AT II ( * stimulates thirst, * increases TPR) → • AT II stimulates release of * AT III and * aldosterone (increases $Na^+$ reabsorption) |

*Table continued on following page*

## Table 1–3. FLUID AND ELECTROLYTE DISORDERS
*Continued*

| Most Common... | Answer and Explanation |
| --- | --- |
| clinical term reflecting volume status | **effective arterial blood volume (EABV)**— EABV represents the total circulating volume of blood that is necessary to stimulate volume receptors |
| mechanism of fluid movement limited to the ECF compartment | **Starling's force abnormality**—if plasma hydrostatic pressure is increased (e.g., RHF) or oncotic pressure (serum albumin) is decreased (e.g., cirrhosis), a transudate (cell/protein-poor fluid) diffuses out of the vascular compartment into the ISF compartment |
| clinical expressions of an alteration in Starling's forces | • **pitting edema**— * transudates contain Na$^+$, * the greater the Na$^+$ concentration in the ISF compartment, the greater the likelihood of pitting edema, * an excess in TBW cannot produce pitting edema, since most of the water is in the ICF compartment and not the ISF compartment, • *body cavity effusions* [**Note:** fluid trapped in the ISF compartment/body cavities decreases venous return to the right heart, which automatically decreases EABV.] |
| sites of low and high pressure baroreceptors | • **low-pressure sites**— * left atrium, * major intrathoracic veins, • **high-pressure sites**— * aortic arch, * carotid sinus [**Note:** baroreceptors are innervated by cranial nerves IX and X.] |
| physiologic events associated with volume depletion | • **stimulation of baroreceptor reflex**—underfilling of the arterial system causes increased sympathetic activity with catecholamine release, • *activation of the RAA system*—see above discussion, • *neural reflexes in the left atrium stimulate ADH release*—increase reabsorption of free water in kidneys, • *decrease in renal blood flow decreases the peritubular capillary hydrostatic pressure* ($P_H$) *and increases the peritubular capillary oncotic pressure* ($P_O$)—the increase in $P_O$ allows the kidneys to reabsorb out of the urine and into the vascular compartment a slightly hypotonic salt solution (more water than salt) |

## Table 1–3. FLUID AND ELECTROLYTE DISORDERS
*Continued*

| Most Common... | Answer and Explanation |
|---|---|
| catecholamine effects associated with volume depletion | • **venoconstriction**—increases venous return to the heart, • **increases cardiac output**—increases the force of contraction, • **increases heart rate**, • **increases TPR**—raises diastolic BP, • **stimulates RAA system** |
| physiologic events associated with an increased EABV (volume excess) | • **stimulus for ANP release**—due to distention of the left/right atrium, • **activation of the baroreceptor reflex**— * cranial nerves IX and X are activated, * there is no sympathetic nervous system response, • **no release of ADH**—inhibited by ANP, • *no activation of the RAA system,* • $P_H > P_O$—decreased proximal reabsorption of salt/water owing to the increase in $P_H$, • **renal loss of a hypotonic solution** |
| functions of ANP | • **suppresses baroreceptor events listed above,** • *vasodilates peripheral vessels,* • *directly inhibits renal $Na^+$ reabsorption* [**Note:** ANP counters an increase in ECF volume and offsets the actions of AT II and aldosterone.] |
| functions of renal prostaglandin $E_2$ | • **inhibits ADH**, • **blocks renal $Na^+$ reabsorption**, • **vasodilates the afferent arterioles** |
| nephron site for $Na^+$ reabsorption | **proximal tubule**— * reabsorbs 60–80% of the filtered $Na^+$, * $P_O$ must be greater than $P_H$ in order to reabsorb $Na^+$ into the peritubular capillaries and into the vascular compartment |

*Table continued on following page*

### Table 1–3. FLUID AND ELECTROLYTE DISORDERS
*Continued*

| Most Common... | Answer and Explanation |
|---|---|
| nephron site for the generation of free water | **thick ascending limb (TAL)** [**Note:** the TAL segment in the medulla contains the $Na^+$-$K^+$-$2Cl^-$ cotransport pump, which produces free water (solute-free water). Obligated water is water that must accompany solute for excretion (20 mL water per mOsm of solute). Up to the TAL segment, all the water in the tubule is obligated water. When urine reaches the $Na^+$-$K^+$-$2Cl^-$ cotransport pump, the obligated water is separated from $Na^+$, $K^+$, and $Cl^-$, the latter entering the interstitium and helping maintain the high osmotic gradient. The water that remains behind in the lumen is now called free water, since it no longer is associated with solutes. For normal dilution to occur, free water must be excreted in the absence of ADH. For normal concentration to occur, free water must be reabsorbed in the presence of ADH. Inability to excrete free water always produces hyponatremia.] |
| MOA of loop diuretics | **blocks $Na^+$-$K^+$-$2Cl^-$ cotransport pump**— * this automatically interferes with the generation of free water: most of the water excreted in the urine is obligated water that must accompany the blocked $Na^+$, $K^+$, and $Cl^-$ solutes, * blocking the generation of free water significantly impairs normal dilution |
| MOA of thiazide diuretics | **blocks the $Na^+/Cl^-$ pump in the cortical segment of the TAL** |
| nephron site where the aldosterone-enhanced ATPase pumps for $Na^+/K^+$ exchange are located | **late distal and collecting tubules**— * aldosterone increases $Na^+$ reabsorption in exchange for either $K^+$ or $H^+$ ions: if $K^+$ is used up in exchanging for $Na^+$, then $H^+$ ions are used for the exchange, which may result in reclamation of bicarbonate and metabolic alkalosis, * this pump is the primary site for $K^+$ secretion: inhibition of this pump may result in hyperkalemia |

## Table 1–3. FLUID AND ELECTROLYTE DISORDERS
*Continued*

| Most Common... | Answer and Explanation |
|---|---|
| nephron site where the aldosterone-enhanced H$^+$/K$^+$ ATPase pump is located | **collecting tubule**— * the H$^+$/K$^+$ pump is the primary site for secreting excess H$^+$ ions, * this pump also regenerates (de novo synthesis) HCO$_3^-$, * blocking this pump causes: ♦ retention of H$^+$ ions (normal AG metabolic acidosis), ♦ an alkaline pH urine (no H$^+$ to combine with HPO$_4^-$ or NH$_3$ ions), ♦ loss of K$^+$ in the urine (hypokalemia), ♦ this is called type I distal RTA |
| cause of hypokalemia with the use of loop or thiazide diuretics | **increased distal delivery of nonreabsorbed Na$^+$ to aldosterone-enhanced Na$^+$/K$^+$ pumps**—* exchange of Na$^+$ for K$^+$ causes K$^+$ loss in the urine, which leads to hypokalemia, * hypokalemia is prevented by the patient taking K$^+$ supplements: enough K$^+$ is available to exchange with Na$^+$, * Na$^+$ exchanges with H$^+$ ions if K$^+$ is used up: this results in increased reclamation of HCO$_3^-$ and metabolic alkalosis |
| acid-base/electrolyte abnormalities associated with loop or thiazide diuretics | • **metabolic alkalosis**, • **hyponatremia**, • **hypokalemia** [**Note:** once tubular K$^+$ is depleted in exchange for Na$^+$, Na$^+$ exchanges with H$^+$ ions. H$^+$ ions increase HCO$_3^-$ reclamation resulting in metabolic alkalosis. Urine Na$^+$ loss is hypertonic (more Na$^+$ lost than water) causing hyponatremia.] |
| MOA of spironolactone | **aldosterone blocker**— * distal/collecting duct diuretic, * block of Na$^+$/K$^+$ pump: ♦ loss of Na$^+$ (hyponatremia), ♦ retention of K$^+$ (potential for hyperkalemia), * block of H$^+$/K$^+$ pump: ♦ retention of H$^+$ ions (metabolic acidosis), ♦ loss of K$^+$ in the urine (offsets retention of K$^+$ from block of the other pump) |
| nephron site for dilution/ concentration | **collecting ducts**— * absence of ADH leads to dilution: loss of free water, * presence of ADH leads to concentration: reabsorption of free water [**Note:** loss of concentration of urine is the first lab alteration in renal failure.] |

*Table continued on following page*

**Table 1–3. FLUID AND ELECTROLYTE DISORDERS**
*Continued*

| Most Common... | Answer and Explanation |
|---|---|
| nephron site for secretion of H⁺ ions | **collecting ducts**— * contain aldosterone-enhanced $H^+/K^+$ ATPase pumps, * $H^+$ ions secreted into urine combine with $HPO_4^-$ to form $NaH_2PO_4$ (titratable acid) and combine with $NH_3$ to form $NH_4Cl$: this acidifies the urine |
| patient parameter that best reflects volume depletion or gain | • **daily weight,** • *records of intake and output*— * intake should equal output in normal fluid homeostasis, * in 24 h, the normal intake of water from liquids in a 70-kg man is 800–1500 mL, water from solids is 500–700 mL, and water from oxidation reactions is 150–200 mL, * the normal intake of sodium is 50–150 mEq/L, * the normal intake of potassium is 50–80 mEq/L |
| types of normal fluid loss | • **sensible loss**— * urine: ♦ water 800–1500 mL, ♦ $Na^+$ 10–80 mEq/L, ♦ $K^+$ 50–80 mEq/L, * sweat: ♦ water 0–100 mL, ♦ $Na^+$ 10–60 mEq/L, ♦ $K^+$ 0–10 mEq/L, * intestine: ♦ water 0–250 mL, $Na^+$ 0–20 mEq/L, • *insensible loss*— * electrolyte free water resulting from evaporation of water from the mucous membranes: 600–900 mL in 24 h from lungs/skin [**Note:** the net fluid losses per 24 h are >1200 mL.] |
| GI sites responsible for significant losses of $Na^+$ | • **bile**— ~145 mEq/L, • *duodenum/ileum/pancreas*— ~140 mEq/L, • *stomach/colon*—60 mEq/L |
| GI sites responsible for significant losses of $K^+$ | • **colon**— ~30 mEq/L, • *stomach/duodenum/ileum/pancreas/bile*— ~5 mEq/L |
| GI sites responsible for significant losses of $Cl^-$ | • **stomach**— ~130 mEq/L, • *bile/ileum*— ~105 mEq/L, • *duodenum*— ~80 mEq/L, • *colon*— ~40 mEq/L |
| GI sites responsible for significant losses of $HCO_3^-$ | • **pancreas**— ~115 mEq/L, • *bile*— ~35 mEq/L, • *ileum*— ~30 mEq/L |

### Table 1–3. FLUID AND ELECTROLYTE DISORDERS
*Continued*

| Most Common... | Answer and Explanation |
|---|---|
| electrolyte abnormalities associated with vomiting | • **serum Na$^+$**— * hyponatremia, * fluid is hypotonic, • **serum K$^+$**—hypokalemia, • **serum Cl$^-$**—hypochloremia, • **serum HCO$_3$$^-$**— * high, * metabolic alkalosis |
| electrolyte abnormalities associated with diarrhea/small bowel fistulas | • **serum Na$^+$**— * usually normal, * isotonic fluid loss: indicates that most cases are a secretory diarrhea, • **serum K$^+$**—hypokalemia, • **serum Cl$^-$**—high, due to replacement of lost HCO$_3$$^-$, • **serum HCO$_3$$^-$**— * low, * normal AG metabolic acidosis: diarrhea is the most common cause |
| organs most sensitive to volume depletion | • **kidneys**— * the renal medulla is most susceptible, since it only receives 10% of the total blood allotted to the kidneys, * the TAL in the medulla is the most sensitive part of the entire nephron to hypoxia, • *brain*—neurons are more susceptible than neuroglial cells, • *heart*—subendocardium is the most susceptible: coronary arteries penetrate the epicardial surface, hence the subendocardium is farthest from the blood supply, • *liver*—hepatocytes around THV are most susceptible: oxygenated blood enters the sinusoids around the portal triad, hence hepatocytes around the THV receive less O$_2$ and nutrients |
| extrarenal losses resulting in volume depletion | • **hemorrhage**, • *cutaneous losses*— * sweat, * burn fluid, • *GI losses*— * vomiting, * diarrhea, • *third spacing*—see below |
| causes of third space loss | • **peripancreatic collection of fluid in acute pancreatitis**, • **burns**, • **soft tissue injury**, • **infarcted bowel**, • **ascites** [Note: third space fluid is sequestered fluid that is unavailable for maintenance of volume in the vascular compartment (nonfunctional ECF). If conditions improve, the third space fluid gains entry back into the vascular compartment and may cause fluid overload.] |

*Table continued on following page*

## Table 1–3. FLUID AND ELECTROLYTE DISORDERS
*Continued*

| Most Common... | Answer and Explanation |
|---|---|
| renal causes of volume depletion | • **use of diuretics,** • *aldosterone deficiency*—e.g., * Addison's disease, * spironolactone, * destruction of the JG apparatus: this is called type IV renal tubular acidosis, • *central/nephrogenic DI,* • *osmotic diuresis*— * glucosuria, * mannitol, • *salt-losing renal disease*—e.g., cystic disease, some cases of chronic renal failure |
| fluids used to restore volume | **isotonic saline/Ringer's lactated solution**—1 of 3 liters remains in the vascular compartment: the other 2 liters diffuse into the ISF |
| solutes present in lactated Ringer's | • **Na$^+$ 130 mEq/L,** • **Cl$^-$ 109 mEq/L,** • **HCO$_3^-$ 28 mEq/L,** • **K$^+$ 4 mEq/L,** • **Ca$^{++}$ 3 mEq/L** [**Note:** lactated Ringer's solution most closely resembles the electrolyte composition of ECF. Lactate is converted into HCO$_3^-$.] |
| clinical conditions in which 0.9% NaCl is preferred over lactated Ringer's | • **hyperkalemia,** • **hypercalcemia,** • **hyponatremia,** • **hypochloremia,** • **metabolic alkalosis** |
| clinical conditions where lactated Ringer's is preferred over 0.9% NaCl | • **replacement of GI losses**—lactated Ringer's best matches the composition of diarrhea fluid, • **hypovolemic shock**—bicarbonate counteracts lactic acidosis from tissue hypoxia, • **initial crystalloid for Rx of fluid losses in third-degree burns** |
| methods of uncovering volume deficits that are clinically undetectable | • **volume challenge with 500 mL of isotonic saline infused over 1–3 hr**—improvement in the BP/heart rate is a positive test, • *tilt test*— * evaluates BP/pulse while lying down and sitting up, * a further drop in BP and increase in pulse when sitting up indicates volume deficit, • *SGC measurement of PCWP* (measure of LVEDP) *and cardiac output*—this is the most precise method |
| group of drugs that should be avoided in a volume depletion state | **NSAIDs**— * NSAIDs inhibit the synthesis of prostaglandin E$_2$, which is the primary vasodilator of the afferent arteriole, * PGE$_2$ counteracts the vasoconstrictive effects of AT II, which is the primary vasoconstrictor of the efferent arterioles |

### Table 1–3. FLUID AND ELECTROLYTE DISORDERS
*Continued*

| Most Common... | Answer and Explanation |
|---|---|
| type of fluid loss with the greatest hemodynamic effect | • **loss of whole blood**—whole blood contains albumin for oncotic pressure and sodium, • *loss of isotonic fluid*—e.g., * diarrhea fluid, * plasma from the skin in third-degree burns, * third spacing, • *loss of solute-free water*— * loss of pure water has very little effect on volume status: ♦ water loss mainly affects the ICF compartment, ♦ examples include diabetes insipidus and insensible water loss, * loss of any $Na^+$ has tremendous effects on volume status since $Na^+$ loss is restricted to the ECF compartment |
| conditions with signs of volume depletion unrelated to obvious fluid losses | • **decreased cardiac output**—e.g., * AMI, * pericardial tamponade, • *increased venous capacitance*—e.g., septic shock, • *fluid shifts into the ISF compartment*—third space shifts (see above discussion) |
| causes of volume excess | • **Starling's force alterations**— * increased hydrostatic pressure and/or decrease in oncotic pressure alters Starling's forces: ♦ a transudate diffuses from the vascular into the ISF compartment, ♦ pitting edema is present, ♦ e.g., CHF, cirrhosis, * decrease in EABV causes the kidney to reabsorb a hypotonic salt solution: ♦ more water is retained than salt, ♦ hyponatremia is present, • *primary mineralocorticoid excess*—e.g., primary aldosteronism, • *primary excess in solute-free water*— e.g., SiADH, • *primary renal retention of salt*—e.g., CRF |
| causes of volume excess secondary to an increase in hydrostatic pressure | • **LHF**—increase in pulmonary vein hydrostatic pressure, • *RHF*— * increase in systemic venous pressure, * most RHF develops from preexisting LHF |

*Table continued on following page*

### Table 1–3. FLUID AND ELECTROLYTE DISORDERS
*Continued*

| Most Common... | Answer and Explanation |
|---|---|
| causes of volume excess secondary to a decrease in oncotic pressure | • **malnutrition**—decreased protein intake, • *nephrotic syndrome*— * loss of albumin in the urine, * MCC in children is minimal change disease, * MCC in adults is membranous glomerulonephritis and focal segmental glomerulosclerosis, • *malabsorption*— * protein loss in stool, * examples include: ♦ celiac disease, ♦ Crohn's disease, ♦ chronic pancreatitis, ♦ bile salt deficiency, • *cirrhosis*— * decreased albumin synthesis, * MCC is alcohol excess |
| cause of volume excess due to increased hydrostatic pressure/decreased oncotic pressure | **cirrhosis**— * decreased oncotic pressure from decreased albumin synthesis, * increased portal vein hydrostatic pressure, since the portal vein blood encounters a reduced number of sinusoids in the liver |
| causes of volume excess due to a primary increase in mineralocorticoids | • **primary aldosteronism,** • *Cushing's syndrome* |
| causes of volume excess due to an increase in solute-free water | • **SiADH**—see below, • *psychogenic polydipsia* |
| causes of volume excess due to primary retention of salt | • **renal failure,** • *salt overload*—e.g., * excess $NaHCO_3$ infusions, * infusion of antibiotics containing sodium (e.g., carbenicillin) |
| Rx of volume excess due to an increase in solute-free water | **restrict water** |
| Rx of volume excess due to an excess in TBNa$^+$ | • **restrict salt,** • *diuretics* |
| Rx of volume excess due to excess TBNa$^+$ and TBW (e.g., CHF, cirrhosis) | • **restrict salt and water,** • *diuretics* |
| Rx of volume excess state due to primary mineralocorticoid excess | • **Rx the underlying condition,** • *aldosterone blockers* |

## Table 1–3. FLUID AND ELECTROLYTE DISORDERS
*Continued*

| Most Common... | Answer and Explanation |
|---|---|
| causes of normonatremia and volume depletion | • diarrhea, • *third degree burns,* • *third spacing of fluid,* • *small bowel fistula,* • *drainage of bile/pancreatic secretions* [**Note:** the above conditions have an isotonic loss of fluid— $\leftrightarrow$ serum $Na^+$ = $\downarrow TBNa^+/\downarrow TBW$. $\downarrow TBNa^+$ produces signs of volume depletion. A random $UNa^+$ is <10 mEq/L due to increased proximal tubule reabsorption of $Na^+$ in response to a decreased EABV.] |
| effect of access to water on serum $Na^+$ concentration in isotonic fluid loss | **produces hyponatremia—** * the TBW increases without any change in $TBNa^+$: dilutional effect on the serum $Na^+$, * e.g., $\downarrow$ serum $Na^+$ = $\downarrow TBNa^+/\uparrow \uparrow$ **TBW (water intake)** |
| cause of normonatremia and volume excess with pitting edema | • **excess infusion of isotonic saline/lactated Ringer's** • *return of third space fluid to vascular compartment* [**Note:** the above conditions have an isotonic gain of fluid— $\leftrightarrow$ serum $Na^+$ = $\uparrow TBNa^+/\uparrow TBW$. The $\uparrow TBNa^+$ produces signs of pitting edema and body cavity effusions. The random $UNa^+$ is >20 mEq/L ($P_H > P_O$) due to reduced proximal reabsorption of $Na^+$ related to an increase in EABV.] |
| electrolyte disturbance in a hospitalized population | **hyponatremia—** * serum $Na^+$ <136 mEq/L, * diuretics are the most common cause of hyponatremia |
| pathophysiologic mechanisms responsible for hyponatremia in the volume depleted state | • **increased release of ADH—** * volume changes override osmolality as a stimulus for ADH release, * ADH increases free water reabsorption in the kidneys, • *increased proximal tubule reabsorption of sodium* ($P_O > P_H$)— * increased proximal reabsorption of $Na^+$ reduces the distal delivery of $Na^+$, * this automatically impairs the generation of free water at the $Na^+$-$K^+$-$2Cl^-$ cotransport pump, • *excessive water intake*—hyponatremia develops due to impaired generation of free water: ◆ remember, if a patient has an increased intake of pure water then the kidney must excrete pure water (free water) in the dilution process, ◆ the excretion of obligated water does not include the excess water that is added to the ECF compartment |

*Table continued on following page*

### Table 1–3. FLUID AND ELECTROLYTE DISORDERS
*Continued*

| Most Common... | Answer and Explanation |
|---|---|
| S/S of hyponatremia | • **mental status abnormalities**—confusion, • *seizures,* • *lethargy,* • *cramps,* • *decreased DTRs* [**Note:** an acute onset of hyponatremia is more likely to be associated with S/S than a slow onset of hyponatremia.] |
| renal causes of hyponatremia with volume depletion | • **diuretics,** • *Addison's disease,* • *salt-losing renal diseases* [**Note:** the above conditions are associated with a hypertonic loss of fluid— ↓ serum Na$^+$ = ↓ ↓ TBNa$^+$/↓ TBW. Signs of volume depletion are present. The random UNa$^+$ is >20 mEq/L.] |
| extrarenal causes of hyponatremia with volume depletion | • **infusion of an excess amount of hypotonic fluid**—e.g., D5W, 0.45% NaCl, • *patient access to water in the presence of a hypotonic/ isotonic loss of fluid*— * sweating (hypotonic loss): ◆ hypernatremia is initially present ( ↑ serum Na$^+$ = ↓ TBNa$^+$/↓ ↓ TBW), ◆ after access to water the patient may develop hyponatremia: ↓ serum Na$^+$ = ↓ TBNa$^+$/ ↑ ↑ **TBW** (excess water intake), * isotonic loss of fluid: ◆ initially the serum Na$^+$ is normal (↔ serum Na$^+$ = ↓ TBNa$^+$/↓ TBW), ◆ after access to water the patient may develop hyponatremia ( ↓ serum Na$^+$ = ↓ TBNa$^+$/ ↑ ↑ **TBW**) |
| formula used to calculate Na$^+$ deficit in volume depletion | **Na$^+$ deficit = 0.6 × weight in kg × (140 − measured serum Na$^+$)**— * e.g., 70-kg-man with serum Na$^+$ 120 mEq/L: Na$^+$ deficit = 0.6 (70) × (140 − 120) = 840 mEq/L, * 0.9% normal saline contains 154 mEq/L—infuse 840/154 or ∼ 5.5 liters [**Note:** on the surface it appears that normal saline is hypertonic when compared with plasma because it contains 154 mEq/L (normal range of sodium is 136–145 mEq/L). However, the 154 mEq/L is distributed in the water phase of plasma, which represents 93% of the total. Therefore 154 × 0.93 = 143 mEq/L, which is isotonic.] |

## Table 1–3. FLUID AND ELECTROLYTE DISORDERS
*Continued*

| Most Common... | Answer and Explanation |
|---|---|
| causes of hyponatremia, with volume excess, pitting edema, decreased EABV | • **CHF,** • *cirrhosis,* • *nephrotic syndrome* [**Note:** CHF, cirrhosis, and the nephrotic syndrome represent edema states with a hypotonic gain of more water than salt ( $\downarrow$ serum $Na^+$ = $\uparrow TBNa^+/\uparrow \uparrow TBW$ ). All these patients have a decreased cardiac output owing to alterations in Starling's forces causing redistribution of fluid (transudate) from the vascular compartment into the ISF compartment and body cavities. A decrease in cardiac output equates with a decrease in EABV. Recall that the kidney reabsorbs a slightly hypotonic fluid back into the vascular compartment, which has slightly more water than salt, hence the hyponatremia in these conditions. Due to alterations in Starling's forces in all these conditions (e.g., increased hydrostatic pressure in CHF, decreased oncotic pressure/increased hydrostatic pressure in cirrhosis, and decreased oncotic pressure in nephrotic syndrome), the reabsorbed fluid from the kidneys is again redistributed into the ISF compartment and/or body cavities rather than remaining in the vascular compartment and helping increase the cardiac output. The increase in TBNa$^+$ due to renal reabsorption of salt is limited to the ISF compartment, hence pitting edema is present. The increase in TBW from renal reabsorption of water is distributed in both the ICF and ECF by osmotic forces related to the hyponatremia. The random UNa$^+$ is <10 mEq/L due to increased proximal tubule reabsorption of Na$^+$ (P$_O$ > P$_H$) unless the patient is on diuretics. Rx is water/salt restriction and diuretics.] |
| cause of hyponatremia with volume excess, pitting edema, increased EABV | **renal failure with salt retention—** * most cases of renal failure result in hyponatremia owing to problems with salt excretion, * salt-retention is primarily within the ECF, hence EABV is increased, * Rx is a loop diuretic or dialysis |

*Table continued on following page*

**Table 1–3. FLUID AND ELECTROLYTE DISORDERS**
*Continued*

| Most Common... | Answer and Explanation |
|---|---|
| cause of hyponatremia with a normal physical exam | • **SiADH,** • *primary polydipsia,* • *reset osmostat*—see below [**Note:** the above conditions have a hypotonic gain of pure water leading to a dilutional hyponatremia ($\downarrow$ serum $Na^+$ = $TBNa^+/\uparrow\uparrow TBW$). The osmotic gradient favors movement of water primarily into the ICF; however, the compartments in the ECF are water overloaded as well. Recall that an increase in TBW without an increase in $TBNa^+$ cannot produce pitting edema, hence the normal skin turgor in the patient. Because the EABV is increased, random $UNa^+$ is >20 mEq/L ($P_H > P_O$). Excessive ADH leads to continual concentration of the urine and reabsorption of free water from the collecting duct back into the ECF.] |
| causes of SiADH | • **small cell carcinoma of lung,** • *other neoplastic diseases*— * leukemia/lymphoma, * pancreatic cancer, • *drugs enhancing ADH production*—e.g., * cyclophosphamide, * phenothiazines, * carbamazepine, * vincristine, • *drugs enhancing ADH activity*—e.g., * oxytocin drip, * NSAIDs, * chlorpropamide, * carbamazepine, • *CNS disease*— * trauma, * infection, • *pulmonary disease*— * TB, * pneumonia, * PEEP therapy |
| lab findings in SiADH | • **severe hyponatremia**—invariably the serum $Na^+$ is <120 mEq/L, • *low serum BUN*— * increased plasma volume has a dilutional effect, * increased plasma volume also increases the GFR, hence more urea is filtered and lost in the urine, * because $P_H > P_O$ from the increase in EABV, urea cannot be reabsorbed in the proximal tubule and is lost in the urine, • *hypouricemia*—uric acid is lost in urine for the same reasons described for urea, • *$UNa^+$ >40 mEq/L*— * $Na^+$ loss in the urine is primarily due to $P_H > P_O$ from the increase in EABV plus the inhibition of the RAA system and lack of aldosterone, * as a rule, not enough $Na^+$ is lost in the urine to produce volume depletion, • *UOsm > POsm*—this is due to the constant concentration of the urine in the continual presence of ADH |

## Table 1–3. FLUID AND ELECTROLYTE DISORDERS
*Continued*

| Most Common... | Answer and Explanation |
|---|---|
| Rx of SiADH | • **restrict water,** • *demeclocycline*— * produces nephrogenic DI, * this drug is primarily used in the Rx of a small cell carcinoma, since the drug is nephrotoxic and the patient prognosis is so poor, • *infusion of 3% hypertonic saline + loop diuretic*— * the loop diuretic produces a loss of both salt and water, * the amount of $Na^+$ lost in urine is measured and replaced with 3% saline: water is lost while salt is replaced, * see the calculation below |
| causes of reset osmostat ("sick cell syndrome") | • **chronic disease**—e.g., * TB, * cirrhosis, • *cachexia/malnutrition* [**Note:** in the reset osmostat syndrome, the hypothalamus is set at a lower level of response to ADH for protecting ECF osmolality. Normally, the osmostat is set for 285 mOsm/kg (~serum $Na^+$ 140 mEq/L). In reset osmostat syndrome, the osmostat is set at ~250 mOsm/kg (~serum $Na^+$ 125 mEq/L). Excess infusion of water in these patients results in normal inhibition of ADH (not true in SiADH) and excretion of free water without any further lowering of serum $Na^+$. Recall that in SiADH, infusion of water further reduces serum $Na^+$, since dilution is impaired by inability to inhibit ADH release.] |
| cause of hyponatremia with a normal POsm | **pseudohyponatremia** |
| causes of pseudohyponatremia | • **hypertriglyceridemia** >1500 mg/dL, • *excess in γ-globulins* [**Note:** because 93% of plasma is water and 7% contains nonaqueous components (lipids, proteins), an increase in the nonaqueous phase further reduces the amount of water (<93%) in plasma. This produces a falsely low serum $Na^+$ for some laboratory instruments. However, POsm is normal, because the total amount of $Na^+$ distributed in plasma water remains normal.] |

*Table continued on following page*

### Table 1–3.  FLUID AND ELECTROLYTE DISORDERS
*Continued*

| Most Common... | Answer and Explanation |
|---|---|
| cause of hyponatremia with an increased POsm | • **hyperglycemia**— * DKA, * HNKC, • *mannitol*— * this is used to reduce intracranial/intraocular pressure, * Rx of hemolytic transfusion reactions, • *glycine*—prostate surgery [**Note:** all the solutes listed above are limited to the ECF and produce a dilutional hyponatremia and an ↑ POsm. They are also osmotic diuretics and lead to polyuria and loss of water and electrolytes in the urine.] |
| CNS disorder due to overzealous infusions of saline in patients with hyponatremia | **central pontine myelinolysis** [**Note:** in hyponatremia, the brain is edematous as water moves into brain cells by osmosis. Brain cells synthesize idiogenic osmoles, which, when secreted into the ISF, draw fluid out of the cells with normalization of brain hydration. Isotonic saline is "hypertonic" when compared with the low osmolality in the brain cells. Hence, rapid administration of isotonic fluids should be avoided owing to the potential for irreversible demyelinating disease (central pontine myelinolysis).] |
| types of fluid losses causing hypernatremia (serum $Na^+$ > 145 mEq/L) | • **pure water loss**— ↑ serum $Na^+$ = $TBNa^+$/↓ ↓ TBW: ♦ note that a loss of water without salt does not produce signs of volume depletion, ♦ this type of fluid loss is called dehydration, • *hypotonic fluid loss with more water than salt*— ↑ serum $Na^+$ = ↓ $TBNa^+$/↓ ↓ TBW: note that with the loss of salt, these patients will have signs of volume depletion, • *hypertonic gain in salt*— ↑ serum $Na^+$ = ↑ ↑ $TBNa^+$/↑ TBW: due to the gain in $TBNa^+$, these patients have pitting edema and body cavity effusions |
| mechanism for producing hypernatremia | **lack of patient access to water**— * e.g., patients who develop hypernatremia are too young, too old, or too sick to have easy access to water, * patients who have access to water will increase TBW, which often converts hypernatremia into either normonatremia or hyponatremia |
| S/S of hypernatremia | • **mental status alterations**—irritability, • *seizures*, • *hyperreflexia*, • *ataxia* |

### Table 1–3.  FLUID AND ELECTROLYTE DISORDERS
*Continued*

| Most Common... | Answer and Explanation |
|---|---|
| causes of hypernatremia with volume depletion | • **osmotic diuresis**— * **DKA,** * mannitol, * urea, • *sweating* [**Note:** there is a hypotonic loss of more water than salt ( ↑ serum $Na^+$ = ↓ $TBNa^+$/ ↓ ↓ TBW). Patients show signs of hypovolemia from salt loss. The random $UNa^+$ is < 10 mEq/L in extrarenal fluid loss (sweating) and > 20 mEq/L in osmotic diuresis.] |
| Rx of hypernatremia due to a hypotonic fluid loss containing salt | **isotonic saline to raise BP into normal range**—once the BP is stabilized, use 0.45% saline (see calculation below) to replace any further fluid losses [**Note:** recall that hypotension should never be treated with hypotonic salt solutions. The closer the crystalloid resembles the tonicity of plasma, the more effective it is in restoring the blood pressure.] |
| causes of hypernatremia with volume excess and pitting edema | • **excessive $NaHCO_3$ infusions,** • *infusion of $Na^+$ salt antibiotics* [**Note:** the above infusions are associated with a hypertonic gain of more salt than water ( ↑ serum $Na^+$ = ↑ ↑ $TBNa^+$/ ↑ TBW). The increase in salt produces pitting edema and body effusions. The random $UNa^+$ is >20 mEq/L owing to decreased proximal tubule reabsorption of $Na^+$ ($P_H > P_O$).] |
| Rx of hypernatremia from a hypertonic gain of salt | • **salt restriction,** • **diuretics** |
| cause of hypernatremia with volume excess and absence of pitting edema | **mineralocorticoid excess states**— * primary aldosteronism, * Cushing's syndrome [**Note:** in chronic mineralocorticoid excess states, the increase in EABV reduces proximal tubule reabsorption of $Na^+$, since $P_H > P_O$. Since the aldosterone $Na^+$/$K^+$ pumps are already at maximal function, they cannot retrieve the $Na^+$ lost from the proximal tubules. Enough $Na^+$ is lost in the urine to offset the amount of $Na^+$ reabsorbed, hence pitting edema does not occur.] |

*Table continued on following page*

## Table 1–3. FLUID AND ELECTROLYTE DISORDERS
*Continued*

| Most Common... | Answer and Explanation |
|---|---|
| causes of hypernatremia with a normal physical exam | • **insensible water loss**— * insensible water loss is due to evaporation of water from mucous membranes without salt: e.g., ♦ fever, ♦ respirators, • *central/nephrogenic DI* [**Note:** the above conditions produce a pure water loss, leading to hypernatremia ( ↑ serum $Na^+$ = $TBNa^+$/ ↓ ↓ TBW). Signs of volume depletion are uncommon, since $TBNa^+$ is normal. The random $UNa^+$ is <10 mEq/L in insensible water loss and >20 mEq/L in DI.] |
| Rx of hypernatremia from pure water loss | **oral administration of water**—if oral hydration is not feasible, infuse D5W |
| formula used to calculate the fluid deficit in hypernatremia associated with volume depletion | **fluid deficit = 0.60 × weight in kg × (measured serum $Na^+$/140 − 1)**— * e.g., 70-kg-man with serum $Na^+$ 160 mEq/L: fluid deficit = 0.6 (70) × (160/140 − 1) = ~6 liters, * if hypernatremia is due to pure water loss, give IV D5W or water by mouth, * if hypernatremia is due to a hypotonic loss of more water than salt, give normal saline first until the blood pressure is stabilized and then infuse 0.45% saline |
| CNS abnormality produced with overzealous infusions of saline in patients with hypernatremia | **cerebral edema leading to herniation** [**Note:** in hypernatremia, brain cells are initially contracted from water loss owing to the osmotic gradient in the ECF favoring the exodus of water from the ICF compartment. Idiogenic osmoles (see above) are manufactured in the brain cells, which draw fluid back into the cells over time, with subsequent rehydration of the brain. In the setting of a normally hydrated brain, a rapid IV infusion may cause cerebral edema and herniation. Hence, IV fluids must be administered slowly over 24–48 hrs. As a rule, serum $Na^+$ should not drop ≥0.5 mEq/L/hr when infusing fluids.] |
| surgical causes of hypokalemia (serum $K^+$ <3.5 mEq/L) | • **GI loss**—random urine potassium ($UK^+$) is <20 mEq/L: e.g., ♦ vomiting/diarrhea, ♦ NG suction, ♦ villous adenoma, • *renal loss*—the random $UK^+$ is >20 mEq/L: e.g., ♦ **diuretics**, ♦ osmotic diuresis, ♦ increased urine anions like $HCO_3^-$ and ketoacids, • *transcellular shifts of $K^+$ into the cells*— see below |

**Table 1–3. FLUID AND ELECTROLYTE DISORDERS**
*Continued*

| Most Common... | Answer and Explanation |
|---|---|
| factors promoting $K^+$ shift into cells (transcellular shift into ICF) leading to hypokalemia | • **insulin**— * insulin enhances the $Na^+/K^+$ ATPase pump, * this reduces $Na^+$ permeability and favors a shift of $K^+$ into cells, • *epinephrine,* • *alkalosis*—cells (e.g., RBCs) are an excellent extrarenal source of $H^+$ ions in alkalotic states: to maintain electroneutrality, $H^+$ ions moving out of cells are counterbalanced by $K^+$ ions moving into the cells, • $\beta_2$-*agonists*—e.g., albuterol: $\beta_2$-agonists enhance the $Na^+/K^+$ ATPase pump, • *aldosterone*—enhances the $Na^+/K^+$ pumps in the distal and collecting tubules, • *refeeding syndrome*—in malnourished patients receiving TPN, $K^+$ rapidly moves into cells that are undergoing mitosis |
| S/S of hypokalemia | • **muscle weakness**—hypokalemia changes the intracellular/extracellular $K^+$ membrane potential, • *constipation,* • *paralytic ileus*—absence of bowel sounds, • *polyuria*—hypokalemia produces a vacuolar nephropathy: ♦ the collecting tubules become resistant to ADH, ♦ acquired nephrogenic DI, • *rhabdomyolysis*—hypokalemia inhibits insulin, which decreases muscle glycogenesis, leading to rhabdomyolysis, • *ventricular arrhythmias*—common finding in patients on digitalis, • *hypokalemia precipitates hepatic encephalopathy in chronic liver disease*—hypokalemia increases renal ammoniagenesis |
| ECG findings in hypokalemia | • **U waves**—the U wave is a positive wave after the T wave, • *sagging ST segment,* • *T wave depression* |
| Rx of hypokalemia | • **oral replacement**—enteric-coated preparations may produce jejunal strictures, • *IV infusion of $K^+$*—add KCl to IV solutions: ♦ the final concentration should be ~40 mEq/L, ♦ infusion rate should not exceed 10–20 mEq $K^+$/h, • *use of aldosterone blockers in patients taking diuretics*—conserves $K^+$ by blocking its secretion, • *dietary $Na^+$ restriction*—less $Na^+$ delivery to the distal tubule/collecting duct reduces the exchange of $K^+$ for $Na^+$ |

*Table continued on following page*

**Table 1–3. FLUID AND ELECTROLYTE DISORDERS**
*Continued*

| Most Common... | Answer and Explanation |
| --- | --- |
| nonpathologic cause of hyperkalemia | **pseudohyperkalemia secondary to iatrogenic hemolysis of RBCs**—pseudohyperkalemia also occurs with an increase in WBCs or platelets |
| pathophysiologic causes of hyperkalemia | • **decreased renal excretion**—e.g., * **renal failure,** * aldosterone deficiency— ♦ Addison's, ♦ hyporeninemic hypoaldosteronism (destruction of the JG apparatus), • *increased tissue release*—e.g., rhabdomyolysis, • *transcellular shift*—see below |
| factors promoting K⁺ shift out of cells, leading to hyperkalemia | • **inorganic metabolic acidoses**—e.g., * renal failure, * intracellular buffering of H⁺ ions causes K⁺ to move out of cells in order to maintain electroneutrality, • *insulin deficiency,* • *hypertonicity*—e.g., hyperglycemia, • *β-antagonists*—e.g., propranolol, • *digitalis toxicity*—inhibits Na⁺-K⁺-ATPase pump, • *succinylcholine*—muscle relaxant |
| S/S of hyperkalemia | • **cardiac arrhythmias**—e.g., * ventricular arrhythmias, * the heart stops in diastole, • *muscle weakness*—hyperkalemia partially depolarizes the cell membrane, which interferes with membrane excitability, • *impairs renal acid excretion, leading to metabolic acidosis*— * K⁺ moves into the distal/collecting duct tubules in exchange for H⁺ ions |
| early ECG finding in hyperkalemia | **peaked narrow T waves**—this is due to accelerated repolarization of cardiac muscle [**Note:** a serum K⁺ between 7 and 8 mEq/L decreases cardiac excitability owing to inactivation of Na⁺ permeability during the initial spike of the action potential. This results in widening of the PR interval and the QRS. Serum K⁺ levels > 8 mEq/L result in cardiac standstill in diastole.] |

### Table 1–3. FLUID AND ELECTROLYTE DISORDERS
*Continued*

| Most Common... | Answer and Explanation |
|---|---|
| Rx of hyperkalemia | • **IV calcium gluconate**— * calcium decreases membrane excitability, hence protecting the heart, * it does not lower the serum K⁺, • *IV NaHCO₃*—creates metabolic alkalosis, which shifts K⁺ into cells, • *insulin + glucose*—shifts K⁺ into ICF, • *β₂-agonists*—shifts K⁺ into ICF, • *cation exchange resins*— * Na⁺ polystyrene promotes Na⁺ exchange for K⁺ in the GI tract, * increases K⁺ excretion, • *loop diuretics*—increase K⁺ excretion |
| functions of PTH | • **increases early distal tubule reabsorption of calcium,** • *decreases proximal tubule reabsorption of phosphate,* • *increases 1α-hydroxylase synthesis in the proximal tubule*—second hydroxylation of vitamin D, • *increases bone resorption to maintain the serum ionized calcium* [**Note:** PTH receptors are on osteoblasts. When activated by PTH, osteoblasts release IL-1 (osteoclast-activating factor). IL-1 stimulates osteoclasts to remove calcium from bone. Estrogen and testosterone have an inhibitory effect on IL-1.] |
| function of vitamin D | **increases jejunal reabsorption of calcium/ phosphorus** |
| causes of hypercalcemia | • **metastasis to bone**—see below, • *primary HPTH,* • *ectopic secretion of PTH-like peptide*—see below, • *hyperthyroidism,* • *sarcoidosis,* • *multiple myeloma,* • *hypervitaminosis D,* • *thiazides* |
| cause of ambulatory hypercalcemia | **primary HPTH**—>50% of cases |
| cause of hypercalcemia in hospitalized patients | **malignancy** |
| mechanisms of malignancy-induced hypercalcemia | • **metastasis to bone**—metastatic tumor releases osteoclast-activating factors (IL-1, prostaglandins), which resorb bone, • *secretion of PTH-like peptide*—increases calcium and decreases phosphorus reabsorption |

*Table continued on following page*

### Table 1–3.  FLUID AND ELECTROLYTE DISORDERS
*Continued*

| Most Common... | Answer and Explanation |
| --- | --- |
| cancer associated with hypercalcemia | **metastatic breast cancer to bone** |
| cancers secreting PTH-like peptide | • **primary squamous carcinoma of lung,** • *renal adenocarcinoma,* • *breast cancer* |
| lab findings in malignancy-induced hypercalcemia | • **hypercalcemia,** • *low PTH*—hypercalcemia suppresses endogenous PTH release [**Note:** assays are available for measuring PTH-like peptide.] |
| mechanism of hypercalcemia in sarcoidosis | **macrophages in granulomas synthesize 1 α-hydroxylase**—increases 1,25[OH]$_2$D synthesis |
| mechanism of hypercalcemia with thiazides | • **increased calcium reabsorption from urine,** • *volume depletion increases proximal tubule reabsorption of calcium,* • *subclinical HPTH is often present, which enhances calcium reabsorption* |
| mechanism of hypercalcemia in multiple myeloma | **intramarrow release of IL-1 (osteoclast-activating factor) from malignant plasma cells** |
| mechanism of hypercalcemia in hypervitaminosis D | • **increased calcium reabsorption from the jejunum,** • *conversion of macrophages in the bone marrow into osteoclasts, leading to increased bone resorption* |
| mechanism of hypercalcemia in thyrotoxicosis | **increased bone resorption** |
| S/S of hypercalcemia | • **renal stones**—hypercalciuria is the most common underlying metabolic abnormality, • *mental status alterations*— * depression, * psychosis, • *acute pancreatitis*—calcium stimulates phospholipase in the pancreas, • *PUD*—calcium stimulates gastrin release, leading to peptic ulcers, • *constipation,* • *diastolic HTN,* • *polyuria*—due to nephrocalcinosis, • *short QT interval* |

## Table 1–3. FLUID AND ELECTROLYTE DISORDERS
*Continued*

| Most Common... | Answer and Explanation |
|---|---|
| Rx of hypercalcemia | • **induce diuresis with isotonic saline and follow up with a loop diuretic**, • *bisphosphonates*— * drug of choice in severe hypercalcemia, * pamidronate is most often used, • *calcitonin*— * calcitonin receptors are located on osteoclasts, * inhibits osteoclastic activity, * blocks renal calcium reabsorption, • *plicamycin*—inhibits osteoclast resorption, • *gallium nitrate*—inhibits osteoclast resorption, • *glucocorticoids*—mainly used for hypercalcemia due to: ♦ hypervitaminosis D (e.g., sarcoidosis), ♦ IL-1 (e.g., multiple myeloma) |
| causes of hypocalcemia | • **hypoalbuminemia**—see below, • *vitamin D deficiency*—renal failure is the MCC, • *acute pancreatitis*, • *post-total thyroidectomy*—hypoparathyroidism, • *acute alkalosis*, • *primary hypoparathyroidism*, • *hypomagnesemia*—see below |
| mechanism of hypocalcemia in hypoalbuminemia | **albumin is binding protein for calcium** — * total calcium is calcium bound to albumin (40%), bound to phosphates/sulfates (13%), and free (47%, ionized, metabolically active calcium), * hypoalbuminemia reduces total calcium without altering the ionized calcium (no tetany) |
| formula used to correct total calcium for hypoalbuminemia | **corrected calcium = (measured calcium − serum albumin) + 4** |
| S/S of hypocalcemia, hypoparathyroidism | • **tetany**— * due to a low ionized calcium: ♦ lowers the threshold potential to a value close to the resting membrane potential, ♦ less stimulus is required to initiate the action potential, * tingling in circumoral area, hands/feet, * Trousseau's sign—carpopedal spasm while measuring blood pressure: thumb adducts into the palm, * Chvostek's sign—facial muscle twitching with tapping of the facial nerve, * laryngeal stridor, * muscle cramping, • *prolonged QT interval* |

*Table continued on following page*

### Table 1–3. FLUID AND ELECTROLYTE DISORDERS
*Continued*

| Most Common... | Answer and Explanation |
| --- | --- |
| cause of tetany when the total calcium is normal | **alkalosis**—alkalosis (respiratory primarily, metabolic less commonly) increases negative charges on albumin, leading to further calcium binding to albumin at the expense of the ionized calcium pool |
| mechanism of hypocalcemia in hypovitaminosis D | **decreased calcium reabsorption from the jejunum** |
| mechanism of hypocalcemia in acute pancreatitis | **enzymatic fat necrosis**— * calcium is consumed by binding to fatty acids, * bad prognostic sign |
| mechanism of hypocalcemia in CRF | • **hypovitaminosis D**—loss of the 1-α-hydroxylating enzyme located in the proximal tubule, • *hyperphosphatemia*—phosphorus drives calcium into soft tissue/bone |
| mechanism of hypocalcemia in malabsorption | **malabsorption of vitamin D** |
| Rx of hypocalcemia | • **oral calcium,** • *IV calcium*—emergency conditions, • *vitamin D*—in hypovitaminosis D |
| causes of hypermagnesemia | • **renal failure,** • *iatrogenic*—e.g., use of $Mg^{++}$ sulfate in Rx of eclampsia |
| S/S of hypermagnesemia | • **depressed DTRs,** • *muscle weakness,* • *hypotension,* • *bradycardia* |
| Rx of hypermagnesemia | • **calcium gluconate**—protect the heart, • **saline infusion followed by a loop diuretic**—similar to Rx of hypercalcemia |
| pathologic cause of hypocalcemia in a hospitalized patient | **hypomagnesemia** |
| mechanisms of hypocalcemia in hypomagnesemia | • **$Mg^{++}$ enhances PTH activity,** • *$Mg^{++}$ increases PTH release from the parathyroids,* • *$Mg^{++}$ is a cofactor for adenylate cyclase*—cAMP is necessary for PTH function |

### Table 1–3. FLUID AND ELECTROLYTE DISORDERS
*Continued*

| Most Common... | Answer and Explanation |
|---|---|
| causes of hypomagnesemia | • **diuretics**, • *vomiting/diarrhea*, • *TPN*—diarrhea, • *alcoholism*—also noted in alcohol withdrawal, • *osmotic diuresis*—e.g., DKA, • *post-AMI*, • *drugs*—e.g., * aminoglycosides, * cisplatin, * cyclosporine, * amphotericin B |
| S/S of hypomagnesemia | • **tetany**—secondary to hypocalcemia, • *hyperreflexia*, • *mental status alterations*, • *ventricular arrhythmias*—related to digitalis Rx |
| Rx of hypomagnesemia | • **oral**—Mg$^{++}$ oxide, • *parenteral* |
| causes of hyperphosphatemia | • **CRF**—decreased excretion of phosphate, • *increased phosphate load*—transfusion of old blood, • *primary hypoparathyroidism*, • *normal childhood* |
| clinical finding associated with hyperphosphatemia | • **metastatic calcification**— * drives Ca$^{++}$ into the kidneys (renal failure due to nephrocalcinosis), skin/soft tissue, • *hypovitaminosis D*— * high PO$_4^{--}$ inhibits 1-α hydroxylase synthesis, which decreases vitamin D synthesis, • *secondary HPTH*—secondary effect of hyperphosphatemia causing hypocalcemia, • *renal osteodystrophy*—due to: ♦ secondary HPTH, ♦ renal failure (metabolic acidosis) |
| Rx of hyperphosphatemia | • **oral calcium bicarbonate with meals**, • *dialysis* |
| acquired causes of hypophosphatemia | • **respiratory/metabolic alkalosis**—alkalosis activates phosphofructokinase (PFK) with enhanced glycolysis and phosphorylation of glucose, • *insulin Rx in DKA*— * glucose must be phosphorylated to remain in adipose/muscle, * phosphate is lost in urine from osmotic diuresis, • *ingestion of phosphate binders*—aluminum/calcium/magnesium antacids, • *phosphaturic drugs*— * diuretics, * corticosteroids, • *hypovitaminosis D*— * malabsorption, * inadequate intake, * decreased sunlight, • *primary HPTH*—phosphaturia, • *burn patients*—phosphaturia associated with fluid mobilization |

*Table continued on following page*

## Table 1–3. FLUID AND ELECTROLYTE DISORDERS
*Continued*

| Most Common... | Answer and Explanation |
|---|---|
| clinical findings in hypophosphatemia | • **muscle weakness**— * respiratory paralysis: occurs with levels <1.0 mg/dL, * low intracellular ATP, • *RBC hemolysis*—spectrin in RBC membrane must be phosphorylated for the RBC to remain in a biconcave state, • *rhabdomyolysis*—muscles need ATP |
| Rx of hypophosphatemia | • **oral replacement**—preferred route, • *parenteral*—for severe depletion |

**Question:** Which of the following clinical situations are associated with signs of volume depletion and a normal AG metabolic acidosis? **SELECT 3**

    (A) DKA
    (B) Addison's disease
    (C) Small bowel fistula
    (D) Nasogastric suction
    (E) Drainage of a pancreatic pseudocyst
    (F) High fever
    (G) Congestive heart failure

**Answers:** **(B), (C), (E):** DKA is associated with volume depletion from osmotic diuresis and loss of $Na^+$. However, the metabolic acidosis of DKA is of the increased AG type (**choice A is incorrect**). In Addison's disease, the loss of aldosterone causes significant renal loss of salt with volume depletion, and $H^+$ ions are retained, causing a normal AG metabolic acidosis (**choice B is correct**). Drainage from a small bowel fistula and drainage of fluid from a pancreatic pseudocyst cause a significant loss of isotonic saline in addition to bicarbonate, the latter leading to a normal AG metabolic acidosis (**choices C and E are correct**). Nasogastric suction causes volume depletion due to loss of salt; however, metabolic alkalosis is the primary metabolic abnormality (**choice D is incorrect**). High fever causes insensible water loss without significant alterations in volume status or acid-base balance (**choice F is incorrect**). CHF is associated with hypervolemia and lactic acidosis (increased AG metabolic acidosis) from tissue hypoxia (**choice G is incorrect**).

## Table 1–3. FLUID AND ELECTROLYTE DISORDERS
### *Continued*

ACE = angiotensin-converting enzyme, ADH = antidiuretic hormone, AG = anion gap, AMI = acute myocardial infarction, ANP = atrial natriuretic peptide, AT I, II, III = angiotensin I, II, III, ATN = acute tubular necrosis, ATP = adenosine triphosphate, cAMP = cyclic adenosine monophosphate, CHF = congestive heart failure, $Cl^-$ = chloride, CRF = chronic renal failure, DCT = distal convoluted tubule, DI = diabetes insipidus, DKA = diabetic ketoacidosis, DM = diabetes mellitus, DTRs = deep tendon reflexes, EABV = effective arterial blood volume, ECF = extracellular fluid, EOsm = effective osmolality, GFR = glomerular filtration rate, $H^+$ = protons, $HCO_3^-$ = bicarbonate, Hct = hematocrit, HNKC = hyperosmolar nonketotic coma, $HPO_4^-$ = monophosphate, HPTH = hyperparathyroidism, HTN = hypertension, ICF = intracellular fluid, IL-1 = interleukin-1, ISF = interstitial fluid, JG = juxtaglomerular, LHF = left heart failure, LVEDP = left ventricular end-diastolic pressure, MCC = most common cause, $Mg^{++}$ = magnesium, MOA = mechanism of action, $NH_3$ = ammonia, $NH_4^+$ = ammonium, NSAIDs = nonsteroidal anti-inflammatory drugs, PCWP = pulmonary capillary wedge pressure, PEEP = positive end-expiratory pressure, PFK = phosphofructokinase, $PGE_2$ = prostaglandin $E_2$, $P_H$ = peritubular capillary hydrostatic pressure, $P_O$ = peritubular capillary oncotic pressure, POsm = plasma osmolality, PTH = parathormone, PUD = peptic ulcer disease, RAA = renin-angiotensin-aldosterone, RBF = renal blood flow, RHF = right heart failure, RTA = renal tubular acidosis, SGC = Swan-Ganz catheter, SiADH = syndrome of inappropriate antidiuretic hormone, S/S = signs and symptoms, TAL = thick ascending limb, $TBK^+$ = total body potassium, $TBNa^+$ = total body sodium, TBW = total body water, THV = terminal hepatic venule, TPN = total parenteral nutrition, TPR = total peripheral resistance, $UK^+$ = urine potassium, $UNa^+$ = urine sodium, UOsm = urine osmolality.

# CHAPTER

# HEMATOLOGIC EVALUATION OF THE SURGICAL PATIENT

## CONTENTS

### Table 2–1. HISTORY AND PHYSICAL FINDINGS IN ANEMIA

| Most Common... | Answer and Explanation |
|---|---|
| anemia in surgical patients | **iron deficiency**—usually due to blood loss from a GI source, e.g., duodenal ulcer: adult, Meckel's diverticulum: child |
| macrocytic anemia in alcoholics | **folate deficiency**—due to a combination of decreased intake and loss of folate in the GI tract |
| anemia in women <50 yrs old | **iron deficiency secondary to menorrhagia** |
| anemia in men <50 yrs old | **iron deficiency secondary to a duodenal ulcer** |

*Table continued on following page*

**47**

## Table 2–1. HISTORY AND PHYSICAL FINDINGS IN ANEMIA *Continued*

| Most Common... | Answer and Explanation |
|---|---|
| anemia in men/women >50 yrs of age | **iron deficiency secondary to colon cancer** |
| anemia associated with pica for clay, ice, or starch | **iron deficiency**—PICA is the term applied to a craving for something unusual |
| anemia in neonates and children | **bleeding Meckel's diverticulum** |
| anemia in malignancy | **anemia of chronic disease (ACD)** [Note: examples of the many other causes of anemia in malignancy include iron deficiency, metastasis to the bone marrow, autoimmune hemolytic anemia.] |
| anemia in CRF | **normocytic anemia secondary to deficiency of erythropoietin**—erythropoietin is synthesized by endothelial cells in the peritubular capillaries |
| anemia in hospitalized patients | **ACD** |
| drugs associated with folate deficiency | • **methotrexate,** • *BCP,* • *phenytoin,* • *TMP/SMX* |
| types of anemia associated with jaundice | **extravascular hemolytic anemias**— * sickle cell anemia, * congenital spherocytosis, * AIHA [Note: the end-product of macrophage destruction of RBCs is unconjugated bilirubin.] |
| anemias associated with calcium bilirubinate stones | **extravascular hemolytic anemias**— * sickle cell disease, * congenital spherocytosis |
| anemias associated with malabsorption | • **iron,** • *folate deficiency,* • $B_{12}$ *deficiency* |
| anemias associated with a Billroth II | • **iron deficiency,** • $B_{12}$ *deficiency* [Note: a Billroth II is a subtotal gastrectomy with anastomosis of the stomach to the jejunum. The duodenum (where iron is primarily absorbed) is left as a blind loop, hence it has no contact with iron in the gastric meal. Decreased acid production interferes with the release of $B_{12}$ from meat.] |

### Table 2–1. HISTORY AND PHYSICAL FINDINGS
### IN ANEMIA *Continued*

| Most Common... | Answer and Explanation |
|---|---|
| anemia associated with terminal ileal disease/resection | $B_{12}$ **deficiency**—site of $B_{12}$ absorption |
| symptoms of anemia | • **dyspnea with exertion,** • *dizziness,* • *palpitations,* • *insomnia,* • *angina*—in people with CAD [**Note:** an Hgb of <7 g/dL is usually associated with symptoms.] |
| anemia associated with spoon nails (koilonychia) | **iron deficiency** |
| cardiovascular signs of anemia | • **pulmonic flow murmur,** • *wide pulse pressure*—reduced viscosity leads to a high-output failure, • *hypotension,* • *tachycardia* |
| cutaneous signs of anemia | • **pallor of palmar creases,** • **jaundice**—if anemia is related to extravascular hemolysis, • **telangiectasia**—Osler-Weber-Rendu disease—GI bleeding leads to iron deficiency, • **petechiae/ecchymoses**—thrombocytopenia and potential for GI blood loss |
| anemias associated with glossitis | • **iron deficiency,** • *$B_{12}$/folate deficiency* |
| anemia associated with dysphagia for solids | **iron deficiency**—esophageal web, part of the Plummer-Vinson syndrome |
| anemia in right-sided colon cancer | **iron deficiency**—"left side obstructs, right side bleeds" |
| anemias associated with peripheral neuropathy | • **$B_{12}$ deficiency,** • *Pb poisoning,* • *sideroblastic anemia associated with $B_6$ deficiency*—$B_6$ deficiency is most commonly due to Rx of TB with isoniazid |
| anemia associated with decreased vibratory sensation and loss of proprioception | $B_{12}$ **deficiency** |

*Table continued on following page*

# 50  MOST COMMONS IN SURGERY

## Table 2–1. HISTORY AND PHYSICAL FINDINGS IN ANEMIA *Continued*

**Question:** Which of the following are associated with iron deficiency?
**SELECT 5**
 (A) Osler-Weber-Rendu disease
 (B) Methotrexate
 (C) Koilonychia
 (D) Peripheral neuropathy
 (E) Plummer-Vinson syndrome
 (F) Terminal ileum resection
 (G) Billroth II
 (H) Internal hemorrhoids
 (I) Meckel's diverticulum

**Answers: (A), (C), (E), (G), (I).** Osler-Weber-Rendu disease is associated with telangiectasias on the skin and throughout the GI tract, the latter site a source for bleeding and iron deficiency (**choice A is correct**). Methotrexate is associated with inhibition of dihydrofolate reductase, which leads to folate deficiency (**choice B is incorrect**). Koilonychia, or spoon nails, is a sign of iron deficiency (**choice C is correct**). Peripheral neuropathy is more often associated with $B_{12}$ deficiency and Pb poisoning than iron deficiency (**choice D is incorrect**). The Plummer-Vinson syndrome is due to iron deficiency. It includes esophageal webs leading to dysphagia for solids, achlorhydria, and glossitis (**choice E is correct**). Terminal ileal resection results in $B_{12}$ deficiency (**choice F is incorrect**). A Billroth II leads to both iron and $B_{12}$ deficiency (**choice G is correct**). Internal hemorrhoids cause bleeding but not iron deficiency (**choice H is incorrect**). A Meckel's diverticulum is the most common cause of iron deficiency in neonates and young children (**choice I is correct**).

ACD = anemia of chronic disease, AIHA = autoimmune hemolytic anemia, BCP = birth control pill, CAD = coronary artery disease, CRF = chronic renal failure, Pb = lead, TMP/SMX = trimethoprim/sulfamethoxazole.

## Table 2–2. COMMON DIAGNOSTIC TESTS IN HEMATOLOGY

| Most Common... | Answer and Explanation |
| --- | --- |
| test used to evaluate erythropoiesis | **PB blood reticulocyte count** [Note: reticulocytes are young RBCs that require 24 h to mature. A supravital stain identifies RNA filaments in the reticulocytes.] |
| formula that corrects PB reticulocyte count for degree of anemia | **(patient Hct ÷ 45) × % reticulocyte count** [Note: for example: Hct 30%, reticulocyte count 15%: (30 ÷ 45) × 15 = 10%. A good BM response to anemia is >3%, whereas a poor response is <2%.] |

## Table 2–2. COMMON DIAGNOSTIC TESTS
## IN HEMATOLOGY *Continued*

| Most Common... | Answer and Explanation |
| --- | --- |
| parameters reported in a CBC (complete blood cell count) | • **cell counts**— \* RBC, \* WBC, \* platelets, • **Hgb/Hct**—the Hgb × 3 should approximately equal the Hct, • **RBC indices**— \* the MCV is the most important index for anemia classification, • **RBC distribution width (RDW)**— \* the RDW is the numerical estimate of size variation of RBCs: another term for this is anisocytosis, \* RDW is increased if both small and large RBCs are present in the peripheral blood, \* RDW is normal if RBCs are uniform in their size, \* iron deficiency is the only microcytic anemia with an increased RDW: normocytic and microcytic cells are present, • **RBC shape abnormalities**—another term for this is poikilocytosis, • **RBC size abnormalities**—anisocytosis, • **platelet morphology,** • **WBC morphology,** • **100 WBC differential count**—% neutrophils, eosinophils, basophils, monocytes, lymphocytes based on a 100-cell count |
| use of the MCV | **classification scheme for anemia**—anemias are classified as: ♦ normocytic, ♦ microcytic, ♦ macrocytic |
| microcytic anemia where the RBC count is normal to increased whereas the Hgb and Hct are decreased | **α- and β-thalassemia** |
| parameters reported in a BM aspirate/core biopsy | • **assessment of cellularity**—normal cellularity is 30% fat, 70% cells, • **myeloid/erythroid (M/E) ratio**—normally 3/1, • **cell morphology,** • **adequacy of megakaryocytes,** • **estimate of iron stores**—a Prussian blue stain is utilized to stain hemosiderin, • **additional uses**— \* R/O metastatic disease, \* culture for work-ups of FUO, \* staging malignant lymphomas |
| anemias requiring iron studies | • **iron deficiency,** • *ACD,* • *sideroblastic anemias* |

*Table continued on following page*

### Table 2–2. COMMON DIAGNOSTIC TESTS
### IN HEMATOLOGY *Continued*

| Most Common... | Answer and Explanation |
|---|---|
| iron studies | • **serum ferritin**— * ferritin is the storage form of iron stored in macrophages located in the marrow, * a small circulating fraction of ferritin parallels iron stores in the bone marrow, * normal ferritin concentration is 20–250 ng/mL, * a serum ferritin is the best overall screen of iron-related disorders, • *serum iron*—50–170 μg/dL, • *TIBC*— * the TIBC is an indirect measure of the transferrin concentration, * normal TIBC is 250–425 μg/dL, * TIBC increases (transferrin synthesis increases) when iron stores are decreased: an inverse relationship exists of transferrin synthesis in the liver with iron stores in the marrow, * TIBC decreases (transferrin synthesis decreases) when iron stores in the marrow are increased, • *% saturation*—calculated as follows: serum Fe ÷ TIBC × 100, * normal iron saturation is 20–50% [**Note:** a problem with ferritin is that it lacks specificity because some ferritin is also stored in hepatocytes and used in the cytochrome P450 system. Any inflammatory condition can falsely increase ferritin derived from the liver rather than the marrow.] |
| hematologic disorders requiring an Hgb electrophoresis for confirmation | **hemoglobinopathies**—examples include: ♦ thalassemias, ♦ sickle cell trait/disease and its variants [**Note:** Hemoglobinopathies are disorders in Hgb synthesis. Hgb electrophoresis reports the percentage of normal Hgbs based on their density when they are electrophoretically separated out on cellulose acetate. Normal values are: HgbA > 97%, HgbA$_2$ < 2.5%, HgbF < 1%. Hgb electrophoresis also identifies abnormal Hgbs (e.g., Hgb H, Hgb E).] |
| causes of an elevated EPO level | • **decreased Hgb concentration**—e.g., iron deficiency, • *tissue hypoxia*—e.g., * high altitude, * hypoxemia in lung disease, * CO poisoning, • *ectopic production*—e.g., * renal disease: renal adenocarcinoma, cysts, * hepatocellular carcinoma |
| causes of a low EPO level | • **chronic renal failure**—decreased synthesis, • *PRV*, • *HIV infection*, • *ACD* |

Table 2–2. **COMMON DIAGNOSTIC TESTS IN HEMATOLOGY** Continued

| Most Common... | Answer and Explanation |
| --- | --- |
| confirmatory test to order when $B_{12}$ levels are nondiagnostic for suspected $B_{12}$ deficiency | **urine for methylmalonic acid**— * $B_{12}$ is a cofactor for the reaction that converts methylmalonyl CoA into succinyl CoA, * $B_{12}$ deficiency causes an increase in methylmalonyl CoA, which is metabolized into methylmalonic acid |
| test used to localize the cause of $B_{12}$ deficiency | **Schilling's test** [Note: if the absorption of orally administered radioactive $B_{12}$ is corrected with the addition of IF, the patient has PA. If $B_{12}$ absorption is corrected after a course of antibiotics, bacterial overgrowth in the small bowel is responsible. If $B_{12}$ reabsorption is corrected after the patient receives pancreatic enzymes, chronic pancreatitis is the cause of $B_{12}$ deficiency. No correction of $B_{12}$ reabsorption with any of the above indicates that terminal ileal disease or other less common causes of $B_{12}$ deficiency must be considered.] |
| types of hemolytic anemia associated with an increase in UCB | **extravascular hemolytic anemias**— * extravascular refers to macrophage removal of RBCs from the circulation, * UCB is the end product of Hgb metabolism in macrophages: UCB binds to albumin and is taken up by the liver and conjugated into CB, * examples of extravascular hemolysis include: ♦ congenital spherocytosis, ♦ HgbS |
| types of anemia associated with a decrease in serum haptoglobin levels | **intravascular hemolytic anemias**— * haptoglobin, synthesized by the liver, binds to free Hgb in plasma to form a haptoglobin-Hgb complex, * the complex is removed and metabolized by macrophages: haptoglobin is also called the suicide protein, because it is metabolized along with Hgb, * low haptoglobin levels indicate intravascular hemolysis: low levels are also noted in chronic liver disease, * examples of intravascular hemolysis include: ♦ ABO-incompatible blood transfusion (e.g., a blood group A patient receives blood group B blood), ♦ microangiopathic hemolytic anemia, ♦ G6PD deficiency, ♦ PNH |

*Table continued on following page*

### Table 2–2. COMMON DIAGNOSTIC TESTS
### IN HEMATOLOGY *Continued*

| Most Common... | Answer and Explanation |
|---|---|
| types of sickle cell screening tests | • **sodium metabisulfite test**— * sodium metabisulfite reduces $O_2$ tension and induces sickling, * the test has high sensitivity/specificity, • *solubility test*— * deoxygenated HgbS is insoluble when compared with other Hgbs, * the test has good specificity but poor sensitivity |
| confirmatory test for a positive sickle screen | **Hgb electrophoresis** |
| test used to confirm congenital spherocytosis | **osmotic fragility of RBCs** [**Note:** RBCs are placed in test tubes with decreasing salt concentration. Spherocytes begin hemolyzing at a concentration of 0.65% (increased fragility), whereas normal RBCs begin hemolyzing at 0.50%.] |
| screening test for warm and cold AIHA | **direct Coombs' test**— * the test detects RBCs coated by IgG or C3b |
| serum test used to identify antibodies | **indirect Coombs' test**—identifies antibodies (e.g., anti-D) in the patient's serum: it is an antibody screen |
| tests to screen/ confirm G6PD deficiency | • **screen**— * Heinz body preparation of peripheral blood RBCs: requires a supravital stain, * usually performed during the acute hemolytic phase, • **confirm**—RBC enzyme assay: usually performed when hemolysis has subsided |
| WBC test used to distinguish a neutrophilic leukemoid reaction (>30,000 cells/μL) from CML | **leukocyte alkaline phosphatase (LAP) score** [**Note:** a leukemoid reaction is an absolute peripheral blood increase in mature leukocytes that may be mistaken for a leukemic process. Mature neutrophils contain LAP, whereas those in neoplastic disorders like CML do not. A high LAP score (the sum total of intensity of the stain from 0–4$^+$ in a 100-cell leukocyte count) in a peripheral blood smear with increased neutrophils rules out CML. CML has a very low score owing to the neoplastic nature of the leukocytes.] |

## Table 2–2. COMMON DIAGNOSTIC TESTS
### IN HEMATOLOGY Continued

| Most Common... | Answer and Explanation |
|---|---|
| test used to diagnose infectious mononucleosis | **heterophile antibody test**—the heterophile antibodies specific for infectious mononucleosis include: antihorse RBC antibodies, antibovine RBC antibodies, and antisheep RBC antibodies |
| test used to identify lymphocyte subtypes | **immunophenotyping**—membrane receptors (e.g., $CD_{21}$ receptor for EBV on B cells) or antigens (e.g., $CD_4$ antigen-marking helper T cells) are identified on lymphocytes by using monoclonal antibodies when the cells pass through a flow cytometer |
| MPD requiring an ABG | **PRV** [**Note:** an ABG classifies the type of polycythemia as appropriate or inappropriate. If the $SaO_2$ is ≤88%, it is an appropriate RBC response mediated by EPO release secondary to tissue hypoxia (e.g., high altitude, COPD). It is an inappropriate polycythemia if the $SaO_2$ is ≥92% (e.g., PRV, ectopic production of EPO).] |
| use of cytogenetic studies in hematology | **Dx of leukemia and malignant lymphomas**—e.g., identification of the t(9;22) in CML or the t(8;14) defect in Burkitt's lymphoma |
| initial screening test for multiple myeloma | **SPE**— * detects a monoclonal spike (85%) in the γ-globulin region: the spike is produced by a single clone of neoplastic plasma cells synthesizing one Ig and its corresponding light chain (κ or λ), * excess light chains are excreted in the urine as BJ protein [**Note:** a serum and urine IEP—these tests specifically identify the Ig involved (e.g., IgG, IgA, IgM) and its light chain in the urine.] |
| confirmatory test for multiple myeloma | **bone marrow aspirate/biopsy** |
| platelet test | **platelet count** |
| platelet function test | **bleeding time** (BT)— * the BT evaluates vessel/platelet number and function up to the formation of a temporary hemostatic plug, * the BT does not evaluate the integrity of the coagulation system (e.g., BT is normal in hemophilia A), * key factors in a normal BT include: ♦ normal platelet count, ♦ presence of vWF (adhesion molecule of the platelet), ♦ platelet synthesis of $TXA_2$ |

Table continued on following page

### Table 2–2. COMMON DIAGNOSTIC TESTS
### IN HEMATOLOGY *Continued*

| Most Common... | Answer and Explanation |
|---|---|
| cause of a prolonged BT | **NSAIDs**—NSAIDs block platelet cyclooxygenase and subsequent production of $TXA_2$ |
| test to measure vWF (von Willebrand's factor) | **ristocetin cofactor assay**— * ristocetin normally aggregates platelets containing vWF and possessing a receptor for vWF, * absence of agglutination indicates a deficiency of either vWF or the platelet receptor for vWF |
| coagulation system tests | • **prothrombin time (PT)**, • *partial thromboplastin time* (PTT), • *mixing studies*, • *thrombin time* (TT) |
| test used to evaluate the extrinsic coagulation system | **PT**— * the PT evaluates the extrinsic system down to the formation of a fibrin clot: VII → X → V → II → I → clot, * the PT is prolonged if one or more of the above factors are <40% of normal: normal factor level is ~100% |
| uses of the PT | • **follow the state of anticoagulation in patients who are taking warfarin**, • *index of severity of liver disease*—a prolonged PT indicates severe disease, • *detecting factor VII, X, V, and II deficiencies* |
| use of International Normalized Ratio (INR) for reporting PT | **follow warfarin anticoagulation**— * the INR standardizes the PT regardless of the reagents used in the test kits, * INR = (patient PT ÷ control PT) × International Sensitivity Index (value assigned to the particular type of protein-lipid tissue factor used in the test kit), * the INR should be between 2 and 3 for adequate anticoagulation |
| test used to evaluate the intrinsic coagulation system test | **PTT**— * the PTT evaluates the intrinsic system down to the formation of a clot: XII → XI → IX → VIII → X → V → II → I → clot, * the PTT is prolonged if one or more of the above factors are below 30–40% of normal |
| uses of the PTT | • **follow patients on heparin anticoagulation**, • *detect factor XII, XI, IX, VIII, X, V, and II deficiencies* |
| use of mixing studies | **differentiate true coagulation factor deficiency from a circulating inhibitor (antibody)**— * patient plasma is mixed 50:50 with normal plasma, * correction of a prolonged PTT and/or PT indicates factor deficiency, * no correction indicates an inhibitor |

## Table 2–2. COMMON DIAGNOSTIC TESTS
### IN HEMATOLOGY *Continued*

| Most Common... | Answer and Explanation |
|---|---|
| uses of TT | • **fibrinogen deficiency,** • *follow heparin Rx* [**Note:** the TT detects abnormalities in the conversion of fibrinogen into a fibrin clot by adding thrombin to the test system.] |
| fibrinolytic system tests | • D-**dimer assay**— * dimers are cross-linked FDPs associated with a fibrin clot: ♦ cross-links indicate factor XIII activity, ♦ the cross-links are detected on D fragments, * dimers are specific for DIC, • **fibrin(ogen) degradation (split) products (FDPs)**— * FDPs are X, Y, D, and E fragments resulting from plasmin degradation of either fibrinogen or clot-associated fibrin, * they are not specific for split products associated with dissolution of a fibrin clot [**Note:** other uses for D-dimer are in the diagnosis of deep vein thrombosis and as an adjunctive screening test for a pulmonary embolus.] |
| ABO blood group tests | • **forward type**—using anti-A and anti-B reagents, the forward type identifies the blood group antigen(s) (e.g., A, B, or AB) on patient RBCs, • *back type*— * using A and B antigen-positive test RBCs, the patient's serum is tested to identify antibodies (isohemagglutinins) corresponding with each blood group: ♦ O patients have anti-A-IgM, anti-B-IgM, anti-A,B-IgG, ♦ A patients have anti-B-IgM, ♦ B patients have anti-A-IgM, ♦ AB patients lack antibodies [**Note:** elderly patients often lose the isohemagglutinins. In some cases, they do not even host an immune reaction against an ABO-incompatible transfusion.] |
| test for detecting Rh antigens | **Rh agglutination reactions**—anti-D, -C, -c, -E, and -e test antisera are reacted against patient RBCs to detect D, C, c, E, or e Rh antigens, respectively: there is no d antigen. [**Note:** a weak variant of D antigen is called Du. It requires further testing for identification. Patients who are D or Du$^+$ are considered Rh positive.] |

*Table continued on following page*

### Table 2–2. COMMON DIAGNOSTIC TESTS
### IN HEMATOLOGY *Continued*

| Most Common... | Answer and Explanation |
|---|---|
| compatibility test for blood transfusion | **major cross-match**—patient's serum is mixed with RBCs from each donor unit to check their compatibility—rules out patient antibodies directed against donor and RBC antigens |
| transfusion reaction work-up tests | • **check for clerical error**, • **visual inspection of patient serum in pre- and post-transfusion specimen**—check for free Hgb in the plasma to rule out intravascular hemolysis of donor RBCs, • **direct Coombs' test**—R/O antibody destruction of donor RBCs, • **urine check for Hgb**—R/O hemoglobinuria [**Note:** a transfusion reaction work-up is requested when a patient receiving a transfusion has any type of reaction, including fever, rash, shock.] |

**Question:** Which of the following clinical disorders is most likely to have an anemia with an increase in the corrected reticulocyte count? **SELECT 4**

- (A) Blood loss >1 week
- (B) Iron deficiency
- (C) Congenital spherocytosis
- (D) Aplastic anemia
- (E) Chronic renal failure
- (F) Anemia of chronic disease
- (G) Autoimmune hemolytic anemia
- (H) Folate deficiency
- (I) $B_{12}$ deficiency under treatment with $B_{12}$ injections

**Answers: (A), (C), (G), (I).** The reticulocyte count is elevated in the peripheral blood when there is no intrinsic bone marrow disease, when RBCs are destroyed outside the bone marrow (e.g., extravascular removal by splenic macrophages), when there is a bleed over 1 week and the marrow has had a chance to produce and release RBCs, or when iron, folate, or $B_{12}$ deficiency is being treated with the missing element. Therefore, a good reticulocyte response is expected in blood loss >1 week, congenital spherocytosis (macrophage removal of RBCs), AIHA (macrophage removal of IgG- and/or C3-coated RBCs), and when $B_{12}$ is being treated with IM $B_{12}$ (**choices A, C, G, and I are correct**). A poor reticulocyte response is noted in iron deficiency (no iron to synthesize Hgb), aplastic anemia (destruction of stem cells in marrow), chronic renal failure (no EPO to stimulate erythroid stem cells), anemia of chronic disease (iron blockaded in macrophages), and folate deficiency (no folate for DNA synthesis) (**choices B, D, E, F, and H are incorrect**).

ABG = arterial blood gas, ACD = anemia of chronic disease, AIHA = autoimmune hemolytic anemia, BJ = Bence Jones, BM = bone marrow, BT = bleeding time, CB = conjugated bilirubin, CD = cluster designation, CML = chronic myelogenous leukemia, CO = carbon monoxide, CoA = coenzyme A, COPD = chronic obstructive pulmonary disease, DIC = disseminated intravascular coagulation, EBV = Epstein-Barr virus, EPO = erythropoietin, FDP = fibrin(ogen) degradation products, FUO = fever of unknown origin, G6PD = glucose 6-phosphate dehydrogenase, Hct = hematocrit, HgbA = adult hemoglobin A, HgbF = fetal hemoglobin, HgbS = sickle hemoglobin, HIV = human immunodeficiency virus, IEP = immunoelectrophoresis, IF = intrinsic factor, Ig = immunoglobulin, IgG = immunoglobulin G, IgM = immunoglobulin M, IM = infectious mononucleosis, INR = International Normalized Ratio, LAP = leukocyte alkaline phosphatase, MCC = most common cause, MCV = mean corpuscular volume, M/E = myeloid/erythroid ratio, MPD = myeloproliferative disease, NSAIDs = nonsteroidal anti-inflammatory drugs, PA = pernicious anemia, Pb = lead, PB = peripheral blood, PNH = paroxysmal nocturnal hemoglobinuria, PRV = polycythemia rubra vera, PT = prothrombin time, PTT = partial thromboplastin time, RDW = RBC distribution width, R/O = rule out, $SaO_2$ = oxygen saturation of arterial blood, SPE = serum protein electrophoresis, t = translocation, TIBC = total iron-binding capacity, TT = thrombin time, $TXA_2$ = thromboxane $A_2$, UCB = unconjugated bilirubin, VWD = von Willebrand disease, vWF = von Willebrand's factor.

### Table 2–3. GENERAL CONCEPTS IN HEMATOPOIESIS AND ANEMIA

| Most Common... | Answer and Explanation |
|---|---|
| site for EPO synthesis | **peritubular capillary endothelial cells in the kidneys**—EPO stimulates the burst-forming unit-erythroid stem cell to produce RBCs |
| stimuli for accelerated erythropoiesis | • **tissue hypoxia secondary to hypoxemia (low $PaO_2$)**—examples: ◆ primary lung disease, ◆ cyanotic congenital heart disease with a right to left shunt, • *severe anemia,* • *left-shifted ODC*—e.g., ◆ CO, ◆ methemoglobinemia |
| mechanism for removal of senescent, abnormally shaped, or IgG/C3-coated RBCs | **extravascular hemolysis by macrophages in the spleen**—the end-product of macrophage destruction of RBCs is UCB, which may produce jaundice |

*Table continued on following page*

Table 2–3. **GENERAL CONCEPTS IN HEMATOPOIESIS AND ANEMIA** *Continued*

| Most Common... | Answer and Explanation |
| --- | --- |
| causes of a left-shifted neutrophil count | • **bacterial infection,** • *sterile inflammation*—e.g., * blood in peritoneal cavity, * AMI [**Note:** left shift implies a shift to immature neutrophils (>10% bands/stabs or younger cells).] |
| effect of corticosteroids on the leukocyte count | • **absolute neutrophilic leukocytosis**—steroids decrease adhesion molecule synthesis, which releases the marginating pool of neutrophils: because the marginating pool is ~50% of the leukocyte pool in the PB, the neutrophil count doubles, • *eosinopenia,* • *lymphopenia* |
| lymphocytes in the PB | • **T cells**— * 60–80%, * CD$_4$ cells outnumber CD$_8$ cells 2/1, • *B cells*—10–20%, • *NK cells*—5–10% |
| adult Hgbs in decreasing concentration | • **HgbA**—2α/2β, • *HgbA$_2$*—2α/2δ, • *HgbF*—2α/2γ |
| definitions of anemia in adult men and women | • **adult men**—*Hgb < 13 g/dL,* • **adult woman**—*Hgb < 12 g/dL* [**Note:** anemia is a sign of an underlying disease rather than a specific diagnosis.] |
| effect of anemia on the PaO$_2$ and SaO$_2$ | **anemia has no effect** [**Note:** the PaO$_2$ and SaO$_2$ are normal, since gas exchange in the lungs is normal. However, the O$_2$ content is decreased in anemia: O$_2$ content = (1.34 × Hgb g/dL) × SaO$_2$ + (0.003 × PaO$_2$). According to the formula, the Hgb concentration has the greatest effect on the amount of O$_2$ that is available for delivery to tissue.] |

### Table 2–3. GENERAL CONCEPTS IN HEMATOPOIESIS AND ANEMIA *Continued*

**Question:** A patient with anemia has jaundice. The total bilirubin concentration is increased, and the predominant fraction is unconjugated bilirubin. Which of the following anemias potentially fall into this category of anemia? **SELECT 3**
  (A) Congenital spherocytosis
  (B) Iron deficiency
  (C) Autoimmune hemolytic anemia
  (D) Pernicious anemia
  (E) Anemia of chronic disease
  (F) Microangiopathic hemolytic anemia
  (G) α- or β-thalassemia minor

**Answers: (A), (C), (D).** Only anemias associated with macrophage removal and destruction of RBCs are associated with jaundice. This includes congenital spherocytosis (**choice A is correct**) and AIHA (**choice C is correct**). Pernicious anemia, the most common cause of B$_{12}$ deficiency, is also associated with jaundice owing to macrophage destruction of megaloblastic RBCs in the bone marrow (**choice D is correct**). Iron deficiency, ACD, microangiopathic hemolytic anemia (intravascular, not extravascular hemolysis), and α- and β-thalassemia minor are not examples of extravascular hemolytic anemias, hence they are not associated with jaundice (**choices B, E, F, G are incorrect**).

ACD = anemia of chronic disease, AIHA = autoimmune hemolytic anemia, AMI = acute myocardial infarction, EPO = erythropoietin, NK = natural killer, ODC = oxygen dissociation curve, PaO$_2$ = partial pressure of oxygen in arterial blood, PB = peripheral blood, PRV = polycythemia rubra vera, SaO$_2$ = oxygen saturation in arterial blood, UCB = unconjugated bilirubin.

### Table 2–4. MICROCYTIC ANEMIAS OF SURGICAL IMPORTANCE

| Most Common... | Answer and Explanation |
|---|---|
| mechanism for producing microcytic anemias | **reduced Hgb synthesis**—Hgb is the combination of heme (iron + protoporphyrin) + globin chains [**Note:** decreased intracellular concentration of Hgb in developing normoblasts in the marrow causes the RBCs to undergo further divisions, hence the presence of microcytosis.] |
| microcytic anemias due to a reduction in heme synthesis | • **iron deficiency,** • *ACD,* • *sideroblastic anemias* |

*Table continued on following page*

### Table 2–4. MICROCYTIC ANEMIAS OF
### SURGICAL IMPORTANCE *Continued*

| Most Common... | Answer and Explanation |
|---|---|
| microcytic anemia due to a reduction in globin chain synthesis | **thalassemia**— * both α- and β-thalassemia are AR diseases, * α-thalassemia is seen in Asians and blacks, * β-thalassemia is present in blacks, Greeks, and Italians |
| causes of iron deficiency | • **neonates/children**—bleeding Meckel's diverticulum, • **women <50 yrs**—menorrhagia, • **men <50 yrs**—bleeding duodenal ulcer, • **men/women >50 yrs**—colon cancer |
| lab findings in iron deficiency | • **decreased serum ferritin**—best screening test, • *low serum iron,* • *increased TIBC,* • *decreased % saturation,* • *increased RDW,* • MCV—starts normocytic and becomes microcytic |
| lab stages of iron deficiency | **loss of BM iron** → *low serum ferritin* (single best test) → *low serum iron, increased TIBC, low % saturation* → *normocytic anemia* → *microcytic anemia* |
| effect of acute hemorrhage on the lab stages of iron deficiency | **Hgb concentration may be decreased before the loss of BM iron stores** |
| Rx of iron deficiency | **oral ferrous sulfate (325 mg, tid)**— * do not Rx the anemia without having a cause for the iron deficiency, * expect an ~0.5–1 Hct point/day increase after a lag period of ~1 wk, * expect black stools, * the Hct should be ~50% of normal by 3 wks, * continue Rx for ~6 mos after Hct returns to normal to ensure an adequate supply in the marrow [**Note:** the first stage of recovery from iron deficiency is a normocytic anemia, then the iron studies return to normal, and then the marrow stores become increased.] |
| cause of no reticulocyte response or increase in Hct after iron Rx | • **noncompliance,** • *poor GI absorption of iron,* • *persistent GI bleed,* • *wrong Dx* |
| mechanism of anemia in ACD | • **decreased synthesis of EPO**— * cytokines IL-1 and TNF block production of EPO, • *cytokines block iron release by macrophages,* • *cytokines inhibit transferrin synthesis in the liver,* • *slightly reduced RBC survival* |

## Table 2–4. MICROCYTIC ANEMIAS OF SURGICAL IMPORTANCE *Continued*

| Most Common... | Answer and Explanation |
|---|---|
| causes of ACD | • **chronic inflammation**—e.g., * liver disease, * inflammatory bowel disease, • *malignancy*—ACD is the most common anemia in malignancy |
| lab findings in ACD | • **high serum ferritin**—due to increased stores of iron in the macrophages + release of ferritin from hepatocytes, • *low serum iron*, • *low TIBC*—due to a decrease in transferrin synthesis, • *low % saturation*, • *normal RDW*, • *MCV*—normal or slightly decreased |
| Rx of ACD | **Rx underlying disease**—EPO has been useful in some cases |
| lab findings in α-thalassemia minor | • **normal Hgb electrophoresis**—HgbA, A$_2$, and F all need α-chains, hence all Hgbs are equally decreased and the percentages remain the same, • *normal iron studies*, • *normal RDW*, • *RBC count >5.0 cells/μL*—this is a very characteristic finding |
| lab findings in β-thalassemia minor | • **abnormal Hgb electrophoresis**—a decrease in β-globin chain synthesis causes: ♦ decrease in HgbA, ♦ increase in HgbA$_2$ and F, • *normal iron studies*, • *normal RDW*, • *RBC count >5.0 cells/μL*—a very characteristic finding |
| Rx of α- and β-thalassemia | **no Rx**—Rx with iron may result in iron overload and should be avoided |
| pathogenesis of the sideroblastic anemias | **defect in synthesizing heme in the mitochondria**— * iron normally enters the mitochondria to combine with protoporphyrin to form heme, * defects in the synthesis of heme (see below) result in iron accumulating in the mitochondria and the production of ringed sideroblasts |
| causes of sideroblastic anemias | • **alcohol excess**— * alcohol is a mitochondrial poison, * iron enters the mitochondria but cannot exit • *pyridoxine (B$_6$) deficiency*—Rx of TB with INH is the most common cause, B$_6$ is a cofactor in the first reaction in heme synthesis: succinyl CoA + glycine + ALA synthase (+ B$_6$) → δ-aminolevulinic acid, • *Pb poisoning*—Pb denatures ferrochelatase, which catalyzes the reaction that combines protoporphyrin + iron to produce heme |

*Table continued on following page*

## Table 2–4. MICROCYTIC ANEMIAS OF
### SURGICAL IMPORTANCE *Continued*

| Most Common... | Answer and Explanation |
|---|---|
| lab abnormalities in the sideroblastic anemias | • **microcytic anemia**—coarse basophilic stippling is noted in RBCs in patients with Pb poisoning: Pb denatures ribonuclease, hence ribosomes are not degraded in peripheral RBCs, • **ringed sideroblasts in a bone marrow aspirate**—it is not necessary to do a marrow aspirate to Dx Pb poisoning, • *iron overload*— * high serum ferritin, * high serum iron, * low TIBC: decreased synthesis of transferrin with increased iron stores, * high % saturation, • *high serum Pb*—screening and confirmatory test for Pb poisoning |

**Question:** Which of the following tests differentiate iron deficiency, ACD, and β-thalassemia? **SELECT 2**

(A) MCV
(B) Serum iron
(C) TIBC
(D) Hemoglobin electrophoresis
(E) RDW
(F) Percent saturation of iron
(G) Serum ferritin
(H) RBC count

**Answers: (C), (G).** A low MCV is present in all the anemias (choice A is incorrect). Serum iron is low in iron deficiency and ACD and normal in β-thalassemias (choice B is incorrect). The TIBC is high in iron deficiency, low in ACD, and normal in β-thalassemias (choice C is correct). The Hgb electrophoresis is normal in both iron deficiency and ACD, and abnormal in β-thalassemia (choice D is incorrect). The RDW is increased in iron deficiency and normal in both ACD and β-thalassemia (choice E is incorrect). The % saturation is low in both iron deficiency and ACD and normal in β-thalassemia (choice F is incorrect). The serum ferritin is low in iron deficiency, high in ACD, and normal in β-thalassemia (choice G is correct). The RBC count is low in both iron deficiency and ACD and high in β-thalassemia (choice H is incorrect).

ACD = anemia of chronic disease, ALA = aminolevulinic acid, AR = autosomal recessive, BM = bone marrow, EPO = erythropoietin, Hct = hematocrit, Hgb = hemoglobin, IL = interleukin, INH = isoniazid, MCV = mean corpuscular volume, Pb = lead, RDW = RBC distribution width, TIBC = total iron binding capacity, TNF = tumor necrosis factor.

## Table 2–5. MACROCYTIC ANEMIAS OF SURGICAL IMPORTANCE

| Most Common... | Answer and Explanation |
|---|---|
| causes of macrocytic anemia | • **folate deficiency**—most commonly occurs in alcoholics, • $B_{12}$ *deficiency*—PA is the most common cause, • *hypothyroidism* |
| sources of folate and $B_{12}$ | • **folate**—present in plant and animal products, • **$B_{12}$**—present only in animal products [**Note:** both are required for DNA synthesis. Deficiency leads to a large immature nucleus and megaloblastic anemia. All nucleated cells in the body are enlarged.] |
| factor required for absorption of $B_{12}$ | **intrinsic factor (IF)**— * IF is synthesized in parietal cells, * salivary gland synthesizes R factor, which complexes with $B_{12}$ to prevent acid destruction in the stomach, * pancreatic enzymes cleave R factor to liberate $B_{12}$, * IF complexes with $B_{12}$ in the duodenum for subsequent reabsorption in the terminal ileum |
| function of $B_{12}$ in relation to folate metabolism | **cleaves the methyl group of $N^5$-methyl FH$_4$ (unconjugated circulating form of folate) to form FH$_4$ (tetrahydrofolate)**— * FH$_4$ is used in synthesizing deoxythymidine monophosphate for DNA synthesis, * methyl-$B_{12}$ (cobalamin) transfers the methyl group to homocysteine, which is converted into methionine, * plasma homocysteine is increased in both $B_{12}$/folate deficiency |
| function of $B_{12}$ in propionate metabolism | **propionate (odd chain fatty acid) is converted to propionyl CoA → methylmalonyl CoA → succinyl CoA, the latter reaction requiring $B_{12}$**—$B_{12}$ deficiency results in a proximal accumulation of methylmalonic acid (excellent screening test for $B_{12}$ deficiency) and propionates, which cause demyelination of the posterior columns and lateral corticospinal tracts |
| causes of folate deficiency | • **nutritional deficiency**—e.g., **alcohol abuse:** excluding beer, which is rich in folates, • *small bowel disease*—e.g., celiac disease, • *drugs*— * phenytoin: blocks intestinal conjugase, hence the polyglutamate form of folate cannot be converted into absorbable monoglutamate, * alcohol/birth control pills: prevent reabsorption of monoglutamate form of folate in the jejunum, * methotrexate/TMP: block dihydrofolate reductase, • *overutilization*—e.g., * cancer, * pregnancy/lactation |

*Table continued on following page*

### Table 2–5. MACROCYTIC ANEMIAS OF
### SURGICAL IMPORTANCE *Continued*

| Most Common... | Answer and Explanation |
|---|---|
| causes of $B_{12}$ deficiency | • **pernicious anemia**—autoimmune destruction of parietal cells/IF in body and fundus, • *pure vegan diet,* • *achlorhydria*—acid is necessary to free $B_{12}$ from food, • *bacterial overgrowth*—e.g., * small bowel diverticula, * Billroth II, • *gastrectomy,* • *chronic pancreatitis*—cannot cleave off R factor, • *fish tapeworm,* • *terminal ileal disease*—cannot reabsorb $B_{12}$-IF complex: e.g., ♦ surgical resection, ♦ Crohn's disease |
| S/S associated with both folate and $B_{12}$ deficiency | • **glossitis**—smooth, sore tongue, • **malabsorption**—small bowel epithelial cells are adversely affected due to lack of DNA |
| S/S of $B_{12}$ alone | • **posterior column disease**— * decreased vibratory sensation, * loss of proprioception, • **lateral corticospinal tract dysfunction**— * upper motor neuron S/S of spasticity, * Babinski's, • *sallow complexion,* • *dementia*—neurologic problems may occur without any anemia or MCV alteration |
| S/S of PA alone | • **achlorhydria,** • **stomach cancer,** • **autoantibodies against parietal cells and IF,** • **correction of $B_{12}$ absorption in the Schilling's test after adding IF to radioactive $B_{12}$** |
| PB findings in $B_{12}$/folate deficiency | • **hypersegmented neutrophils**—>5 nuclear lobes, • *pancytopenia*—this is due to extrasinusoidal macrophage destruction of megaloblastic cells, • *macroovalocytes*—egg-shaped RBCs |
| lab findings in folate deficiency | • **low serum folate and RBC folate**—RBC folate is a more accurate assessment of folate stores, • *high plasma homocysteine,* • *high serum LDH*—BM destruction of RBCs releases LDH in hematopoietic cells, • *slightly high UCB*—BM macrophage destruction of RBCs causes increased release of UCB from macrophages |

### Table 2–5. MACROCYTIC ANEMIAS OF
### SURGICAL IMPORTANCE *Continued*

| Most Common... | Answer and Explanation |
|---|---|
| lab findings in PA | • **low serum B$_{12}$**, • *high plasma homocysteine,* • *high urine methylmalonic acid*—most sensitive test, • *high LDH*, • *slightly high UCB*, • *Schilling's test*—correction of B$_{12}$ reabsorption with the addition of IF (see Table 2–2), • *high serum folate*—absence of B$_{12}$ causes methyl-FH$_4$ in cells to leak back into the blood |
| Rx of folate and B$_{12}$ deficiency | • **folate deficiency**—folic acid, • **B$_{12}$ deficiency**—intramuscular B$_{12}$ [NOTE: Rx with folate corrects the hematologic problems in B$_{12}$ deficiency, but not the neurologic problems.] |

**Question:** Which of the following are laboratory tests or clinical findings that distinguish B$_{12}$ deficiency caused by pernicious anemia from other causes of B$_{12}$ deficiency and folate deficiency? **SELECT 4**
  (A) Urine methylmalonic acid
  (B) MCV
  (C) Plasma homocysteine
  (D) Antiparietal cell antibodies
  (E) Hypersegmented neutrophils
  (F) Neurologic exam
  (G) Achlorhydria
  (H) Serum gastrin levels
  (I) Schilling's test corrected with IF

**Answers: (D), (G), (H), (I).** An increase in urine methylmalonic acid is present in any cause of B$_{12}$ deficiency but is not present in folate deficiency **(choice A is incorrect).** The MCV is increased in all of them **(choice B is incorrect).** Plasma homocysteine levels are increased in all of them **(choice C is incorrect).** Antiparietal cell antibodies are present only in PA and not the other types of B$_{12}$ or folate deficiency **(choice D is correct).** Hypersegmented neutrophils are present in all of them **(choice E is incorrect).** The neurologic exam is abnormal in any cause of B$_{12}$ deficiency, but it is normal in folate deficiency **(choice F is incorrect).** Achlorhydria and the concomitant increase in serum gastrin levels are unique to PA **(choices G and H are correct).** A Schilling's test that is corrected with the addition of IF is unique to PA **(choice I is correct).**

BM = bone marrow, CoA = coenzyme A, FH$_4$ = tetrahydrofolate, IF = intrinsic factor, LDH = lactate dehydrogenase, MCV = mean corpuscular volume, PA = pernicious anemia, PB = peripheral blood, S/S = signs/symptoms, TMP = trimethoprim, UCB = unconjugated bilirubin.

### Table 2–6. NORMOCYTIC ANEMIAS OF SURGICAL IMPORTANCE/SEPSIS

| Most Common... | Answer and Explanation |
|---|---|
| initial effect of acute blood loss on the Hgb concentration | **no effect**— * an equal amount of RBCs and plasma is lost, hence Hgb and Hct remain normal, * plasma is initially replaced and uncovers the RBC deficit in a few hours to a few days |
| hematologic effect of infusion of 0.9% NaCl in acute blood loss | **uncovers the RBC deficit**—since 0.9% NaCl is limited to the ECF, it uncovers the RBC deficit, hence lowering Hgb, Hct, and RBC count |
| cause of acute blood loss | **GI bleed**—most GI bleeds are due to peptic ulcer disease (e.g., duodenal ulcer) |
| known causes of aplastic anemia | • **drugs**—e.g., * busulfan, * phenylbutazone, * propylthiouracil, • *infection*—e.g.,* HCV, * NANB hepatitis, • *radiation* |
| S/S in aplastic anemia | • **mucosal bleeding and petechia/ecchymoses**—due to thrombocytopenia, • **fever**—due to infection from neutropenia, • **fatigue**—due to anemia |
| lab findings in aplastic anemia | • **normocytic anemia**—corrected reticulocyte count <2%, • **pancytopenia**, • **hypocellular BM** |
| Rx for aplastic anemia | • **BM transplantation for patients <50 yrs old**, • *antithymocyte/antilymphocyte globulins,* • *cyclosporine,* • *corticosteroids,* • *growth factors*—e.g., * EPO, * CSF-GM,* thrombopoietin |
| cause of anemia in renal disease | **EPO deficiency** |
| hematologic lab findings in renal disease | • **normocytic anemia**—corrected reticulocyte count < 2%, • *prolonged BT*— * qualitative platelet defect: defect in platelet factor 3 (phospholipid), * reversible with dialysis |
| Rx of anemia in renal disease | **EPO** |
| anemias in malignancy | • **ACD,** • *iron deficiency*—usually GI blood loss, • *marrow invasion by tumor*—this is called myelophthisis, • *chemotherapy*—BM suppression, • *hemolytic anemia*—e.g., HUS triggered by mitomycin C, • *folate deficiency*—overutilization by tumor |

## Table 2–6. NORMOCYTIC ANEMIAS OF SURGICAL
## IMPORTANCE/SEPSIS *Continued*

| Most Common... | Answer and Explanation |
|---|---|
| general mechanisms of hemolysis in hemolytic anemias | • **extravascular**—macrophage-induced, • *intravascular* [**Note:** see Table 2–2 for discussions on lab differentiation of extravascular from intravascular hemolysis.] |
| types of intrinsic (RBC defect) hemolytic anemias | • **membrane defects**—e.g., * **congenital spherocytosis,** * hereditary elliptocytosis, * PNH, • *abnormal Hgb*—e.g., **sickle cell disease** and its variants, • *deficient enzymes*—**G6PD deficiency** |
| types of extrinsic (defect outside the RBC) hemolytic anemias | • **AIHA**—e.g., * **collagen vascular disease: SLE,** * drugs, * *malignancy,* • *microangiopathic hemolytic anemias*—e.g., * **DIC,** * TTP, * HUS, • *macroangiopathic hemolytic anemia*—e.g., * **calcific aortic stenosis,** * prosthetic heart valves |
| lab findings in hemolytic anemias | **see Table 2–2 discussions** |
| hemolytic anemias with predominantly extravascular hemolysis | • **congenital spherocytosis,** • *congenital elliptocytosis,* • *sickle cell disease,* • *warm AIHA* |
| hemolytic anemias with predominantly intravascular hemolysis | • **microangiopathic hemolytic anemia,** • *cold AIHA,* • *G6PD deficiency,* • PNH |
| defect in congenital spherocytosis | **AD disease with a defect in spectrin and band 4.1 in the RBC membrane—** * the RBC has reduced membrane (decreased surface to volume ratio) leading to formation of a sphere, * spherocytes are extravascularly removed by macrophages in the cords of Billroth |
| clinical triad in congenital spherocytosis | • **splenomegaly,** • **anemia,** • **jaundice—** * UCB type of jaundice, * jet-black calcium bilirubinate stones lead to cholecystitis (55–75%) |

*Table continued on following page*

Table 2–6. NORMOCYTIC ANEMIAS OF SURGICAL
IMPORTANCE/SEPSIS *Continued*

| Most Common... | Answer and Explanation |
|---|---|
| lab findings in congenital spherocytosis | • **increased osmotic fragility**–see Table 2–2, • *spherocytes in PB,* • *high MCHC*— * loss of RBC membrane concentrates Hgb in the RBC, * there is no central area of pallor, • *reticulocytosis*—corrected reticulocyte count >3% |
| Rx of congenital spherocytosis | **splenectomy**— * splenectomy is recommended in patients with an Hgb <11 g/dL and a corrected reticulocyte count > 6%, * splenectomy is normally performed in children after 6 yrs of age, * Pneumovax/Hib type b vaccines are recommended before splenectomy, * US is recommended before surgery to R/O gallstones, * spherocytes remain after splenectomy |
| cause of persistent hemolytic anemia postsplenectomy for congenital spherocytosis | **failure to identify and remove an accessory spleen** |
| defect in hereditary elliptocytosis | **AD disease with defects in spectrin** |
| lab findings in hereditary elliptocytosis | • **elliptocytes (ovalocytes) >25% of PB RBCs,** • *reticulocytosis,* • *compensated hemolytic anemia*—BM production keeps pace with hemolysis |
| Rx of hereditary elliptocytosis | **usually none**—splenectomy is reserved for severe cases |
| Hgb disorder in blacks | • **sickle cell trait,** • *sickle cell disease,* • α- *and* β-*thalassemia* [**Note:** the sickle cell gene occurs in ~8% of blacks.] |
| defect in sickle cell disease | **AR disease with a point mutation**—there is a substitution of valine for glutamic acid at the 6th position of the β-globin chain |
| cause of sickling of RBCs in HgbSS | • **increased amount of sickle Hgb**—>60%, • *reduced $O_2$ tension*— * high altitude, * renal medulla, • *presence of other Hgbs*—e.g., HgbC, • *volume depletion,* • *acidosis*—right shifts in the ODC with release of more $O_2$ |

## Table 2–6. NORMOCYTIC ANEMIAS OF SURGICAL IMPORTANCE/SEPSIS *Continued*

| Most Common... | Answer and Explanation |
|---|---|
| Hgb that inhibits sickling | **HgbF**—presence of HgbF in RBCs plus the reduced amount of HgbS in the RBCs of neonates prevents sickling for ~6–9 mos |
| S/S of sickle cell trait | • **microscopic/macroscopic hematuria**— * the low O₂ tension in the renal medulla induces sickling in the peritubular capillaries, * consequences of sickling include: ♦ microinfarctions/hematuria, ♦ isosthenuria (inability to concentrate/dilute urine), ♦ renal papillary necrosis, • *potential for sudden death with vigorous exercise,* • *splenic infarction at altitudes >10,000 feet,* • *bacteriuria,* • *pyelonephritis in pregnancy* |
| problems in sickle cell disease (HgbSS) | • **vaso-occlusive disease**— * sickle cells block the microcirculation, leading to tissue hypoxia and organ dysfunction, * nonsickled cells adhere to the endothelium, • *chronic hemolytic anemia*—primarily extravascular hemolysis |
| initial site for a vaso-occlusive crisis in HgbSS | • **hands/feet (dactylitis)**—this usually occurs in a 6- to 9-mo-old infant, • *brain*—strokes, particularly in children, • *lungs*—acute chest syndrome, • *liver*—liver cell necrosis, • *bone marrow*— * aplastic crisis, * no reticulocytes are present in the PB, * usually precipitated by a parvovirus infection, • *spleen*—sequestration crisis, • *penis*—priapism |
| manifestation of HgbSS | **vaso-occlusive painful crises**— * this commonly occur in the limbs, back, and chest, * it is not associated with hemolysis |
| S/S and lab findings of the acute chest syndrome | • **fever,** • **chest pain,** • **pulmonary infiltrates,** • **neutrophilic leukocytosis,** • **hypoxemia** |
| bone complications in HgbSS | • **aseptic necrosis of the femoral head**—bone infarction, • *osteomyelitis*— * most often due to *Salmonella* species, * less commonly, *Staphylococcus aureus,* • *aplastic crisis* |

*Table continued on following page*

### Table 2–6. NORMOCYTIC ANEMIAS OF SURGICAL IMPORTANCE/SEPSIS *Continued*

| Most Common... | Answer and Explanation |
|---|---|
| spleen complications in HgbSS | • **painful splenomegaly,** • *splenic dysfunction*— * usually complete by 2–3 yrs of age, * the presence of Howell-Jolly bodies in the PB is a good sign of splenic dysfunction: Howell-Jolly bodies are remnants of nuclear material in mature RBCs, • *autosplenectomy*—usually occurs in late adolescence or in young adults, • *splenic sequestration*— * sickled cells are trapped in the spleen, * the reticulocyte count is elevated in the PB |
| complications of chronic hemolysis in HgbSS | • **jaundice,** • *calcium bilirubinate stones,* • *iron overload owing to a heavy transfusion requirement* |
| lab findings in sickle cell trait | • **Hgb electrophoresis**— * HgbS ~40%, * HgbA ~60%, • **normal CBC** |
| lab findings in sickle cell disease | • **Hgb electrophoresis**— * HgbSS 85–98%, * HgbF 5–15%, * there is no HgbA, • **hematologic findings**— * sickle cells, * target cells, * Howell-Jolly bodies, * reticulocytosis: ♦ present in splenic sequestration crisis, ♦ absent in aplastic crisis, * neutrophilic leukocytosis, * thrombocytosis: due to a dysfunctional or autosplenectomized spleen |
| Rx of painful crises in HgbSS | • **hydration**— * use 0.9% NaCl, * avoid blood transfusion, • *morphine sulfate*—analgesic of choice, • *oxygen* |
| COD in children <5 yrs old who have HgbSS disease | **sepsis**—usually due to *Streptococcus pneumoniae,* * less commonly due to *Haemophilus influenzae* [**Note:** this underscores the importance of Pneumovax and Hib vaccination plus prophylactic antibiotics.] |
| COD in adults with HgbSS | • **acute chest syndrome,** • *stroke,* • *infection* |
| pathogenesis of hemolysis in G6PD deficiency | **absence of GSH**— * the production of GSH requires the presence of G6PD, the primary enzyme of the hexose monophosphate shunt: deficiency of the enzyme is an SXR trait, * GSH normally neutralizes peroxide, * peroxide left unneutralized denatures Hgb to form Heinz bodies and also damages the RBC membrane, * primarily intravascular hemolysis |

## Table 2–6. NORMOCYTIC ANEMIAS OF SURGICAL IMPORTANCE/SEPSIS *Continued*

| Most Common... | Answer and Explanation |
|---|---|
| precipitating factors leading to hemolysis in G6PD deficiency | • **infections,** • *oxidizing drugs*—e.g., * primaquine, * dapsone, * trimethoprim, • *fava beans*—occurs only with the Mediterranean variant |
| defect in the black versus the Mediterranean variant of G6PD deficiency | • **black variant**— * defective G6PD is present only in older RBCs, * less severe hemolysis, • **Mediterranean variant**— * G6PD defective/deficient in young and old RBCs, * more severe hemolysis |
| PB findings in G6PD deficiency | • **Heinz bodies**—product of oxidant damage of peroxide on Hgb, • *bite cells*—macrophage removes part of RBC membrane |
| tests used to Dx G6PD deficiency | • **Heinz body preparation in the acute hemolytic phase,** • **enzyme assay in the nonhemolytic phase** [Note: see Table 2–2 for further discussion.] |
| Rx of G6PD deficiency | • **avoid drugs known to precipitate hemolysis,** • *adequate hydration,* • *splenectomy is not indicated* |
| types of AIHA | • **warm AIHA secondary to collagen vascular disease**— * SLE, * warm AIHA refers to IgG-mediated hemolysis, • *drug-induced AIHA*— * penicillin/cephalosporins, * methyldopa, * immunocomplex disease (e.g., quinidine), • *cold AIHA*— * cold AIHA refers to IgM-mediated hemolysis, * e.g., *Mycoplasma pneumoniae* |
| S/S of AIHA | • **fever,** • **jaundice**—increased UCB, • **generalized painful lymphadenopathy,** • **hepatosplenomegaly** |
| tests used to identify an AIHA | **direct/indirect Coombs' test**—see Table 2–2 for a further discussion |
| Rx of warm AIHAs | • **if possible, avoid transfusion**—RBCs will be hemolyzed, • **corticosteroids**—first step, • *splenectomy*—second step if corticosteroids are unsuccessful, • *alkylating agents*—last resort |

*Table continued on following page*

## Table 2-6. NORMOCYTIC ANEMIAS OF SURGICAL IMPORTANCE/SEPSIS *Continued*

| Most Common... | Answer and Explanation |
|---|---|
| Rx of cold AIHA | **alkylating agents** |
| Rx of drug-induced AIHA | **withdraw drug** |
| Rx of life-threatening AIHA unresponsive to above Rx | **IV gamma globulin**— * IgG binds to Fc receptors on macrophages and prevents them from phagocytosing sensitized RBCs, * this is a temporary Rx |
| PB finding in micro/macroangiopathic hemolytic anemias | **schistocytes**—fragmented RBCs |
| lab findings in micro/macroangiopathic hemolytic anemias | **those of intravascular hemolysis**—see Table 2–2 |
| anemias in alcoholics | • **ACD**—80%, • *folate deficiency*—30%, • *acute blood loss*—25%, • *sideroblastic anemia*— * 25%, • *iron deficiency*—13% [**Note:** ~50% have a single cause for anemia, 30% have 2 causes, and 20% have 3 or more causes, hence these unusual percentages.] |
| anemias in AIDS | • **ACD,** • *hemolytic*—immune mechanisms, • *microangiopathic*—usually due to disseminated cancer or DIC |
| types of blood cultures | • **aerobic,** • **anaerobic** |
| factor improving isolation of blood-borne pathogens | **volume of blood drawn into the culture containers**— * volume of blood is more important than timing of when blood is drawn, * 10 mL is the minimal amount to draw into each culture container (aerobic/anaerobic), * 1 mL of blood is the minimal amount to draw into the containers in children |
| contaminants in blood culture | • ***Staphylococcus epidermidis***—coagulase-negative, • *Corynebacterium* species, • *Bacillus* species [**Note:** always suspect contamination if the blood culture drawn in the other arm is negative.] |

## Table 2–6. NORMOCYTIC ANEMIAS OF SURGICAL IMPORTANCE/SEPSIS Continued

| Most Common... | Answer and Explanation |
|---|---|
| findings in the systemic inflammatory response syndrome (SIRS) | • **fever >38°C or <36°C,** • *heart rate >90/min*—exception is sinus bradycardia in typhoid fever, • *respiratory rate >20/min,* • *hypoxemia,* • *lethargy,* • *increased/decreased WBC count*—e.g., * the WBC count is increased in *Staphylococcus aureus* septicemia, * the WBC count is decreased in *E. coli* septicemia: endotoxins increase adhesion molecule synthesis and increase the marginating neutrophil pool, • *left-shifted smear*—* band neutrophils >10%, * left-shifted even with low WBC counts, particularly in the elderly |
| cause of pneumonia/ sepsis in the ICU | ***Pseudomonas aeruginosa*—**this is related to contaminated water in respirators |
| hospital risk factor for sepsis | • **indwelling urinary catheter**—this predisposes to *E. coli* sepsis, • *indwelling line in place >48 hrs*— * *S. aureus* sepsis is the most common pathogen, * Rx with IV vancomycin, • *intravenous lipid emulsion*—usually *Staphylococcus epidermidis* or *Malassezia furfur,* Rx with vancomycin for former pathogen and amphotericin B for latter |
| patient risk factors for sepsis | • **immunosuppression from cancer Rx**—usually gram-negative sepsis, • *chronic illness,* • *DM,* • *therapeutic procedure*—e.g., * indwelling urinary catheter, * respirator, • *angiography* |
| diseases predisposing to sepsis | • **pneumonia**—*Streptococcus pneumoniae* is most common pathogen, • *AIDS,* • *pyelonephritis*—*E. coli* most common, • *burns*— * *Pseudomonas aeruginosa* most common, * *Staphylococcus aureus,* • *trauma,* • *pancreatitis,* • *biliary tract infection*—*E. coli* most common pathogen, • *sickle cell disease*—*S. pneumoniae* most common, • *splenectomy*—*S. pneumoniae* most common, • *peritonitis*— * *E. coli,* * *Bacteroides fragilis,* • *ascites*—spontaneous peritonitis due to *E. coli* in adults and *S. pneumoniae* in children, • *absolute neutropenia with WBC count <500 cells/μL*—usually *P. aeruginosa* sepsis |

*Table continued on following page*

## Table 2–6. NORMOCYTIC ANEMIAS OF SURGICAL IMPORTANCE/SEPSIS *Continued*

| Most Common... | Answer and Explanation |
|---|---|
| clinical findings in candidemia | • **predisposing cause**— * indwelling catheters for TPN, * broad-spectrum antibiotics, * neutropenia, • **clinical**— * 5–10% nosocomial septicemias, * nodular skin lesions: metastatic abscess, * fluffy white chorioretinal exudates: endophthalmitis, * fever unresponsive to empirical antibacterial agents, • **Rx**— * replace/culture tip of indwelling catheter, * amphotericin B or high-dose fluconazole |

**Question:** Which of the following normocytic anemias are likely to have anemia with a corrected reticulocyte count >3%? **SELECT 4**

    (A) Chronic renal failure
    (B) Blood loss <5 days
    (C) Anemia of chronic disease
    (D) Congenital spherocytosis
    (E) Aplastic anemia
    (F) Warm AIHA
    (G) Malignancy
    (H) Sickle cell trait
    (I) G6PD deficiency
    (J) Severe calcific aortic stenosis

**Answers:** (D), (F), (I), (J). Normocytic anemias without an appropriate reticulocyte response are chronic renal failure (EPO deficiency, **choice A is incorrect**), blood loss < 5 days (insufficient time for erythropoiesis, **choice B is incorrect**), ACD (macrophage trapping of iron, **choice C is incorrect**), aplastic anemia (hypocellular marrow, **choice E is incorrect**), and malignancy (ACD most common cause of anemia, **choice G is incorrect**). Sickle cell trait does not have anemia, hence reticulocytosis is not expected (**choice H is incorrect**). In most instances, hemolytic anemias, whether extravascular or intravascular, are associated with an appropriate corrected reticulocyte response > 3%. Therefore, congenital spherocytosis, warm AIHA, and G6PD deficiency have an appropriate response (**choices D, F, I are correct**). Severe calcific aortic stenosis is the most common cause of macroangiopathic hemolytic anemia with schistocytes (**choice J is correct**).

ACD = anemia of chronic disease, AD = autosomal dominant, AIHA = autoimmune hemolytic anemia, AR = autosomal recessive, BM = bone marrow, BT = bleeding time, COD = cause of death, CRF = chronic renal failure, CSF-G = colony-stimulating factor–granulocytes, CSF-GM = colony-stimulating factor–granulocytes/macrophages, DIC = disseminated intravascular coagulation, DM = diabetes mellitus, ECF = extracellular fluid, EPO = erythropoietin, ESR = erythrocyte sedimentation rate, G6PD = glucose 6-phosphate dehydrogenase, GSH = glutathione, Hct = hematocrit, HCV = hepatitis C virus, Hgb = hemoglobin, HgbSS = sickle cell anemia, Hib = *Haemophilus influenzae* type b vaccine, HUS = hemolytic uremic syndrome, ICs = immunocomplexes, ICU = intensive care unit, MCHC = mean corpuscular hemoglobin concentration, MCV = mean corpuscular volume, NANB = non-A, non-B hepatitis, ODC = oxygen dissociation curve, PB = peripheral blood, PNH = paroxysmal nocturnal hemoglobinuria, R/O = rule out, SIRS = systemic inflammatory response syndrome, SLE = systemic lupus erythematosus, S/S = signs/symptoms, SXR = sex-linked recessive, TPN = total parenteral nutrition, TTP = thrombotic thrombocytopenic purpura, UCB = unconjugated bilirubin, US = ultrasonography.

## Table 2–7. BENIGN WBC DISORDERS OF SURGICAL IMPORTANCE

| Most Common... | Answer and Explanation |
|---|---|
| causes of absolute neutrophilic leukocytosis (>7000 cells/μL) | • **bacterial infection**—e.g., * acute appendicitis/diverticulitis/cholecystitis, * cellulitis, * peritonitis, • *decreased adhesion molecule synthesis*—e.g., * corticosteroids, * catecholamines, • *sterile inflammation*—e.g., * blood in peritoneal cavity,* postoperative atelectasis [**Note:** a medically significant absolute neutrophil count is >14,000 cells/μL (% neutrophils in the differential × total WBC count).] |
| PB findings in acute bacterial infections | • **absolute neutrophilic leukocytosis,** • *toxic granulation*—prominence of azurophilic granules, • *left shift*— * >10% band neutrophils, * any neutrophil younger than a band |
| causes of a leukemoid reaction | • **infection**—e.g., TB, • *malignancy*—e.g., renal adenocarcinoma [**Note:** a leukemoid reaction is a benign increase in WBCs >30,000 cells/μL). They may involve any cell type (e.g., **neutrophils,** lymphocytes, eosinophils).] |

*Table continued on following page*

### Table 2-7. BENIGN WBC DISORDERS OF SURGICAL IMPORTANCE *Continued*

| Most Common... | Answer and Explanation |
|---|---|
| cause of a leukoerythroblastic reaction | **bone metastasis**—e.g., breast cancer: most common malignancy of bone [**Note:** a leukoerythroblastic smear refers to peripheralization of immature WBCs (e.g., myeloblasts, progranulocytes) and RBCs (e.g., NRBCs) due to a space-occupying lesion(s) in the BM. Metastasis is the most common cause of a leukoerythroblastic smear. Other causes include myelofibrosis and leukemia.] |
| cause of absolute neutropenia (<1500 cells/μL) | • **decreased production of neutrophils due to drugs**—e.g., * chemotherapy agents, * see aplastic anemia in Table 2-6, • *increased marginating pool*—e.g., * normal in blacks, * endotoxins, • *infection*—e.g., typhoid, • *neutrophil destruction*—e.g., * Felty's syndrome (autoimmune neutropenia + splenomegaly + RA), * AIDS [**Note:** less than 500 cells/μL requires prophylactic antibiotics (IV vancomycin + parenteral third-generation cephalosporin).] |
| cause of absolute lymphocytosis (adults: >4000 cells/μL) | • **viral infections**—e.g., infectious mononucleosis, • *bacterial infections*—e.g., TB, • *Graves' disease,* • *drugs*—e.g., phenytoin |
| cause of atypical lymphocytosis | • **infectious mononucleosis,** • *viral hepatitis,* • *CMV,* • *toxoplasmosis,* • *HIV,* • *phenytoin* [**Note:** atypical lymphocytes are antigenically stimulated lymphocytes. Atypical lymphocytosis is significant if they are >10% of the total WBC count.] |
| method of transmission of infectious mononucleosis | • **kissing**— * EBV is present in saliva, * replicates in the oropharynx, * infects B cells: $CD_{21}$ receptor for EBV, • *blood transfusion,* • *sexual transmission* |
| S/S of infectious mononucleosis | • **fever**—>90%, • *pharyngitis*— * often exudative, * palatal petechiae, • *generalized painful lymphadenopathy*—80-90%, • *rash with ampicillin,* • *hepatomegaly*—10-15%, *splenomegaly*— * 50-60%, * spontaneous rupture rare, * rupture is usually secondary to contact sports |

### Table 2–7. BENIGN WBC DISORDERS OF SURGICAL IMPORTANCE *Continued*

| Most Common... | Answer and Explanation |
|---|---|
| lab findings noted in infectious mononucleosis | • **atypical lymphocytosis**—the atypical lymphocytes are T cells reacting against infected B cells, • *positive heterophile antibody test*—Monospot, • *elevated transaminases*— * 80–90%, * anicteric hepatitis in most cases |
| causes of absolute lymphopenia (<1500 cells/$\mu$L) | • **viral infection**—initial phase, • *drugs*—e.g., corticosteroids, • *immunodeficiency syndromes*—e.g., AIDS |
| causes of eosinophilia (>700 cells/$\mu$L) | • **type I hypersensitivity reactions**—e.g., * **drug reaction**, * hay fever, * asthma, • *invasive helminthic diseases*—this does not include pinworms (noninvasive), • *Addison's disease*—decreased cortisol levels increase the eosinophil count, • *Hodgkin's disease*, • *polyarteritis nodosum* |
| causes of eosinopenia | • **corticosteroids**, • *Cushing's syndrome* |
| causes of monocytosis (>800 cells/$\mu$L) | • **chronic inflammation**, • *autoimmune disease*, • *malignancy* |
| clues suggesting a phagocytic disorder | • **history of a delayed separation of the umbilical cord**—$\beta_2$-integrin ($CD_{11}$/$CD_{18}$ glycoprotein) adhesion molecule defect, * no marginating neutrophils and no neutrophils present in umbilical cord tissue, * poor wound healing, • **unusual pathogens**—e.g., * *Serratia marcescens*, * *Staphylococcus epidermidis*, • **child is always sick**, • **chronic periodontitis and loss of teeth**, • **"cold" soft tissue abscesses**— * no inflammatory response, * probable chemotaxis problem |
| phagocytic defects in DM | • **impaired chemotaxis**, • **impaired phagocytosis**, • **impaired intracellular killing of bacteria** [Note: hyperglycemia is responsible for these defects, hence the importance of good glycemic control.] |
| phagocytic defects in AIDS | **defective neutrophil and monocyte chemotaxis** |

*Table continued on following page*

### Table 2–7. BENIGN WBC DISORDERS OF SURGICAL IMPORTANCE *Continued*

| Most Common... | Answer and Explanation |
|---|---|
| PB WBC findings in AIDS | • **lymphopenia**— * 70–95%, * this is due to the direct HIV lymphocytotoxic effect on CD₄ T helper cells, • *neutropenia*— * 45–75%, * immune-mediated, • *pancytopenia*—35–40% |

**Question:** Absolute neutrophilic leukocytosis is expected in which of the following disorders? **SELECT 3**
- (A) Viral hepatitis
- (B) Acute diverticulitis
- (C) Acute small bowel infarction
- (D) Cutaneous drug reaction to penicillin
- (E) Corticosteroids
- (F) Tuberculosis
- (G) Pinworm infestation

**Answers:** **(B), (C), (E)**. Viral hepatitis is associated with an atypical lymphocytosis (**choice A is incorrect**). Acute diverticulitis, acute small bowel infarction, and corticosteroids are associated with absolute neutrophilic leukocytosis (**choices B, C, and E are correct**). A cutaneous drug reaction due to penicillin produces eosinophilia (**choice D is incorrect**). TB is associated with a lymphocytosis and monocytosis (**choice F is incorrect**). A pinworm infection is not associated with any inflammatory reaction, since it is noninvasive (**choice G is incorrect**).

BM = bone marrow, CMV = cytomegalovirus, EBV = Epstein-Barr virus, HIV = human immunodeficiency virus, NRBCs = nucleated RBCs, PAN = polyarteritis nodosa, PB = peripheral blood, RA = rheumatoid arthritis.

### Table 2–8. NEOPLASTIC WBC DISORDERS OF SURGICAL IMPORTANCE

| Most Common... | Answer and Explanation |
|---|---|
| MPDs | • **PRV**, • *CML*, • *AMM*, • *ET* |
| type of polycythemia | **relative polycythemia**— * e.g., loss of volume increases the RBC count (reported as cells/μL), * the total number of RBCs when reported as mL/kg (RBC mass) is normal, because the BM is not producing more RBCs |

### Table 2–8. NEOPLASTIC WBC DISORDERS OF SURGICAL IMPORTANCE *Continued*

| Most Common... | Answer and Explanation |
|---|---|
| appropriate absolute polycythemia | **hypoxia-induced secondary polycythemia—** e.g., * COPD, * high altitude, * right to left shunt in the heart [**Note:** appropriate polycythemia refers to an $SaO_2$ ≤88% leading to EPO-induced RBC BM hyperplasia. The term *absolute* indicates that both the RBC count and RBC mass are increased.] |
| inappropriate absolute polycythemias | • **PRV,** • *ectopic production of EPO—* * renal disease: renal adenocarcinoma, cysts, hydronephrosis, * hepatocellular carcinoma [**Note:** inappropriate absolute polycythemia refers to a nonhypoxic stimulus ($SaO_2$ ≥92%) for an increase in RBC mass.] |
| cause of PRV | **clonal expansion of multipotential myeloid stem cell—**there is an increased production of RBCs, WBCs (not lymphocytes), platelets |
| clinical findings of PRV | • **hyperviscosity signs—**predisposes to thrombosis, leading to AMI, stroke, bowel infarction, • *hypervolemia—*PRV is the only MPD with an increased plasma volume, • *hyperuricemia—* * increased cell turnover causes the release of purines, which are metabolized into uric acid, * PRV is commonly associated with gout, • *histaminemia—* * histamine is released from the increased number of mast cells/basophils, * histamine causes vasodilatation (plethoric face, headache) and pruritus after bathing |
| lab findings of PRV | • **category A—** * high RBC mass: not RBC count, * $SaO_2$ ≥92%, * splenomegaly, • **category B—** * platelet count >400,000 cells/$\mu$L, * leukocytosis >12,000 cells/$\mu$L, * LAP score >100 (see Table 2–2), * serum $B_{12}$ >900 pg/mL (WBCs carry transcobalamin I), • *PRV criteria for Dx—* * all 3 category A are present, * high RBC mass along with either of the other category A criteria plus 2 of the 4 category B criteria, • *miscellaneous findings—* * normal/high plasma volume, * low EPO: EPO is suppressed due to the elevated $O_2$ content, * hyperuricemia, * low MCV: secondary to iron deficiency from bleeding or phlebotomy, * Hct >58% in men and >52% in women |

*Table continued on following page*

### Table 2–8.  NEOPLASTIC WBC DISORDERS OF
### SURGICAL IMPORTANCE *Continued*

| Most Common... | Answer and Explanation |
|---|---|
| Rx of PRV in asymptomatic/ symptomatic patients | • **asymptomatic patients**—phlebotomy: ♦ decreases RBC mass, ♦ produces iron deficiency: decreases RBC production, • **symptomatic patients**— * **hydroxyurea,** * anagrelide, * $^{32}$P, * alkylating agents and radioactive phosphorus increase the risk for leukemic transformation |
| lab findings present in absolute polycythemia associated with tissue hypoxia | • **high RBC mass,** • *normal plasma volume,* • *$SaO_2$ ≤88%,* • *high EPO* [**Note:** examples include COPD, high altitude, hypoventilation syndromes (obstructive sleep apnea), cyanotic CHD, methemoglobinemia, and CO poisoning.] |
| lab findings present in absolute polycythemia with an $SaO_2$ ≥92% | • **high RBC mass,** • *normal plasma volume,* • *$SaO_2$ ≥92%,* • *high EPO* [**Note:** examples include renal disorders (renal adenocarcinoma, Wilms' tumor, cysts, hydronephrosis [e.g., uterine leiomyoma pressing on the ureter], and hepatocellular carcinoma).] |
| S/S of CML | • **hepatosplenomegaly**—leukemic infiltration, • *hypermetabolic state*— * fever, * weight loss, * sweating, • *generalized lymphadenopathy,* • *myeloblast or lymphoblast crisis after ~2–3 yrs* |
| lab findings of CML | • **leukoerythroblastic smear**—50,000–150,000 cells/μL, • *normocytic/macrocytic anemia*—increased cell turnover may cause folate deficiency and a macrocytic anemia, • *basophilia/eosinophilia,* • *thrombocytosis*— * 40–50%, * CML is the only leukemia that is commonly associated with thrombocytosis, • *myeloblasts <10% in BM and PB,* • *low LAP score*—see Table 2–2, • *Philadelphia chromosome*— * t9;22, * present in 95%, * poor prognosis if absent, • *positive bcr-fusion gene study in 100%* |
| S/S of AMM | • **massive splenomegaly**— * hallmark of the disease, * splenomegaly is due to extramedullary hematopoiesis, • *abdominal pain*— * splenic infarctions, * friction rubs are often present, as well as left-sided pleural effusions |

## Table 2–8. NEOPLASTIC WBC DISORDERS OF
## SURGICAL IMPORTANCE *Continued*

| Most Common... | Answer and Explanation |
|---|---|
| lab findings of AMM | • **leukoerythroblastic smear**—hematopoietic cells are directly released into the blood through the splenic sinusoids, • *normocytic anemia,* • *thrombocytosis,* • *marrow fibrosis,* • *tear drop RBCs in PB*—very characteristic, • *increased LAP score,* • *absent Philadelphia chromosome* |
| S/S of ET | • **venous thrombosis,** • *bleeding*— * usually GI, * platelets are defective even though they are increased, • *splenomegaly* |
| lab findings of ET | • **thrombocytosis**—>600,000 cells/μL, • *iron deficiency anemia*—from GI bleeding, • *neutrophilic leukocytosis,* • *abnormal megakaryocytes in BM* |
| leukemia in neonates to 14 yrs old | **ALL**—this is the most common overall cancer and leukemia in children |
| leukemia in 15- to 39-yr-old age bracket | **AML** |
| leukemia in 40- to 60-yr-old age bracket | • **AML,** • *CML* |
| leukemia in > 60-yr-old age bracket | **CLL**— * also the most common cause of generalized lymphadenopathy in patients >60 yrs old, * CLL is the most common overall leukemia |
| method of distinguishing acute from chronic leukemia | • **acute leukemia**— * BM blast count >30%: e.g., myeloblasts, lymphoblasts, monoblasts, erythroblasts, * PB demonstrates thrombocytopenia and circulating blasts, * normocytic/slightly macrocytic anemia, • **chronic leukemia**— * BM blast count <30%, * evidence of maturation of WBCs in the PB, * thrombocytopenia present: CML is an exception, * normocytic/macrocytic anemia |
| causes of leukemia | • **chromosomal abnormalities**—e.g., Down syndrome, • **radiation**—particularly CML, • **alkylating agents**— * **melphalan,** * cyclophosphamide, * chlorambucil, • **benzene,** • **immunodeficiency syndromes,** • **viruses**—e.g., HTLV-1 |

*Table continued on following page*

### Table 2–8. NEOPLASTIC WBC DISORDERS OF SURGICAL IMPORTANCE *Continued*

| Most Common... | Answer and Explanation |
|---|---|
| S/S of leukemia | • **fever**— * usually due to gram-negative infections, * hypermetabolic state, • **hepatosplenomegaly**, • **petechiae/ecchymoses/ bleeding**—due to thrombocytopenia, • **generalized lymphadenopathy**, • **DIC**—particularly acute progranulocytic leukemia: M3, • **bone pain**—expansion of the bone marrow with leukemic cells, • **gum infiltration**—acute monocytic leukemia: M5 |
| initial step in a leukemia work-up | **BM aspirate and biopsy**—the Dx of leukemia must be made on a bone marrow aspirate/biopsy |
| cell type of CLL | **virgin B cells**—neoplastic B cells are unable to produce plasma cells: hypogammaglobulinemia |
| complications associated with CLL | • **hypogammaglobulinemia**—50%, • *AIHA warm and cold*, • *second malignancies*— * lung, * skin: BCC and squamous, • *transformation into a malignant lymphoma*— this is called Richter's syndrome |
| lab findings in CLL | • **lymphocytosis**— * 15,000–200,000 cells/μL, * "smudge" cells are present: fragile neoplastic B cells, • *normocytic anemia*, • *thrombocytopenia*, • *diffuse BM infiltration*, • *monoclonal IgM spike*, • *hypogammaglobulinemia* |
| COD in CLL | **infections** |
| acute nonlymphocytic leukemia | **FAB classification**—M2: AML with maturation |
| cytoplasmic abnormality in AML | **Auer rods**—these are present only in acute leukemias arising from neutrophils |
| COD in leukemia | • **infections**—usually gram-negatives, • *bleeding* |

## Table 2–8. NEOPLASTIC WBC DISORDERS OF SURGICAL IMPORTANCE *Continued*

**Question:** Which of the following differentiate PRV from other causes of absolute polycythemia? **SELECT 4**
(A) SaO₂
(B) Plasma volume
(C) EPO
(D) Platelet count
(E) Leukemic transformation
(F) RBC mass

**Answers:** (B), (C), (D), (E). The SaO₂ is normal in PRV and inappropriate EPO-producing disorders (e.g., renal adenocarcinoma) and low in hypoxia-induced polycythemia (**choice A is incorrect**). PRV is the only polycythemia with a high plasma volume (**choice B is correct**). The EPO in polycythemia is low and high in both inappropriate EPO-producing and hypoxia-induced polycythemias (**choice C is correct**). The platelet count is elevated in PRV (**choice D is correct**) and normal in the other types of polycythemia. Leukemic transformation (**choice E is correct**) is unique to PRV, which is a myeloproliferative disorder. The RBC mass is increased in all the absolute polycythemias (**choice F is incorrect**).

AIHA = autoimmune hemolytic anemia, ALL = acute lymphoblastic leukemia, AMI = acute myocardial infarction, AML = acute myelogenous leukemia, AMM = agnogenic myeloid metaplasia, BCC = basal cell carcinoma, bcr = break cluster region, BM = bone marrow, CHD = congenital heart disease, CLL = chronic lymphocytic leukemia, CML = chronic myelogenous leukemia, CO = carbon monoxide, COD = cause of death, COPD = chronic obstructive lung disease, DIC = disseminated intravascular coagulation, EPO = erythropoietin, ET = essential thrombocythemia, FAB = French-American-British, Hct = hematocrit, HTLV-1 = human T cell lymphotropic virus, LAP = leukocyte alkaline phosphatase, MCV = mean corpuscular volume, MPD = myeloproliferative disease, PB = peripheral blood, PRV = polycythemia rubra vera, SaO₂ = oxygen saturation of arterial blood, S/S = signs and symptoms.

## Table 2–9. LYMPH NODE DISORDERS OF SURGICAL IMPORTANCE

| Most Common... | Answer and Explanation |
| --- | --- |
| causes of generalized tender lymphadenopathy | • **infections**—e.g., * HIV, * infectious mononucleosis, * secondary syphilis, • *drugs*—e.g., phenytoin, • *autoimmune disease*—e.g., * SLE, * RA |
| cause of cat-scratch disease | ***Bartonella henselae***—organisms are identified in lymph nodes with silver stains |

*Table continued on following page*

Table 2–9. LYMPH NODE DISORDERS OF
SURGICAL IMPORTANCE *Continued*

| Most Common... | Answer and Explanation |
|---|---|
| S/S of cat-scratch disease | **isolated skin lesion, usually on the hands → regional, painful lymphadenopathy**—granulomatous microabscesses |
| Rx of cat-scratch disease | **antibiotics**— * azithromycin, * S/S usually resolve without Rx in 2–6 mos |
| benign nodal disorder mistaken for HD | **lymph nodes in infectious mononucleosis**—infected B cells transform into plasmacytoid immunoblasts that resemble Reed-Sternberg cells |
| drug producing generalized lymphadenopathy and atypical lymphocytosis in the PB | **phenytoin**— * fever, * generalized lymphadenopathy, * skin rash, * eosinophilia |
| benign nodal disorder associated with malignancy | **sinus histiocytosis**—in breast cancer, a favorable prognostic sign |
| malignancy associated with Virchow's node | **stomach adenocarcinoma**— * Virchow's nodes are left supraclavicular nodes, which drain the abdominal cavity, * other malignancies that metastasize to these nodes include pancreas, colon adenocarcinomas, and cervical cancer |
| malignancies associated with para-aortic lymph node enlargement | • **primary malignant lymphomas**, • *metastatic testicular cancers* |
| causes of hilar lymph node enlargement | • **primary lung cancer**—this is the most common initial site of metastasis, • *sarcoidosis*, • *TB*, • *systemic fungal infections*— * histoplasmosis is the most common pathogen, * multiple calcifications are very characteristic: particularly in lungs and spleen |
| cause of nontender unilateral epitrochlear node enlargement | **NHL** |

Table 2–9. LYMPH NODE DISORDERS OF
SURGICAL IMPORTANCE *Continued*

| Most Common... | Answer and Explanation |
|---|---|
| causes of generalized nontender lymphadenopathy | • **acute and chronic leukemias,** • *NHL* |
| cause of lymphadenopathy in a patient <30 yrs old | **benign disease in ~80%**—e.g., infection |
| cause of lymphadenopathy in a patient >30 yrs old | **malignancy**—most often metastatic disease |
| types of malignant lymphoma | • **non-Hodgkin's malignant lymphoma (NHL),** • *Hodgkin's disease* (HD) |
| extranodal site for a primary malignant lymphoma | **stomach**— * the majority arise in mucosa-associated lymphoid tissue (MALT), * most are high-grade malignancies |
| bacteria associated with NHL in the stomach | ***Helicobacter pylori***—this pathogen is the cause of a low-grade B cell lymphoma in MALT |
| cause of increased incidence of primary CNS NHL | **AIDS** |
| malignancy of lymph nodes | **metastasis**—e.g., * breast cancer, * primary lung cancer |
| organ metastasized to | **lymph nodes**—carcinomas generally drain to regional lymph nodes |
| CD antigen marker for malignant lymphomas | **CD$_{45}$**—this marker identifies ~90% of malignant lymphomas |
| translocation associated with malignant lymphoma | • **t(14;18) in B cell follicular lymphomas** • *t(8;14) in Burkitt's lymphoma* |
| causes for the increase in NHL in the United States | • **increase in HIV-positive patients,** • *immunosuppressive Rx*—alkylating agents, • *congenital immunodeficiencies*—e.g., Wiskott-Aldrich syndrome, • *autoimmune disease*—e.g., Sjögren's syndrome, • *EBV infections* |

*Table continued on following page*

### Table 2–9. LYMPH NODE DISORDERS OF
### SURGICAL IMPORTANCE *Continued*

| Most Common... | Answer and Explanation |
|---|---|
| classification scheme for NHL that utilizes pattern and size of the cells | **Rappaport classification—** * patterns are nodular or diffuse, * lymphoma cell size is based on its comparison with that of endothelial cells, * cells smaller than endothelial cells are called lymphocytic; those larger are called histiocytic, * nodular lymphomas more favorable than diffuse, * lymphocytic lymphomas more favorable than histiocytic |
| classification scheme based on marker studies | **Lukes-Collins classification—** * this classification system is more accurate than the Rappaport system, * more expensive and difficult to diagnose lymphomas with this system |
| classification scheme that groups NHL by clinical features, morphology, immunophenotype, and genotype | **Revised European-American Classification of Lymphoid Neoplasms (REAL)—**this system was developed to replace the deficiencies noted in the **Working Formulation for Clinical Usage** system that divided lymphomas into low, intermediate, and high grades |
| NHL | **peripheral B-cell neoplasm: follicular lymphoma cytologic grade I—**this type of B cell lymphoma is associated with a t(14;18), with inactivation of the apoptosis gene causing the B cells to become immortal |
| clinical features of cytologically low-grade non-Hodgkin's lymphomas | • **incurable,** • *involve older patients,* • *stage III/IV disease at onset*—BM involvement is common, • *can respond to chemotherapy,* • *long survival even after relapse*—median survival of ~8 yrs |
| clinical features of cytologically high-grade non-Hodgkin's lymphomas | • **potentially curable,** • **often progress to a more aggressive lymphoma,** • **length of survival is short in those who do not go into remission** |
| S/S of cytologically low-grade NHLs | **painless lymphadenopathy** |
| S/S of cytologically high-grade NHLs | • **fever,** • **drenching night sweats,** • **weight loss,** • **abdominal pain**—typical for American Burkitt's lymphoma |

## Table 2–9. LYMPH NODE DISORDERS OF SURGICAL IMPORTANCE Continued

| Most Common... | Answer and Explanation |
|---|---|
| NHL in children | **Burkitt's lymphoma—** * malignant B cell lymphoma, * cytologically a high-grade lymphoma |
| site for Burkitt's lymphoma | **abdominal cavity—** * most often occurs in Peyer's patches of the small intestine in boys, * most often occurs in the pelvic organs in girls, * relationship with EBV |
| work-up of NHL | • **chest x-ray, • CT of abdomen/pelvis, • bilateral BM aspirates/biopsies—** * BM involvement is more common in cytologically low-grade than high-grade NHLs, * BM involvement is automatically stage IV disease |
| features more often associated with HD than NHL | • **younger patient,** • *fever,* • *rarely involves Waldeyer's ring*—tonsils/adenoids, • *localized rather than generalized nodal involvement,* • *pain in an involved lymph node after alcohol ingestion* |
| cell required to Dx HD | **RS cells—** * RS cells are the neoplastic cell in HD: marker studies indicate that they are either B or T cells, * single cell with two or more nuclei or nuclear lobes with a large red nucleolus surrounded by a clear halo ("owl-eye" appearance) |
| virus associated with HD | **EBV**—PCR detection of EBV is noted in 60–80% of cases |
| subtypes of HD in order of increasing number of RS cells, decreasing survival, and increasing age | • **lymphocyte predominant (LP)—** * male dominant, * 5%, • *nodular sclerosing (NS)—* * female dominant, * most common type: 40–70%, • *mixed cellularity (MC)—* * male dominant, * 20–40%, • *lymphocyte depletion (LD)—* * male dominant, * rare |
| HD subtype with mediastinal involvement | **NS/HD**—the usual clinical scenario is a young woman with a single lymph node group in the axilla or cervical or supraclavicular area, plus involvement of the anterior mediastinum |

*Table continued on following page*

### Table 2–9. LYMPH NODE DISORDERS OF
### SURGICAL IMPORTANCE Continued

| Most Common... | Answer and Explanation |
|---|---|
| factors determining prognosis of HD | • **clinical stage,** • *type of HD*— * LP best, * LD worst |
| initial work-up of HD | • **history/physical exam,** • **chest x-ray,** • **CT**— * thorax, * abdomen, * pelvis, • **bipedal lymphangiography,** • **CBC with differential,** • **bilateral BM aspiration/biopsy,** • **serum albumin,** • **serum calcium,** • **serum LDH,** • **liver function tests** |
| stage at initial presentation of HD | • **stage IIA**— * refers to involvement of 2 or more lymph node regions on the same side of diaphragm, * large case letter **A** indicates absence of fever >38°C, drenching night sweats, and weight loss >10% of body weight within preceding 6 mos: **B** indicates the presence of the above S/S, • *stage I*—single lymph node region, • *stage III*—nodal involvement above/below the diaphragm, • *stage IV*—disseminated disease involving liver/BM |
| Rx of HD | • **localized disease (stage IA, IIA)**—radiation, • *intermediate disease (stage IIB, IIIA)*—combination chemotherapy: doxorubicin, bleomycin, vincristine, dacarbazine, • *disseminated disease (stage IIIB, IV)*—intensive chemotherapy with high doses of doxorubicin, bleomycin, vincristine, dacarbazine |
| complication of Rx of HD | • **second malignancies related to alkylating agents**—e.g., * acute nonlymphocytic leukemia, * B cell NHL, • *solid tumors related to radiation*—cancers of thyroid, breast, skin, stomach, head/neck, • *infertility,* • *hypothyroidism*—radiation effect, • *sepsis*—*Streptococcus pneumoniae* in splenectomized patients, • *congestive cardiomyopathy*—doxorubicin effect |

**Table 2–9.  LYMPH NODE DISORDERS OF
SURGICAL IMPORTANCE** *Continued*

**Question:** Which of the following lymph node enlargements **MOST
LIKELY** represent a malignant lymph node disorder? **SELECT 4**
  (A)  Cervical lymph node enlargement in a patient exposed to
       head/neck radiation
  (B)  Painful axillary lymph node enlargement in a veterinarian
  (C)  Left supraclavicular lymph node enlargement in a patient
       with sudden outcropping of seborrheic keratoses
  (D)  Para-aortic lymph enlargement in a 19-yr-old man with a
       history of cryptorchid testis
  (E)  Generalized lymphadenopathy in an HIV-positive patient
  (F)  Painless axillary lymph node enlargement in a 55-yr-old
       woman with a normal mammogram

**Answers: (A), (C), (D), (F).** A patient with radiation to the head/
neck and cervical lymph node enlargement most likely has metastatic
papillary adenocarcinoma of the thyroid gland **(choice A is correct).**
A veterinarian with painful axillary lymph nodes most likely has cat-
scratch disease **(choice B is incorrect).** Involvement of Virchow's node
is most likely a patient with metastatic adenocarcinoma of the stomach. Sudden outcroppings of seborrheic keratoses is called the Leser-
Trélat sign and often harbingers a stomach adenocarcinoma **(choice C
is correct).** A testicular mass in a young man with para-aortic nodal
involvement and a history of cryptorchidism is most likely due to
metastatic seminoma **(choice D is correct).** Generalized lymphadenopathy is a common benign finding in HIV-positive patients and does
not represent malignancy **(choice E is incorrect).** Axillary nodes in a
woman over 50 yrs old is metastatic breast cancer regardless of the
mammogram results **(choice F is correct).** The lymph node should
be excised.

ALL = acute lymphoblastic leukemia, BM = bone marrow, CD = cluster
designation, CLL = chronic lymphocytic lymphoma, CNS = central
nervous system, CT = computed tomography, EBV = Epstein-Barr virus,
HD = Hodgkin's disease, HIV = human immunodeficiency virus, LD =
lymphocyte depleted, LDH = lactate dehydrogenase, LP = lymphocyte
predominant, MALT = mucosa-associated lymphoid tissue, MC = mixed
cellularity, NHL = non-Hodgkin's lymphoma, NS = nodular sclerosis, PB
= peripheral blood, PCR = polymerase chain reaction, RA = rheumatoid
arthritis, RS = Reed Sternberg cells, SLE = systemic lupus erythematosus, S/S = signs/symptoms.

### Table 2–10. PLASMA CELL AND SPLENIC DISORDERS OF SURGICAL IMPORTANCE

| Most Common... | Answer and Explanation |
|---|---|
| monoclonal gammopathy (MG) | **MGUS**— * > MGUS accounts for 50% of all cases of MG, * it most commonly occurs in the elderly, * ~25% develop MM or related disorder over the next 20 yrs |
| location for a monoclonal spike on an SPE | **γ-globulin region**— * the majority of monoclonal gammopathies involve IgG (60%) followed by IgM and IgA, * immunoglobulins are located in the γ-globulin region of an SPE |
| primary malignancy of bone | **multiple myeloma (MM)**— * MM accounts for ~20% of all cases of MG, * median age ~60 yrs, * women > men, * blacks > whites |
| S/S of MM | • **bone pain**— * ~65%, * back/ribs, • *pathologic fractures*— * osteolytic lesions occur in the axial skeleton: skull, spine, ribs, proximal long bones, * osteoporosis, • *renal failure*— ~50%, • *fatigue*—due to anemia, • *recurrent infections*—particularly *Streptococcus pneumoniae,* • *spinal cord compression*—compression fractures of the vertebral column |
| lab findings of MM | • **abnormal serum immunoelectrophoresis (SIEP) and urine immunoelectrophoresis (UIEP)**— * the predominant immunoglobulin involved produces abnormal arcs when compared with the normal control, whereas the other immunoglobulins are suppressed, * UIEP is useful in confirming the presence of BJ protein: BJ protein is excess light chains that spill into the urine, • *monoclonal (M) protein ≥3 g/dL,* • *sheets of malignant plasma cells (>10%) are present in the BM,* • *BJ proteinuria*— * best detected by urine electrophoresis, * a negative dipstick reaction for protein but a strongly positive test with sulfosalicylic acid (SSA): ♦ the standard urine dipstick detects only albumin in the urine, ♦ SSA detects both albumin and globulins, ♦ BJ protein is a globulin, • *hypercalcemia*—due to increased osteoclastic activity related to secretion of osteoclast-activating factor (interleukin-1) from the malignant plasma cells, • *high ESR,* • *prolonged BT*—qualitative platelet defect, • *radionuclide bone scans*—not useful because lesions are lytic and have no osteoblastic response |

### Table 2–10. PLASMA CELL AND SPLENIC DISORDERS OF SURGICAL IMPORTANCE *Continued*

| Most Common... | Answer and Explanation |
| --- | --- |
| COD in MM | **infection** |
| locations for solitary plasmacytomas of bone | • **vertebrae,** • *ribs,* • *pelvis* [**Note:** MM must be excluded before this Dx can be made. ~75% of solitary plasmacytomas of bone progress into MM. Rx is radiation.] |
| location for extramedullary plasmacytoma | **upper respiratory tract**— * 85% occur in the upper respiratory tract, * sites include: ♦ nasopharynx, ♦ larynx, ♦ sinuses, * the majority of extramedullary plasmacytomas do not progress into MM, * they are potentially curable with radiation |
| functions of the spleen | • **filter blood**—the spleen removes: ♦ senescent RBCs, ♦ parasites, ♦ encapsulated bacteria, • *immunologic function*—antigen trapping for macrophages, • *platelet storage,* • *hematologic*—site for extramedullary hematopoiesis |
| causes of massive splenomegaly in United States | • **MPDs**— * AMM, * PRV, * CML, • *CLL* |
| complications of splenomegaly | • **LUQ pain**— * pain is due to stretching of the capsule, * infarction, • *hypersplenism*—see below |
| nontraumatic indication for splenectomy | **hematologic disorders**—e.g., * congenital spherocytosis, * ITP, * AIHA, * NHL, * HD, * β-thalassemia major |
| traumatic indication for splenectomy | • **trauma,** • *surgery*—spleen is commonly injured during stomach or pancreatic surgery |
| complication of splenectomy | **atelectasis** |
| clinical effects of splenectomy | • **predisposition to infection**— * particularly *Streptococcus pneumoniae,* * *Haemophilus influenzae* to a lesser extent, * drop in IgM activity decreases production of C3b (opsonizing agent), * 80% of infections occur in first 2 yrs after surgery, • *hematologic effects*— * thrombocytosis, * HJ bodies are present in the peripheral blood, * target cells are present in the peripheral blood |

*Table continued on following page*

### Table 2–10. PLASMA CELL AND SPLENIC DISORDERS OF SURGICAL IMPORTANCE *Continued*

| Most Common... | Answer and Explanation |
|---|---|
| causes of hypersplenism | • **portal HTN**—most often a complication of alcoholic cirrhosis, • *Felty's syndrome*—triad of: ♦ RA, ♦ splenomegaly, ♦ neutropenia, • *Gaucher's disease*—AR lysosomal storage disease [**Note:** hypersplenism is an exaggeration of normal splenic function, leading to cytopenias involving single or multiple cell lines.] |
| parasitic disease of spleen | **Echinococcosis**—calcifications are commonly seen on x-ray |
| primary splenic tumor | **benign hemangiomas** |
| splenic malignancy | **metastatic NHL** |
| cause of multifocal calcifications in spleen | **histoplasmosis** |

**Question:** Which of the following abnormalities occur in multiple myeloma? **SELECT 4**
- (A) Secondary amyloidosis
- (B) Elevated alkaline phosphatase
- (C) Pathologic fractures
- (D) Generalized lymphadenopathy
- (E) IgM monoclonal spike
- (F) Renal failure
- (G) Secondary hyperparathyroidism
- (H) Light chains in urine
- (I) Punched-out lesions in skull

**Answers: (C), (F), (H), (I).** Primary amyloidosis with conversion of light chains into amyloid protein is associated with MM. Secondary amyloidosis is due to chronic inflammation and conversion of serum-associated amyloid into amyloid protein (**choice A is incorrect**). Alkaline phosphatase is usually normal in MM, since the bone lesions are osteolytic rather than osteoblastic (**choice B is incorrect**). Pathologic fractures due to osteolytic lesions and osteoporosis are the rule in MM (**choice C is correct**). Generalized lymphadenopathy is not a feature of MM and is more often noted in Waldenström's macroglobulinemia (**choice D is incorrect**). An IgM monoclonal spike is most often associated with Waldenström's macroglobulinemia (**choice E is incorrect**). Renal failure is a common COD in MM (**choice F is correct**). Secondary hyperparathyroidism implies hypocalcemia stimulating the release of PTH. MM is associated with hypercalcemia (**choice G is incorrect**). Bj protein (light chains) are characteristically present in the urine in MM (**choice H is correct**). Punched-out skull lesions representing osteolytic activity are commonly observed in MM (**choice I is correct**).

AIHA = autoimmune hemolytic anemia, AMM = agnogenic myeloid metaplasia, AR = autosomal recessive, BJ = Bence Jones, BM = bone marrow, BT = bleeding time, CLL = chronic lymphocytic lymphoma, CML = chronic myelogenous leukemia, COD = cause of death, EPO = erythropoietin, ESR = erythrocyte sedimentation rate, HD = Hodgkin's disease, HJ = Howell-Jolly, HTN = hypertension, ITP = idiopathic thrombocytopenic purpura, LUQ = left upper quadrant, M = monoclonal, MG = monoclonal gammopathy, MGUS = monoclonal gammopathy of undetermined significance, MM = multiple myeloma, MPD = myeloproliferative disease, NHL = non-Hodgkin's lymphoma, PRV = polycythemia rubra vera, PTH = parathormone, RA = rheumatoid arthritis, SAA = serum-associated amyloid, SIEP = serum immunoelectrophoresis, SPE = serum protein electrophoresis, S/S = signs/symptoms, SSA = sulfosalicylic acid, UIEP = urine immunoelectrophoresis.

## Table 2–11. GENERAL CONCEPTS OF HEMOSTASIS

| Most Common... | Answer and Explanation |
|---|---|
| components of the hemostasis system | • **blood vessels,** • **platelets,** • **coagulation system,** • **fibrinolytic system** |
| endothelial cell–derived anticoagulants | • **tissue plasminogen activator (tPA)**—activates plasminogen to produce plasmin, • **heparin-like products**—enhance antithrombin III (AT III) activity, • **prostacyclin (PGI$_2$)**— * inhibits platelet aggregation, * vasodilator |
| liver-derived anticoagulants | • **AT III**—inhibits coagulation factors that are serine proteases: e.g., thrombin, factor X, • **proteins C and S**— * enhance fibrinolytic activity, * inactivate factors V and VIII |
| endothelial cell–derived procoagulants | • **VIII:Ag**—antigenic determinant of VIII:C, • **VIII:vWF**—initial adhesion agent for platelets in endothelial injury, • **VIII:RCo**—activity necessary for platelet aggregation due to ristocetin, • **tissue thromboplastin**—activates factor VII in the extrinsic coagulation system |
| platelet-derived procoagulants | • **thromboxane A$_2$ (TXA$_2$)**— * platelet aggregator, * vasoconstrictor, * bronchoconstrictor, • *VIII:vWF*— * synthesized by megakaryocytes and stored in α-granules within platelets, * circulates as multimers, • *ADP*— platelet aggregator located in platelet-dense bodies |

*Table continued on following page*

## Table 2–11. GENERAL CONCEPTS OF HEMOSTASIS
### *Continued*

| Most Common... | Answer and Explanation |
|---|---|
| liver-derived procoagulants | **all the coagulation factors except VIII:vWF and VIIIC:Ag** |
| site of platelet production | **BM—** * produced by cytoplasmic fragmentation of megakaryocytes, * platelets live ~10 days, * ~one-third of the platelets are stored in the spleen |
| platelet enzyme blocked by aspirin and NSAIDs | **platelet cyclooxygenase—** * cyclooxygenase converts arachidonic acid into $PGG_2$, * $PGG_2$ is converted into $PGH_2$, * $PGH_2$ is converted by thromboxane synthetase into $TXA_2$ [**Note:** endothelial cell cyclooxygenase is less affected by NSAIDs than platelet cyclooxygenase. Dipyramidole blocks thromboxane synthase.] |
| binding agent for the vitamin K–dependent factors | **calcium—** * calcium specifically binds vitamin K–dependent factors: ♦ II (prothrombin), ♦ VII, ♦ IX, ♦ X, ♦ protein C/S to platelet factor 3 ($PF_3$), * the vitamin K–dependent factors must be $\gamma$-carboxylated by vitamin K1 for calcium to bind them to $PF_3$ |
| sequence of reactions used by the extrinsic coagulation system down to the final common pathway | **factor VII → factor X → factor V → factor II → factor I (fibrinogen) → clot**—VIIa also activates factor IX in the intrinsic pathway |
| sequence of reactions used by intrinsic coagulation system down to final common pathway | **factor XII (Hageman's factor) → factor XI → factor IX → factor VIII → factor X → factor V → factor II → factor I (fibrinogen) → clot** |
| sequence of reactions in the formation of a stable clot | **factor II (prothrombin) → thrombin cleaves fibrinogen into a fibrin monomer + fibrinopeptides A and B → fibrin monomers form fibrin aggregates → soluble fibrin (urea-soluble) → insoluble fibrin (urea-insoluble clot) with strong covalent cross-links (factor XIII) → stable clot** |

### Table 2–11. GENERAL CONCEPTS OF HEMOSTASIS
*Continued*

| Most Common... | Answer and Explanation |
|---|---|
| coagulation factors consumed in forming a fibrin clot | • **factor I**—fibrinogen, • **factor II**—pro-thrombin, • **factor V**, • **factor VIII** [Note: these factors are absent in serum and present in plasma.] |
| activators of plasminogen in the fibrinolytic pathway | • **tPA**, • **XII**, • **streptokinase**, • **urokinase** [Note: tPA, streptokinase, and urokinase are clinically used to activate the fibrinolytic system to dissolve clots.] |
| initial vessel response in small vessel injury (e.g., bleeding time) | **vasoconstriction**—this reduces blood flow to facilitate platelet adhesion |
| platelet response in small vessel injury: step 1 | **platelet adhesion to exposed VIII:vWF in injured endothelial cells via platelet GPIb receptors →** |
| platelet response in small vessel injury: step 2 | **platelet release reaction of ADP**—begins platelet aggregation |
| platelet response in small vessel injury: steps 3, 4 | **step 3: platelet synthesizes TXA$_2$** (further enhances platelet aggregation/vasoconstrictor) **→ step 4: platelet aggregation with cessation of bleeding (temporary hemostatic plug)—** * platelets are held together by fibrinogen cross-links between subjacent GPIIb/IIIa platelet fibrinogen receptors, * the platelet plug is unstable and easily broken apart, * fibrinogen must be converted into fibrin before the platelet plug is stable: thrombin must be present from activation of the coagulation system for this to occur |
| sequence involved in bleeding time (BT) | **small vessel injury → temporary hemostatic plug—** * the BT evaluates only the small vessel and platelet component in forming the temporary hemostatic plug, * the BT does not evaluate the coagulation system component, * see Table 2–2 |

*Table continued on following page*

## Table 2–11. GENERAL CONCEPTS OF HEMOSTASIS
*Continued*

| Most Common... | Answer and Explanation |
|---|---|
| coagulation system response in small vessel injury | **injury of tissue causes the initial release of tissue thromboplastin, which activates the extrinsic pathway → exposure of factor XII to collagen causes activation of the intrinsic system (both extrinsic/intrinsic systems generate thrombin) → thrombin converts platelet-associated fibrinogen into fibrin → stable platelet plug—** * the coagulation system via production of thrombin converts the fibrinogen, which is holding the platelet plug together, into fibrin, * fibrin stabilizes the platelet plug |
| fibrinolytic system response in small vessel injury | **plasminogen is activated by tPA and activated factor XII—** * plasmin is released, * the stable platelet plug is dissolved: plasmin breaks the fibrin strands holding the platelets together, * blood flow is re-established |
| tests evaluating hemostasis | **see Table 2–2** |

**Question:** Which of the following disorders will prolong the bleeding time? **SELECT 3**
- (A) Factor VIII: coagulant deficiency
- (B) Factor VIII:vWF deficiency
- (C) Factor VII deficiency
- (D) Thrombocytopenia
- (E) Factor XII deficiency
- (F) NSAIDs

**Answers: (B), (D), (F):** Factor deficiencies in the extrinsic (VII) and intrinsic (VIII, XII) systems do not alter the bleeding time; however, they are important in the production of a stable platelet plug (**choices A, C, and E are incorrect**). Deficiency of VIII:vWF, the platelet adhesion factor, prolongs the BT and is one of the hemostatic abnormalities in von Willebrand's disease (**choice B is correct**). Thrombocytopenia prolongs the BT (**choice D is correct**). NSAIDs are the most common cause of a prolonged BT and do so by inhibiting platelet cyclooxygenase and production of TXA₂ (**choice F is correct**).

ADP = adenosine diphosphate, AT III = antithrombin III, BM = bone marrow, BT = bleeding time, HMWK = high molecular weight kininogen, NSAIDs = nonsteroidals, PF₃ = platelet factor 3, PG = prostaglandin, PGI₂ = prostacyclin, tPA = tissue plasminogen activator, TT = thrombin time, TXA₂ = thromboxane A₂, VIII:Ag = antigenic determinant of VIII:C, VIII:C = VIII coagulant, VIII:RCo = von Willebrand factor activity with ristocetin, VIII:vWF = von Willebrand factor.

### Table 2–12. SELECTED VASCULAR AND PLATELET DISORDERS

| Most Common... | Answer and Explanation |
|---|---|
| S/S associated with vessel/platelet disorders | • **epistaxis**—nosebleeds, • *petechiae*—1–3 mm, red, nonblanching, nonpalpable hemorrhages on skin/mucous membranes,• *ecchymoses*—purpuric lesions about the size of a quarter, • *easy or spontaneous bruising,* • *bleeding from superficial scratches*—no temporary hemostatic plug is present to prevent bleeding, • *spontaneous mucous membrane bleeding* |
| genetic vascular disorders | • **hereditary hemorrhagic telangiectasia (Osler-Weber-Rendu disease)**— * AD disease, * vascular ectasias in the mouth (tongue, lips), GI tract (produces iron deficiency), and skin, • *Marfan syndrome*—AD defect in fibrillin, • *Ehlers-Danlos syndrome*—multifactorial disease with defects in collagen |
| age-dependent vessel disease in the elderly | **senile purpura**— * senile purpura is due to atrophy of perivascular support tissue, * purpura is located on extensor surfaces of hands/forearms: these are normal areas of trauma |
| nutritional vascular disease | **scurvy**— * vitamin C deficiency, * structurally weak collagen |
| metabolic vascular disease | **excess glucocorticoids**—steroids interfere with collagen synthesis |
| causes of thrombocytopenia | **increased destruction**—e.g., **immune,** • decreased production—e.g., BM suppression, • *abnormal sequestration*—e.g., splenomegaly, • consumption—DIC, TTP, HUS |
| cause of thrombocytopenia in adults | **immune thrombocytopenia**— * IgG antibodies develop against platelets with extravascular removal by macrophages: ♦ type II hypersensitivity reaction, ♦ same mechanism for thrombocytopenia in children, * immune thrombocytopenia is common in SLE |
| lab findings in immune thrombocytopenia in adults | • **thrombocytopenia,** • *prolonged bleeding time,* • *IgG antibodies against platelets* |

*Table continued on following page*

Table 2–12. SELECTED VASCULAR AND
PLATELET DISORDERS *Continued*

| Most Common... | Answer and Explanation |
|---|---|
| Rx of immune thrombocytopenia in adults | • **initially corticosteroids**— * 70% response, * if no response → • *splenectomy*— * 75% response, * definitive Rx, * if no response → • *danazol*— * blocks macrophage Fc receptor sites, * if no response → • *immunosuppressive agents*—e.g., * vincristine, * vinblastine, * azathioprine, * cyclophosphamide, * cyclosporin, if life-threatening → • *IV γ-globulin plus platelet transfusions*—IV γ-globulin blocks IgG Fc receptor sites on macrophages |
| mechanism for drug-induced thrombocytopenia | **type III immunocomplex destruction** |
| drugs associated with immune thrombocytopenia | • **heparin**—see below, • *quinidine,* • *H₂ blockers,* • *sulfonamides,* • *thiazides,* • *procainamide,* • *rifampin* [**Note:** withdrawal of the drug reverses the disease in 4–14 days.] |
| drug associated with immune thrombocytopenia in a hospitalized patient | **heparin**— * type III immunocomplex reaction, * antibodies develop in 10% of patients |
| heparin variant associated with early destruction | **type I variant**— * occurs early, * transient, * not immune-mediated |
| variant associated with thrombocytopenia/ thrombosis | **type II variant**— * immune-mediated, * platelet destruction: median time 10 days post Rx, * bleeding is uncommon, * platelet release reaction of thrombogenic agents results in venous (more common) or arterial thromboses |
| virus-associated immune thrombocytopenias | **HIV**— * thrombocytopenia is the most common coagulation abnormality in AIDS: 30–45% of patients, * it is not an AIDS-defining disorder |
| mechanism of post-transfusion purpura | **PLᴬ¹-negative patient with previous exposure to PLᴬ¹-positive platelets develops IgG antibodies and on re-exposure to PLᴬ¹-positive platelets develops severe thrombocytopenia ~5–7 days after the transfusion**— * both donor and patient platelets are destroyed, * mortality is 10–15% |

### Table 2–12. SELECTED VASCULAR AND PLATELET DISORDERS *Continued*

| Most Common... | Answer and Explanation |
|---|---|
| cause of primary thrombocytosis | **myeloproliferative disease**— * examples include: ♦ PRV, ♦ essential thrombocythemia, * thrombocytosis is associated with thrombosis and bleeding |
| cause of platelet sequestration | **congestive splenomegaly**—this most commonly occurs in patients with portal HTN secondary to cirrhosis |
| causes of secondary thrombocytosis | • **malignancy**— * 35%, • *infection*—e.g., TB, • *rebound after thrombocytopenia*, • *chronic iron deficiency*, • *splenectomy* |
| Rx of postsplenectomy thrombocytosis | **aspirin**—aspirin is used if the count is >1,000,000 cells/μL |
| acquired causes of a qualitative platelet defect with a normal platelet count and prolonged BT | • **patient taking aspirin or NSAIDs**— * effect of aspirin on platelet cyclooxygenase is irreversible, * other NSAIDs produce a reversible defect when the patient is off the drug for 48 hrs, • *uremia*, • *cardiopulmonary bypass*, • β-*lactam antibiotics* [**Note:** desmopressin or conjugated estrogens can reverse qualitative defects in the above conditions.] |
| time frame to discontinue aspirin prior to surgery | **7 days** |
| genetic cause of a qualitative platelet defect | **VWD**—see below |
| platelet abnormality in uremia | **platelet dysfunction**—uremia produces a defect in platelet adhesion/aggregation |
| Rx of platelet abnormality in uremia | • **dialysis**, • *desmopressin*, • *combined estrogen/progestin pills* |

*Table continued on following page*

### Table 2–12. SELECTED VASCULAR AND PLATELET DISORDERS *Continued*

**Question:** Immune mechanisms are involved in the pathogenesis of which of the following causes of thrombocytopenia? **SELECT 3**
  (A) HIV
  (B) von Willebrand's disease
  (C) Uremia
  (D) DIC
  (E) Heparin
  (F) Idiopathic thrombocytopenic purpura
  (G) NSAIDs

**Answers: (A), (E), (F).** Thrombocytopenia associated with HIV, heparin, and ITP are all immune-mediated (**choices A, E, and F are correct**). Von Willebrand's disease is associated with absence of VIII:vWF, hence platelets cannot adhere to damaged endothelium (**choice B is incorrect**). Uremia produces a qualitative platelet defect causing problems with adhesion and aggregation (**choice C is incorrect**). DIC involves the consumption of platelets and clotting factors in the formation of fibrin clots (**choice D is incorrect**). NSAIDs inhibit platelet cyclooxygenase (**choice G is incorrect**).

AD = autosomal dominant, BM = bone marrow, DIC = disseminated intravascular coagulation, HIV = human immunodeficiency virus, ITP = idiopathic thrombocytopenic purpura, NSAIDs = nonsteroidal anti-inflammatory drugs, PL = platelet, PRV = polycythemia rubra vera, SLE = systemic lupus erythematosus, S/S = signs/symptoms, VIII:vWF = von Willebrand factor, VWD = von Willebrand's disease.

### Table 2–13. COAGULATION, FIBRINOLYTIC, THROMBOEMBOLIC DISORDERS OF SURGICAL IMPORTANCE

| Most Common... | Answer and Explanation |
| --- | --- |
| signs of a coagulation disorder | • **delayed bleeding**—e.g., after appendectomy: a temporary hemostatic plug is present but not a stable platelet plug, hence bleeding occurs when the patient begins moving around, • *hemarthroses*—only in severe hemophilia A/B, • *bleeding into spaces*—only severe hemophilia A/B, • *hematuria*, • *GI bleeds*, • *menorrhagia* |

**Table 2–13. COAGULATION, FIBRINOLYTIC,
THROMBOEMBOLIC DISORDERS OF
SURGICAL IMPORTANCE** *Continued*

| Most Common... | Answer and Explanation |
|---|---|
| causes of a coagulation deficiency | • **decreased production**— * e.g., **acquired:** ♦ liver disease, ♦ vitamin K deficiency, * hereditary, • *increased consumption*— e.g., DIC, • *increased destruction*—e.g., circulating anticoagulants: antibodies, inhibitors, • *combinations of the above* |
| SXR hereditary coagulation disorders | • **hemophilia A**— * affected man does not transmit disease to his sons, * all his daughters are asymptomatic female carriers, * female carriers transmit the disease to 50% of their sons, • *hemophilia B—factor IX deficiency* |
| method of detecting asymptomatic female carriers of hemophilia A or B | **DNA techniques with identification of the abnormal locus on the X chromosome**—a ratio of VIII:C/VIII:Ag <0.75 suggests a carrier state: VIII:Ag is normal in hemophilia A, while VIII:C is deficient |
| factor determining the severity of hemophilia A | **factor VIII:C concentration** |
| clinical findings in severe hemophilia A | • **spontaneous hemarthroses,** • *subcutaneous hematomas,* • *atrophied muscles,* • *hematomas in GI/GU tract* [**Note:** the above findings occur when the factor VIII:C level is <1% of normal.] |
| bleeding sites in severe hemophilia A | • **joints,** • *muscle,* • *GI tract* [**Note:** severe hemophiliacs bleed spontaneously and do not require trauma or a surgical insult to bleed. 50% of male neonates bleed at circumcision.] |
| lab findings in hemophilia A | • **low factor VIII:C,** • *prolonged PTT,* • *normal PT,* • *normal platelet count,* • *normal BT,* • *normal VIII:Ag,* • *normal VIII:vWF,* • *infusion of products containing factor VIII:C causes an immediate nonsustained increase in de novo synthesis of factor VIII:C that is not in excess of the amount infused* |

*Table continued on following page*

### Table 2–13. COAGULATION, FIBRINOLYTIC, THROMBOEMBOLIC DISORDERS OF SURGICAL IMPORTANCE *Continued*

| Most Common... | Answer and Explanation |
|---|---|
| Rx of hemophilia A | • **mild hemophilia**— * factor VIII:C levels range from 6–25%, * Rx with desmopressin: increases the synthesis of all factor VIII components, * ε-aminocaproic acid: inhibits fibrinolysis and keeps factor VIII:C levels high, • **moderate/severe**— * factor VIII:C levels range between 1 and 5%,* initial trial of desmopressin for moderate hemophilia, * factor VIII infusion is required for most moderately severe and all severe hemophiliacs, * a new factor VIII product is produced by monoclonal antibodies or recombinant DNA techniques: no risk for transmitting HIV, HBV, or HCV [**Note:** ~75% of patients treated with factor VIII concentrates before 1985 (before screening was available) became infected with HIV.] |
| hereditary coagulation disorder | **classical VWD**— * AD disorder, * accounts for 70–80% of cases of VWD, * VWD variants are uncommon |
| S/S of VWD | **signs of platelet and coagulation defects**— * epistaxis, * menorrhagia: main problem in women, * ecchymoses, * bleeding from superficial scratches, * bleeding from tooth extractions, * GI bleeding, * easy bruisability, * bleeding exacerbated by aspirin |
| GI association with VWD | **angiodysplasia**— * dilated vessels that bleed, * occurs in the stomach/small intestine in younger patients and in the cecum in older patients [**Note:** angiodysplasia is second to diverticulosis as the most common cause of hematochezia in adults.] |
| lab findings in classical VWD | • **low VIII:RCo**— * this is the best overall test, * see Table 2–2, • *low VIII:Ag,* • *low VIII:vWF,* • *low VIII:C,* • *prolonged BT—* ~50%, • *prolonged PTT,* • *normal PT,* • *infusion of products containing factor VIII produces a slow but sustained increase in de novo synthesized factor VIII:C in excess of the amount infused* |

### Table 2–13. COAGULATION, FIBRINOLYTIC, THROMBOEMBOLIC DISORDERS OF SURGICAL IMPORTANCE *Continued*

| Most Common... | Answer and Explanation |
|---|---|
| Rx for VWD with minor bleeding problems | • **desmopressin**—contraindicated in type IIb VWD, • *oral contraceptives for menorrhagia*—estrogen increases the synthesis of all the factor VIII components |
| Rx for VWD with moderately severe bleeding problems | **intermediate purity factor VIII concentrate (Humate P)**—is rich in HMW multimers of VIII:vWF |
| Rx for VWD when contemplating minor surgery | **desmopressin 1 hr preop**—daily for 2–3 days postop |
| Rx for VWD when contemplating major surgery | • **monitor VIII:C/VIII:RCo levels,** • infusion of desmopressin is given at more frequent intervals [**Note:** cryoprecipitate was the previous gold standard of Rx of VWD. However, being a blood product, it can transmit HIV and hepatitis. Cryoprecipitate contains all the factor VIII components (highest concentration of all blood products), fibrinogen, and factor XIII.] |
| circulating anticoagulant | **factor VIII antibodies**— * this most commonly occurs in the Rx of hemophilia A, * a prolonged PTT does not correct with the addition of normal plasma: true VIII deficiency does correct, * see Table 2–2 for discussion of mixing studies, * additional causes include: ♦ postpartum state, ♦ chlorpromazine |
| circulating anticoagulant against platelet PF$_3$ | **lupus anticoagulant (LA)**— * prolongs the PTT (90%) and less commonly the PT (20%), * it is an IgG, IgM, or IgA antibody |
| causes of LA | • **SLE,** • *procainamide,* • *hydralazine,* • *HIV,* • *quinidine* |
| circulating anticoagulant producing a false-positive RPR or VDRL | **anticardiolipin antibody (ACA)**—the test substrate used in the RPR/VDRL is beef cardiolipin: ACAs react against this substrate, leading to a FP test result |
| syndrome associated with LA and/or ACA | **antiphospholipid syndrome**— * both antibodies are present in 60% of cases, * one antibody is present in 40% |

*Table continued on following page*

**Table 2–13. COAGULATION, FIBRINOLYTIC, THROMBOEMBOLIC DISORDERS OF SURGICAL IMPORTANCE** *Continued*

| Most Common... | Answer and Explanation |
|---|---|
| coagulation abnormalities associated with APL | • **venous thrombosis**— * placental bed thrombosis: spontaneous abortion, * hepatic vein: Budd-Chiari syndrome, * DVTs, * cutaneous skin necrosis, * renal vein thrombosis, • *arterial thrombosis*— * CNS: stroke, * coronary artery: acute myocardial infarction, * renal artery, • *recurrent spontaneous abortions*—thrombosis of placental bed, • *premature delivery,* • *livedo reticularis,* • *multiinfarct dementia* |
| mechanism of thrombosis in APL | **APL antibodies react against phospholipids in endothelial cells, resulting in damage and subsequent thrombosis** |
| Rx/prevention of thrombosis in APL syndrome | • **heparin followed by warfarin**—keep the INR >3, • *prednisone*—rapidly eliminates LA, • *pregnancy*—low-dose aspirin + heparin |
| vitamin deficiency resulting in a coagulation disorder | **vitamin K deficiency**— * $K_1$ is active and $K_2$ is inactive: $K_2$ is synthesized by colon bacteria, * epoxide reductase converts $K_2$ to $K_1$ |
| adult causes of vitamin K deficiency | • **warfarin anticoagulation**— * warfarin inactivates epoxide reductase, * liver-synthesized vitamin K–dependent factors are nonfunctional: they must be γ-carboxylated by $K_1$ to be bound to a clot by calcium, • *malabsorption*— * pancreatic disease, * bile salt deficiency, * celiac disease, • *broad-spectrum antibiotics*—e.g., * third-generation cephalosporins, * neomycin |
| clinical scenario for adult vitamin K deficiency | **postop patient on antibiotics who is not eating properly** |
| mechanism of DIC | **thrombohemorrhagic disorder**— * intravascular clotting causes the consumption of clotting factors, * secondary fibrinolysis |
| causes of DIC | • **malignancy**— * leukemia, * prostate cancer, * lung cancer, • *septicemia*—particularly gram-negatives like *E. coli,* • *surgery/trauma,* • *obstetric problems*—e.g., * amniotic fluid embolism, * retained dead fetus, • *HTR,* • *snake envenomation* |

### Table 2–13. COAGULATION, FIBRINOLYTIC, THROMBOEMBOLIC DISORDERS OF SURGICAL IMPORTANCE *Continued*

| Most Common... | Answer and Explanation |
|---|---|
| factors consumed in DIC | • **fibrinogen,** • **II,** • **V,** • **VIII,** • **platelets,** • **AT III**—it is used up in neutralizing serine proteases |
| S/S of acute DIC | • **oozing of blood from wounds/venipuncture sites,** • *hypovolemic shock*— * the complement system is activated by plasmin with release of anaphylatoxins, * blood loss, • *widespread ecchymoses*—due to platelet dysfunction from FDPs and thrombocytopenia, • *widespread organ dysfunction*—e.g., * renal failure, * intracranial hemorrhage [**Note:** in chronic DIC, thrombosis is more common than bleeding.] |
| lab findings in DIC | • **positive D-dimers/FDPs**— * D-Dimers are the best all-around screen, * see Table 2–2, • *thrombocytopenia*—sensitivity of 90%, • *prolonged PT*—sensitivity of 90%, • *prolonged PTT,* • *low fibrinogen*— * sensitivity of 70%, * serial assays show a progressive drop in concentration, • *normocytic anemia,* • *schistocytes,* • *low AT III,* • *increased fibrinopeptide A*—cleavage product of fibrinogen, • *increased PF_4*—indicates platelet activation |
| Rx of DIC | • **Rx the underlying cause of the DIC,** • *blood components*— * temporary solution because they are consumed as well, * packed RBCs, * FFP, * platelet concentrates, * cryoprecipitate, • *heparin*—targets the thrombosis part of the syndrome by inactivating thrombin: this reduces platelet/coagulation factor consumption |
| mechanisms of coagulation deficiency in liver disease | • **multiple factor deficiencies**— * decreased production, * malabsorption of vitamin K due to bile salt deficiency, * factor VII deficiency: first factor to decrease in liver disease, • *increased fibrinolysis*—less clearing of plasminogen activator owing to decreased production of $\alpha_2$-antiplasmin, • *dysfibrinogenemia*—dysfunctional fibrinogen is synthesized, • *platelet dysfunction*—due to increased FDPs, which interfere with platelet aggregation, • *thrombocytopenia*—decreased BM production |

*Table continued on following page*

### Table 2–13. COAGULATION, FIBRINOLYTIC, THROMBOEMBOLIC DISORDERS OF SURGICAL IMPORTANCE *Continued*

| Most Common... | Answer and Explanation |
|---|---|
| causes of multiple factor deficiencies | • **severe liver disease**, • *DIC*, • *vitamin K deficiency*, • *anticoagulation with heparin/warfarin* |
| cause of secondary fibrinolysis | **DIC**—activation of factor XII leads to plasminogen activation and plasmin release |
| causes of primary fibrinolysis | • **radical prostatectomy**—release of urokinase from damaged tissue, • *metastatic prostate cancer*, • *open heart surgery* [**Note:** serious bleeding is likely to occur once $\alpha_2$-plasmin inhibitor is used up in neutralizing excess plasmin.] |
| lab findings in primary fibrinolysis | • **increased FDPs**, • *absent D-dimers*—recall that D-dimers are present only if a fibrin clot has been degraded, • *low fibrinogen*, • *prolonged PTT/PT*— * FDPs interfere with clotting, * coagulation factors are degraded by plasmin, • *normal platelet count* |
| lab findings that differentiate primary from secondary fibrinolysis | • **D-dimer assay**—absent in primary and increased in secondary fibrinolysis, • *platelet count*—normal in primary and low in secondary fibrinolysis |
| Rx of primary fibrinolysis | • **ε-aminocaproic acid (EACA)**, • *aprotinin* |
| MOA of EACA | **binds to plasminogen and plasmin**—prevents plasmin from degrading fibrinogen and other clotting factors |
| MOA of aprotinin | **inhibits plasmin and kallikrein** |
| MOA of heparin | **enhances AT III activity**— * heparin complexes with AT III and is then reused, * AT III primarily inactivates thrombin, Xa, IXa, * synthesized in the liver |
| blood components in an arterial thrombus | **platelets held together by fibrin strands**—platelet thrombi develop in areas of rapid arterial blood flow where there is endothelial damage (e.g., components in cigarette smoke) or turbulence (e.g., **atherosclerotic plaque**, branching points in arteries) |

### Table 2–13. COAGULATION, FIBRINOLYTIC, THROMBOEMBOLIC DISORDERS OF SURGICAL IMPORTANCE *Continued*

| Most Common... | Answer and Explanation |
|---|---|
| blood components in a venous thrombus | • **coagulation factors**— * fibrinogen, * V, * VIII, * II, • *fibrin,* • *platelets,* • *entrapped RBCs* [**Note:** venous clots develop in areas of stasis (e.g., venous system) or in hypercoagulable states (e.g., AT III deficiency).] |
| risk factors for venous thrombosis | • **stasis**—e.g., **postoperative state,** • *CHF*— decreased venous return to the heart, • *obesity,* • *oral contraceptives*—decreased AT III, • *smoking,* • *orthopedic surgery*—particularly hip surgery, • *malignancy,* • *sepsis,* • *varicose veins* |
| risk factors for arterial thrombosis | • **age**— * men >45 yrs old, * women >55 yrs old, • *LDL >160 mg/dL,* • *HDL <35 mg/dL,* • *DM,* • *HTN,* • *smoking,* • *family Hx of premature CAD/stroke,* • *high plasma homocysteine levels*— * homocysteine damages vessel endothelium, * folate deficiency is the MCC, • *oral contraceptives,* • *malignancy,* • *PRV* |
| hereditary causes of a hypercoagulable state | • **factor V Leiden mutation**— * AD trait, * facytor V Leiden is resistant to degradation by activated protein C, • *protein C deficiency*—AD trait, • *protein S deficiency*—AD trait, • *AT III deficiency*—AD trait |
| clues suggesting a hereditary hypercoagulable state | • **recurrent DVTs with/without PE,** • *family Hx of above,* • *DVTs/PE at early age,* • *unusual sites for venous thrombosis*—e.g., * axilla, * dural sinuses |
| clinical findings in factor V Leiden mutation | **recurrent venous thrombosis**— * heterozygotes have a 30-fold risk for DVTs, * homozygotes have an 80-fold risk for DVTs |
| Rx of factor V Leiden mutation | **heparin/warfarin** |
| causes of protein C deficiency | • **acquired**— * warfarin Rx: protein C is a vitamin K–dependent factor, * DIC, * L-asparaginase, * liver disease, * malignancy, • *hereditary*— * homozygotes usually die in infancy of neonatal purpura fulminans, * S/S in heterozygotes occur in mid to late teens |

*Table continued on following page*

Table 2–13. COAGULATION, FIBRINOLYTIC,
THROMBOEMBOLIC DISORDERS OF
SURGICAL IMPORTANCE *Continued*

| Most Common... | Answer and Explanation |
|---|---|
| clinical/lab findings in protein C deficiency | • **recurrent DVTs**— * ~65%, • *PE*— ~40%, • *hemorrhagic skin necrosis*—see below, • *recurrent superficial thrombophlebitis,* • *lab findings*— * low protein C by functional/immunologic tests, * normal BT, * normal PTT/PT |
| cause of hemorrhagic skin necrosis in a patient placed on warfarin | **heterozygote carrier with protein C deficiency**— * carriers have 30–60% protein C, * warfarin creates a "homozygous" state: ♦ the existing protein C that has been γ-carboxylated becomes nonfunctional in 6–8 hrs after warfarin has been given, ♦ this predisposes patients to vessel thrombosis before they are fully anticoagulated,* thrombosis occurs primarily in cutaneous vessels, * the same disorder may occur with protein S deficiency |
| Rx of DVTs due to protein C deficiency | **heparin followed by warfarin**— * first, fully anticoagulate the patient with heparin before starting warfarin, * warfarin is then given at lower doses than normal to prevent skin necrosis, * patients must be on warfarin for life |
| clinical/lab findings in protein S deficiency | **similar to findings in protein C deficiency** |
| causes of AT III deficiency | • **acquired**— * oral contraceptives, * DIC, * severe liver disease, * heparin Rx, * *hereditary* |
| clinical findings in AT III deficiency | • **recurrent DVTs/PE,** • *mesenteric artery/vein thrombosis,* • *no prolongation of PTT at standard doses of heparin*—this is often the first clue for Dx, • *lab findings*—low AT III levels for both immunologic/functional assays |
| Rx of AT III deficiency | • **acute Rx**— * **FFP/cryoprecipitate** or * AT III concentrate + heparin, * much higher doses must be given than normal, * pregnant women with AT III deficiency should be on low-dose heparin, • *warfarin*—patients are sent home on warfarin |

## Table 2–13. COAGULATION, FIBRINOLYTIC, THROMBOEMBOLIC DISORDERS OF SURGICAL IMPORTANCE *Continued*

| Most Common... | Answer and Explanation |
|---|---|
| renal disease with an increased risk of venous thrombosis | **nephrotic syndrome**—patients lose AT III, protein C/S in urine |
| site of origin of emboli to the lungs | **femoral veins**—femoral/iliac vein thrombosis is usually the result of propagation from a thrombosis in the deep veins of the lower leg |
| site of origin of emboli into the arterial system | **clots/vegetations dislodged from the left side of the heart**—e.g., * mural thrombus, * vegetations on the aortic or mitral valve |
| arrhythmia predisposing to arterial embolization | **atrial fibrillation** |
| cause of paradoxical embolization | **thromboembolism from the venous system through a patent foramen ovale into the systemic circulation** |
| cause of phlebothrombosis | **stasis of blood flow**— * phlebothrombosis is thrombosis of a vein without inflammation, * causes include: ♦ postpartum, ♦ postop, particularly after hip/pelvic surgery |
| location for phlebothrombosis | **deep veins of the calf**— * most clots resolve spontaneously, * ~20% propagate into the proximal femoral vessels, * ~50% of DVTs involving the proximal vessels (femoral, popliteal, iliac veins) embolize to the lungs |
| tests used to document DVTs in lower legs | • **duplex ultrasonography**—modification of Doppler ultrasound, • *impedance plethysmography,* • *invasive venography*—gold standard [**Note:** both duplex US and impedance plethysmography detect DVTs in the femoral veins. Invasive venography is more sensitive in locating DVTs in deep veins of the calf.] |
| nonpharmacologic technique used in preventing DVTs in the hospital | • **early ambulation,** • *graded stockings*—method of choice in low-risk elective surgery, • *intermittent pneumatic compression*—method of choice in GU/neurosurgery |

*Table continued on following page*

Table 2–13. COAGULATION, FIBRINOLYTIC,
THROMBOEMBOLIC DISORDERS OF
SURGICAL IMPORTANCE *Continued*

| Most Common... | Answer and Explanation |
|---|---|
| drug prevention for surgical patients at risk for DVTs in the hospital | • **low-dose heparin**— * low doses of heparin are recommended in low to moderate risk patients scheduled for major surgery: 5000 units SC of low-dose heparin (LDH) started 2 hrs before surgery and continued q12h postop, * in high-risk surgical patients (not including hip/knee replacement): LDH q8h + intermittent pneumatic compression, • *warfarin*—patients undergoing total hip/knee surgery are started on warfarin from preop day 1 to the time of ambulation (high risk of postop bleeding) [**Note:** patient risk factors—>40 yrs old, previous DVTs, malignancy, CHF, obesity. Surgery risk factors include hip/knee replacement, prostate surgery, and GU/neurosurgery.] |
| initial anticoagulant used in the Rx of proximal DVTs | **intravenous heparin**— * initial dose is usually between 5000–10,000 units, with a PTT between 50 and 80 sec, * warfarin is started on day 1 with heparin and continued for ~3 days, * heparin is discontinued when the INR for warfarin Rx is therapeutic (2.0–3.0) for ~48 hrs, * it requires ~3–5 days before a patient on warfarin is fully anticoagulated: ♦ time that is necessary for all the previously γ-carboxylated vitamin K–dependent factors to be eliminated, ♦ factor VII half-life is the shortest and factor II half-life is the longest |
| cancer associated with migratory superficial thrombophlebitis | **pancreatic carcinoma**—this is called Trousseau's sign |
| cause of fat embolization | **fractures of long bones and/or pelvis**—microglobules of fat enter the circulation from the disrupted marrow and the fat surrounding fractures |
| clinical findings in fat embolism | • **S/S**— * occur within 3 days, * mental status alterations, * dyspnea, * petechiae limited to the upper half of the torso, • **lab findings**— * hypoxemia < 60 mmHg, * thrombocytopenia < 15,000 cells/μL: platelets adhere to fat globules, * high serum lipase, * lipiduria: uncommon |

## Table 2–13. COAGULATION, FIBRINOLYTIC, THROMBOEMBOLIC DISORDERS OF SURGICAL IMPORTANCE *Continued*

| Most Common... | Answer and Explanation |
|---|---|
| Rx of fat embolism | • **$O_2$ delivered with PEEP**, • **corticosteroids** [**Note:** the mortality is ~10%.] |
| mechanism of heparin clearance from the blood | **macrophage uptake in liver with subsequent degradation into inactive products that are excreted in the urine**— * the half-life of heparin is ~90 min, * liver/renal disease alters its metabolism, * heparin does not cross placenta: anticoagulant of choice in pregnancy |
| complications of heparin therapy | • **bleeding**—5–10%, • *hypersensitivity reactions*— * chills, * fever, * urticaria,* shock, • *thrombocytopenia*— * see Table 2–12, * 10% develop antiplatelet antibodies, • *osteoporosis*—may occur if the patient is on heparin for > 2 mos, • *paradoxical venous/arterial thrombosis*— * due to platelet release of $PF_4$ (heparin neutralizing agent) and serotonin, which cause platelet aggregation, * arterial thrombosis of the aorta and iliac artery commonly occur, • *skin necrosis* |
| cause of heparin resistance | • **low AT III levels**— * **acquired**, * hereditary, • *high levels of factor VIII*, • *high levels of heparin-binding proteins*—e.g., $PF_4$ |
| Rx of significant bleeding secondary to heparin | **protamine sulfate** |
| surgical uses of heparin | • **anticoagulation in DVT**, • *pulmonary embolus*, • *post-thrombolytic therapy*, • *Rx of DIC*, • *prevention of DVTs prior to orthopedic procedures* |
| method of monitoring heparin therapy | **PTT**—the PTT should be kept between 1.5 and 2.5 times normal |
| MOA of low molecular weight (fractionated) heparin | **primarily inactivates factor Xa**— * LMW heparin has a longer half-life than unfragmented heparin, * is more predictable acting, * does not require lab monitoring: does not prolong the PTT, * has less risk for heparin-induced thrombocytopenia |
| MOA of warfarin | **inhibits epoxide reductase** |

*Table continued on following page*

Table 2–13. COAGULATION, FIBRINOLYTIC,
THROMBOEMBOLIC DISORDERS OF
SURGICAL IMPORTANCE *Continued*

| Most Common... | Answer and Explanation |
| --- | --- |
| complications of warfarin Rx | • **bleeding**— * 10–20%, * INR >5 is at increased risk for patient bleeding, • *drug interactions*—see below, • *hemorrhagic skin necrosis*—see above, • *urticaria,* • *alopecia,* • *teratogenic*— * nasal hypoplasia, * CNS abnormalities, * contraindicated in the first trimester |
| conditions potentiating warfarin activity (need less warfarin, it prolongs the PT) | • **drugs producing vitamin K deficiency**—broad-spectrum antibiotics kill the colonic bacteria that synthesize vitamin K, • **drug displacing plasma-bound warfarin**—phenylbutazone, • **competitive inhibition for hepatic degradation**—phenytoin, • **enhanced affinity for hepatic receptor sites**— * high-dose salicylates, * quinidine, • **drugs inhibiting platelet function**—aspirin, • *liver disease,* • *CHF,* • **vitamin E toxicity**—inhibits liver synthesis of vitamin K–dependent factors |
| conditions antagonizing warfarin activity (need more warfarin, lowers PT) | • **drugs inducing the hepatic cytochrome system**— * alcohol, * barbiturates, * rifampin, * griseofulvin, • **diuretics**—thiazides, • **decrease GI absorption**—cholestyramine, • **oral contraceptives,** • **administration of vitamin K** |
| surgical uses of warfarin | • Rx/prophylaxis for DVT/PE, • *prevention of thrombi on mechanical valves,* • *prevention/Rx of thrombi in hereditary thrombotic conditions*— * AT III deficiency, * protein C/S deficiency |
| method of monitoring warfarin Rx | INR— * see Table 2–2, * the INR is usually kept between 2 and 3, * kept at a higher value for mechanical valves: 2.5–3.5 |
| reason why heparin/warfarin are started simultaneously | **heparin immediately anticoagulates the patient, whereas warfarin requires 3–5 days for full anticoagulation owing to the different half-lives of vitamin K–dependent factors that have already been $\gamma$-carboxylated**— * protein C and factor VII have the shortest half-lives: 4–6 hrs, * factor II has the longest half-life: 72 hrs |

**Table 2–13. COAGULATION, FIBRINOLYTIC,
THROMBOEMBOLIC DISORDERS OF
SURGICAL IMPORTANCE** *Continued*

| Most Common... | Answer and Explanation |
|---|---|
| Rx of life-threatening hemorrhage in a patient on warfarin | **infusion of fresh-frozen plasma (FFP)**— * FFP contains functional coagulation factors, * oral or intramuscular vitamin K is recommended for less serious bleeds |
| coagulation lab findings in patients on warfarin or heparin | • **prolonged PTT/PT,** • **normal platelet count,** • **normal BT** [Note: PT has most of the vitamin K–dependent factors (II, VII, X, not IX), hence it provides a better monitor for warfarin therapy than the PTT. PTT has most of the serine proteases inhibited by AT III (XII, XI, IX, X, II, thrombin), hence it provides a better monitor for heparin than warfarin.] |
| platelet inhibitors | • **low-dose aspirin**— * irreversibly blocks platelet cyclooxygenase, • **ticlopidine**—this is used if patients are allergic to aspirin, • *dipyridamole* |
| MOA of ticlopidine | **alters the platelet membrane**— * this prevents platelet aggregation, * may cause neutropenia |
| MOA of dipyridamole | **inhibits platelet adhesion to thrombogenic surfaces**—it also inhibits thromboxane synthase |
| fibrinolytic agents used in surgery | • **tPA,** • *streptokinase* |
| uses of fibrinolytic therapy in surgery | • **iliofemoral deep venous thrombosis,** • **axillary vein thrombosis,** • **SVC thrombosis,** • **large PA embolus in unstable patient,** • **re-establish patency in vascular graft occlusions,** • **re-establish patency of acute thrombosis of SMA and peripheral arteries** |

*Table continued on following page*

### Table 2–13. COAGULATION, FIBRINOLYTIC, THROMBOEMBOLIC DISORDERS OF SURGICAL IMPORTANCE *Continued*

**Question:** Which of the following tests differentiate classic von Willebrand's disease from hemophilia A? **SELECT 3**
- (A) Platelet count
- (B) PTT
- (C) Bleeding time
- (D) VIII:RCo
- (E) VIII:Ag
- (F) VIII:C
- (G) PT

**Answers: (C), (D), (E):** In both hemophilia A and VWD, the platelet count is normal, PTT is prolonged, VIII:C is prolonged, and the PT is normal **(choices A, B, F, G are incorrect)**. Lab abnormalities unique to VWD include a prolonged bleeding time **(choice C is correct)**, low VIII:RCo **(choice D is correct)**, and low VIII:Ag **(choice E is correct)**.

ACA = anticardiolipin antibody, AD = autosomal dominant, AMI = acute myocardial infarction, APL = antiphospholipid, AT III = antithrombin III, BM = bone marrow, BT = bleeding time, CAD = coronary artery disease, CHF = congestive heart failure, DIC = disseminated intravascular coagulation, DM = diabetes mellitus, DVT = deep venous thrombosis, EACA = $\epsilon$-aminocaproic acid, FDPs = fibrin(ogen) degradation products, FFP = fresh-frozen plasma, FP = false-positive, HBV = hepatitis B virus, HCV = hepatitis C virus, HDL = high-density lipoprotein, HIV = human immunodeficiency virus, HMW = high molecular weight, HTN = hypertension, HTR = hemolytic transfusion reaction, INR = International Normalized Ratio, LA = lupus anticoagulant, LDH = low-dose heparin, LDL = low-density lipoprotein, LMW = low molecular weight, MCC = most common cause, MOA = mechanism of action, PA = pulmonary artery, PE = pulmonary embolus, PEEP = positive end-expiratory pressure, $PF_3$ = platelet factor III, $PF_4$ = platelet factor 4, PRV = polycythemia rubra vera, PT = prothrombin time, PTT = partial thromboplastin time, RPR = rapid plasma reagin, SLE = systemic lupus erythematosus, SMA = superior mesenteric artery, S/S = signs/symptoms, SVC = superior vena cava, SXR = sex-linked recessive, tPA = tissue plasminogen activator, US = ultrasonography, VIII:Ag = antigenic determinant of VIII:C, VIII:C = factor VIII coagulant, VIII:vWF = von Willebrand factor, VIII:RCo = von Willebrand factor activity with ristocetin, VDRL = Venereal Disease Research Laboratory, VWD = von Willebrand's disease.

## Table 2–14. IMMUNOHEMATOLOGY

| Most Common... | Answer and Explanation |
|---|---|
| ABO blood group | **blood group O**—O RBCs have no A or B antigens |
| universal recipient | **blood group AB**—AB patients have no isohemagglutinins (anti-A or anti-B) in their plasma to attack A or B antigens on other RBCs |
| blood group that can be transfused only with blood group O | **blood group O**—O patients have anti-A-IgM, anti-B-IgM, and anti-A,B-IgG, hence they can receive only RBCs that are negative for A and B antigens |
| universal donor | **blood group O**—anti-A-IgM from B patients and anti-B-IgM from A patients cannot destroy O RBCs since they lack A and B antigens: ♦ transfusion of blood group O–packed RBCs confers immunity to destruction, ♦ transfusion of O whole blood would produce mild hemolysis owing to the presence of anti-A IgM, anti-B IgM, and anti A,B-IgG in O plasma |
| blood groups with a high incidence of duodenal ulcer and gastric cancer | **blood group O and blood group A, respectively** |
| Rh antigen | **D antigen**— * 85% of people are positive for D antigen: patients are designated Rh-positive, * other Rh antigens include: ♦ C, ♦ c, ♦ E, ♦ e (no d antigen) |
| clinically significant antibody in clinical medicine | **anti-D antibodies**— * strong IgG antibodies, * they produce a brisk hemolytic anemia when attached to D-positive RBCs |
| cold (IgM) antibodies of clinical significance | • **anti-I**—hemolytic anemia in *Mycoplasma pneumoniae* infections, • **anti-i**—hemolytic anemia in infectious mononucleosis |
| naturally occurring antibody | **anti-Lewis-IgM antibodies**— * weak antibodies: they do not produce hemolytic anemia, * have no clinical significance |

*Table continued on following page*

## Table 2–14. IMMUNOHEMATOLOGY *Continued*

| Most Common... | Answer and Explanation |
|---|---|
| tests performed on donor blood in the blood bank | • **ABO group**, • **Rh**—presence or absence of D antigen: not the other Rh antigens, • **ABS**—indirect Coombs', looking for antibodies, • **RPR or VDRL**, • **HBsAg**, • **anti-HCV antibodies**, • **anti-HIV-1/HIV-2 antibodies**, • **anti-HTLV I/II antibodies** |
| antibody in the United States | **anti-CMV antibodies** |
| infection transmitted by blood transfusion | **CMV**— * CMV is present in donor lymphocytes, * CMV-negative blood must be transfused into neonates, immunocompromised patients, and those with T cell immunodeficiency states (e.g., AIDS) [**Note:** irradiation of the blood kills lymphocytes and any CMV within lymphocytes.] |
| infection rates post-transfusion for HBV, HCV, HTLV I/II, and HIV | • **HBV**—*1:200,000 per unit*, • **HCV**—*1:3300 per unit*, • **HTLV I/II**—*1:200,000 per unit*, • **HIV**—*1:676,000 per unit* |
| infection rate post-needle stick from blood drawn from an HIV-positive patient | **1:300** |
| Rx for above person with needle stick | • **HIV testing**—periodically up to 6 mos, • **drugs**—triple therapy for 6 mos: AZT + another reverse transcriptase inhibitor + protease inhibitor |
| cause of post-transfusion hepatitis | **HCV**—90% of all cases of post-transfusion hepatitis |
| preservative used in the blood bank | **CPDA1**—represents * **c**itrate: anticoagulant that binds calcium, * **p**hosphate: ♦ maintain 2,3 BPG level, ♦ 100% levels of 2,3 BPG during the first week, * **d**extrose: fuel for RBCs, * **a**denine: substrate for ATP, * shelf life of CPDA1 blood is ~35 days |
| pretransfusion tests performed on a patient | • **ABO**, • **Rh**, • **ABS**—looking for atypical antibodies, • **direct Coomb's**—looking for antibodies attached to the patient's RBCs, • **major cross-match**— * patient serum is reacted against donor RBCs, * the goal of a major cross-match is not having antibodies that will attack donor RBC antigens |

**Table 2–14. IMMUNOHEMATOLOGY** *Continued*

| Most Common... | Answer and Explanation |
|---|---|
| components of a type and screen | **all the above standard tests except the major cross-match with the donor unit**—if the patient's ABS is negative, the chance of having an incompatible cross-match with a donor unit is negligible, * type/screen is used to conserve blood and decrease patient cost |
| method of preventing GVH and CMV infection in the recipient of a blood transfusion | **irradiation of the unit**— * radiation kills donor lymphocytes that could cause GVH and also kills lymphocytes containing CMV, * using leukocyte-depleting filters is a less expensive way of eliminating WBCs that could transmit CMV or produce GVH |
| risks when transfusing blood | • **development of antibodies against foreign antigens,** • *transmitting infection*—e.g., * CMV, * HBV, * HCV, * HIV, * HTLV I/II, * *Yersinia enterocolitica,* • *transfusion reactions*—see below, • *volume overload,* • *noncardiogenic pulmonary edema*—see below, • *GVH reaction* |
| target tissues involved in the acute GVH reaction | • **skin**— * maculopapular rash, * involves the trunk, palms, soles, • *bile duct epithelium*—epithelial cell necrosis of small bile ducts leads to jaundice and an elevated ALP, • *GI tract*—mucosal ulceration with bloody diarrhea |
| bacterial contaminant in packed RBCs | *Yersinia enterocolitica* |
| component with the highest rate of infection | **platelet concentrates**—usually stored at room temperature |
| type of RBC transfusion that eliminates all risks | **autologous transfusion**—refers to the process of collecting, storing, and reinfusing the patient's own blood |
| method of transfusing RBCs | **unit is infused with a Y-shaped catheter, the other arm of which contains 0.9% normal saline (cannot use any other mixing solution) and a macroaggregate filter, which removes clumps of RBCs and debris** [Note: blood should be infused within 4 hrs.] |

*Table continued on following page*

**Table 2–14. IMMUNOHEMATOLOGY** *Continued*

| Most Common... | Answer and Explanation |
|---|---|
| indication for washed RBCs | • **patient with a previous febrile reaction,** • *patient with IgA deficiency* [**Note:** leukocyte-depleting filters are a less expensive way of removing leukocytes that are responsible for febrile reactions (see below).] |
| problem encountered when transfusing IgA-deficient patients | **anaphylactic reactions**— * 1:100,000 risk, * shock may occur if IgA-deficient patients with anti-IgA antibodies are infused plasma products containing IgA |
| S/S of transfusion anaphylaxis | • **bronchospasm**—wheezing, • **urticaria,** • **angioedema,** • **hypotension** |
| Rx of transfusion anaphylaxis | • **maintain the airway,** • *1:1000 subcutaneous aqueous epinephrine,* • *corticosteroids*—for resistant cases |
| indication for transfusing whole blood | **patients who have lost massive amounts of whole blood** |
| indication for transfusing packed RBCs | **symptomatic anemia that cannot be adequately corrected by medical Rx**— * 1 unit of packed RBCs raises the Hgb by 1 g/dL and Hct by 3% in a 70-kg patient, * in general, patients with an Hgb <7 g/dL should be transfused, since the $O_2$-carrying capacity of blood is significantly compromised at this level of Hgb |
| indications for transfusing platelet concentrates | • **platelet count < 20,000 cells/μL,** • **platelet count < 50,000 cells/μL with clinical evidence of bleeding, or candidate for surgery or invasive procedure**—patients with counts > 50,000 cells/μL rarely require platelets except for major surgery where the count should be > 100,000 cells/μL, • **excessive blood transfusions**—>10 units packed RBCs usually requires a platelet count to see whether platelets are necessary, • **functional platelet defect with clinically significant bleeding**—e.g., patient on aspirin [**Note:** in general, 1 unit of platelets raises the platelet count by 5000 cells/μL.] |
| indication for transfusing granulocytes | • **patients with severe sepsis,** • **WBC count < 500 cells/μL that has not responded appropriately to antibiotics** |

### Table 2–14. IMMUNOHEMATOLOGY *Continued*

| Most Common... | Answer and Explanation |
|---|---|
| indication for infusion of FFP | **multiple coagulation deficiencies**— * examples include: ♦ cirrhosis, ♦ DIC, ♦ patient over-anticoagulated with warfarin, * FFP should never be used as a volume expander |
| blood component with the highest concentration of VIII–vWF multimers | **cryoprecipitate** |
| indication for infusion of cryoprecipitate | • **DIC,** • *afibrinogenemia* [**Note:** desmopressin has replaced cryoprecipitate for the Rx of mild to moderate VWD and hemophilia A owing to the risk of transmitting infection with the cryoprecipitate.] |
| indication for ISG | • **prevention of HAV in a patient exposed to an active HAV infection**—should be given within 10 days of exposure, • *B cell immunodeficiencies*—e.g., * Bruton's agammaglobulinemia, * CLL, • *temporary prevention of hemolysis or thrombocytopenia in AIHA and autoimmune thrombocytopenia*—IgG blocks macrophage Fc receptors for IgG, hence preventing macrophage removal of RBCs or platelets sensitized by IgG |
| transfusion reaction | **mild allergic reactions**— * 1:100 chance of a reaction, * patient has IgE antibodies against plasma proteins: type I hypersensitivity reaction, * S/S range from urticaria to fever and an anaphylactic reaction, * Rx with antihistamines |
| mechanism of a febrile reaction | **patient anti-HLA antibodies are directed against donor leukocyte HLA antigens**— * this is a type II hypersensitivity reaction, * patients must be exposed to human blood products to develop anti-HLA antibodies, * leukocyte-depletion filters are excellent in removing leukocytes and preventing these reactions, * Rx with antipyretics |
| types of HTRs | • **intravascular,** • *extravascular* [**Note:** the risk of an HTR per unit of blood is 1:6000.] |

*Table continued on following page*

**Table 2–14. IMMUNOHEMATOLOGY** *Continued*

| Most Common... | Answer and Explanation |
| --- | --- |
| mechanism of intravascular HTR | **ABO mismatch between the recipient and the donor**— * e.g., if a blood group A patient receives B blood, anti-B-IgM antibodies in the recipient will attach to donor B cells (type II hypersensitivity), activate complement, and cause complement destruction of the RBCs, * this is most often due to human error (~50%): the person hanging the blood probably did not check the number of the patient's blood bank bracelet and compare it to the number on the unit of blood |
| mechanism of extravascular HTR | **presence of previously undetected antibodies in the recipient directed against a donor antigen**— * RBCs are removed extravascularly by macrophages: type II hypersensitivity reaction, * common antibodies include: ♦ Kell, ♦ Duffy, ♦ Kidd antibodies |
| mechanism of delayed HTR | **extravascular hemolysis**— * may occur 1–4 wks after transfusion: ♦ titers of antibodies in the patient may have been below the sensitivity of an ABS or major cross-match, ♦ when the patient is transfused, re-exposure of the antigen to the patient's memory B cells causes renewed synthesis of antibody, which may take a few hours to a few weeks to develop, * common antibodies include: ♦ Kidd, ♦ Rh, * this reaction is more common in women: sensitized from previous pregnancies |
| S/S of an HTR | • **pain at infusion site or in the back, abdomen, or chest,** • **fever,** • **drop in Hgb/Hct,** • **hypotension,** • **oliguria,** • **jaundice**—UCB type, • **bleeding**—secondary to DIC |
| lab tests and findings in HTRs | **see Table 2–2** |
| Rx of HTRs | • **immediate termination of transfusion**—keep the IV open with 0.9% NaCl, • *administer a loop diuretic to keep urine flowing*—some use mannitol, • *alkalinize the urine*—give patient sodium bicarbonate [**Note:** the fatality rate of an HTR per unit is 1:100,000.] |

## Table 2–14. IMMUNOHEMATOLOGY *Continued*

| Most Common... | Answer and Explanation |
|---|---|
| complications of massive transfusions | • **coagulopathies**—due to coagulation and platelet deficiencies, • *hypothermia*— * precipitates arrhythmias, * use a blood warmer to prevent hypothermia, • *citrate toxicity*— * hypocalcemia may occur, * IV calcium is recommended after transfusion of 10 units, • *electrolyte abnormalities*— * hyperkalemia may occur from leakage of $K^+$ from old transfused RBCs, * metabolic acidosis [**Note:** a massive transfusion of RBCs is one that is greater in volume than the patient's blood volume in < 24 hrs.] |
| cause of transfusion-associated ARDS | **possibly anti-HLA antibodies against donor WBCs (granulocytes and/or lymphocytes)**—risk per unit is 1:10,000 |
| S/S of post-transfusion ARDS | • **occurs within** ~6 hrs, • **fever**, • **dyspnea**, • **pulmonary infiltrates**— * noncardiogenic pulmonary edema, * PCWP < 18 mm Hg, which R/O circulatory overload or LHF |
| Rx of post-transfusion ARDS | • $O_2$, • **PEEP**, • **furosemide**, • **dopamine** [**Note:** recovery usually occurs within 24–48 hrs.] |

**Question:** A 22-yr-old woman develops fever, chills, jaundice, and fatigue 1 week after delivering a baby boy. She received 2 units of packed RBCs postdelivery owing to uterine atony. Her ABS prior to transfusion was negative, and the major cross-match was compatible for both units. Laboratory tests reveal a drop in hemoglobin and a positive direct and indirect Coombs' test. Which of the following is the most likely diagnosis? **SELECT 1**
    (A) Febrile reaction
    (B) Sepsis
    (C) Post-transfusion hepatitis
    (D) ABO mismatch from previous transfusion
    (E) Delayed hemolytic transfusion reaction

**Answer: (E):** The patient has a classic delayed HTR (**choice E is correct**). A drop in Hgb, jaundice, and a positive direct and indirect (antibody screen) Coombs' test would not be expected in a febrile reaction, sepsis, or post-transfusion hepatitis (**choices A, B, C are incorrect**). An ABO mismatch is unlikely, since the reaction occurs immediately owing to complement activation by IgM antibodies (**choice D is incorrect**).

*Table continued on following page*

ABO = blood groups A, B, and O; ABS = antibody screen, AIHA = autoimmune hemolytic anemia, ALP = alkaline phosphatase, ARDS = adult respiratory distress syndrome, ATP = adenosine triphosphate, BPG = bisphosphoglycerate, CLL = chronic lymphocytic leukemia, CMV = cytomegalovirus, CPDA = citrate/phosphate/dextrose/adenine, DIC = disseminated intravascular coagulation, FFP = fresh-frozen plasma, GVH = graft versus host, HAV = hepatitis A virus, HBsAg = hepatitis B surface antigen, HBV = hepatitis B, Hct = hematocrit, HCV = hepatitis C, HDN = hemolytic disease of the newborn, Hgb = hemoglobin, HIV = human immunodeficiency virus, HLA = human leukocyte antigen, HTLV = human T cell lymphotropic virus, HTR = hemolytic transfusion reaction, ISG = immune serum globulin, LHF = left heart failure, PCWP = pulmonary capillary wedge pressure, PEEP = positive end-expiratory pressure, RhIG = Rh immune globulin, RPR = rapid plasma reagin, S/S = signs/symptoms, UCB = unconjugated bilirubin, VDRL = Venereal Disease Research Laboratory, VWD = von Willebrand's disease.

# CHAPTER 3

# ACUTE RESPIRATORY FAILURE, SHOCK, MECHANICAL VENTILATION, SWAN-GANZ CATHETERS

## CONTENTS

### Table 3–1. ACUTE RESPIRATORY FAILURE, MECHANICAL VENTILATION, ARDS

| Most Common... | Answer and Explanation |
|---|---|
| types of ARF | • **hypoxic ARF** (HARF)— * $PaO_2$ is <60 mmHg that is not corrected after breathing 50% $O_2$, * $PaCO_2$ is normal or <33 mmHg, * tissue hypoxia refers to inadequate oxygenation of tissue, * low $PaO_2$ is called hypoxemia, • *hypercapnic-hypoxic ARF (HHARF)*— * $PaO_2$ is <60 mmHg, * $PaCO_2$ is >45 mmHg, * pH is <7.35—respiratory acidosis |
| causes of ARF | • **cardiogenic pulmonary edema,** • *cardiopulmonary arrest,* • *pneumonia,* • *ARDS,* • *sepsis* |
| pathophysiologic mechanisms of HARF | • **intrapulmonary shunting (ventilation defect)**— * intrapulmonary shunting is due to massive atelectasis, * e.g., ARDS, • *diffusion abnormality*— * problem with gas exchange at alveolar/capillary interface, * e.g., pulmonary edema, • *V/Q mismatch (perfusion defect)*— * increased alveolar dead space, e.g., * PE |
| cause of HARF | **ARDS**—$PaCO_2$ eventually increases |
| pathophysiologic mechanisms of HHARF | • **respiratory center depression**—e.g., * primary intracranial disease, * drug overdose, • *upper airway obstruction*—e.g., angioedema, • *chest bellows disease*—e.g., * flail chest, * diaphragm paralysis, • *metabolic derangements*—e.g., * sepsis, * hypokalemia, * hypophosphatemia, * hypomagnesemia |

*Table continued on following page*

**125**

### Table 3-1. ACUTE RESPIRATORY FAILURE, MECHANICAL VENTILATION, ARDS *Continued*

| Most Common... | Answer and Explanation |
|---|---|
| clinical findings in HARF | • **dyspnea,** • *tachypnea*—>35 breaths/minute, • *cyanosis,* • *tachycardia,* • *restlessness,* • *hypotension/hypertension,* • *mental status alterations,* • *lactic acidosis* |
| clinical findings in HHARF | • **dyspnea,** • *tachypnea*—<30 breaths/min, • *headache*—due to cerebral edema from vasodilation secondary to respiratory acidosis, • *papilledema*—intracerebral HTN, • *cyanosis,* • *conjunctival hyperemia,* • *lethargy/coma,* • *asterixis*—flapping tremor |
| S/S of partial versus complete upper airway obstruction | • **partial**— * patient can cough, talk, breathe, * let patient dislodge foreign body with forceful coughing, • **complete**— * cannot cough, talk, or breathe, * initiate the Heimlich maneuver, * cardiac arrest may occur in 4 min, * irreversible brain injury occurs in 3–5 min |
| causes of upper airway obstruction without ventilation in adults | • **food**—cafe coronary, • *angioedema* |
| lab findings in ARF | • **low PaO$_2$**—present in HARF/HHARF, • *low/normal PaCO$_2$*—HARF, • *high PaCO$_2$ (respiratory acidosis)*—HHARF, • *lactic acidosis*—HARF, • *increased A–a gradient*— * due to primary lung disease in both HARF/HHARF, * see below |
| causes of an increased alveolar-arterial (A–a) gradient | • **perfusion without ventilation**—e.g., * **ARDS,** * PaO$_2$ does not significantly increase after 100% O$_2$, • *ventilation without perfusion*—e.g., * PE, * PaO$_2$ increases with 100% O$_2$: parts of the lung that are perfused can make up the difference and increase the PaO$_2$, • *diffusion abnormalities*—e.g., pulmonary edema [**Note:** the A–a gradient is the difference between the PAO$_2$ (A = Alveolar) and the PaO$_2$ (a = arterial). Normally the A–a is <15 mmHg.] |
| causes of hypoxemia with normal A–a gradient | • **depression of the respiratory center**—see above, • *upper airway obstruction*—see above, • *chest bellows disease*—see above, • *high altitude*—the O$_2$ is still 21% but the atmospheric pressure is decreased |

## Table 3–1. ACUTE RESPIRATORY FAILURE, MECHANICAL VENTILATION, ARDS *Continued*

| Most Common... | Answer and Explanation |
|---|---|
| formula used to calculate the A–a gradient | **PAO$_2$ = % oxygen (713) − PaCO$_2$/0.8.** [Note: using normal values, PAO$_2$ = 0.21 (713) − 40/0.8 = 100 mmHg. If the patient is on a respirator, the % oxygen is used rather than room air (e.g., 0.30 (713) − PaCO$_2$/0.8). A medically significant value set for high specificity is an A–a gradient ≥30 mmHg. Elderly patients normally can have up to a 30 mmHg A–a gradient.] |
| factors to consider in Rx of ARF | • **ventilation**—this refers to the O$_2$ inhaled and the CO$_2$ expired, • **arterial oxygenation**—e.g., how well is PAO$_2$ transferred into the mixed venous blood in the pulmonary capillaries returning from the tissue in exchange for CO$_2$, • **O$_2$ transport**—e.g., * cardiac output, * Hgb concentration, * SaO$_2$, * PaO$_2$, • *O$_2$ extraction/utilization at the tissue level*—e.g., * location of the ODC, * mitochondrial function: are there any problems with oxidative/phosphorylation (e.g., cyanide inhibition of cytochrome oxidase) |
| factors right-shifting ODC | • **increased RBC concentration of 2,3 BPG,** • *acidosis*, • *fever* [Note: a right-shifted ODC refers to increased release of O$_2$ (low affinity) from Hgb.] |
| factors left-shifting ODC | • **decreased RBC concentration of 2,3 BPG,** • *alkalosis*, • *hypothermia*, • *CO*, • *methemoglobin*—iron in the ferric condition: cannot bind O$_2$, • *Hgb F* [Note: a left-shifted ODC refers to decreased release of O$_2$ (high affinity) from Hgb.] |
| method of assessing ventilation | **measure PaCO$_2$** |
| method of assessing arterial oxygenation | • **measure PaO$_2$,** • *measure/calculate SaO$_2$* [Note: calculation of the A–a gradient determines whether hypoxemia is related to primary lung disease (increased A–a) or CNS, upper airway, chest bellows disease (normal A–a).] |

*Table continued on following page*

**Table 3–1. ACUTE RESPIRATORY FAILURE, MECHANICAL VENTILATION, ARDS** *Continued*

| Most Common... | Answer and Explanation |
|---|---|
| methods of assessing $O_2$ transport/extraction | • **measure or calculate $SaO_2$**—$SaO_2$ is measured directly with a pulse oximeter or is calculated from the $PaO_2$, • *measure $MVO_2$ with SGC*— * this is the best index of tissue hypoxia, * a sample of blood is taken from the PA, * it assesses the adequacy of $O_2$ delivery to tissue, adequacy of cardiac index, and adequacy of the systemic arterial $O_2$ content |
| noninvasive method for measuring $SaO_2$ | **pulse oximeter**— * it measures the differential absorption of two wavelengths of light (oxy- and deoxyHgb) in pulsatile fashion: this reflects the $SaO_2$ of Hgb, * it is dependent on: ♦ blood flow (e.g., vasoconstriction alters readings), ♦ position of the ODC, ♦ type of Hgb present (e.g., falsely elevated with CO or metHgb) |
| general management principles in Rx of ARF | • **improve ventilation**— * mechanical ventilation: see below, * endotracheal intubation: e.g., provides a closed system for mechanical ventilation and delivery of high fractions of inspired $O_2$, * reduce dead space: e.g., remove secretions, * naloxone: reverses the effects of respiratory depression from narcotic overdose, • **improve arterial oxygenation**— * incentive spirometry: deep breathing to prevent atelectasis, * antibiotics: Rx of pneumonia, sepsis, * upright position: prevent atelectasis, * administer $O_2$: e.g., ♦ nasal prongs, ♦ Venturi mask, ♦ CPAP, ♦ PEEP, * transfuse packed RBCs: Rx of anemia |
| cause of chronic respiratory failure | **COPD with end-stage fibrosis**—honeycomb lung |
| general types of mechanical ventilation | • **volume ventilator**—volume ventilators are set for: ♦ tidal volume, ♦ rate of ventilation, ♦ inspired $O_2$ concentration ($FiO_2$), ♦ level of end-expiratory pressure (PEEP), • **pressure ventilator**—pressure ventilators deliver a preset pressure to determine: ♦ flow, ♦ tidal volume, ♦ inspiratory time, ♦ frequency |
| differences between nasal prongs and Venturi mask | • **nasal prongs**— * the exact concentration of $O_2$ is not known, * e.g., 1 liter flow = ~$FiO_2$ 24%, * each additional liter ~4% increase, • **Venturi mask**—known $O_2$ concentration ranging from 24–50% |

## Table 3–1. ACUTE RESPIRATORY FAILURE, MECHANICAL VENTILATION, ARDS *Continued*

| Most Common... | Answer and Explanation |
|---|---|
| indications for mechanical ventilation | • **acute hypoxemia or acute hypercapnia not responding to appropriate Rx,** • *clinical instability,* • *apnea* |
| goals for mechanical ventilation | • **FiO₂ ≤0.50,** • **SaO₂ >92%—equivalent to PaO₂ of ≥60 mmHg,** • **airway pressure ≤40 cm H₂O,** • **mean airway pressures ≤30 cm H₂O,** • **arterial pH between 7.35 and 7.50** |
| use of continuous positive airway pressure (CPAP) | **decrease the work of breathing**—positive pressure is maintained throughout the breathing cycle |
| use of PEEP therapy | **improve oxygenation**— * PEEP keeps the terminal bronchioles open during the expiratory cycle (decreases intrapulmonary shunting), * maintains/increases FRC: FRC is the volume remaining in the lung after a resting expiration, * FRC = ERV: ERV is that part of the FRC that is expelled with forceful deflation of the lung plus the residual volume (that part not expelled with forceful deflation) |
| complication of PEEP therapy | • **decreases CO**— * the positive intrathoracic pressures compress the thin-walled RV, RA, and SVC entering the right heart, * positive pressure expands lungs (increases lung compliance), leading to compression of interalveolar blood vessels, • *barotrauma,* • *hypotension,* • *potential for pneumothorax* |
| cause of barotrauma with mechanical ventilation | **increasing TV**—if more ventilation is required, it is safer to increase the rate of breathing than to increase the TV |
| effects of increasing or decreasing the minute volume (ventilatory rate per minute x TV) | • **increasing minute volume**— * produces respiratory alkalosis, * alkalosis causes vasoconstriction of the cerebral blood vessels, * useful in the Rx of cerebral edema, • **decreasing minute volume**— * produces respiratory acidosis, * vasodilates the cerebral blood vessels: predisposes to cerebral edema, * vasoconstricts the pulmonary arterioles |
| complications associated with barotrauma | • **subcutaneous emphysema**—Hamman's crunch is heard with a stethoscope, • *pneumomediastinum,* • *pneumothorax,* • *systemic gas embolization* |

*Table continued on following page*

### Table 3–1. ACUTE RESPIRATORY FAILURE, MECHANICAL VENTILATION, ARDS *Continued*

| Most Common... | Answer and Explanation |
|---|---|
| danger of an $FiO_2$ $\geq 0.50$ | **oxygen free radical damage of lung tissue** |
| causes of ARDS | • **gram-negative sepsis,** • *aspiration of gastric contents,* • *nonpulmonary trauma,* • *shock,* • *near-drowning,* • *multiple blood transfusions,* • *DIC,* • *drug overdose* |
| pathophysiologic abnormality in ARDS | **massive intrapulmonary shunting from widespread atelectasis—** * atelectasis is due to neutrophil-related injury of type II pneumocytes: they contain surfactant within lamellar bodies, * emigration of neutrophils into the alveoli produces leaky capillaries and deposition of a protein-rich edema fluid forming hyaline membranes |
| S/S of ARDS | • **rapid onset of dyspnea within 24–48 hrs of the initiating event,** • *tachypnea,* • *inspiratory crackles* |
| chest x-ray findings in ARDS | • **bilateral pulmonary infiltrates with an initial interstitial pattern followed by an alveolar pattern,** • *air bronchograms*—this is present in 80% of cases, • *absence of vessel redistribution*—no upper lung venous engorgement is present as in CHF, • *normal heart size,* • *absence of pleural effusions in uncomplicated cases* |
| lab abnormalities in ARDS | • **severe hypoxemia—** * $PaO_2$ <50 mmHg while on $FiO_2$ >60%: this is a sign of intrapulmonary shunting, * *increased A–a gradient—* * due to intrapulmonary shunting, * diffusion abnormalities: from hyaline membranes, • *PCWP ≤18 mmHg—>18* mmHg is noted in cardiogenic pulmonary edema, • *respiratory acidosis* (alkalosis initially) |
| Rx of ARDS | • **PEEP + oxygen—** * this improves oxygenation, * no improvement in survival, • *placement of an SGC*—measures $MVO_2$: see Table 3–2, * find the lowest PCWP to maintain an adequate cardiac output, • *drugs are of questionable benefit—* * ? inhalation of NO: potent vasodilator, * ? ketoconazole effect in inhibiting lipoxygenase and $TXA_2$ |

## Table 3–1. ACUTE RESPIRATORY FAILURE, MECHANICAL VENTILATION, ARDS *Continued*

| Most Common... | Answer and Explanation |
|---|---|
| COD in ARDS | **nonpulmonary multiple organ failure**—mortality rate is >50% and >90%, if sepsis is the cause of the ARDS |

**Question:** Which of the following are associated with hypoxemia and an increased A–a gradient? **SELECT 4**
  (A) Paralysis of the diaphragms
  (B) COPD
  (C) Flail chest
  (D) Laryngeal edema
  (E) ARDS
  (F) Pulmonary edema
  (G) Intracranial injury
  (H) Teralogy of Fallot

**Answers: (B), (E), (F), (H).** Only those disorders that primarily affect the lungs and those that produce right to left shunts in the heart cause hypoxemia and an increase in the A–a gradient. In the lungs, ventilation defects, perfusion defects, and diffusion defects increase the A–a gradient and cause hypoxemia. COPD, ARDS, pulmonary edema, and tetralogy of Fallot prolong the A–a gradient and produce hypoxemia **(choices B, E, F, and H are correct).** Hypoxemia without an increase in the A–a gradient occurs with CNS depression, upper airway obstruction, or dysfunction of the chest bellows. Hence, paralysis of the diaphragms, flail chest, laryngeal edema, and intracranial injury do not increase the A–a gradient but do cause hypoxemia **(choices A, C, D, and G are incorrect).**

A–a = Alveolar-arterial, ARDS = adult respiratory distress syndrome, ARF = acute respiratory failure, BPG = bisphosphoglycerate, COPD = chronic obstructive pulmonary disease, CPAP = continuous positive airway pressure, DIC = disseminated intravascular coagulation, ERV = expiratory reserve volume, $FiO_2$ = inspired oxygen concentration, FRC = functional residual capacity, HARF = hypoxic acute respiratory failure, HHARF = hypercapnic-hypoxic acute respiratory failure, HTN = hypertension, ILD = interstitial lung disease, metHgb = methemoglobin, $MVO_2$ = mixed venous oxygen content, NO = nitrous oxide, ODC = oxygen dissociation curve, PA = pulmonary artery, $PaCO_2$ = partial pressure of arterial carbon dioxide, $PaO_2$ = partial pressure of arterial oxygen, $PAO_2$ = partial pressure of alveolar oxygen, PCWP = pulmonary capillary wedge pressure, PE = pulmonary embolus, PEEP = positive end-expiratory pressure, RA = right atrium, RV = right ventricle, $SaO_2$ = oxygen saturation in arterial blood, SGC = Swan-Ganz catheter, S/S = signs/symptoms, SVC = superior vena cava, TV = tidal volume, $TXA_2$ = thromboxane $A_2$, V/Q = ventilation/perfusion ratio.

### Table 3–2. SHOCK, SWAN-GANZ CATHETERS

| Most Common... | Answer and Explanation |
|---|---|
| types of shock | • **hypovolemic**—e.g., * **hemorrhage**, * pancreatitis, • *cardiogenic*—e.g., * **AMI**, * dysrhythmia, • *distributive*—e.g., * **sepsis**, * anaphylactic, • *obstructive*—e.g., * **cardiac tamponade**, * tension pneumothorax |
| pathophysiologic effect of shock | **tissue hypoxia**—inadequate oxygenation of tissue |
| factors to monitor in shock | • **arterial BP**, • **heart rate**, • **pulse pressure**—difference between the systolic and diastolic BP, • **respiratory rate**, • **cardiac output**, • **mental status**, • **urine output**, • **skin temperature** |
| findings in stage I shock or compensated shock | • **arterial pressure**— * normal to −1, * catecholamine release causes peripheral vasoconstriction (cool skin), which may "normalize" the BP, • **heart rate**—+1, • **narrow pulse pressure**— * −1, * initially, this is due to the catecholamine effect of arteriolar vasoconstriction with an increase in diastolic BP, * later, the systolic BP decreases, which further decreases the pulse pressure, • **respiratory rate**—normal, • **cardiac output**— * −1, * may be +1 in early septic shock, • **mental status**—restlessness due to inadequate brain perfusion, • **urine output**— * normal to −1, * decreased cardiac output will decrease the glomerular filtration rate, • **skin**—cool: catecholamine effect, • **comments**—vigorous Rx often reverses this stage |
| findings in stage II shock or decompensated shock | • **arterial pressure**—−2, • **heart rate**—+2, • **pulse pressure**—−2, • **respiratory rate**—+2, • **cardiac output**—−2, • **mental status**—obtunded, • **urine output**— * −2, * oliguric, • **skin**—mottled, • *comments*— * compensatory mechanisms include: ♦ peripheral vasoconstriction, ♦ activation of the RAA system, ♦ venoconstriction, ♦ increased renal reabsorption of salt/water, * compensatory mechanisms are insufficient to maintain perfusion of vital organs, * myocardial depressant factor is released from the underperfused pancreatic tissue |

### Table 3–2. SHOCK, SWAN-GANZ CATHETERS *Continued*

| Most Common... | Answer and Explanation |
|---|---|
| findings in stage III shock or irreversible shock | • **arterial pressure**—$-3$, • **heart rate**—$+3$ to $-3$, • **pulse pressure**—$-3$, • **respiratory rate**—$+3$ to $-3$, • **cardiac output**—$-3$, • **mental status**—comatose, • **urine output**—anuric, • **skin**— * cold, * cyanotic, • **comments**—irreversible organ injury is due to: ♦ mitochondrial dysfunction (decreased ATP), ♦ intracellular release of lysosomal enzymes, ♦ activation of the complement system, ♦ release of TNF (cachectin) from macrophages, ♦ generation of FRs, ♦ endothelial cell damage |
| bacterial causes of septic shock | **gram-negative sepsis**— * *Escherichia coli*—related to indwelling urinary catheters, * *Klebsiella pneumoniae*, * *Pseudomonas aeruginosa*—related to respirators |
| sources of gram-negative sepsis | • **GU tract**—indwelling urinary catheters, • *GI tract*, • *wounds*, • *respirators*, • *intravenous catheters* |
| causes of gram-positive septic shock | • *Staphylococcus aureus*—related to indwelling venous catheters, • *Streptococcus* species |
| S/S of endotoxic shock | • *fever*, • *tachycardia*, • *variable BP*, • *warm, dry skin*, • *mental confusion* |
| mechanisms involved in endotoxic shock | • **activation of the alternative complement pathway by endotoxins**— * release of anaphylatoxins: ♦ C3a, C5a, ♦ anaphylatoxins directly stimulate mast cell/basophil release of histamine, * arteriolar vasodilatation: warm skin, • *damage to endothelial cells by endotoxins*—release of nitric oxide and $PGI_2$: ♦ both are potent vasodilators, ♦ vasodilatation decreases the total peripheral resistance, • *tissue hypoxia*—arteriolar vasodilatation increases blood flow and decreases tissue extraction of $O_2$, • *increased venous return to heart*— * due to arteriolar vasodilatation, * increases cardiac output: high-output failure, * increases $MVO_2$: tissues cannot extract $O_2$ owing to increased blood flow through the microcirculation |

*Table continued on following page*

**Table 3–2. SHOCK, SWAN-GANZ CATHETERS** *Continued*

| Most Common... | Answer and Explanation |
|---|---|
| stages of septic shock | **warm shock → cold shock → MOFS**—see below |
| clinical complications of shock | • **ischemic acute tubular necrosis**— * due to decreased renal perfusion, * the renal medulla normally receives only 10% of the renal blood flow and is most subject to ischemic ATN, • *DIC*— * most commonly due to gram-negative sepsis, * DIC leads to: ♦ generalized ischemic damage of organs, ♦ bleeding, ♦ renal cortical necrosis, • *ARDS*—most commonly due to gram-negative sepsis, • *stress bleeding from the GI tract,* • *gut-mucosal function abnormalities*—bacteria from the GI tract enter the blood stream, leading to sepsis, • *hepatic dysfunction* |
| types of shock associated with spinal injuries | • **spinal cord shock,** • **neurogenic shock** |
| clinical findings in spinal shock | • **it occurs soon after either complete or partial spinal cord injuries,** • **absence of motor, sensory, autonomic function below level of injury,** • **spinal shock disappears in 1–3 days,** • **previously flaccid muscle becomes spastic, DTRs are exaggerated, and Babinski's sign is positive** |
| clinical findings in neurogenic shock | • **dysfunction of the descending sympathetic pathways,** • *heart/BV do not respond to sympathetic responses*— * no compensatory tachycardia, * bradycardia is present, • *vasomotor tone is decreased*—causes pooling of blood |
| differences between neurogenic and hypovolemic shock | • **neurogenic shock**—hypotension + sinus bradycardia, • **hypovolemic shock**—hypotension + sinus tachycardia |
| COD in shock | **MOFS**—this is the postshock syndrome |
| clinical findings in MOFS | **multiple organ dysfunctions**— * ARDS, * GI bleeding, * sepsis, * hepatic dysfunction, * 75% mortality rate |
| uses of SGC in monitoring shock | **evaluates preload, afterload, and the cardiac index**—it is an intravascular catheter |

## Table 3–2. SHOCK, SWAN-GANZ CATHETERS *Continued*

| Most Common... | Answer and Explanation |
|---|---|
| parameters measured by the SGC | • **central venous pressure**—CVP = 0–4 mmHg, • **PA systolic (15–30 mmHg) and diastolic (3–12 mmHg) pressures**, • **mean arterial pressure (MAP)**—85–95 mmHg, • **MVO₂**— * 15 mL/dL, * this is the best index of tissue hypoxia, • **CO**—4–8 L/min, • **cardiac index**— * CI = CO ÷ body surface area, * 2.5–4 L/min/m², • **PCWP**— * assesses preload in the LA/LV, * 12–15 mmHg, • **SVR**— * indicates the afterload the LV must contract against, * SVR = [MAP − CVP ÷ CO] × 80 = 900–1400 dynes/sec/cm² |
| hemodynamic pattern in hypovolemic shock | • **CVP**—decreased, • **CI**—decreased, • **SVR**—increased, • **PCWP**—decreased, • **MVO₂**—decreased |
| hemodynamic pattern in cardiogenic shock | • **CVP**—increased, • **CI**—decreased, • **SVR**—increased, • **PCWP**— * increased, * decreased in hypovolemic shock, • **MVO₂**—*decreased* |
| hemodynamic pattern in early septic shock | • **CVP**—increased, • **CI**— * increased, * decreased in hypovolemic/cardiogenic shock, • **SVR**— * decreased: vasodilatation, * increased in hypovolemic/cardiogenic shock, • **PCWP**—decreased, • **MVO₂**— * increased, * decreased in hypovolemic/cardiogenic shock |
| hemodynamic pattern in late septic shock | • **CVP**—decreased, • **CI**—decreased, • **SVR**—increased: vasoconstriction of arterioles, • **PCWP**—decreased, • **MVO₂**—increased or decreased |
| lab findings in shock | • **increased anion gap metabolic acidosis**—anaerobic glycolysis → lactic acidosis, • *hyperglycemia*—release of cortisol, glucagon, and catecholamines increase glycogenolysis, • *neutrophilic leukocytosis*—in hypovolemic/cardiogenic shock: cortisol and catecholamines decrease adhesion molecule synthesis with release of marginating neutrophil pool into the circulating pool, • *absolute neutropenia*—endotoxins decrease neutrophil count by increasing adhesion molecule synthesis |

*Table continued on following page*

**Table 3–2. SHOCK, SWAN-GANZ CATHETERS** *Continued*

| Most Common... | Answer and Explanation |
|---|---|
| effect of acute blood loss on Hgb and Hct | **no change**—see Table 2–6 |
| effect of acute blood loss when crystalloids are infused | **drop in Hgb/Hct concentration**—see Table 2–6 |
| parameters to monitor in all types of shock | • **cerebral status**—sensitive indicator of cerebral perfusion, • **urine output**— * **most important parameter of adequate tissue perfusion,** * should be at least 0.5 mL/per kg of body weight each hr, • **arterial pH/serum lactate**— * metabolic acidosis secondary to elevated lactate levels indicates tissue hypoxia, * unlike lactate in Ringer's lactated solution, which is converted into bicarbonate, the lactate associated with tissue hypoxia produces metabolic acidosis, • **measurement of SaO$_2$**— * measure of oxygenation, * O$_2$ is given to maintain the SaO$_2$ ≥ 92% and PaO$_2$ ≥60 mmHg, • **Hgb concentration**—should be ≥ 10 g/dL to maintain an adequate O$_2$ content, • **volume status**— * Ringer's lactated solution is the mainstay in the Rx of hypovolemic shock, * packed RBCs are recommended if the Hgb falls < 10 g/dL or Hct <30%, • **heart rate**—ECG monitoring, • **cardiac output**—use cardiotonic agents (see below) |
| Rx of hypovolemic shock | • **volume replacement**— * crystalloid solutions (e.g., lactated Ringer's) or blood depending on the cause of volume depletion, * replace volume until the increase in CVP and PCWP does not further benefit CO or BP, • *place the patient in Trendelenburg position*—elevate legs above level of heart |
| Rx of cardiogenic shock | • **inotropic agents**— * dopamine, * use intra-aortic balloon pump if there is no improvement, • *diuretics*—decrease preload |
| Rx of septic shock | • **vigorous volume resuscitation**— * crystalloid infusion, * monitor CO and PCWP with a SGC, • *increase peripheral vascular tone*— * dopamine, * phenylephrine, * norepinephrine, • *Rx underlying sepsis* |

## Table 3-2. SHOCK, SWAN-GANZ CATHETERS *Continued*

| Most Common... | Answer and Explanation |
|---|---|
| Rx of neurogenic shock | **similar to septic shock except for antibiotics** |
| metabolic problem associated with infusing 0.9% NaCl in shock | **hyperchloremic normal anion gap metabolic acidosis**— * normal saline contains 154 mEq/L of NaCl, * infusion of large quantities of saline dilutes the bicarbonate concentration, * Ringer's lactated solution is the preferred crystalloid: replaces bicarbonate |
| cardiotonic agents used in the Rx of shock | • **dopamine**— * doses 2–3 µg/kg/min increase renal/splanchnic blood flow, * doses 4–5 µg/kg/min increase cardiac contractility, • *dobutamine*—inotropic vasodilator, • *amrinone*— * noncatecholamine that inhibits phosphodiesterase III, * inotropic vasodilator • *nitroprusside*—vasodilator that decreases SVR: decreases afterload |
| Dx and Rx of decreased CI, decreased PCWP, decreased/increased SVR | • **Dx**—volume depletion, • **Rx**—crystalloid solutions: lactated Ringer's or blood depending on the cause of volume depletion |

**Question:** Which of the following distinguish early septic shock from hypovolemic shock? **SELECT 5**
- (A) CI
- (B) SVR
- (C) Skin temperature
- (D) MVO$_2$
- (E) PCWP
- (F) CVP
- (G) Urine output

**Answers: (A), (B), (C), (D), (F).** In early septic shock, the CI is increased (low in hypovolemic shock), SVR is decreased (increased in hypovolemic shock), the skin is warm (cold and clammy in hypovolemic shock), the MVO$_2$ is increased (decreased in hypovolemic shock), and the CVP is increased (decreased in hypovolemic shock) **(choices A, B, C, D, and F are correct).** The PCWP is decreased in both early septic and hypovolemic shock **(choice E is incorrect).** The urine output is reduced in both types of shock **(choice G is incorrect).**

AMI = acute myocardial infarction, ARDS = adult respiratory distress syndrome, ATN = acute tubular necrosis, ATP = adenosine triphosphate, BP = blood pressure, BV = blood vessel, CI = cardiac index, CO = cardiac output, COD = cause of death, CVP = central venous pressure, DIC = disseminated intravascular coagulation, DTRs = deep tendon reflexes, FR = free radicals, LA = left atrium, LV = left ventricle, MAP = mean arterial pressure, MOSF = multiple organ system failure, $MVO_2$ = mixed venous oxygen, PA = pulmonary artery, PCWP = pulmonary capillary wedge pressure, $PGI_2$ = prostacyclin, RAA = renin-angiotensin-aldosterone, $SaO_2$ = oxygen saturation of arterial blood, SGC = Swan-Ganz catheter, S/S = signs/symptoms, SVR = systemic vascular resistance, TNF = tumor necrosis factor.

# CHAPTER

**4**

## PERIOPERATIVE EVALUATION, POSTOPERATIVE COMPLICATIONS, SURGICAL WOUNDS

### CONTENTS

### Table 4–1. PREOPERATIVE CARE

| Most Common... | Answer and Explanation |
|---|---|
| phases of management of surgical patient | • **preoperative care,** • **anesthesia/surgery,** • **postoperative care** |
| components of preoperative care | • **diagnostic work-up**—cause/effect of present illness, • **preoperative evaluation**— * see below, * see Table 4–2 for nutritional evaluation, • **preoperative preparation**— * procedures, * specific interventions |
| components of preoperative evaluation | • **history**— * ?pre-existing medical conditions: e.g., DM, heart disease, * ?smoker, * ?alcohol, * ?drugs: including over-the-counter drugs such as NSAIDs, • **physical exam,** • **diagnostic testing**—see below, • **risk classification**—see below |
| recommendations for preoperative chest radiograph | **recommended for those at risk for pulmonary complications**— * see below, * it is not a routine procedure |
| recommendations for preoperative ECG | • **men >40 yrs old,** • **women >50 yrs old,** • **Hx suggesting angina/arrhythmia** [Note: risk of CAD increases with age. See risk factors for cardiovascular complications below.] |

*Table continued on following page*

**Table 4–1. PREOPERATIVE CARE** *Continued*

| Most Common... | Answer and Explanation |
|---|---|
| preoperative recommendations for CBC | • **major surgery with an expected blood loss**—e.g., hip surgery, • **patients with chronic disease,** • **patients with a positive FOBT** [**Note:** a CBC is not routine for minor surgery. An Hgb of ≥10 g/dL is considered safe for operation.] |
| recommendations for preoperative hemostasis testing | • **patients with a family history of bleeding,** • **patients who have had bleeding problems after a molar extraction**—this imposes a great stress on hemostasis, • **patients with liver disease**— * the PT is the best indicator of severity of liver disease, * preoperative IM vitamin K is recommended [**Note:** tests for patients at risk should include a PT, PTT, platelet count, and BT. Patients on aspirin/ NSAIDs should be off these drugs for 7 days before surgery.] |
| recommendations for preoperative chemistries | **patients at risk who require electrolytes, BUN, creatinine**— * >60 yrs old, * known CAD, * on diuretics, * DM, * liver disease, * renal disease, * chronic diarrhea [**Note:** pre-operative chemistries are not a routine procedure. Medically significant values include a serum $K^+$ <3.0 mEq/L, a serum BUN >50 mg/dL, and a serum creatinine >3 mg/dL.] |
| preoperative fluid disorder | **volume depletion**—secondary to: ♦ diarrhea, ♦ vomiting, ♦ hemorrhage |
| preoperative sodium disorder | **hyponatremia**—due to: ♦ diuretics, ♦ GI losses, ♦ edema states (e.g., CHF, cirrhosis, CRF), ♦ SiADH |
| preoperative cause of hypernatremia | **insensible water loss due to fever**—fever causes increased evaporation of pure water from mucous membranes |
| preoperative causes of hypokalemia | • **diuretics,** • *vomiting,* • *diarrhea* |
| preoperative cause of hyperkalemia | **renal disease** |
| preoperative causes of metabolic alkalosis | • **vomiting,** • *diuretics* |

### Table 4–1. PREOPERATIVE CARE *Continued*

| Most Common... | Answer and Explanation |
|---|---|
| preoperative causes of metabolic acidosis | • **lactic acidosis**—most often associated with shock, • *diarrhea*—normal AG type of metabolic acidosis, • *renal failure*—increased AG type of metabolic acidosis |
| preoperative tests routinely performed on women of child-bearing age | • **pregnancy test,** • *cervical Pap smear if >30 yrs old* |
| preoperative recommendations for urinalysis | • **patients with urinary tract symptoms,** • **patients scheduled for surgery involving the urinary tract** [**Note:** a urinalysis is not a routine test.] |
| classification scheme for assessing patient risk | • **category I**— * healthy, * 0.01% mortality, • **category II**— * mild systemic disease, • **category III**— * severe systemic disease limiting activity, • **category IV**— * systemic disease that threatens the patient's life, * ~18% mortality, • **category V**— * moribund patient not likely to survive without operation, * 50% mortality [**Note:** the categories have been established by the American Society of Anesthesiologists. Risks double in categories I, II, III if the patient must undergo emergency surgery.] |
| risk factors for infection | • **poor host immune defense**— * B/T cell disorders, * corticosteroids, * prolonged use of antibiotics, * previous radiation, • *malnutrition*—see Table 4–2, • *DM,* • *renal failure* |
| risk factors for cardiovascular complications | • **S₃ gallop/jugular venous distention**—these are signs of CHF, • *AMI within the last 6 mos*— * there is an increased risk of reinfarction, * patients are particularly at risk if it was a non-Q wave type of AMI, • **age**—>70 yrs old, • *>5 PVCs/min,* • *significant degree of aortic stenosis*—evaluate with echocardiography, • *DM*—independent risk factor, • *peripheral vascular disease*—independent risk factor, • *ABG status*—risk factor if $PaO_2$ <60 mmHg, $PaCO_2$ >50 mmHg, • *HTN*—not an established risk factor for perioperative cardiac morbidity [**Note:** the above criteria are part of the Goldman index.] |

*Table continued on following page*

**Table 4–1. PREOPERATIVE CARE** *Continued*

| Most Common... | Answer and Explanation |
|---|---|
| types of surgery with greatest cardiac risk | • **emergency surgery,** • *right upper quadrant abdominal surgery,* • *thoracic surgery* |
| preoperative testing for those at high risk for cardiovascular complications | • **dipyridamole thallium imaging—** * best predictive test, * greater sensitivity (>90%) than specificity (>60%), * dobutamine stress test also has excellent sensitivity: 100%, • *ECG—see above,* • *cardiac catheterization—* * for very-high-risk patients determined by the Goldman index, * positive noninvasive tests |
| clinical predictor of postoperative complications | **Hx of productive cough** |
| risk factors for pulmonary complications | • **COPD**—encourage the patient to stop smoking 1 mo before surgery, • *type of surgery—* * RUQ surgery is the most dangerous, * thoracic surgery, • *obesity,* • *duration of surgery >2hrs* |
| preoperative tests of pulmonary function in those at risk | • **PFTs—** * FVC: high risk if <25–30% of predicted (normal >80%), * $FEV_{1sec}$: high risk if <25–30% of predicted (normal > 80%), * $FEV_{1sec}/FVC$: high risk if <30% of predicted (normal 70–80%), • *ABGs—* * $PaCO_2$ > 45 mmHg is a high risk (normal 33–45 mmHg), * $PaO_2$ <60 mmHg is a high risk (normal 75–105 mmHg), • *chest x-ray*—identifies parenchymal and/or pleural disease |
| preoperative management for those at risk for pulmonary complications | • **incentive spirometry**—reduces the risk for atelectasis, • *smoking*—stop smoking for 1 month prior to surgery if not forever, • *drugs—* * bronchodilators for COPD: e.g., $\beta_2$-agonist medihaler such as albuterol, * corticosteroids for severe COPD/asthma, * antibiotics are not recommended |
| risk factors for stroke | • **Hx of TIAs**—~40% risk for stroke in noncarotid surgery, * see below, • *elderly,* • *HTN*—reducing BP has its greatest effect on reducing mortality due to stroke, • *DM,* • *smoking* |

**Table 4–1. PREOPERATIVE CARE** *Continued*

| Most Common... | Answer and Explanation |
|---|---|
| steps in the preoperative management of carotid artery disease | • **arterial duplex scanning**—evaluates the degree of stenosis, • *criteria for endarterectomy prior to surgery*— * asymptomatic with >50% stenosis and ulcerated plaque or symptoms persist with aspirin, * asymptomatic with >60% stenosis, * symptomatic with >70% stenosis |
| risk factors for thromboembolism | • **type of surgery**— * **total hip surgery is the greatest risk,** * pelvic surgery, * neurosurgery, • *obesity,* • *age*—>45 yrs old, • *CHF,* • *previous Hx of thrombosis,* • *hypercoagulable state*— * cancer, * on oral contraceptives, * hereditary condition: see Table 2–13 |
| preoperative management to prevent venous thrombosis | **see Table 2–13** |
| risk factors for ARF | • **type of surgery**— * **abdominal aortic aneurysm repair is the greatest risk,** * cardiac surgery, • *pre-existing azotemia*— * BUN >50 mg/dL, * creatinine >3 mg/dL, • *CHF,* • *elderly*—creatinine clearance/GFR normally decrease with age, • *drugs*—e.g., aminoglycosides are nephrotoxic, • *DM,* • *pre-existing volume depletion,* • *sepsis,* • *previous intravenous pyelogram (IVP)* |
| preoperative management to prevent ARF | • **volume expansion**—crystalloids, • *if a previous IVP has been performed*—consider the use of: ♦ mannitol, ♦ furosemide, ♦ dopamine, • *nephrotoxic drugs*—eliminate or adjust the doses |
| preoperative evaluation of patients with known liver disease | • **establish the severity of the hemostasis risk**— * prolonged PT is a poor risk, * a serum albumin < 3.0 g/dL is a poor risk, • *risk assessment*—Child's criteria: see below, • *viral hepatitis*— * acute hepatitis is a contraindication to surgery, * chronic HBV/HCV poses no increased risk, • *alcoholic hepatitis*—associated with a high operative mortality |

*Table continued on following page*

**Table 4–1. PREOPERATIVE CARE** *Continued*

| Most Common... | Answer and Explanation |
|---|---|
| causes of hyperglycemia prior to surgery | • **DM,** • *presence of infection,* • *stress/ trauma*—raises catecholamines (increases glycogenolysis) and cortisol (increases gluco- neogenesis), • *patient on corticosteroids,* • *bedridden patients*—become resistant to in- sulin |
| perioperative problems encountered in DM | • **infectious complications**— * wound infec- tions, * pneumonia, * UTIs, • *renal*— * ARF, * urinary retention, • *silent AMI,* • *DKA* |
| recommendations for diabetics the day before major surgery | • **major surgery in type I or II DM**— * IV infusion of 1 liter of D5W at a rate of 50 mL/hr, * D/C long-acting sulfonylureas 1 day before surgery, * D/C short-acting sulfonyl- ureas on morning of surgery, • **mix 50 units of regular human insulin with 250 mL of 0.9 mL normal saline**— * hang the infusion as a "piggyback" to the D5W solution, * the infu- sion rate of insulin/hr = plasma glucose mg/ dL/100: use 150 in the denominator if the patient is not on corticosteroids or is thin, • **measure plasma glucose every 3 hrs**— * use the above formula to adjust the insulin infusion rate if necessary, * maintain glucose between 100 and 200 mg/dL: do not exceed a glucose of 250 mg/dL |
| recommendations for diabetics on the day of major surgery | • **continue D5W infusion at rate of 50 mL/hr,** • **use nonglucose infusions for management of all fluid and electrolyte abnormalities,** • **obtain plasma glucose q 2hrs during surgery**—use the above formula to set the in- sulin infusion rate, • **measure plasma glucose q 2hrs for the remaining 24-hr period**—adjust the infusion rate as necessary |
| recommendations for diabetics after day 1 of major surgery | • **continue D5W infusion rate of 50 mL/hr,** • **measure daily fasting and afternoon plasma glucose**—use the above formula to adjust insulin infusion rate, • **if the patient is able to tolerate solids**— * stop the D5W infusion, * return patient back to original schedule |

## Table 4–1. PREOPERATIVE CARE *Continued*

| Most Common... | Answer and Explanation |
|---|---|
| factors evaluated with the Child's criteria in patients with liver disease | • **encephalopathy**—none → mild → moderate/severe, • **serum albumin**—>3.5 g/dL → 3.0–3.5 g/dL → <3.0 g/dL, • **ascites**—none → mild → moderate/severe, • **serum bilirubin**—<2.0 mg/dL → 2.0–3.0 mg/dL → >3.0 mg/dL |

**Question:** Which of the following correctly describe smoking as a preoperative risk factor? **SELECT 4**
  (A) Decreases mucociliary clearance
  (B) Increases the risk for bleeding
  (C) Reduces the A–a gradient
  (D) Increases the risk for ARF
  (E) Increases the risk for thromboembolism
  (F) Increases the risk for atelectasis
  (G) Decreases the risk for stroke

**Answers:** (A), (D), (E), (F). Smoking increases the risk for postoperative atelectasis (**choice F is correct**) owing to a reduction in mucociliary clearance (**choice A is correct**). Smoking does not increase the risk for bleeding (**choice B is incorrect**); however, it does increase the risk for thromboembolism (**choice E is correct**), and stroke (**choice G is incorrect**), because chemicals in smoke damage endothelial surfaces. Smoking increases the A–a gradient because of COPD (**choice C is incorrect**) and has a deleterious effect on increasing the risk for ARF postoperatively (**choice D is correct**).

A–a gradient = Alveolar-arterial gradient, ABG = arterial blood gas, AG = anion gap, AMI = acute myocardial infarction, ARF = acute renal failure, BP = blood pressure, BT = bleeding time, BUN = blood urea nitrogen, CAD = coronary artery disease, CHF = congestive heart failure, COPD = chronic obstructive pulmonary disease, CRF = chronic renal failure, DKA = diabetic ketoacidosis, DM = diabetes mellitus, D5W = 5% dextrose and water, $FEV_{1sec}$ = forced expiratory volume in 1 sec, FOBT = fecal occult blood test, FVC = forced vital capacity, GFR = glomerular filtration rate, HBV = hepatitis B virus, HCV = hepatitis C virus, Hgb = hemoglobin, HTN = hypertension, IVP = intravenous pyelogram, NSAIDs = nonsteroidal anti-inflammatory drugs, PFTs = pulmonary function tests, PT = prothrombin time, PTT = partial thromboplastin time, PVCs = premature ventricular contractions, RUQ = right upper quadrant, SiADH = syndrome of inappropriate antidiuretic hormone, TIAs = transient ischemic attacks, UTIs = urinary tract infections.

**Table 4–2. NUTRITIONAL ASSESSMENT IN SURGERY, PROTEIN-CALORIE MALNUTRITION (PCM), ENTERAL AND PARENTERAL THERAPY, TRACE METAL DEFICIENCY**

| Most Common... | Answer and Explanation |
|---|---|
| macronutrients | • **protein**— * important for the synthesis of: ♦ structural proteins, ♦ enzymes, ♦ immunoglobulins, * most protein is located in muscle, * there is no storage form for protein, • *fat*—primary energy source during fasting and starvation, • *carbohydrates*—primary energy source for the brain and RBCs |
| sites for protein digestion/absorption | • **sites for digestion**— * pepsin begins protein digestion in the stomach, * pancreatic proteases assist digestion in the duodenum: amino acids and dipeptides are produced, • **site of reabsorption**—entire small bowel: 50% of reabsorption is in the duodenum |
| site for protein turnover | **loss of enterocytes and digestive enzymes in GI tract** |
| disorders associated with protein loss | • **GI losses**— * draining secretions: e.g., ileostomy, * malabsorption, • *third-degree burns*—loss of plasma, • *draining wounds* [**Note:** ingestion of CHO spares protein breakdown.] |
| number of calories supplied by protein | **4 kcal/g**—protein accounts for ~15% of the normal body expenditure of energy |
| sites for CHO digestion/absorption | • **sites for digestion**— * mouth: salivary amylase, * proximal small intestine: pancreatic amylase, * amylase breaks CHO into: ♦ α-limit dextrans, ♦ maltose (2 glucoses), ♦ maltotriose (3 glucoses), * brush border disaccharidases hydrolyze the above into: ♦ glucose (>75%), ♦ galactose, ♦ fructose, • **site of reabsorption**— * small intestine, * glucose/galactose cotransport with Na$^+$: for oral replacement of electrolytes, glucose or galactose must be added to the solution for Na$^+$ to be reabsorbed, * fructose is reabsorbed by facilitated diffusion |
| sites for glycogen storage | • **liver,** • *muscle,* • *kidneys* [**Note:** fasting for > 24 hrs depletes glycogen stores.] |

**Table 4–2. NUTRITIONAL ASSESSMENT IN SURGERY, PROTEIN-CALORIE MALNUTRITION (PCM), ENTERAL AND PARENTERAL THERAPY, TRACE METAL DEFICIENCY** *Continued*

| Most Common... | Answer and Explanation |
|---|---|
| number of calories supplied by CHO | **4 kcal/g**— * CHO account for ~30–40% of the total calories in a normal diet, * increased CHO intake produces fatty liver: glycerol 3-phosphate, an intermediate in glycolysis, is the primary substrate for VLDL synthesis |
| sites for lipid digestion/absorption | • **site for digestion**— * small intestine: ♦ pancreatic lipases, ♦ cholesterol esterase, * saturated dietary fat is hydrolyzed into fatty acids and 2-monoglycerides, * bile salts must be present for micelle formation in order to reabsorb fats, • **site of reabsorption**—small bowel |
| cause of lipolysis | **stress**—release of catecholamines, cortisol, glucagon enhances hormone-sensitive lipase in adipose tissue: releases FAs and glycerol |
| number of calories supplied by lipids | **9 kcal/g**— * lipids supply ~25–45% of total calories in a normal diet, * fats are primarily used by skeletal and cardiac muscle for energy |
| CHO events in fasting state (first 24 hrs) | • **gluconeogenesis**— * glucagon is the primary gluconeogenic hormone, * there is increased muscle breakdown to supply alanine: converted into pyruvate by transaminases that remove the amino group, • *glycogenolysis*— * glucagon/catecholamine-mediated , * glycogen is depleted in 24 hrs, • *brain/RBCs use glucose primarily for fuel*—brain uses ketone bodies in starvation |
| protein events in the fasting state | • **increased protein catabolism**—alanine is used as a substrate for gluconeogenesis, • **increased production of urea**—due to increased metabolism of amino acids in the liver urea cycle |
| lipid events in the fasting state | • **lipolysis**—activation of hormone-sensitive lipase in the adipose tissue by glucagon/catecholamines causes the release of FAs and glycerol, • **increased β-oxidation of fatty acids**, • **ketogenesis**—acetyl CoA from FA oxidation is used by the liver to produce AcAc and β-OHB |

*Table continued on following page*

### Table 4–2. NUTRITIONAL ASSESSMENT IN SURGERY, PROTEIN-CALORIE MALNUTRITION (PCM), ENTERAL AND PARENTERAL THERAPY, TRACE METAL DEFICIENCY
*Continued*

| Most Common... | Answer and Explanation |
| --- | --- |
| differences in starvation from the fasting state | • **decreased gluconeogenesis**— * muscle breakdown is spared, * glucose that is produced goes to the RBCs, • **greater increase in β-oxidation of FAs**—muscle primarily uses fat for fuel, • **decreased urea production**— * due to less muscle breakdown, • **the brain uses ketone bodies for fuel** |
| biochemical effects of surgical trauma/ sepsis | • **increased catabolism of protein**— * increased urea production, * hormones involved: ♦ glucagon, ♦ catecholamines, ♦ cortisol, • *early anabolic phase*— * variable time-frame, * cortisol decreases, * positive nitrogen balance with weight gain, • *late anabolic phase*—adipose stores are replaced |
| micronutrients | • **vitamins**, • **minerals**, • **trace elements** |
| formula used to estimate the basal energy expenditure (BEE) | **Harris-Benedict equation**— * separate equations for men and women, * the equation is based on sex, height, weight, and age, * the calculation is further multiplied by a stress factor (0.8–1.8) |
| formula to calculate BEE via a Swan-Ganz catheter | **Fick equation**—the equation includes: ♦ measured oxygen saturation in arterial and venous blood, ♦ cardiac output, ♦ Hgb |
| causes of increased metabolic rate | • **fever**, • *sepsis*, • *burns*, • *massive trauma*, • *hyperthyroidism* |
| formula used to measure body weight | **body mass index (BMI)**— * BMI is the body weight in kg divided by the height in $m^2$, * a BMI >30 $kg/m^2$ is obesity, * a BMI >40 $kg/m^2$ is morbid obesity |
| test to evaluate total body fat composition | **caliper skinfold measurements at multiple sites**—e.g., triceps skin fold |
| tests to evaluate immune competence | • **cutaneous hypersensitivity reactions to common antigens**—lack of response to common antigens indicates anergy and poor cellular immunity, • *total lymphocyte count*— * <1200/$mm^3$ is a poor sign, * T cells are mainly decreased |

### Table 4–2. NUTRITIONAL ASSESSMENT IN SURGERY, PROTEIN-CALORIE MALNUTRITION (PCM), ENTERAL AND PARENTERAL THERAPY, TRACE METAL DEFICIENCY
*Continued*

| Most Common... | Answer and Explanation |
|---|---|
| measurement for skeletal muscle mass | **midarm muscle circumference** |
| tests to evaluate lean body mass | • **urine creatinine**—metabolic product of creatine in muscle, • **urine 3-methylhistidine**—component of actin and myosin in muscle |
| tests to evaluate visceral protein mass | • **albumin**—half-life 18–20 days, • **transferrin**—half-life 8–10 days, • *retinol-binding protein*—1 day half-life, • *prealbumin*—half-life 2–3 days [**Note:** the shorter the protein half-life, the more accurate the correlation with protein mass. Serial measurements are better than isolated measurements.] |
| causes of PCM in the United States | • **postoperative state,** • *malabsorption,* • *sepsis,* • *AIDS,* • *malignancy* |
| sign of macronutrient deficiency | **progressive weight loss**— * it is defined as a 10% unintended weight loss in 6 mos or a 5% unintended weight loss in 1 mo |
| physical findings of macronutrient deficiency | • **muscle wasting**— * temporal area, * thenar atrophy, * extremity muscles, • *loss of subcutaneous fat* |
| effect of PCM on nitrogen balance | **negative nitrogen balance**—intake (protein intake 24 hrs/6.25); excretion (urine urea nitrogen 24 hrs + 4/total urine volume in liters) [**Note:** normal individuals should have a nitrogen balance approaching zero.] |
| causes of PCM | • **inadequate protein intake,** • *nutrient losses,* • *increased nutrient requirements* |
| effect of PCM on hepatic function | **decreased protein synthesis** |
| effect of PCM on the heart | **myofiber atrophy with subsequent decrease in cardiac output** |
| effect of PCM on the lungs | • **atrophy of muscles of respiration**—decreases VC and TV, • *decreased mucociliary clearance*—prone to infections |

*Table continued on following page*

Table 4–2. NUTRITIONAL ASSESSMENT IN SURGERY,
PROTEIN-CALORIE MALNUTRITION (PCM), ENTERAL
AND PARENTERAL THERAPY, TRACE METAL DEFICIENCY
*Continued*

| Most Common... | Answer and Explanation |
|---|---|
| effect of PCM on the GI tract | • **loss of brush border enzymes**—"use it or lose it," • **loss of villi**—malabsorption, • **pancreatic insufficiency**—malabsorption |
| effect of PCM on the immune system | • **decreases total lymphocyte count**— * <1200/mm³, * decreased CD₄ T cells, • *decreased C3 and factor B,* • *abnormal phagocytic function*—e.g., * chemotaxis, * phagocytosis, • *decreased secretory IgA* |
| effect of PCM on wound healing | **all phases are adversely affected**—adverse effects on: ♦ neutrophil function, ♦ collagen deposition, ♦ granulation tissue formation, ♦ remodeling of collagen |
| clinical findings in marasmus | • **total reduction in caloric intake,** • *muscle wasting,* • *loss of subcutaneous fat,* • *"broomstick extremities,"* • *decreased arm muscle circumference,* • *normal visceral protein stores,* • *normal immune function,* • *good response to nutritional Rx* |
| clinical findings in kwashiorkor | • **inadequate amount of protein**— * normal total caloric intake, * mainly CHO intake, • *hypoalbuminemia*— * <3.0 g/dL, * decrease in plasma oncotic pressure → pitting edema and ascites, • *decreased liver apolipoprotein synthesis*—hepatomegaly with fatty change, • *"flaky paint" dermatitis,* • *diarrhea*— * loss of brush border enzymes, * parasitic diseases, * malabsorption, • *anemia,* • *decreased immune response*— * <1200/mm³ total lymphocytes, * anergy, • *reddish hair*— * flag sign, * sign of copper deficiency, • *normal to low arm muscle circumference,* • *response to nutritional Rx*— * persistent hypoalbuminemia, * ?restoration of lean body mass, * restoration of immune competence |

**Table 4–2. NUTRITIONAL ASSESSMENT IN SURGERY, PROTEIN-CALORIE MALNUTRITION (PCM), ENTERAL AND PARENTERAL THERAPY, TRACE METAL DEFICIENCY**
*Continued*

| Most Common... | Answer and Explanation |
|---|---|
| lab findings in kwashiorkor | • **hypoalbuminemia/low transferrin**— * <3.0 g/dL of albumin, * <200 mg/dL of transferrin, * decrease in plasma oncotic pressure → pitting edema and ascites, • anemia, • *decreased immune response*— * <1200/mm³ total lymphocytes, * anergy |
| recommendation for number of kcal to lose, maintain, gain weight | • **lose**—25 kcal/kg, • **maintain**—30 kcal/kg—stressed patients require 25–35 kcal/kg, • **gain**—>35 kcal/kg |
| estimates for protein intake/day in nonstressed versus stressed patients | • **nonstressed**—0.8 g/kg, • **stressed**—1.5 g/kg |
| modes of feeding | • **oral supplementation**— * preferable mode, * less expensive, * fewer complications, • *enteral*— * tube feeding, * maintains mucosal integrity, * less translocation of bacteria from GI lumen to blood: less risk for sepsis, * preferred over the parenteral route, • *parenteral*— * peripheral IV for short-term Rx <10 days, * TPN via a catheter in the internal jugular/subclavian vein if >10 days is anticipated for nutritional support, * danger of infection: ♦ *Staphylococcus aureus* most common, ♦ *Candida* sepsis |
| contraindications for enteral feeding | • **short bowel syndrome**, • **intestinal obstruction**, • **severe vomiting/diarrhea**, • **enterocolitis**, • **GI fistula** |
| complications of enteral feeding | • **diarrhea**, • *electrolyte imbalance*— * hypo/hyperkalemia, * hypo/hypernatremia, * hypomagnesemia, * hypophosphatemia, • *hyperglycemia*—particularly in diabetics and septic patients, • *aspiration*, • *bowel motility dysfunction* |

*Table continued on following page*

Table 4–2. NUTRITIONAL ASSESSMENT IN SURGERY,
PROTEIN-CALORIE MALNUTRITION (PCM), ENTERAL
AND PARENTERAL THERAPY, TRACE METAL DEFICIENCY
*Continued*

| Most Common... | Answer and Explanation |
|---|---|
| complications of TPN | • **diarrhea**— * normal AG metabolic acidosis, * hypokalemia, * hypomagnesemia, • *liver dysfunction*— * fatty liver: due to excessive CHO and synthesis of VLDL, * transaminasemia, * gallstones: usually acalculous type, • *trace element deficiencies*—see below, • *essential fatty acid deficiency*—see below, • *increased serum BUN*—due to excess protein in the TPN mixture, • *hyperglycemia*— * often due to HNKC: there is enough insulin to prevent ketosis but not enough to prevent hyperglycemia, * hyperglycemia may be a sign of early sepsis, • *catheter infection*— * *Staphylococcus aureus* is the most common pathogen, * *Candida* is the most common fungal pathogen: culture blood and the catheter tip, • *pneumothorax*— * related to catheter placement, * always order a chest x-ray postcatheter placement |
| essential fatty acids | • **linolenic**— * ω-3 fatty acid, * cardioprotective: ♦ decreases platelet aggregation, ♦ limits the size of a myocardial infarction, * inhibits the synthesis of $TXA_2$ by platelets: ♦ decreases thrombogenesis, ♦ produces $TXA_3$, which is less thrombogenic, * ω-3 FAs are present in: ♦ canola oil, ♦ fish oil, • **linoleic**— * ω-6 fatty acid, * it is involved in the synthesis of arachidonic acid: increases the synthesis of inflammatory types of prostaglandins, * ω-6 FAs are present in: ♦ corn oil, ♦ safflower oil, ♦ sunflower oil, ♦ soybean oil |
| S/S of essential fatty acid deficiency | • **eczematous rash**, • *alopecia*, • *thrombocytopenia*, • *poor wound healing*, • *decreased intraocular pressure*—due to decreased linoleic acid and decrease in prostaglandin synthesis |
| S/S of zinc deficiency | • **perioral pustular rash**, • *darkening in skin creases*, • *dysgeusia*—decreased taste, • *decreased wound healing*—cofactor for collagenase in remodeling wounds, • *impaired cellular immunity* |

**Table 4–2. NUTRITIONAL ASSESSMENT IN SURGERY,
PROTEIN-CALORIE MALNUTRITION (PCM), ENTERAL
AND PARENTERAL THERAPY, TRACE METAL DEFICIENCY**
*Continued*

| Most Common... | Answer and Explanation |
|---|---|
| S/S of copper deficiency | • **microcytic anemia**—cofactor for ferroxidase: converts iron to ferric state in order to bind to transferrin, • *neutropenia,* • *poor wound healing*—cofactor in lysyl oxidase: responsible for producing the cross-bridging of collagen |
| S/S of chromium deficiency | • **hyperglycemia**—chromium is part of the glucose tolerance factor: enhances insulin activity, • *peripheral neuropathy,* • *encephalopathy* |
| S/S of selenium deficiency | • **myopathy,** • *cardiomyopathy* [**Note:** selenium is an antioxidant that neutralizes peroxide and enhances production of glutathione.] |
| S/S of manganese deficiency | • **dermatitis,** • *impairs the synthesis of vitamin K–dependent clotting factors* |
| nutritional problems in renal failure | • **inability to handle a urea load**—must restrict protein intake to ~0.5 g/kg, • *increased incidence of DM,* • *hyperphosphatemia,* • *negative nitrogen balance* |
| nutritional problems in liver disease | • **hepatic encephalopathy**—accumulation of ammonia and false neurotransmitters, • *malabsorption*— * due to bile salt deficiency, * leads to: ♦ fat-soluble deficiencies, ♦ iron/folate deficiency, • *retention of salt/ water*—due to secondary aldosteronism [**Note:** branched-chain amino acids are utilized in the Rx of liver disease. Muscle has enzymes to metabolize these amino acids. Medium-chain fatty acids are also administered, since they can be reabsorbed without digestion.] |
| nutritional problems in cancer | • **anorexia**—?deranged CNS satiety center, • **cachexia**— * due to tumor necrosis factor-α, * poor intake and utilization |
| nutritional problems in DM | • **hyper/hypoglycemia**— * hyperglycemia predisposes to sepsis, * hypoglycemia may precipitate seizures/shock, * insulin requirements increase with stress, • *trace metal deficiencies*—zinc in particular, • *poor wound healing* |

*Table continued on following page*

**Table 4–2. NUTRITIONAL ASSESSMENT IN SURGERY, PROTEIN-CALORIE MALNUTRITION (PCM), ENTERAL AND PARENTERAL THERAPY, TRACE METAL DEFICIENCY**
*Continued*

**Question:** Which of the following clinical/laboratory findings are more often associated with kwashiorkor than marasmus? **SELECT 4**
- (A) Decreased total caloric intake
- (B) Normal midarm muscle circumference
- (C) Anemia
- (D) Low serum albumin/transferrin
- (E) Normal cutaneous hypersensitivity
- (F) Broomstick extremities
- (G) Severe thenar/temporal atrophy
- (H) Total lymphocyte count <1200 mm³

**Answers:** (B), (C), (D), (H). Kwashiorkor patients usually have a normal midarm muscle circumference (**choice B is correct**), anemia (**choice C is correct**, multifactorial), low serum albumin/transferrin (**choice D is correct**), and a low total lymphocyte count (**choice H is correct**). Patients with kwashiorkor have a normal total caloric intake; however the protein intake is decreased (**choice A is incorrect**). Marasmus patients are more likely to have a decreased total caloric intake. Marasmus rather than kwashiorkor patients are more likely to have a normal cutaneous hypersensitivity (**choice E is incorrect**), broomstick extremities (**choice F is incorrect**), severe thenar/temporal atrophy (**choice G is incorrect**), and a normal total lymphocyte count.

AcAc = acetoacetic acid, AG = anion gap, BEE = basal energy expenditure, BMI = body mass index, BUN = blood urea nitrogen, CAD = coronary artery disease, CH = cholesterol, CHO = carbohydrate, CoA = coenzyme A, DM = diabetes mellitus, FA = fatty acid, Hgb = hemoglobin, HNKC = hyperosmolar nonketotic coma, LDL = low density lipoprotein, β-OHB = β-hydroxybutyric acid, PCM = protein-calorie malnutrition, S/S = signs/symptoms, TG = triglyceride, TPN = total parenteral nutrition, TV = tidal volume, $TXA_2/A_3$ = thromboxane $A_2/A_3$, VC = vital capacity, VLDL = very low density lipoprotein.

**Table 4–3. INTRAOPERATIVE AND POSTOPERATIVE COMPLICATIONS**

| Most Common... | Answer and Explanation |
|---|---|
| intraoperative causes of fever | • **pre-existing infection,** • *malignant hyperthermia,* • *hemolytic transfusion reaction*— see Table 2–14 |
| mechanism of malignant hyperthermia | • **AD disorder**—variable penetrance, • **triggers**— * succinylcholine, * volatile anesthetics, • **pathogenesis**—hypermetabolic disorder due to movement of calcium into skeletal muscle, leading to rapid consumption of ATP |

### Table 4–3. INTRAOPERATIVE AND POSTOPERATIVE COMPLICATIONS *Continued*

| Most Common... | Answer and Explanation |
|---|---|
| clinical findings in malignant hyperthermia | • **fever**— * 40–42°C: 104–108°F, * temperature increases 1–2°C q5min, * intraoperative or postoperative complication, • *trismus of the masseter muscle*—early premonitory sign, • *respiratory acidosis/hypoxemia*—early finding, • *tachycardia,* • *tachypnea,* • *HTN,* • *hyperkalemia,* • *rhabdomyolysis/myoglobinuria,* • *DIC,* • *ATN* |
| Rx of malignant hyperthermia | **dantrolene**—reduces the movement of calcium into muscle |
| causes of postop tachycardia | • **pain/fear/anxiety,** • *fever,* • *"relative hypotension" in a patient who is normally hypertensive* |
| causes of postop tachypnea | • **atelectasis,** • *pneumonia,* • *PE,* • *decreased lung capacity*— * ileus, * pleural effusion |
| causes of postop hypoxemia | • **pulmonary**— * **atelectasis,** * aspiration, * ARDS, * hypoventilation: e.g., anesthesia, * obesity: poor diaphragm excursion, • *cardiovascular*— * heart failure, * blood loss: tissue hypoxia, normal $PaO_2$ |
| anatomic sites for the origin of postop fever | • **lungs,** • *wound,* • *visceral compartments,* • *urinary tract,* • *intravascular devices* |
| causes of postop fever | • **atelectasis**— * most common cause of fever in first 24–36 hrs, ◆ occurs in ~25% of patients, ◆ RUQ surgery most hazardous, * aspiration, • *fever 2–7 days*— * **pneumonia** (3–10 days), * catheter-related sepsis/phlebitis (2–3 days), * UTI (3–5 days), * PE (5–7 days), * wound infection ( ◆ see Table 4–4, ◆ 5th–10th day), • *fever >7 days*— * intra-abdominal abscess, * DTR (see Table 2–14), * drug allergy, * DVT, * halothane hepatotoxicity |
| causes of atelectasis postoperatively | • **anesthesia**—dry secretions, • *systemic analgesic effects,* • *painful upper abdominal incisions* [**Note:** these all reduce tidal volume, which predisposes to atelectasis.] |

*Table continued on following page*

Table 4–3. **INTRAOPERATIVE AND POSTOPERATIVE COMPLICATIONS** Continued

| Most Common... | Answer and Explanation |
| --- | --- |
| S/S of atelectasis | • **fever**—not related to infection, • *cyanosis*—if widespread, • *dyspnea/tachypnea*— * hypoxemia, * respiratory acidosis, • *elevation of diaphragm*—loss of lung mass on ipsilateral side, • *inspiratory lag on inspiration on ipsilateral side,* • *decreased breath sounds,* • *increased tactile fremitus* |
| Rx of atelectasis | • **incentive spirometry,** • $O_2$ |
| complication of postoperative atelectasis | **pneumonia**—particularly if atelectasis is >3 days |
| causes of postoperative aspiration | • **during intubation/altered level of consciousness,** • *type of surgery*—thoracic or abdominal surgery, • *recovering from anesthesia* |
| S/S of gastric aspiration | **acute-onset dyspnea, wheezing, tachypnea**— * 2–3 hrs postaspiration, * due to a chemical pneumonia, * pH < 2.5 increases damage to bronchi, vessels, and alveoli, • *signs of bronchial obstruction*—due to food particles |
| method of Dx of gastric aspiration | • **recovery of gastric contents after suctioning the endotracheal tube,** • *ABGs*—severe hypoxemia, • *chest x-ray*—patchy alveolar infiltrates at both lung bases |
| complications of gastric aspiration | • **ARDS,** • *pneumonia,* • *lung abscess* |
| Rx of gastric aspiration | • **supportive**— * $O_2$, * antibiotics, if pneumonia develops: usually develops after 2–3 days, * administer TPN or enteral tubes distal to the pylorus, * corticosteroids are controversial, • **prognosis**—mortality 50% |
| cause of fever after 3 days | **pneumonia** |
| causes of pneumonia | • **atelectasis,** • *aspiration,* • *excessive secretions* |

### Table 4–3. INTRAOPERATIVE AND POSTOPERATIVE COMPLICATIONS *Continued*

| Most Common... | Answer and Explanation |
|---|---|
| risk factors for pneumonia | • **ventilatory support**— * increased risk for *Pseudomonas aeruginosa* from respirators, * lack of cough reflex, • *peritonitis—ileus* causes bowel distention → atelectasis/aspiration, • *medications that suppress cough reflex,* • *dysfunctional alveolar macrophages*—due to: ♦ $O_2$, ♦ edema, ♦ corticosteroids |
| S/S pneumonia | • **sudden onset of high fever with productive cough,** • *dyspnea/tachypnea,* • *pleuritic chest pain,* • *decreased percussion,* • *inspiratory rales,* • *increased tactile fremitus* |
| organisms producing pneumonia | **nosocomial organisms colonizing upper airways**— * *Escherichia coli,* * *P. aeruginosa:* respirators, * *Staphylococcus aureus* |
| Rx of pneumonia | • **antibiotics**— * based on the Gram stain/culture, * empiric Rx of nosocomial pneumonia: IV imipenem cilastatin, or IV meropenem, * prophylactic antibiotics do not reduce the risk of gram-negative pneumonia, • $O_2$, • *clear secretions*—encourage patient to cough |
| COD following surgery | **pneumonia** |
| organisms involved in intravascular catheter sepsis | • ***Staphylococcus aureus,*** • *Staphylococcus epidermidis,* • *Candida* |
| S/S of catheter-related sepsis | **sudden development of a high, spiking fever**—a positive blood culture with *Staphylococcus aureus* is invariably catheter-related |
| clinical findings in candidemia | • **predisposing cause**— * indwelling catheters for TPN, * broad-spectrum antibiotics, * neutropenia, • **clinical**— * accounts for 5–10% of nosocomial septicemias, * nodular skin lesions: metastatic abscesses, * fluffy white chorioretinal exudates: endophthalmitis, * fever unresponsive to empirical antibacterial agents, • **Rx**— * replace indwelling catheter, * amphotericin B or high-dose fluconazole |

*Table continued on following page*

Table 4–3. INTRAOPERATIVE AND POSTOPERATIVE
COMPLICATIONS *Continued*

| Most Common... | Answer and Explanation |
|---|---|
| Rx of catheter-related sepsis | • **remove IV catheter**— * culture tip with rolling method across media, * >15 colonies correlates with infection, • **antibiotics**— * vancomycin for staphylococci, * amphotericin B or fluconazole for *Candida* |
| source of postop UTI | **indwelling urinary catheter**—organisms are more resistant to Rx than are community-acquired uropathogens |
| Rx of postop UTI | • **remove indwelling catheter as soon as possible**, • **antibiotics**— * uncomplicated infection: TMP/SMX, * complicated infection: ampicillin + gentamicin |
| risks for intra-abdominal abscess | • **penetrating trauma of the gut**, • *patients with complications following elective GI procedure*, • *emergency operations for spontaneous GI perforations* |
| S/S of intra-abdominal abscess | • **fever**— * intermittent spiking or sawtooth pattern, * usually occurs within 5–7 days, • *abdominal pain/tenderness*—pelvic abscess can be felt on rectal exam, • *neutrophilic leukocytosis* |
| test of choice to R/O intra-abdominal abscess | **CT scan of abdomen/pelvis** |
| Rx of intra-abdominal abscess | • **drainage of abscess**, • *surgical exploration in patients with persistent fever/high risk*, • *antibiotics*—e.g., * cefoxitin + gentamicin or imipenem alone |
| time-frame for postop PE | **5–7 days**—see Table 4–1 for risk factors |
| site of origin for most PE | **proximal deep veins of thigh**— * femoral, iliac, popliteal, * see Table 2–13 |
| pathophysiologic effects of a PE | • **perfusion defect in first 24–48 hrs**—this produces increased dead space, • **low PaO$_2$**—hypoxemia causes generalized vasoconstriction of pulmonary vessels: this further exacerbates the perfusion defect, • **segmental atelectasis after 24–48 hrs**— * surfactant is decreased, * segmental atelectasis causes intrapulmonary shunting of blood |

## Table 4–3. INTRAOPERATIVE AND POSTOPERATIVE COMPLICATIONS *Continued*

| Most Common... | Answer and Explanation |
|---|---|
| site in the lungs for a PE | **right lower lobe**—perfusion is greater than ventilation in this lung area |
| initial S/S of a PE | • **tachypnea (sign)/dyspnea (symptom),** • *pleuritic chest pain,* • *cough,* • *leg pain—DVT,* • *hemoptysis,* • *fever,* • *wheezing*—TXA$_2$ released from platelets in embolus has bronchoconstrictive effects |
| chest x-ray findings in a PE | • **parenchymal infiltrate with or without a pleural effusion**— * ~45% have this finding, * 10% of patients have a normal chest x-ray, • *area of hypovascularity*—called Westermark's sign: appears as an area of hyperlucent lung, • *pleural-based wedge-shaped density*—called Hampton's hump: represents area of infarction |
| initial step in Dx of a PE | **ventilation/perfusion scan**— * normal scan rules out a PE, * a high probability scan has a high predictive value for PE, * a low probability scan does not exclude PE and requires pulmonary angiography: gold standard test [**Note**: most centers are also ordering a D-dimer along with the ventilation/perfusion scan to increase overall sensitivity. Some centers are using spiral CT and D-dimers.] |
| lab and ECG abnormalities in PE | • **respiratory alkalosis**—PaCO$_2$ < 33 mmHg: normal is 33–45 mmHg, • *PaO$_2$ < 80 mmHg*— * 85% of cases, * due to the perfusion defect, • *increased A–a gradient*–see Table 3–1, • D-*dimers in large emboli*—cross-linked fibrin monomers indicating plasmin breakdown of a fibrin clot, • *ECG*— * RV strain pattern in massive emboli: S$_1$Q$_3$T$_3$, * nonspecific ST-T wave changes, * sinus tachycardia in ~80% |
| Rx of PE | • **anticoagulation**— * IV heparin with PTT 1.5–2.5 × control value, * warfarin is started coincident with heparin: INR 2.0–3.0, * patients are sent home on warfarin, • *supplemental O$_2$,* • *thrombolytic therapy*—for patients with massive emboli and hypotension |

*Table continued on following page*

## Table 4–3. INTRAOPERATIVE AND POSTOPERATIVE COMPLICATIONS *Continued*

| Most Common... | Answer and Explanation |
|---|---|
| causes of chest pain postop | • **ischemia**— * 0.4% have an AMI, * > 50% are asymptomatic: ? effect of anesthesia in blunting the pain response, • *atelectasis,* • *pneumonia,* • *pneumothorax,* • *PE*—see above |
| causes of postop spontaneous pneumothorax | • **insertion of a subclavian catheter,** • *PEEP therapy,* • *type of surgery*— * adrenalectomy, * nephrectomy |
| S/S of a spontaneous pneumothorax | • **sudden onset of severe pleuritic chest pain with dyspnea,** • *hyperresonance to percussion,* • *absent tactile fremitus,* • *ipsilateral tracheal deviation,* • *elevation of ipsilateral hemidiaphragm* |
| S/S of a tension pneumothorax | • **respiratory failure/cardiovascular collapse**— * movement of mediastinal structures to the contralateral side by expanding pressure in the ipsilateral pleural cavity: compression atelectasis of the lung from increased positive pressure in the pleural cavity, * air enters the pleural cavity through a pleural tear: ♦ flap opens on inspiration and causes air to enter the cavity, ♦ flap closes on expiration, which results in a continual build-up of positive pressure in the cavity, • *hypotension*—decreased venous return, • *bulging of intercostal muscles,* • *depression of ipsilateral diaphragm,* • *tracheal deviation to contralateral side* |
| x-ray appearance of a pneumothorax | • **pleural shadow separates from the chest wall in spontaneous pneumothorax,** • **Dx of a tension pneumothorax is clinically made** |
| Rx of a spontaneous pneumothorax | **depends on the size of the pneumothorax**—a symptomatic pneumothorax requires chest tube placement under water seal drainage, with suction to re-expand the lung: must re-create the negative intrathoracic pressure to re-expand lungs |
| Rx of tension pneumothorax | **needle decompression**— * a large-bore needle is inserted into the 2nd ICS in the midclavicular line: this relieves excess positive pressure, * a chest tube is inserted |

### Table 4–3. INTRAOPERATIVE AND POSTOPERATIVE COMPLICATIONS *Continued*

| Most Common... | Answer and Explanation |
|---|---|
| causes of arrhythmias | • **induction of anesthesia**—majority are atrial arrhythmias, • *electrolyte imbalance*— * hypokalemia, * metabolic alkalosis, • *hypoxemia*— * atelectasis, * pneumonia |
| COD following carotid endarterectomy | **AMI** |
| cause of shock postop | **bleeding**—usually hemoperitoneum post-abdominal surgery: usually due to a slipped ligature |
| cause of fever and parotid pain postop | **acute sialadenitis**— * this complication usually occurs in elderly, intubated patients with poor oral hygiene, * dry secretions prompt infections, * usually occurs 1 wk postop, * pathogen is usually *Staphylococcus aureus* |
| Rx of acute sialadenitis | **drainage + antibiotics** |
| causes of postop N/V | • **combination of surgery itself + anesthesia**—N/V most commonly occurs when drugs act directly on the CTZ area in the brain, • *AMI*, • *ileus*— * paralytic, * mechanical, • *intra-abdominal abscess* |
| Rx of postop N/V | • **R/O obstruction**—order an obstruction GI series, • **NG suction**, • **medication**—use central-acting antiemetics, • **gastric motility agents**— * metoclopramide, * cisapride |
| causes of postop abdominal pain | • **incisional pain**, • *intra-abdominal sepsis*— * fever, * neutrophilic leukocytosis, * >5 days postop, • *acute pancreatitis*—most often post CBD exploration, • *perforated duodenal ulcer*, • *ischemia/bowel infarction*— * bloody diarrhea, * pain out of proportion to physical findings, * lactic acidosis |
| causes of ileus postop | • **combination of abdominal surgery + anesthesia**—e.g., commonly associated with the use of morphine for postop pain, • *inflammation*— * peritonitis, * pancreatitis, • *electrolyte abnormalities*—e.g., hyperkalemia, • *pain* |

*Table continued on following page*

### Table 4–3. INTRAOPERATIVE AND POSTOPERATIVE
### COMPLICATIONS *Continued*

| Most Common... | Answer and Explanation |
|---|---|
| time-frame for the return of peristalsis in the small bowel | **24 hrs** |
| time-frame for the return of peristalsis in the stomach and right colon | **48 hrs** |
| time-frame for the return of peristalsis in the left colon | **72 hrs** |
| causes of postop bowel obstruction | • **paralytic ileus**— * nonmechanical cause of ileus: e.g., metabolic disturbances (see ileus discussion), * inflammation, * ischemia, • *mechanical obstruction*— * adhesions, * internal hernia |
| cause of an anastomotic leak | **technical complication**— * it is usually a well-localized leak, * complications: ♦ pericolic abscess, ♦ enterocutaneous fistula, ♦ diffuse peritonitis |
| causes of postop jaundice | • **hepatocellular insufficiency**—due to hepatic cell necrosis from anesthesia drugs, • *extensive hepatic resection,* • *CBD obstruction*— * stone, * direct surgical injury, • *acute acalculous cholecystitis*— * one-third have jaundice, * common in patients with prolonged ICU stays |
| causes of postop hyponatremia | • **iatrogenic**—excessive infusion of hypotonic fluids, • *SiADH*— * stress-induced, * medications: e.g., morphine, • *GI losses of fluid* |
| causes of postop hypernatremia | • **iatrogenic**—infusion of sodium-rich TPN, • *insensible water loss*—fever |
| cause of postop hypokalemia | **GI fluid loss**— * diarrhea, * N/V, * NG suction |
| causes of postop hyperkalemia | • **renal failure,** • *crush injuries*—release of $K^+$ from damaged tissue, • *massive transfusions* |
| metabolic abnormality postop | **metabolic alkalosis**— * N/V, * NG suction |

### Table 4–3. INTRAOPERATIVE AND POSTOPERATIVE COMPLICATIONS *Continued*

| Most Common... | Answer and Explanation |
|---|---|
| causes of postop metabolic acidosis | • **renal failure,** • *diarrhea*—due to TPN |
| causes of postop respiratory alkalosis | • **anxiety related to pain,** • *excessive mechanical ventilation,* • *PE* |
| causes of postop respiratory acidosis | • **hypoventilation**—*anesthesia,* • *COPD patient,* • *ARDS* |
| causes of postop shock | **see Table 3–2** |
| causes of postop oliguria | • **prerenal azotemia**—see below, • *renal azotemia*—see below, • *postrenal azotemia*—see below [**Note:** oliguria is defined as a urine flow <400 mL/day or <20 mL/hr.] |
| tests used to evaluate oliguria | • **FENa$^+$,** • **random UNa$^+$,** • **UOsm,** • **serum BUN/creatinine ratio,** • **urinalysis (UA)** |
| causes of an increased serum BUN | • **decreased GFR**—e.g., * CHF, * shock, * hypovolemia, • *renal failure*—e.g., ischemic ATN, • *postrenal obstruction*—e.g., stone, • *increased intake of protein*—bacterial ureases convert urea into ammonia, which is reabsorbed and converted into urea in the liver urea cycle, • *TPN,* • *GI bleed*—blood is protein and protein is converted by ureases into ammonia [**Note:** a decrease in GFR leads to an increased proximal reabsorption of urea (called prerenal azotemia).] |
| causes of a low serum BUN | • **chronic liver disease**—dysfunctional urea cycle, • *pregnancy*— * dilutional effect of increased plasma volume, * increased renal clearance, • *SiADH*— * dilutional effect of excess water added to the ECF, * increased renal clearance of urea, • *malnutrition*—decreased protein intake |
| pathologic causes of an elevated creatinine | • **prerenal azotemia**—decreased GFR reduces clearance of creatinine, • *renal failure*—cannot excrete creatinine, • *postrenal obstruction*— * cannot excrete creatinine, * decreases GFR |

*Table continued on following page*

**Table 4–3. INTRAOPERATIVE AND POSTOPERATIVE
COMPLICATIONS** *Continued*

| Most Common... | Answer and Explanation |
|---|---|
| effect of prerenal azotemia on the serum BUN/ creatinine ratio | **BUN/creatinine ratio > 15/1** [**Note:** in prerenal azotemia, a decrease in GFR leads to an increase in proximal tubule reabsorption of urea. Creatinine also increases owing to reduced renal clearance; however, it is not reabsorbed in the kidneys as urea is. The normal BUN/creatinine ratio is 10/1. In prerenal azotemia, a disproportionate increase in urea over creatinine leads to >15/1 ratio. For example, if the serum BUN is 80 mg/dL and the serum creatinine is 2 mg/dL, the ratio is 40/1.] |
| effect of renal failure on serum BUN/ creatinine ratio | **BUN/creatinine ratio remains ~10/1** [**Note:** in the presence of intrinsic renal disease, the serum BUN and creatinine are equally affected, hence they both increase at the same rate. For example, if the serum BUN is 80 mg/dL, the serum creatinine increases proportionately (e.g., 8 mg/dL), hence the ratio remains ~10/1.] |
| effect of postrenal obstruction on the serum BUN/ creatinine ratio | **BUN/creatinine ratio is >15/1** [**Note:** in postrenal azotemia related to obstruction to urine flow behind the kidneys, there is a back diffusion of urea from the urine into the blood and in addition a decrease in GFR. This results in a disproportionate increase in the serum BUN over the serum creatinine, leading to a ratio that is >15/1.] |
| lab abnormality in early tubular dysfunction | **inability to concentrate urine** |
| use of the UOsm in the work-up of oliguria | **UOsm is an index of the concentrating capacity of the kidneys**— * a UOsm <350 mOsm/kg indicates tubular dysfunction, * a UOsm >500 mOsm/kg indicates intact tubular function |
| use of the $FENa^+$ in the work-up of oliguria | **$FENa^+$ is an index of tubular function**— * $FENa^+ = (UNa^+/PNa^+) \div (UCr/PCr) \times 100$, * a value <1 indicates intact tubular function, * a value >1 (usually >2) indicates tubular dysfunction |

### Table 4–3. INTRAOPERATIVE AND POSTOPERATIVE
### COMPLICATIONS *Continued*

| Most Common... | Answer and Explanation |
|---|---|
| use of the random urine Na⁺ in the work-up of oliguria | **random UNa⁺ is an index of tubular function—** * a $UNa^+$ <20 mEq/L indicates good tubular function, * a $UNa^+$ >40 mEq/L indicates poor tubular function |
| use of the UA in the work-up of oliguria | • **dipstick reactions—** * R/O proteinuria, * R/O hematuria, • **sediment exam**—cast identification: e.g., ♦ renal tubular casts are the key casts in ATN, ♦ RBC cast is the key cast in oliguria secondary to glomerulonephritis |
| profile for good tubular function | • **$FENa^+$ <1,** • **UOsm >500 mOsm/kg,** • **random $UNa^+$ <20 mEq/L,** • **BUN/serum creatinine ratio >15/1,** • **UA without renal tubular casts or proteinuria** |
| profile for poor tubular function | • **$FENa^+$ >1**—usually >2, • **UOsm <350 mOsm/kg,** • **random $UNa^+$ >40 mEq/L,** • **BUN/serum creatinine ratio <15/1,** • **UA with renal tubular casts/proteinuria** |
| surgical cause of prerenal azotemia | **hypovolemia—** * hemorrhage, * fluid losses |
| profile for prerenal azotemia | • **$FENa^+$: <1,** • **$UNa^+$: <20**—unless the patient is taking a diuretic, • **UOsm: >500 mOsm/kg,** • **BUN/creatinine: >15/1,** • **UA: normal** |
| Rx of prerenal azotemia | • **flush the urinary catheter to R/O obstruction of catheter,** • **fluid challenge**—use 500 mL 0.45% NaCl, • **insert SGC**—measure CVP and PCWP, * give fluids to restore volume: monitor CVP and PCWP to avoid overhydration |
| causes of ARF of surgical importance | • **hypovolemia**—e.g., * hemorrhage, * leads to ischemic ATN, • *AMI/CHF,* • *ureteral obstruction*—e.g., * blood clot, * least common cause of ARF, * this is the most treatable cause of ARF: emphasizes the importance of bladder catheterization as an early part of an oliguria work-up, • *tubular injury*—e.g., * drugs, * IVP dye, • *tubulointerstitial disease*—e.g., drugs |

*Table continued on following page*

**Table 4–3.  INTRAOPERATIVE AND POSTOPERATIVE COMPLICATIONS** *Continued*

| Most Common... | Answer and Explanation |
|---|---|
| patterns of ATN | • **ischemic ATN**— * oliguric, * polyuric: >800 mL/day, • *nephrotoxic ATN* |
| cause of ischemic ATN | **prerenal azotemia**—see below |
| causes of nephrotoxic ATN | • **drugs**—e.g., * **aminoglycosides,** * cyclosporine, • *radiocontrast agents*—patients at risk include: ♦ **DM,** ♦ multiple myeloma, ♦ old age, ♦ volume depleted, ♦ SLE, • *crush injuries with myoglobinuria* |
| mechanisms of oliguria in ATN | • **vasoconstriction of the afferent arterioles,** • **sloughed-off tubular cells block the lumen,** • **increased interstitial pressure from fluid leaking through damaged tubular BMs,** • **decreased glomerular permeability** |
| profile for ATN | • **FENa$^+$—>1,** • **UNa$^+$—>40,** • **UOsm—<350 mOsm/kg,** • **BUN/creatinine—<15/1,** • **UA—** * pigmented renal tubular casts, * "dirty urine" |
| sodium/water problems associated with ARF | **sodium/water retention**—correlates with: ♦ weight gain (Na$^+$ retention), ♦ hyponatremia (water retention) |
| acid-base problems in ARF | **increased AG metabolic acidosis**—decreased excretion of H$^+$ ions |
| electrolyte problems in ARF | • **hyponatremia/hypernatremia**— * hyponatremia occurs if the gain in water is greater than the gain in salt, * hypernatremia occurs if the gain of salt is greater than the gain in water, • *hyperkalemia*—decreased renal excretion |
| hematologic problems in ARF | • **normocytic anemia**—decreased EPO, • *GI bleeding*—hemorrhagic gastritis |
| metabolic problems in ARF | • **high serum creatinine**—increases when GFR is <40% of normal, * increases 0.5–1.0 mg/dL/day, • **high serum BUN**—increases 10–20 mg/dL/day, • **hyperphosphatemia**—decreased excretion, • **hypocalcemia**—decreased renal synthesis of 1,25-dihydroxy-vitamin D, • **hyperuricemia**—decreased excretion |

### Table 4–3. INTRAOPERATIVE AND POSTOPERATIVE COMPLICATIONS *Continued*

| Most Common... | Answer and Explanation |
|---|---|
| systemic problems in ARF | • **uremic pericarditis**— * usually hemorrhagic, * may produce cardiac tamponade, • *uremic syndrome*—accumulation of toxic products with multiorgan dysfunction |
| phases of ARF | • **oliguric phase**— * lasts 1–2 wks, * azotemia, * hyperkalemia, * metabolic acidosis, • **diuretic phase**— * usually occurs during the 3rd week, * hypokalemia may occur, * severe hypercalcemia may occur if ATN is secondary to rhabdomyolysis, • **recovery phase**—GFR improves over subsequent 3–12 mos |
| Rx of ARF | • **fluid challenge**—useful in oliguric patients if they are not already volume overloaded, • *loop diuretic*— * used to convert an oliguric into a nonoliguric ARF (also called polyuric ARF), * flushes tubular cells out of the lumen, • **keep the patient hemodynamically stable**— * Rx volume depletion with 0.45 saline, * Rx volume excess with loop diuretics, • **low-dose dopamine**—renal vasodilator, • **daily weight**—restrict sodium if weight increases, • **limit dietary protein**— * 0.5 g/kg/day, * reduces the urea load presented to the kidneys, • **Rx hyperphosphatemia**—see Table 1–3, • **Rx hyperkalemia**— * see Table 1–3, * Rx when the serum $K^+$ is >6.5 mEq/L or the ECG is abnormal, • **Rx metabolic acidosis**—Rx if bicarbonate is < 15–16 mEq/L, • **avoid all nephrotoxic drugs**, • **uses of dialysis**— * keep serum BUN < 100 mg/dL, * Rx hemorrhagic pericarditis, * Rx peripheral neuropathy, * Rx for volume overload resistant to diuretics, * Rx hyperkalemia/hyperphosphatemia when medical management is inadequate |
| COD in ARF | • **infection**—sepsis, • *cardiopulmonary disease* |
| time-frame for aminoglycoside-induced ATN | **5–10 days**— * some degree of ARF occurs in 10–15% of patients, * gentamicin/amikacin are the most toxic: streptomycin is least toxic, * usually produces polyuric ATN, * $K^+$/$Mg^{++}$ wasting are common |

*Table continued on following page*

Table 4–3. **INTRAOPERATIVE AND POSTOPERATIVE COMPLICATIONS** *Continued*

| Most Common... | Answer and Explanation |
|---|---|
| type of nephrotoxic ATN in which alkalinization of urine is helpful | **rhabdomyolysis**—heme pigments produce intrarenal vasoconstriction and tubular obstruction |
| clinical findings in myoglobin-induced ATN | • **clinical settings**— * **crush injuries,** * alcoholism, • **usually polyuric type of ATN,** • **lab findings**—similar to those of ATN |
| Rx of myoglobin-induced ATN | • **forced diuresis**—mannitol is used to remove heme pigments, • **alkalinize the urine** |
| mechanisms of ARF due to radiocontrast dyes | • **intrarenal vasoconstriction,** • **tubular lumen obstruction,** • **direct tubular toxicity** [Note: patients become oliguric in 1–2 days after administration of the dye. $FENa^+$ is <1. It is usually reversible within a week.] |
| preventive methods to avoid radiocontrast dye-induced ARF | • **decrease dose of dye,** • **forced diuresis with normal saline,** • **adequate hydration** |
| surgical causes of postrenal azotemia | • **ureteral injury associated with surgery**— e.g., * **TAH,** * **colectomy,** • *BPH,* • *indwelling catheter obstruction,* • *cervical cancer* |
| profile for postrenal azotemia | • **$FENa^+$—>1,** • **$UNa^+$—>40,** • **UOsm—<350 mOsm/kg,** • **BUN/creatinine—<15/1,** • **UA—** normal, • **other**—renal US may demonstrate hydronephrosis or a stone |
| Rx of postrenal azotemia | • **flush the indwelling urinary catheter to R/ O catheter obstruction,** • **consult a urologist** |
| psychiatric complications postop | • **delirium tremens (DTs)**—complication in alcoholics, • **acute Wernicke's encephalopathy**—complication in alcoholics, • **intensive care syndrome,** • **postoperative psychosis** |
| causes of DTs during surgery | • **hyperventilation with production of respiratory alkalosis,** • **pre-existing nutritional deficiencies in patient** |

**Table 4–3. INTRAOPERATIVE AND POSTOPERATIVE COMPLICATIONS** *Continued*

| Most Common... | Answer and Explanation |
|---|---|
| S/S of DTs | • **tremulousness,** • **disorientation,** • **visual hallucinations,** • **agitation,** • **β-adrenergic signs**— * tachycardia, * sweating, * fear, * tachypnea, * HTN, • **incontinence,** • **seizure activity**—may dehisce wound |
| Rx of DTs | • **IV diazepam,** • *IV thiamine*—to prevent or Rx Wernicke's syndrome |
| cause of acute Wernicke's encephalopathy | **thiamine deficiency in an alcoholic** |
| S/S of Wernicke-Korsakoff syndrome | • **Wernicke's syndrome**— * confusion, * ataxia, * nystagmus, * external ophthalmoplegia, * multiple cranial nerve palsies, * peripheral neuropathy, * tachycardia, * often precipitated by infusion of glucose-containing electrolyte solutions: ♦ uses up the remaining thiamine as pyruvate is converted into acetyl CoA, ♦ always administer IV thiamine before infusing glucose, • **Korsakoff's syndrome**— * targets the limbic system, * inability to form new memories (anterograde amnesia) or recall old ones (retrograde amnesia), * confabulation |
| Rx of acute Wernicke's encephalopathy | **IV thiamine** |
| clinical features of intensive care syndrome | • **type of delirium,** • **combination of bright lights, noise, and sleep deprivation** |
| clinical features of postop psychosis | • **elderly patient with chronic disease**— * often with pre-existing mood disorder, * postabdominal or post-thoracic surgery, • *contributing factors*— * stress, * drugs, * high β-endorphins, • *delirium in 20%* |
| types of procedures predisposing to air embolism | • **head/neck surgery,** • *insertion of a central venous line* |

*Table continued on following page*

## Table 4–3. INTRAOPERATIVE AND POSTOPERATIVE
## COMPLICATIONS *Continued*

| Most Common... | Answer and Explanation |
| --- | --- |
| mechanism of air embolism | **suction of air into the venous system—** * ~100 mL of air can be fatal, * air mixes with blood in the right heart, causing frothy material to block blood into PA |
| S/S of air embolism | • **hypotension,** • **tachycardia,** • **tachypnea** |
| Rx of air embolism | • **position the patient right-side-up and head down (Trendelenburg) to trap air outside the lungs,** • *supplemental $O_2$,* • *mechanical ventilation if necessary* |

**Question:** An afebrile postoperative patient, who had a repair of a ruptured aortic aneurysm, develops oliguria. He has a serum BUN of 80 mg/dL and serum creatinine of 8 mg/dL. What additional findings would you expect in this patient? **SELECT 4**

(A) FENa$^+$ > 1
(B) UOsm > 500 mOsm/kg
(C) Normal urine sediment
(D) Random UNa$^+$ > 40 mEq/L
(E) Hypophosphatemia
(F) Normal arterial pH
(G) Hypocalcemia
(H) Normocytic anemia
(I) Hypokalemia

**Answers: (A), (D), (G), (H)**. The patient has developed ischemic ATN secondary to volume depletion from his ruptured aortic aneurysm. The BUN/creatinine ratio is 10/1 (80/8 = 10/1), indicating intrinsic renal disease. The FENa$^+$, UOsm, and random UNa$^+$ are markers of tubular function. In tubular dysfunction, the FENa$^+$ is > 1 (**choice A is correct**), UOsm < 350 mOsm/kg (**choice B is incorrect**), and the random UNa$^+$ is > 40 mEq/L (**choice D is correct**). The urine sediment should contain numerous pigmented renal tubular casts (**choice C is incorrect**). With renal disease, vitamin D synthesis is reduced, hence hypocalcemia is expected (**choice G is correct**). Reduced renal function leads to hyperphosphatemia (**choice E is incorrect**), an increased AG metabolic acidosis (**choice F is incorrect**), a normocytic anemia due to EPO deficiency (**choice H is correct**), and hyperkalemia (**choice I is incorrect**).

A–a = Alveolar-arterial, ABG = arterial blood gas, AD = autosomal dominant, AG = anion gap, AMI = acute myocardial infarction, ARDS = adult respiratory distress syndrome, ARF = acute renal failure, ATN = acute tubular necrosis, ATP = adenosine triphosphate, BPH = benign prostatic hyperplasia, BUN = blood urea nitrogen, CBD = common bile duct, CHF = congestive heart failure, CoA = coenzyme A, COD = cause of death, COPD = chronic obstructive pulmonary disease, CTZ = chemoreceptor trigger zone, CVP = central venous pressure, DIC = disseminated intravascular coagulation, DM = diabetes mellitus, DTs = delirium tremens, DTR = delayed transfusion reaction, DVT = deep venous thrombosis, ECF = extracellular fluid, EPO = erythropoietin, $FENa^+$ = fractional excretion of sodium, GFR = glomerular filtration rate, HTN = hypertension, ICS = intercostal space, INR = International Normalized Ratio, IVP = intravenous pyelogram, NG = nasogastric, N/V = nausea/vomiting, PA = pulmonary artery, PCr = plasma creatinine, PCWP = pulmonary capillary wedge pressure, PE = pulmonary embolus, PEEP = positive end-expiratory pressure, $PNa^+$ = plasma sodium, PTT = partial thromboplastin time, RUQ = right upper quadrant, RV = right ventricle, SiADH = syndrome of inappropriate antidiuretic hormone, SLE = systemic lupus erythematosus, S/S = signs/symptoms, TAH = total abdominal hysterectomy, TMP/SMX = trimethoprim/sulfamethoxazole, TPN = total parenteral nutrition, $TXA_2$ = thromboxane $A_2$, UA = urinalysis, UCr = urine creatinine, $UNa^+$ = urine sodium, UOsm = urine osmolality, UTI = urinary tract infection.

### Table 4–4. SURGICAL WOUNDS, BITES, BURNS, AND COLD INJURIES

| Most Common... | Answer and Explanation |
| --- | --- |
| types of wound healing | • **primary intention**— * approximation of edges of the wound: e.g., sutures, * wound should be <4 hrs old, • *secondary intention*— * the wound is left open to close by itself, * wound >4 hrs old, * wound is obviously infected, • *delayed primary closure*— * wound approximation after wound is left open, * bacterial contamination risk drops after 4–5 days |
| general phases of wound healing | • **inflammation**— ~24 hrs, • *epithelial regeneration*— ~48 hrs, • *fibroplasia*— * collagen synthesis, * ~3 days to 6 wks, • *wound contraction*—after 5 days |

*Table continued on following page*

Table 4–4. SURGICAL WOUNDS, BITES, BURNS, AND
COLD INJURIES *Continued*

| Most Common... | Answer and Explanation |
|---|---|
| sequential reactions in healing by primary intention | • **wound fills with fibrin clot**—fibrin is cross-linked with fibronectin for stability → • *neutrophils emigrate into the wound*— * 24 hrs → • *basal epithelial cells divide and migrate below the clot and form a continuous lining*— * 1–2 days, * wound is watertight → • *macrophages replace neutrophils in the wound*— * fibronectin is chemotactic to macrophages and opsonizes bacteria, * fibrin clot begins to lyse → • *granulation tissue begins forming + myofibroblasts migrate into the wound*— * 3–4 days, * vascular tissue buds from existing venules, * fibroblasts produce type III collagen: binds to fibronectin → • *granulation tissue peaks*— * 5 days, * beginning of wound contraction → • *tensile strength of the wound is ~10%*—7–10 days → *maximal tensile strength of 70–80%*— * greatest remodeling first 2–3 mos, * plateaus 1 yr, * type III collagen is degraded/replaced by type I collagen, * collagenases secreted by macrophages and fibroblasts: collagenase contains zinc as a cofactor, * tensile strength correlates with cross-linking of collagen |
| sign of a properly healing surgical wound | **healing ridge**— * palpable thickening extending 0.5 cm on each side of the incision after first week, * absence of this finding indicates deficient wound healing |
| functions of EGF and TGF-α | • **stimulate cell proliferation**— * **keratinocytes,** * fibroblasts, endothelial cells, • **angiogenesis,** • **collagen synthesis** |
| functions of TGF-β | • **most important factor in stimulating collagen synthesis,** • *angiogenesis,* • *high concentration in platelets* |
| functions of FGFs | **strongly angiogenic**—stimulate endothelial cell proliferation |
| functions of PDGF | • **cell proliferation**— * fibroblasts, * smooth muscle, • *chemotaxis*— * monocytes, * fibroblasts |

## Table 4–4. SURGICAL WOUNDS, BITES, BURNS, AND COLD INJURIES *Continued*

| Most Common... | Answer and Explanation |
|---|---|
| functions of MDGF | **cell proliferation**— * fibroblasts, * endothelial cells, * smooth muscle, * fibronectin stimulates monocytes to release cytokines |
| functions of IL-1 | • **chemotactic to fibroblasts**—also stimulates fibroblast proliferation, • **stimulates angiogenesis** [**Note:** IL is a cytokine secreted by monocytes.] |
| functions of fibronectin | • **insoluble glycoprotein of extracellular matrix**—major importance in early stages of wound healing, • **molecular glue**— * cross-links with: ♦ itself, ♦ collagen, ♦ fibrin, * fibronectin is a transglutaminase-like factor XIII: produces cross-links, • **chemotactic**— * macrophages, * fibroblasts, * endothelial cells |
| causes of poor wound repair | • **infection,** • *foreign body,* • *malnutrition,* • *sepsis*— * leukocyte dysfunction, * poor wound contraction, • *scurvy*— * reduces wound contractility, * poor granulation tissue formation and collagen deposition, * absence of cross-bridges between collagen fibrils, • *anemia*— * tissue hypoxia, * must be < 5 g/dL, • *zinc deficiency*—zinc is a cofactor in collagenase, • *corticosteroids*—inhibit collagen synthesis, • *chemotherapy*— * interferes with early stages of healing, * delay for 1 wk postop, • *DM*— * glucose is a culture medium for bacteria, * ischemia, * impaired chemotaxis, • *AIDS*—all stages of wound healing are impaired, • *local risk factors*— * edema, * obesity, * recent radiation, * site of wound: ♦ poor around tibia where skin adheres to bone, ♦ excellent on the face, which is more vascular |
| environmental factor accelerating wound healing | **UV light** |
| vitamin that reverses corticosteroid effects in a wound | **retinoic acid** |

*Table continued on following page*

Table 4–4. SURGICAL WOUNDS, BITES, BURNS, AND COLD INJURIES *Continued*

| Most Common... | Answer and Explanation |
|---|---|
| clinical features of a keloid versus hypertrophic scar | • **mechanism of a keloid**— * "maturation arrest" of normal healing, * rate of collagen production is greater than that of collagen degradation, * type III is greater than type I collagen, * broad bands of collagen are present, * irregular collagen bundles, • **gross**— * keloid: ♦ tumor-like mass that progresses beyond the site of initial injury, ♦ tends to recur after excision, • **hypertrophic scar**— * localized to the site of initial injury, * does not recur after excision |
| complications associated with deficient scar formation | • **wound dehiscence,** • *incisional hernia* |
| method for wound irrigation | **normal saline** |
| cleansing agents for surrounding skin | • **povidone-iodine,** • **hexachlorophene,** • **chlorhexidine gluconate** |
| classification used for surgical wounds | • **clean,** • **clean-contaminated**—minimal contamination, • **contaminated,** • **dirty** |
| features of a clean surgical wound | • **refers to elective surgery with no entry into**— * GI, * GU, * respiratory tract, * oropharynx, * vagina, • **nontraumatic,** • **examples** — * mastectomy, * herniorrhaphy, * thyroidectomy, • **infection rate**—2% |
| features of clean-contaminated surgical wound | • **wound not usually associated with trauma,** • **entry into GI, GU, respiratory tract but minimal contamination,** • **examples**— * gastrectomy, * hysterectomy, * appendectomy, • **infection rate**—3–7% |
| features of a contaminated surgical wound | • **entry into unprepared part of body with large number of endogenous microflora,** • **open, traumatic wound,** • **uncontrolled spillage from a hollow viscus,** • **minor break in sterile technique,** • **examples**— * unprepared colon surgery, * resection of obstructed/necrotic bowel, * ruptured appendix, • **infection rate**—20% |

## Table 4–4. SURGICAL WOUNDS, BITES, BURNS, AND COLD INJURIES *Continued*

| Most Common... | Answer and Explanation |
|---|---|
| features of a dirty surgical wound | • **open, traumatic, dirty wound,** • **traumatic, perforated hollow viscus,** • **evidence of pus in surgical field,** • **examples—** * intestinal fistula resection, * intra-abdominal abscess, • **infection rate—30–70%** |
| patient risk factors for infection | • **age**—>60 yrs old, • *DM,* • *obesity,* • *malnutrition,* • *chronic disease,* • *pre-existing infection,* • *immunocompromised* |
| surgical risk factors for infection | • **abdominal surgery,** • **surgery >2 hrs,** • **contamination of wound during surgery** |
| time-frame for antibiotic prophylaxis | • **few hours prior to surgery,** • **q6–8h during surgery,** • **24–48 hrs after surgery** |
| antibiotic used for prophylaxis | **cefazolin** |
| cardiovascular surgery requiring antibiotic prophylaxis | • **prosthetic valve replacement,** • **peripheral artery/aorta bypass surgery with prosthetic graft** |
| orthopedic surgery requiring antibiotic prophylaxis | • **total joint replacement,** • **internal fixation of fractures,** • **traumatic wound** |
| GI surgery requiring antibiotic prophylaxis | • **biliary,** • **colorectal,** • **appendectomy,** • **ruptured viscus** |
| GYN surgery requiring antibiotic prophylaxis | • **vaginal/abdominal hysterectomy,** • **cesarean section** |
| causes of wound hematoma | • **inadequate wound hemostasis,** • *anticoagulants,* • *NSAIDs* |
| cause of wound seroma | **creation of large subcutaneous space—** collection of lymphatic fluid and/or serum |
| gross appearance of a wound hematoma/ seroma | • **swelling/pain in the wound,** • **draining of blood (hematoma) from suture line,** • **draining of nonhematogenous fluid (seroma)** |

*Table continued on following page*

Table 4–4. SURGICAL WOUNDS, BITES, BURNS, AND
COLD INJURIES *Continued*

| Most Common... | Answer and Explanation |
|---|---|
| natural history of wound hematomas/seromas | • **usually spontaneously resolve,** • *may become infected* |
| time-frame for wound dehiscence | **5th–8th postop day**—wound is weakest at this point |
| initial sign of wound dehiscence | **discharge of serosanguineous fluid from wound** |
| systemic risk factors for wound dehiscence | • **age**—>60 yrs old, • *DM,* • obesity, • *uremia,* • *immunosuppression,* • *jaundice,* • *corticosteroids* [**Note:** wound dehiscence is a partial or complete disruption of any or all layers of the operative wound. Evisceration may occur.] |
| local risk factors for wound dehiscence | • **inadequate closure**— * inadequate number of sutures, * sutures too close to edge of fascia, • *increase in intra-abdominal pressure*— e.g., * ileus, * COPD, * coughing, • *deficient wound healing*— * infection, * presence of drains/hematomas/seromas |
| Rx of wound dehiscence | • **without evisceration**— * elective reclosure of incision, * wrap abdomen with binder, • **with evisceration**— * cover exposed bowel with sterile moist towels, * elective surgery with full-thickness retention sutures |
| complications of wound dehiscence | • **infection,** • *incisional hernia,* • *increased mortality*—10% with evisceration |
| time-frame for wound infections | **4–7 days postop**—infection can occur within 24 hrs if organisms are *Streptococcus* or *Clostridium perfringens* |
| organisms producing wound infections | • ***Staphylococcus aureus,*** • *enteric gram-negatives*—bowel surgery, • streptococci |
| S/S of wound infection | • **fever**—4th–7th day postop, • *neutrophilic leukocytosis with left shift,* • *wound tenderness/erythema/swelling,* • *purulent discharge* |
| Rx of wound infection | • **open/drain wound,** • *debride devitalized tissue,* • *antibiotics*— * only if extensive cellulitis, * cefazolin is drug of 1st choice |

## Table 4–4. SURGICAL WOUNDS, BITES, BURNS, AND COLD INJURIES *Continued*

| Most Common... | Answer and Explanation |
|---|---|
| cause of myonecrosis | ***Clostridium perfringens***—gram-positive bacillus |
| cutaneous findings associated with *C. perfringens* | • **sudden pain/edema in wound site,** • *prostration,* • *foul-smelling, bloody brown serous discharge,* • *discolored skin/soft tissue,* • *crepitance in tissue due to gas* |
| Rx of *C. perfringens* myonecrosis | • **debridement,** • *clindamycin + penicillin G,* • *hyperbaric* $O_2$ |
| cause of persistent fever after opening and draining surgical wound infection | • **wound is not completely drained,** • *devitalized tissue remains,* • *if abdominal surgery*—consider coexistent intra-abdominal abscess due to same organism |
| recommendation for tetanus and diphtheria (Td) immunization | **Td vaccine series**— * Td series should be completed in adults who have not had the primary series (0, 2, and 8–14 mos) and periodic boosters at least once every 10 yrs, * nonimmunized adults should receive two doses of Td 1–2 mos apart followed by a booster dose 6–12 mos later, * Td is given to patients ≥7yrs of age, * DTP is for children <7yrs of age |
| recommendation for clean wound in immunized and non-immunized patient | • **immunized**— * clean wound, * no booster if the last booster was within 10 yrs, • **nonimmunized**— * clean wound, * give Td [**Note:** quaternary ammonium compounds are used for cleaning wounds.] |
| recommendation for dirty wound in immunized and non-immunized patient | • **immunized**— * clean wound, * if the last booster is within 5 yrs, no Td booster is necessary, * if the last booster is >5 yrs, give Td booster, • **nonimmunized**— * clean wound, * give ½ dose of immune globulin (passive immunization) into the wound and ½ in another site, * give Td: active immunization |
| types of human bites | • **hand (usually knuckle) laceration from punching the mouth of another person,** • *patient bitten by another person* |

*Table continued on following page*

**Table 4–4. SURGICAL WOUNDS, BITES, BURNS, AND
COLD INJURIES** *Continued*

| Most Common... | Answer and Explanation |
| --- | --- |
| organisms associated with human bites | • *Eikenella corrodens,* • *Streptococcus viridans,* • *Staphylococcus epidermidis,* • *Corynebacterium* spp, • *S. aureus* • *Bacteroides* spp, • *Peptostreptococcus* spp |
| organisms associated with cat bites | • *Pasteurella multocida*—causes infection within 24 hrs, • *S. aureus* [**Note:** cats tend to produce puncture wounds.] |
| organisms associated with dog bites | • *S. viridans,* • *Pasteurella multocida* [**Note:** dogs tear and crush tissue.] |
| initial Rx of bites | • **cleaning**— * quaternary ammonium compounds, * water, • *irrigation,* • *debridement* |
| bites requiring antimicrobial prophylaxis | • **human bites**— * most serious bite, * wounds are best left open, • *cat bites*— * danger of tenosynovitis, * they can be closed if properly irrigated, • *high-risk dog bites*—e.g., * hand: order an x-ray to R/O fracture, * puncture wounds, * bites older than 6–12 hrs, • *wild animals*— * bats, * raccoons, * skunks |
| antibiotic prophylaxis recommended for human, cat, dog, wild animal bites | • **amoxicillin/clavulanate**—expensive, • *penicillin V*— * cheaper, * good alternative drug |
| poisonous spider bites | • **brown recluse (*Loxosceles reclusa*)**— * common in South/Midwest, * also called the "violin spider" or "fiddler": violin-shaped mark is located on the dorsum of cephalothorax, * bites occur at night while patient is in bed or when putting on old clothes, • *black widow (Latrodectus mactans)*— * common throughout United States, * red hourglass on the ventral undersurface, * females envenomate, * bites occur when: ♦ picking up wood from wood pile, ♦ moving boxes in a dark basement, ♦ sitting down in an outdoor privy |

### Table 4–4. SURGICAL WOUNDS, BITES, BURNS, AND COLD INJURIES *Continued*

| Most Common... | Answer and Explanation |
|---|---|
| S/S of a brown recluse spider bite | **painless bite followed by intense local pain in 2–6 hrs** $\rightarrow$ **bulla/pustule surrounded by erythema ("bull's eye" lesion)** $\rightarrow$ **expanding necrotic ulcer**— * necrotoxin, * systemic findings: ♦ ATN, ♦ petechiae, ♦ hemolytic anemia |
| Rx of brown recluse bite | • **ulcer should be debrided**—some recommend early total excision of wound to reduce spreading necrosis, • *drugs*— * colchicine and dapsone, * some recommend broad-spectrum antibiotic, • *tetanus prophylaxis is recommended* |
| S/S of a black widow spider bite | • **sharp prick is followed by muscle spasms in the thighs and abdomen**— * neurotoxin, * systemic signs: ♦ chest pain, ♦ respiratory arrest, ♦ ptosis, ♦ skin rash |
| Rx of black widow bite | • **antivenin**—antivenin is recommended in children <6 yrs old, • *calcium gluconate*— reduces muscle spasms, • *tetanus prophylaxis recommended* |
| S/S associated with poisonous scorpion bites | • **paresthesias at the envenomation site,** • *HTN,* • *respiratory paralysis*—most common COD [**Note:** only 1 species is poisonous in the United States (*Centruroides* species seen in deserts of Arizona).] |
| COD due to a venomous bite in the United States | **anaphylaxis secondary to a bee sting** |
| poisonous snake envenomation in the United States | • **rattlesnake envenomation**— * rattlesnakes, copperheads, and water moccasins are pit vipers (heat-sensitive organ), * pit viper venom has phospholipase A as its main component, • *coral snake*—red and yellow colors abut each other, * type of cobra, * venom is a neurotoxin |
| S/S or rattlesnake envenomations | • **localized pain, swelling, redness**—due to the cytolytic nature of the venom, • *hypotension,* • *anaphylaxis*—histamine release, • *DIC*— * there is a drop in Hgb concentration and the platelet count, * prolonged PT and PTT, • *pulmonary edema,* • *cardiotoxicity* |

*Table continued on following page*

### Table 4–4. SURGICAL WOUNDS, BITES, BURNS, AND COLD INJURIES *Continued*

| Most Common... | Answer and Explanation |
|---|---|
| "do nots" in rattlesnake envenomations | • **tight tourniquets**—only the lymphatic flow should be occluded, • **running or excessive movement**—these increase the distribution of the venom, • **ice application**—this damages tissue and causes even greater dissemination of the venom when the tissue thaws, • **cutting into the wound to remove venom**—nerves, tendons, and muscles are frequently injured |
| Rx of rattlesnake envenomations | • **bring the patient to a hospital ASAP,** • **polyvalent crotalin antivenin**— * use antivenin if systemic signs appear, * a type I IgE-mediated hypersensitivity reaction may initially occur with horse serum antivenin: a skin test is usually performed before administering antivenin, * serum sickness: type III IC disease often occurs as a late complication, • **ceftriaxone,** • **tetanus prophylaxis** |
| S/S of coral snake envenomation | **neurologic findings**— * increased salivation, * paresthesias, * ptosis, * muscle weakness, * respiratory arrest |
| Rx of coral snake envenomation | **coral snake antivenin** |
| causes of foot ulcers in DM | • **peripheral neuropathy**— * 80%, * patients cannot feel pressure, • *pressure ulcers are complicated by:* ♦ ischemia (60%), ♦ infection of soft tissue, * osteomyelitis (R/O with an x-ray) |
| Rx of foot ulcers in DM | • **debridement,** • **culture**—tissue biopsy, • **antibiotics**—IV antibiotics: clindamycin, • **correct maldistribution of pressure on the foot**—no weight bearing is mandatory, • **improve peripheral circulation** |
| sites for pressure ulcers | • **sacrum,** • *greater trochanter,* • *ischial tuberosity,* • *calcaneus,* • *lateral malleolus* |
| risk factors for pressure ulcers | • **immobility,** • *urinary/fecal incontinence,* • *nutritional deficiency*—e.g., zinc, • *age-related changes* |

## Table 4–4.  SURGICAL WOUNDS, BITES, BURNS, AND COLD INJURIES *Continued*

| Most Common... | Answer and Explanation |
|---|---|
| causes of pressure ulcers | • **pressure**— * produces tissue ischemia by compressing capillaries, * predisposes to ulceration, • *shearing force/friction*—e.g., * patient is dragged across the bed, * angulates and occludes subcutaneous vessels, • *moisture*— * causes tissue maceration, * urine is a common offender |
| complications of pressure ulcers | • **infection**—obtain the culture from deep tissue, not the surface of the ulcer, • *osteomyelitis*— * suspect osteomyelitis when the wound does not heal, * a bone biopsy is the gold standard for culture/diagnosis in suspected osteomyelitis |
| Rx of pressure ulcers | • **rotate the patient q2h,** • *pressure-reducing mattresses,* • *debride dead tissue,* • *control urinary incontinence,* • *nutritional support,* • *antibiotics for infections* |
| factors determining burn severity | • **depth of the burn,** • *surface area,* • *burn site,* • *whether inhalation has occurred* |
| types of burns | • **partial-thickness**— * limited to the epidermis and superficial (sometimes deep) dermal layers, * this corresponds with first- and second-degree burns, • *full-thickness*— * all layers of skin are involved: subcutaneous tissue, adnexal structures, and nerves are destroyed, * this corresponds with third- and fourth-degree burns |
| characteristics of first-degree burns | • **pain, erythema, edema in epidermis**— * focal epidermal necrosis, * examples of first-degree burns: ♦ scalding, ♦ sunburn, • **healing**— * complete, * no scarring, * heals in 3–4 days |
| characteristics of second-degree burns | • **pain, erythema, edema, blister formation**— * superficial type involves the entire epidermis and the superficial dermis, * deep type involves the deep (reticular) dermal tissue and is insensitive to pain, • **healing**— * occurs by regeneration of epithelium from edge of the burn and residual adnexal epithelium, * no scarring occurs in the superficial type: heals in 10–20 days, * scarring occurs in the deep type: ♦ heals in > 20 days, ♦ can become a third-degree burn if it becomes infected |

*Table continued on following page*

Table 4–4. SURGICAL WOUNDS, BITES, BURNS, AND COLD INJURIES *Continued*

| Most Common... | Answer and Explanation |
|---|---|
| characteristics of third-degree burns | • **multicolored, dry, insensitive to pain,** • **healing**— * requires grafts for healing, * extensive dermal scarring is often associated with keloid formation |
| characteristics of fourth-degree burns | **burn wound involves fat, fascia, muscle, or bone** |
| rules applied to determining the extent of burns in adults | • **small area**—1% for palms, genitals, • **large area**—rule of 9's: ♦ 9% for head/neck and each arm, ♦ 18% for anterior trunk, posterior trunk, and each leg |
| rules applied to determining extent of burns in infants | • **9% for each arm,** • **14% for each leg,** • **18% for head/neck, anterior trunk, posterior trunk** |
| examples of minor burns | • **second-degree burn <15% BSA in adults or <10% in infants,** • **third-degree burn <2% BSA** |
| examples of major burns | • **second-degree burn >25% BSA in adults/ infants,** • **third-degree burn >10% BSA,** • **burns involving hands, face, eyes/ears, feet, or perineum,** • **poor-risk person with burns,** • **inhalation injury, electrical burn, major trauma** |
| metabolic response to major burns | • **secretion of hormones**— * cortisol, * ADH, * AT II, * catecholamines, * glucagon, * aldosterone, • **sodium/water retention,** • **glycogenolysis,** • **hypermetabolism**—twice that of basal conditions in severe burns, • **increased O₂ consumption,** • **water evaporation**—major heat loss, • **hypovolemia**— * massive edema in burned/nonburned tissue, * weeping of plasma from burn tissue |
| immunologic response to major burns | • **depressed B cell function**—drop in all immunoglobulins, • **T cell dysfunction**— * homografts/xenografts survive longer, * dysfunction is due to a drop in IL-2 production by CD₄ T helper cells, * increased T cell suppressor activity: predicts sepsis and a fatal outcome, • **leukocyte dysfunction** |
| complications in burns | • **wound infection**— * *Pseudomonas aeruginosa,* * *S. aureus,* • *sepsis* |

## Table 4–4. SURGICAL WOUNDS, BITES, BURNS, AND COLD INJURIES *Continued*

| Most Common... | Answer and Explanation |
| --- | --- |
| features of *P. aeruginosa* infection | • **onset**—a rapid onset in 12–36 hrs, • **appearance**—no wound granulation, • **CNS changes**—deterioration, • **temperature**—elevated, • **absolute neutrophil count**—high, • **hypotension**—moderate, • **mortality rate**—high |
| features of *Staphylococcus aureus* infection | • **onset**—slow over 2–5 days, • **appearance**—black, patchy distribution, • **CNS changes**—minimal, • **temperature**—variable, • **absolute neutrophil count**—high or low, • **hypotension**—severe, • **mortality rate**—moderate |
| method of determining whether an invasive burn infection is present | **tissue biopsy**— * >10$^6$ count is presumptive evidence for an invasive infection, * must be histologic evidence of invasion of living tissue |
| viral wound infection | *Herpes simplex* |
| GI abnormality associated with burns | **Curling's stress ulcers in the stomach**—incidence is decreasing due to the use of antacids |
| respiratory abnormality in burns | **inhalation injury**— * edema of the upper airway due to heat, CO, and chemical irritants, * pulmonary edema, * ARDS |
| S/S of pulmonary injury due to a fire | • **singed nasal vibrissae**, • **soot in sputum**, • **pharyngitis**, • **hoarseness** [Note: early fiberoptic bronchoscopy is recommended when the above are present. An endotracheal tube is necessary if impending airway obstruction is suspected. Distal airway injury is difficult to evaluate.] |
| COD in burns | • **infection associated with *P. aeruginosa*,** • *ARDS,* • *severe volume depletion,* • *multiorgan failure* |
| poisonings in a house fire | • **CO,** • *cyanide poisoning*—cyanide gas originates from polyurethane in upholstery and other items |

*Table continued on following page*

Table 4–4. SURGICAL WOUNDS, BITES, BURNS, AND
COLD INJURIES *Continued*

| Most Common... | Answer and Explanation |
|---|---|
| target organs susceptible to CO poisoning | **heart and brain**—CO: * blocks cytochrome oxidase, * left shifts the ODC: less $O_2$ released, * decreases $SaO_2$ |
| S/S of CO poisoning | • **mild (<20% carboxyHgb)**— * headache: earliest sign, * dyspnea, * visual changes, * confusion, • **moderate (20–40%)**— * dizziness, * impaired judgment, * nausea, * fatigue, • **severe (40–60%)**— * hallucinations, * ataxia, * collapse, * coma, • **fatal (>60%)**—respiratory and cardiac arrest [**Note:** CO produces a cherry red color of the skin and lips that masks the presence of cyanosis.] |
| lab findings in CO poisoning | • **increased carboxyHgb**— * direct measurement, * cannot be detected with a pulse oximeter, • *low $SaO_2$*— * if directly measured, * $SaO_2$ is normal if it is calculated from the $PaO_2$: $PaO_2$ is normal in CO poisoning, • *increased AG metabolic acidosis*—lactic acidosis from tissue hypoxia |
| chronic effects of CO poisoning | • **accelerates atherosclerosis,** • *Parkinson's disease*—causes necrosis of the globus pallidus |
| Rx of CO poisoning | **100% $O_2$** |
| S/S cyanide poisoning | • **headache,** • *almond smell to the breath,* • *dizziness,* • *seizures,* • *coma,* • *death* |
| lab findings in cyanide poisoning | • **increased AG metabolic acidosis**—due to an accumulation of lactate from tissue hypoxia, • **increased $MVO_2$**—cytochrome oxidase block also blocks the tissue uptake of $O_2$ |
| Rx for cyanide poisoning | • **nitrites**— * crushed amyl nitrite pearls are used initially followed by IV sodium nitrite: this produces metHgb, which competes with cytochrome oxidase for CN to form cyanmetHgb, • **thiosulfate is administered**—this combines with CN in cyanmetHgb to form harmless thiocyanate |
| COD in a fire | **smoke inhalation** |
| Rx of second-degree burns | • **debride,** • **apply topical antibiotics** |

## Table 4–4. SURGICAL WOUNDS, BITES, BURNS, AND COLD INJURIES *Continued*

| Most Common... | Answer and Explanation |
|---|---|
| Rx of major burns | • **fluid replacement,** • **debridement,** • **topical antimicrobials,** • **grafting of deep second-/third-degree burns** |
| fluid replacement in burns | • **lactated Ringer's solution for the first 24 hrs**—may require as much as 14 liters in a 70-kg person, • **after 24 hrs, replace fluid losses with colloid solution**—5% albumin to increase oncotic pressure |
| topical antimicrobials used in Rx of burns | • **silver sulfadiazine**— * soothing, * poor penetration, * transient granulocyte marrow depression, * may precipitate hemolysis in G6PD deficiency, * is not effective against *P. aeruginosa* or *S. aureus*, • *mafenide*— * painful, * more potent antimicrobial activity, * good penetration, * carbonic anhydrase inhibitor → produces a normal AG metabolic acidosis, * can be used if the wound is infected, • *silver nitrate*—* poor penetration, * used if the patient is allergic to sulfadiazine, * loss of electrolytes, * skin discoloration [**Note:** all topical antimicrobials delay wound healing.] |
| types of skin grafts used in burns | • **temporary skin grafts**— * xenograft: porcine, * homograft (allograft): cadaver skin, * grafts are preferred over topical antibacterials in clean, noninfected burns, • **permanent graft**—autograft: patient's own skin |
| types of electrical current | **alternating**—primarily used in households in United States, • *direct current*— * lightning, * batteries |
| type of current involved in electrocutions | **AC**—it produces tonic contractions of the hand and inability to release the object transmitting the current |
| variable responsible for electrocution | **current is more important than voltage in electrocutions**— * Ohm's law states that I (current) = E (volts)/R (resistance), * as R decreases (wet skin), I increases, * when current passes through the heart or brain, it produces cardiorespiratory arrest, * the most dangerous route is from the left arm to the right leg: the current passes through the heart, leading to ventricular fibrillation |

*Table continued on following page*

Table 4–4. SURGICAL WOUNDS, BITES, BURNS, AND COLD INJURIES *Continued*

| Most Common... | Answer and Explanation |
|---|---|
| tissue resistances to electrical injury from low to high | • **nerve,** • *blood vessels*— * blood is an excellent conductor, * current follows blood vessels, * vessel thrombosis is common, • *muscle*— * myoglobinuria, * hyperkalemia from tissue release, • *skin*— * high voltage often produces third-degree burns, * deeper tissue takes longer to cool off, • *tendon,* • *fat,* • *bone* |
| complications of electrical burns | • **cardiopulmonary arrest**—most commonly occurs with AC, • *vessel thrombosis,* • *spinal cord injury,* • *rhabdomyolysis*— * myoglobinuria, * increased risk for polyuric ARF, • *third-degree burns,* • *cataracts* |
| COD in electrocution | **cardiorespiratory arrest** |
| causes of hypothermia (core temperature <35°C [95°F]) | • **intoxicated alcoholic exposed to cold temperatures,** • *cold water immersion* [**Note:** cold temperatures uncouple oxidative phosphorylation, with eventual progression into circulatory failure.] |
| cardiovascular effects associated with hypothermia | • **decreased CO,** • **prolonged QT interval,** • **sinus bradycardia,** • **classic Osborne waves on ECG**—J-point elevation |
| Rx of hypothermia | • **rewarming patient**— * heated $O_2$, * warm blankets, • *thiamine*—if the patient is an alcoholic |
| clinical findings in immersion foot | • **immersion of foot in water/mud above the freezing point of water,** • **sequential changes**— * vasoconstriction → * localized ischemia → * fixed vasodilatation → * permanent damage to microcirculation → * vessel thrombosis and gangrene |
| clinical findings in frostbite | • **temperatures are at or below the freezing point of water,** • **intracellular formation of ice leading to microvascular occlusion,** • **sites most often involved**— * fingers, * toes, * ears |

### Table 4–4. SURGICAL WOUNDS, BITES, BURNS, AND COLD INJURIES *Continued*

| Most Common... | Answer and Explanation |
|---|---|
| Rx of frostbite | • **rapid rewarming of tissue**—use 40°C water, • **apply dry dressings,** • **elevate injured tissue and keep warm,** • **observe**—a line of demarcation between viable and nonviable tissue takes several days to occur |

**Question:** Arrange the following events in normal surgical wound healing into the proper sequence:
  (A) Granulation tissue peaks
  (B) Fibrin clot
  (C) Acute inflammation
  (D) Type III collagen is converted into type I collagen
  (E) Epithelial regeneration with a watertight wound
  (F) Wound contraction begins

**Answers: (B), (C), (E), (A), (F), (D).** A fibrin clot (**choice B**) initially fills in the wound site and is cross-linked by fibronectin. Neutrophils emigrate into the wound in the first 24 hrs (**choice C**). Epithelial regeneration produces a watertight seal by 48 hrs (**choice E**). Granulation tissue peaks at 5 days (**choice A**). Wound contraction begins by myofibroblasts begins after 5 days (**choice F**). Type III collagen is replaced by type I collagen over the ensuing months (**choice D**) to produce a mature scar with a tensile strength of 70–80%.

AC = alternating current, ADH = antidiuretic hormone, AG = anion gap, ARDS = adult respiratory distress syndrome, ARF = acute renal failure, ASAP = as soon as possible, AT II = angiotensin II, ATN = acute tubular necrosis, BSA = body surface area, carboxyHgb = carboxyhemoglobin, CN = cyanide, CNS = central nervous system, CO = carbon monoxide, COD = cause of death, COPD = chronic obstructive lung disease, DC = direct current, DIC = disseminated intravascular coagulation, DM = diabetes mellitus, DTP = diphtheria-tetanus-pertussis, EGF = epidermal growth factor, FGF = fibroblast growth factor, G6PD = glucose 6-phosphate dehydrogenase, Hgb = hemoglobin, HTN = hypertension, IC = immunocomplex, IL = interleukin, MDGF = macrophage-derived growth factor, metHgb = methemoglobin, $MVO_2$ = mixed venous oxygen content, NSAIDs = nonsteroidal anti-inflammatory drugs, ODC = oxygen dissociation curve, $PaO_2$ = partial pressure of oxygen, PDGF = platelet-derived growth factor, PT = prothrombin time, PTT = partial thromboplastin time, $SaO_2$ = oxygen saturation, S/S = signs/symptoms, Td = tetanus/diphtheria, TGF = transforming growth factor, UV = ultraviolet.

# CHAPTER

## 5

# CARDIOVASCULAR SURGERY

## CONTENTS

### Table 5–1. SIGNS/SYMPTOMS AND DIAGNOSTIC PROCEDURES IN CARDIOVASCULAR DISEASE

| Most Common... | Answer and Explanation |
|---|---|
| symptom of heart failure | **dyspnea**—sensation of difficulty with breathing [**Note:** dyspnea is due to stimulation of J receptors (e.g., fluid) innervated by the vagus nerve in the interstitium of the lung. Orthopnea refers to dyspnea when recumbent. PND is a choking sensation that wakens a patient at night. It is relieved by sitting or standing.] |
| symptom of ischemic heart disease (IHD) | **chest pain** [**Note:** angina usually subsides in <3 min. An AMI has more prolonged chest pain. In a myocardial infarction, the chest pain is described as pressure or tightness in the retrosternal area. Radiation may occur to the jaw, inner aspect of the left arm, upper abdomen (simulating PUD or GERD), or shoulders. Unlike angina, pain is not relieved with nitroglycerin.] |
| causes of calf claudication | • **atherosclerotic peripheral vascular disease (PVD) involving the femoral artery**— * claudication is crampy muscular pain that occurs with exercise and is relieved by resting, * aortofemoral disease refers pain into the buttocks, • *isolated popliteal artery atherosclerosis* |

*Table continued on following page*

**Table 5–1. SIGNS/SYMPTOMS AND DIAGNOSTIC
PROCEDURES IN CARDIOVASCULAR DISEASE** *Continued*

| Most Common... | Answer and Explanation |
|---|---|
| cardiac cause of dependent pitting edema | **right heart failure (RHF)**— * blood builds up in the venous system behind the failed right side of the heart, * the increase in hydrostatic pressure leads to pitting edema: a transudate leaks into the interstitial space from the vascular compartment |
| valvular cause of cardiac-induced dizziness/syncope | **calcific AS** [**Note:** IHSS is also a cause of dizziness and syncope; however, the obstruction is due to occlusion of the outflow tract by the anterior leaflet of the mitral valve against an asymmetrically hypertrophied interventricular septum.] |
| cardiac-induced cause of dysphagia for solids but not liquids | **LA enlargement secondary to MS**— * the left atrium (LA) is the most posteriorly located heart chamber, * when enlarged, it compresses the esophagus |
| method to evaluate the LA | **transesophageal ultrasound** |
| sites for auscultation of MV, AV, TV, PV | • **MV**—apex, • **AV**—2nd right ICS, • **TV**—left parasternal, • **PV**—2nd ICS |
| heart sound corresponding with the carotid pulse | $S_1$ **heart sound** |
| cause of the $S_1$ heart sound | **closure of the MV and TV during systole**—the MV closes before the TV |
| cause of $S_2$ | **closure of the AV and PV during diastole**— * normally, there is a split during inspiration and a single sound during expiration, * blood is drawn into the right side of the heart with inspiration by an increase in negative intrathoracic pressure: the PV closes later than the AV, because there is more blood in the right side of the heart during inspiration |
| cause of an accentuated/ decreased $A_2$ | • **accentuated $A_2$**—essential HTN, • **decreased $A_2$**—severe calcific AS |
| cause of an accentuated/ decreased $P_2$ | • **accentuated $P_2$**—pulmonary HTN, • **decreased $P_2$**—increased AP chest diameter due to COPD |

**Table 5–1. SIGNS/SYMPTOMS AND DIAGNOSTIC PROCEDURES IN CARDIOVASCULAR DISEASE** *Continued*

| Most Common... | Answer and Explanation |
|---|---|
| mechanism of an $S_3$ heart sound | **blood from the atrium enters a volume-over-loaded ventricle in early diastole**—this causes vibration of the ventricle and the $S_3$ |
| pathologic causes of an $S_3$ | • **LHF**— * an $S_3$ is the earliest cardiac finding in LHF, * left-sided $S_3$ is heard loudest during expiration, • *RHF*—right-sided $S_3$ is heard loudest during inspiration, • *valvular regurgitation*—e.g., * AV/PV, * MV/TV |
| mechanism of an $S_4$ heart sound | **reduced compliance (decreased filling) of the ventricle in late diastole**—decreased compliance may be due to hypertrophy and/or volume overload of the ventricle |
| causes of a left-sided/right-sided $S_4$ | • **left-sided $S_4$**— * **LVH secondary to essential hypertension,** * LHF, * AS, * patients > 60 yrs old, • *right-sided $S_4$*— * RVH secondary to PH, * RHF |
| causes of a systolic ejection click | **MVP**— * click occurs as the MV balloons into the LA and is suddenly restrained by the chordae tendineae, * click and murmur is closer to $S_1$ with the following: ♦ standing, ♦ anxiety, * click and murmur is closer to $S_2$ with the following: ♦ lying down, ♦ Valsalva, ♦ sustained hand grip, • *congenital bicuspid aortic valve with AS,* • *aortic sclerosis*— * normal finding in the elderly population, * the AV is sclerotic but not hemodynamically abnormal, * the murmur is shorter than in AS and has no radiation into the carotid artery |
| cause of an OS | **MS**— * the OS occurs when the nonpliable valve finally opens in diastole owing to increased LA pressure, * the closer the OS is to $S_2$, the worse the stenosis, * the farther away the OS is from $S_2$, the less the stenosis |
| cause of a pathologic murmur | • **structural disease**—e.g., * stenotic AV/PV, * regurgitant flow through an incompetent valve: e.g., MV regurgitation, • *shunting of blood from a high to low pressure chamber through an abnormal opening*—e.g., VSD |

*Table continued on following page*

**Table 5–1. SIGNS/SYMPTOMS AND DIAGNOSTIC PROCEDURES IN CARDIOVASCULAR DISEASE** *Continued*

| Most Common... | Answer and Explanation |
|---|---|
| method of grading heart murmurs | **grades 1 through 6—** * grades 1–2 murmurs are difficult to hear, * grade 3 murmurs are heard by most physicians, * grade 6 murmurs are audible without a stethoscope |
| stenosis murmurs that are heard during systole | **AV/PV stenosis—** * stenosis relates to problems with opening the valve, * AV/PV stenosis murmurs are heard during systole when the AV and PV normally open, * they are ejection-type murmurs: crescendo/decrescendo |
| stenosis murmurs that are heard during diastole | **MV/TV stenosis—** * the MV/TV open in diastole, * they begin with an OS and are followed by a mid-diastolic rumble when the blood finally enters the ventricle |
| regurgitation murmurs that are heard during systole | **MV/TV regurgitation—** * regurgitation (insufficiency) murmurs are due to problems in closing the valves, * MV/TV regurgitation murmurs occur during systole, * they are pansystolic: extend through $S_1$ and $S_2$ |
| regurgitation murmurs heard during diastole | **AV/PV regurgitation—** * the AV/PV close during diastole, * they are high-pitched blowing murmurs heard immediately after $S_2$, * volume overload of the ventricles |
| effect of inspiration/ expiration on heart murmur intensity | • **inspiration**—increases the intensity of right-sided murmurs and abnormal heart sounds (e.g., $S_3$ and $S_4$) due to the increase in blood in the right side of the heart secondary to the increase in negative intrathoracic pressure, • **expiration**—increases the intensity of left-sided murmurs and abnormal heart sounds due to the increase in positive intrathoracic pressure |
| cause of a left parasternal heave | **RVH secondary to PH**—the RV lies behind the sternum |
| cause of a laterally displaced PMI | **LVH—** * LVH is most often associated with essential HTN, * there is a sustained PMI during systole |
| mechanisms of ventricular hypertrophy | • **increased afterload**—produces concentric hypertrophy of the ventricle, • *increased preload*—produces dilatation and hypertrophy |

### Table 5–1. SIGNS/SYMPTOMS AND DIAGNOSTIC PROCEDURES IN CARDIOVASCULAR DISEASE *Continued*

| Most Common... | Answer and Explanation |
|---|---|
| causes of LVH | • **essential HTN**—due to increased TPR, • *AS* |
| cause of a pericardial knock | **constrictive pericarditis**— * when the chambers begin to fill up with blood during diastole, they have a premature impact on the thickened parietal pericardium, * a knock does not occur if the pericardium is filled with fluid: e.g., pericardial effusion |
| causes of a pericardial friction rub | • **fibrinous pericarditis secondary to viral pericarditis,** • *transmural AMI,* • *uremia,* • *SLE* [**Note:** a pericardial friction rub has a scratchy sound. Three components may be heard—ventricular systole (most common), early ventricular diastole, and atrial systole.] |
| causes of a narrow pulse pressure | • **AS,** • *tachycardia,* • *pericardial effusion,* • *constrictive pericarditis* [**Note:** the pulse pressure is the difference between systolic and diastolic pressure (normally 30–40 mmHg). Owing to a decreased SV in AS, the systolic pressure is decreased, hence decreasing the pulse pressure.] |
| valvular causes of an increased pulse pressure | • **essential HTN,** • *aortic regurgitation*—volume overload of the LV leads to an increase in SV from Frank-Starling forces, • *hyperthyroidism*—increases systolic pressure owing to an increase in the force of contraction, • *coarctation of the aorta*—due to widening of the AV ring leading to aortic regurgitation and volume overload of the LV, • *high-output failure*—e.g., * thiamine deficiency, * AV fistulas, * severe anemia |
| cause of an increase in systolic BP in elderly people | **loss of compliance of the aorta secondary to atherosclerosis, which decreases vessel elasticity**—loss of aortic compliance is also operative in producing systolic HTN in the elderly |
| components of an arterial pulse wave | • **upstroke**— * due to systolic blood flow, * measure of vessel compliance: elasticity, * peak of the wave corresponds with the peak systolic pressure, • **downstroke**—measure of vessel recoil: elasticity, • **dicrotic wave at the end of ventricular systole**—due to blood refluxing back against the closed AV, * usually nonpalpable |

*Table continued on following page*

**Table 5–1. SIGNS/SYMPTOMS AND DIAGNOSTIC PROCEDURES IN CARDIOVASCULAR DISEASE** *Continued*

| Most Common... | Answer and Explanation |
|---|---|
| cause of a bounding ("water hammer") pulse | **increase in pulse pressure due to essential HTN**—rapid upstroke and downstroke |
| valvular causes of a weak pulse | • **AS,** • *hypovolemic/cardiogenic shock,* • *severe CHF* |
| causes of a bisferiens (dicrotic) pulse | • **IHSS,** • *AS + regurgitation* [**Note:** a bisferiens pulse has a double systolic peak. The usually nonpalpable dicrotic wave is palpable in the above conditions.] |
| mechanism of pulsus paradoxus | **restricted filling of the right side of the heart** [**Note:** there is a normal drop in systolic BP of <10 mmHg during inspiration. Diaphragm contraction does the following: (1) expands the lungs, (2) increases negativity of the intrapleural pressure (normally $-5$ cm $H_2O$, usually $-8$ cm $H_2O$ after inspiration), (3) increases inflow of blood into the right side of the heart (excess blood in the RV pushes against the IVS and reduces LV volume), (4) expands the pulmonary vessels (increases their capacitance) to accommodate the excess RV outflow, (5) reduces LV volume (combination of items 3 and 4), which produces a slight drop in the systolic BP on inspiration. The combination of restriction of blood flow into the right side of the heart and inspiratory expansion of the pulmonary vasculature delivers even less blood to the LV than normal, hence producing a drop in systolic BP that is >10 mmHg, which is called pulsus paradoxus.] |
| causes of pulsus paradoxus | • **pericardial effusion,** • *decreased lung compliance in severe bronchial asthma* |
| mechanism of Kussmaul's sign | **restricted filling of the right side of the heart leads to neck vein distention on inspiration**—neck veins should collapse on inspiration owing to filling of the right side of the heart |
| causes of Kussmaul's sign | • **pericardial effusion,** • *tricuspid stenosis/regurgitation,* • *PH* |

## Table 5–1. SIGNS/SYMPTOMS AND DIAGNOSTIC PROCEDURES IN CARDIOVASCULAR DISEASE *Continued*

| Most Common... | Answer and Explanation |
|---|---|
| uses of a chest radiograph | • **detect aortic abnormalities**—e.g., widening of the aortic shadow in a dissecting aortic aneurysm, • **detect PH**—e.g., pruning of the pulmonary vessels, • **detect LHF**, • **identify calcifications**—e.g., * mitral annulus, * coronary atherosclerosis, * old healed infarct, • **evaluate heart and chamber size**—ECHO is a better test, • **detect a pericardial effusion**— * ECHO is a better test, * "water bottle" configuration |
| uses of an ECG | • **Dx of**— * arrhythmias, * AMI, * LVH, * RVH, * pericarditis, * atrial hypertrophy, electrolyte abnormalities: e.g., ♦ peaked T wave in hyperkalemia, ♦ U wave of hypokalemia, ♦ short QT interval of hypercalcemia, * effects of cardiac drugs, • **assessment of**— * IHD, * syncope/dizziness/palpitations |
| use of a stress ECG | **evaluation of exercise-induced ischemia and hypotension**—this is not a good screen in an asymptomatic patient |
| uses of an ECHO | • **assess heart and chamber size**, • *identify vegetations*, • *evaluate LV wall movement*, • *measure ejection fraction*—EF = SV ÷ LVEDV, • *detect mural thrombi*, • *detect cardiac myxoma*, • *detect pericardial effusion*, • *assess valve abnormalities*—e.g., MVP, • *Dx IHSS*, • *detect an aortic dissection*, • *detect intracardiac shunts* |
| use of radioactive thallium scanning | **assess myocardial perfusion in exercise testing of IHD**— * diminished perfusion shows up as a "cold" spot, * reperfusion when exercise ends indicates reversible ischemia |
| use of technetium pyrophosphate scintigraphy | **detect an acute AMI**— * radionuclide deposits in the area of infarction, * most useful 2–3 days post-AMI |
| use of stress testing with dipyridamole | **stimulates angina in patients who are unable to exercise for a stress test** |
| uses of radionuclide ventriculography | • **calculate ejection fraction**—see above, • **evaluate ventricular function** |

*Table continued on following page*

### Table 5–1. SIGNS/SYMPTOMS AND DIAGNOSTIC PROCEDURES IN CARDIOVASCULAR DISEASE *Continued*

| Most Common... | Answer and Explanation |
|---|---|
| uses of dobutamine stress echocardiography | • **estimates the ejection fraction**—see above,<br>• **evaluates ventricular function** |
| uses of cardiac catheterization | **evaluate both right side/left side heart disease**—e.g., * shunts, * valvular disease, * selective coronary arteriograms, * angioplasty [**Note:** 70% of people with CAD have 2 or more vessels with significant stenosis (>50% narrowing of lumen).] |

**Question:** Which of the following are more likely associated with left-sided heart failure (LHF) than with right-sided heart failure (RHF)? **SELECT 4**

(A) $S_3$ heart sound on expiration
(B) Pansystolic murmur increasing on inspiration
(C) Pillow orthopnea
(D) Bibasilar inspiratory rales
(E) Neck vein distention
(F) $S_4$ heart sound on inspiration
(G) Dependent pitting edema
(H) Decreased ejection fraction

**Answers:** (A), (C), (D), (H). In LHF, there is volume overload of the LV with a backup of blood into the lungs. In RHF, there is a backup of blood into the venous system. The $S_3$ heart sound increases on expiration, since positive intrathoracic pressures increase all left-sided sounds and murmurs **(choice A is correct)**. Volume overload of the LV stretches the MV ring causing mitral regurgitation (pansystolic murmur), which should increase on expiration **(choice B is incorrect, TV regurgitation would increase in inspiration)**. Pillow orthopnea is a feature of LHF **(choice C is correct)**. It is due to increased venous return to the heart while in the recumbent state and reflux of blood back into the lungs. Bibasilar inspiratory rales are a feature of LHF as the pulmonary venous hydrostatic pressure overrides the oncotic pressure of the pulmonary capillaries **(choice D is correct)**. Neck vein distention and dependent pitting edema from an increase in venous hydrostatic pressure are both signs of RHF **(choices E and G are incorrect)**. Since right-sided sounds and murmurs increase on inspiration, an increase in $S_4$ on inspiration is due to RHF **(choice F is incorrect)**. The ejection fraction (EF = SV ÷ LVEDV) is decreased in both LHF and RHF **(choice H is correct)**.

AMI = acute myocardial infarction, AS = aortic stenosis, AV = aortic valve, BP = blood pressure, CAD = coronary artery disease, CHF = congestive heart failure, COPD = chronic obstructive pulmonary disease, ECHO = echocardiogram, EF = ejection fraction, GERD = gastroesophageal reflux disease, HTN = hypertension, ICS = intercostal space, IHD = ischemic heart disease, IHSS = idiopathic hypertrophic subaortic stenosis, IVS = interventricular septum, JVP = jugular venous pulse, LA = left atrium, LBBB = left bundle branch block, LHF = left-sided heart failure, LV = left ventricle, LVEDV = left ventricular end-diastolic volume, LVH = left ventricular hypertrophy, MS = mitral stenosis, MV = mitral valve, MVP = mitral valve prolapse, OS = opening snap, PA = pulmonary artery, PH = pulmonary hypertension, PMI = point of maximal impulse, PND = paroxysmal nocturnal dyspnea, PUD = peptic ulcer disease, PV = pulmonic valve, PVD = peripheral vascular disease, RA = right atrium, RHF = right-sided heart failure, RV = right ventricle, RVH = right ventricular hypertrophy, $S_1$, $S_2$, $S_3$, $S_4$ = first, second, third, and fourth heart sounds, SLE = systemic lupus erythematosus, SV = stroke volume, TPR = total peripheral resistance, TV = tricuspid valve, VSD = ventricular septal defect.

### Table 5–2. VASCULAR DISORDERS OF SURGICAL IMPORTANCE

| Most Common... | Answer and Explanation |
|---|---|
| risk factors for atherosclerosis | • **age,** • *male sex,* • *family history,* • *DM,* • *HTN,* • *LDL > 160 mg/dL,* • *HDL < 35 mg/dL,* • smoking, • *obesity* |
| causes of endothelial damage leading to atherosclerosis | • **cigarette smoke**— * CO, * ammonia, • **native/oxidized LDL,** • **turbulence at vessel bifurcations,** • **immunologic injury,** • **viral/** ***Chlamydia pneumoniae*** **injury,** • **increased plasma homocysteine levels** |
| sites for atherosclerosis in descending order | • **abdominal aorta,** • *coronary artery,* • *popliteal artery,* • *descending thoracic aorta,* • *internal carotid* |

*Table continued on following page*

## Table 5–2.  VASCULAR DISORDERS OF SURGICAL IMPORTANCE *Continued*

| Most Common... | Answer and Explanation |
|---|---|
| complications of atherosclerosis in the abdominal aorta | • **aneurysm formation,** • *embolization*— * embolization to the SMA may result in small bowel infarction, * embolization to vessels in the lower legs may lead to digital infarction, • *mesenteric angina*—severe pain at the splenic flexure: ♦ this is the overlap area between the SMA and inferior mesenteric artery, ♦ like any overlap area, it is more subject to ischemic damage, • *small bowel infarction*—thrombosis over an atheromatous plaque in the proximal SMA, • *renovascular HTN*— * atherosclerotic plaque obstructing the renal artery, * MCC of secondary HTN |
| complications of atherosclerosis in the peripheral vascular system | • **gangrene,** • *claudication*—superficial femoral artery in the adductor canal is the MC vessel involved, • *aneurysms*—e.g., popliteal artery |
| coexisting diseases in patients with peripheral vascular disease | • **CAD**—~20% have previous AMI, • *cerebrovascular disease*—~7% have a history of previous stroke, • *abdominal aortic aneurysm*—20% have a popliteal artery aneurysm |
| complications of atherosclerosis in the coronary artery | • **angina,** • *AMI,* • *sudden cardiac death,* • *chronic ischemic heart disease* |
| complications of atherosclerosis in the internal carotid artery | • **TIA,** • *atherosclerotic stroke,* • *embolic stroke* |
| complication of atherosclerosis in the renal artery | **renovascular HTN** |
| causes of aneurysms | • **atherosclerosis**—abdominal aorta, • *congenital*— * berry aneurysm of circle of Willis, * Marfan syndrome: defect in fibrillin, * Ehlers-Danlos syndrome: defect in collagen, • *inflammation*—mycotic aneurysm, • *HTN*— HTN predisposes to the development of Charcot-Bouchard aneurysms in the lenticulostriate vessels, • *traumatic* |

## Table 5–2. VASCULAR DISORDERS OF SURGICAL
## IMPORTANCE *Continued*

| Most Common... | Answer and Explanation |
|---|---|
| aneurysm | **abdominal aortic aneurysm**—~95% occur below the orifices of the renal arteries (absence of vasa vasorum) [**Note:** according to the Law of Laplace, as the diameter of a hollow structure increases, wall stress increases. Hence, once a vessel begins to dilate, it must continue to dilate owing to a greater increase in wall stress.] |
| cause of an abdominal aortic aneurysm | • **atherosclerosis,** • *genetic*— * familial clustering, * biochemical alterations in the structural matrix of a vessel |
| S/S of an abdominal aortic aneurysm | • **the majority are asymptomatic**—75%, • *rupture*—most common symptomatic presentation, • *midabdominal to lower back pain,* • *pulsatile mass,* • *epigastric bruit*—50%, • *thromboembolic event,* • *renovascular HTN,* • *impotence*—Leriche syndrome, • *hydronephrosis*—compressed ureters |
| complication of an abdominal aortic aneurysm | **rupture**—the majority rupture posteriorly into the retroperitoneum |
| risk factor for rupture of an abdominal aortic aneurysm | **size**— * <4 cm: 2% risk, * 4–5 cm: 3–12% risk, * >5 cm: 25–40% risk |
| S/S of a ruptured abdominal aortic aneurysm | • **sudden onset of left flank pain**—hemorrhage into the retroperitoneum, • **hypotension**—blood loss, • **pulsatile abdominal mass**—aneurysm [**Note:** this is called the rupture triad.] |
| tests used to identify an abdominal aortic aneurysm | • **ultrasound**—gold standard test, • *CT*—100% sensitivity but more expensive than an ultrasound, • *MRI*—sensitive test but too expensive, • *abdominal x-ray*—identifies calcifications in the aortic wall, • *aortography*— * provides information for the potential of aortic reconstruction, * R/O mesenteric artery, peripheral vascular, renal artery disease |

*Table continued on following page*

Table 5–2. VASCULAR DISORDERS OF SURGICAL
IMPORTANCE *Continued*

| Most Common... | Answer and Explanation |
|---|---|
| indications for elective surgery of an abdominal aortic aneurysm | • **any symptomatic aneurysm**—regardless of size, • *aneurysm >5 cm*— * asymptomatic or symptomatic, * sharp increase in rupture if >6 cm, • *4–5 cm*— * controversial |
| contraindications to elective surgery | • **acute AMI in last 6 mos,** • **intractable CHF/ angina,** • **severe dyspnea at rest,** • **severe renal insufficiency,** • **life expectancy <2 yrs** |
| early complications postoperatively for abdominal aortic aneurysm | • **cardiac disorders**— * ischemia, * arrhythmias, * CHF, • *pulmonary insufficiency*— * respiratory failure, * ARDS, • *renal damage,* • *bleeding*—blood salvage techniques are utilized, • *prolonged paralytic ileus*—diarrhea, • *thromboembolism*— * cutaneous ischemia, * digital infarctions, • *bowel infarction,* • *paraplegia*—ischemia to spinal cord |
| late postoperative complications of abdominal aortic aneurysms | • **prosthetic graft infection,** • **aortoenteric fistula,** • **graft occlusion** |
| cause of a thoracic aortic aneurysm | • **dissecting aortic aneurysm,** • *atherosclerosis,* • *trauma,* • *tertiary syphilis* |
| catastrophic disorder of the aorta | **dissecting aortic aneurysm** |
| risk factors for a dissecting aortic aneurysm | • **hypertension**—supplies the shearing force to the structurally weak aorta that is required to produce an intimal tear, • *Marfan's syndrome*— * MC COD, * ~10% of patients with dissections have Marfan's syndrome, • *Ehlers-Danlos syndrome*—MC COD, • *pregnancy*—~50% of dissections in women occur during pregnancy, • *coarctation of the aorta*— * 20%, * 50% if associated with a congenital bicuspid AV, • *congenital bicuspid AV*—5%, • *trauma* [**Note:** dissecting aortic aneurysms are not true aneurysms. True aneurysms are dilatations of vessels where the wall of the dilated vessel forms the wall of the aneurysm.] |
| pathologic changes in the aorta in dissecting aortic aneurysms | • **elastic tissue fragmentation,** • *medial degeneration* [**Note:** ~60% of intimal tears occur in the ascending aorta ~1–2 cm above the AV, 35% occur in the descending aorta, and the remainder occur in the abdominal aorta.] |

### Table 5–2. VASCULAR DISORDERS OF SURGICAL IMPORTANCE *Continued*

| Most Common... | Answer and Explanation |
| --- | --- |
| types of dissecting aortic aneurysm | • **type I**—ascending aorta, arch, descending aorta, • **type II**—ascending aorta, • **type III**—descending aorta below the ligamentum arteriosum |
| type of dissecting aortic aneurysm | **type II** |
| S/S of a dissecting aortic aneurysm | • **acute onset of severe chest pain**—usually in association with HTN: HTN is uncommon in an AMI, • *radiation of pain down the back,* • *unequal pulses in the upper extremity*—this occurs in ~50% of those with involvement of ascending aorta, • *aortic regurgitation*— * ~60%, * due to widening of the aortic root |
| tests used to screen for a dissecting aortic aneurysm | • **chest x-ray**—reveals widening of the superior mediastinum: dilated aortic knob in ~80%, • *transesophageal echocardiogram*—greater sensitivity (~98%) than a chest x-ray, • *CT scan*— * confirms the presence and extent of a dissection, * does not identify the intimal tear or the presence of aortic regurgitation, • *arteriography*—gold standard confirmatory test |
| initial step in treating a dissecting aortic aneurysm | **lower BP**— * nitroprusside prevents further dissection: ♦ danger of thiocyanate toxicity, ♦ must monitor thiocyanate levels, * propranolol lowers the pulse rate |
| types of dissecting aortic aneurysms requiring immediate surgery | **types I and II**—in most cases, type III dissections are treated medically |
| COD in a dissecting aortic aneurysm | **rupture**—site of rupture is usually opposite the intimal tear— * **hemopericardium,** * left pleural space for those distal to ligamentum arteriosum [**Note:** in rare cases they may re-enter the aorta, creating a double-barreled aorta.] |
| cause of traumatic disruption of the aorta | **MVA** |

*Table continued on following page*

### Table 5–2. VASCULAR DISORDERS OF SURGICAL
### IMPORTANCE *Continued*

| Most Common... | Answer and Explanation |
|---|---|
| site for traumatic disruption of aorta | • **proximal to the ligamentum arteriosum**—70%, • *ascending aorta*—10%, • *descending aorta*—20% |
| aneurysms of the peripheral vascular system | • **popliteal artery aneurysm**— * 70%, * 20% associated with abdominal aortic aneurysm, * often bilateral, • *femoral artery aneurysm* |
| S/S of popliteal artery aneurysm | • **embolization**—danger of gangrene, • *thrombosis*— * nonpulsatile, * danger of gangrene, • *claudication*, • *pulsatile mass*—patent |
| differential for a popliteal mass | • **popliteal artery aneurysm**, • *Baker's cyst*—synovial cyst often associated with rheumatoid arthritis |
| Rx of popliteal artery aneurysm | **surgical removal**—danger of gangrene if left untreated |
| S/S of femoral artery aneurysm | • **pulsatile groin mass**, • *thromboembolism*, • *claudication* |
| causes of a subarachnoid hemorrhage | • **ruptured congenital berry (saccular) aneurysm**— * 80% of all causes, * usually located at the junction of the anterior communicating artery with the ACA: ♦ all people have absent internal elastic lamina and smooth muscle at the juncture of communicating branches with the main vessel, ♦ HTN of any cause can result in development of a berry aneurysm, • *ruptured AVM*, • *rupture of a fusiform aneurysm*—atherosclerotic, • *trauma* |
| cause of a berry aneurysm in the circle of Willis | **congenital absence of the internal elastic membrane and muscle wall at the bifurcation of the communicating arteries with their corresponding cerebral arteries**—all people have this defect |
| risk factors for a subarachnoid hemorrhage due to a berry aneurysm | • **HTN of any cause**—e.g., * essential HTN, * adult polycystic kidney disease, • *adult coarctation of the aorta*, • *Marfan's disease*, • *Ehlers-Danlos disease*, • *previous history of a berry aneurysm*—one-third have multiple aneurysms |

## Table 5–2. VASCULAR DISORDERS OF SURGICAL
IMPORTANCE *Continued*

| Most Common... | Answer and Explanation |
|---|---|
| S/S of a subarachnoid hemorrhage | **sudden onset of a severe occipital head-ache**—50% have a sentinel bleed with a warning headache: "worst headache I have ever had," • *N/V,* • *loss of consciousness,* • *CN III deficits,* • *nuchal rigidity* |
| time-frame for vasospastic injury following subarachnoid hemorrhage | **4–14 days after bleed**— * vasospastic injury with further neurologic deficits occurs in ~75% of patients, * release of TXA$_2$ from platelets in the clot material contributes to vasospasm |
| complications associated with a subarachnoid bleed | • **rebleeding**—20% rebleed within a 2-wk time-span, • *myocardial ischemia*—this is due to outpouring of catecholamines from the reticular activating system in the CNS, • *communicating hydrocephalus*—blockage of arachnoid granulations with blood clot prevents reabsorption of spinal fluid, • *SiADH,* • *seizures,* • *hyperglycemia*—catecholamine effect, • *delirium,* • *neutrophilic leukocy-tosis*—catecholamine effect |
| diagnostic tests to document subarachnoid hemorrhage | • **CT within 24–48 hrs of bleed**—this is diagnostic in 90% of cases, • *lumbar puncture if CT cannot identify blood,* • *cerebral angiography*— * confirmatory test, * FN rate 10–20% |
| Rx of ruptured berry aneurysm | • **surgical clipping,** • *nimodipine*—helps prevent vasospasm |
| prognostic factors associated with subarachnoid hemorrhage | **prognosis depends on the level of consciousness when the patient initially presents**— * ~25% die from the initial bleed, * an additional 25–35% die from a rebleed by the end of one year, * ~25% have permanent neurologic deficits |
| symptomatic vascular anomaly in CNS | **AVM**—AVMs are tangles of arteries directly connected to veins |
| complications associated with AVMs | • **subarachnoid bleeds,** • *focal epileptic seizures,* • *progressive neurologic deficits* |

*Table continued on following page*

Table 5–2. VASCULAR DISORDERS OF SURGICAL
IMPORTANCE *Continued*

| Most Common... | Answer and Explanation |
|---|---|
| diagnostic tests used to identify AVMs | • **MRI**, • *CT scan,* • *angiography*—definitive test |
| splanchnic artery aneurysms in descending order | • **splenic**, • *hepatic,* • *SMA,* • *celiac* |
| clinical findings in splenic artery aneurysms | • **increased incidence in women**—increased with multiparity, • **pathogenesis**— * increased arterial blood volume in pregnancy, * fibrodysplasia, * PH, • **complication**—rupture in 5–10%: 95% during pregnancy, • **Dx**— * x-ray with a signet ring–like calcification, * CT-sensitive, * angiography confirmatory |
| Rx of splenic artery aneurysms | **surgery** |
| clinical findings of hepatic artery aneurysms | • **increased incidence in men,** • **pathogenesis**— * **atherosclerosis**, * cystic medial necrosis, * trauma, • **complications**— * **rupture,** * compression of CBD with jaundice, • **Dx**—angiography |
| Rx of hepatic artery aneurysm | **surgery**—high mortality with intraperitoneal rupture |
| cause of a cystic artery aneurysm | **polyarteritis nodosa** |
| types of infected aneurysms in descending order | • **post-traumatic infected false aneurysm,** • *microbial vasculitis,* • *infection of a pre-existing aneurysm,* • *mycotic aneurysm* |
| overall pathogen causing an infected aneurysm | ***Staphylococcus aureus*** |
| cause/pathogen in a post-traumatic infected false aneurysm | • **causes**— * narcotic addiction, * trauma, • **pathogen**—*Staphylococcus aureus* |
| cause/pathogen in microbial vasculitis | • **cause**—persistent bacteremia, • **pathogen**—*Salmonella* species |
| cause/pathogen in an infected pre-existing aneurysm | • **cause**—bacteremia, • **pathogens**— * *Staphylococcus aureus/epidermidis,* * *Escherichia coli* |

## Table 5–2. VASCULAR DISORDERS OF SURGICAL IMPORTANCE *Continued*

| Most Common... | Answer and Explanation |
|---|---|
| cause/pathogen in a mycotic aneurysm | • **cause**—infective endocarditis, • **pathogen**—*Staphylococcus aureus* |
| type of infected aneurysm with the highest mortality | **infection of a pre-existing aneurysm** |
| causes of ischemia of lower extremity | • **atherosclerosis**, • *fibromuscular dysplasia*, • *embolization*, • *vasculitis*— * Takayasu's vasculitis, * thromboangiitis obliterans [**Note:** S/S of atherosclerotic disease parallel the degree of development of collateral vessels.] |
| causes of acute arterial ischemia of the lower extremity | • **embolization**— * most are clots in the left atrium dislodged by atrial fibrillation, * others: ♦ vegetations, ♦ mural thrombi in AMI, ♦ atrial myxoma, ♦ clots from prosthetic heart valves, ♦ marantic vegetations in malignancy, • *thrombosis*, • *descending aortic dissection*, • *trauma* |
| site of embolic occlusion of a peripheral vessel | **bifurcation of common femoral artery—** 35–50% |
| clinical findings of acute arterial ischemia | • **five P's**— * pain: shooting pain followed by numbness and weakness, * pallor: progresses to mottled cyanosis, * pulselessness: below the area of occlusion, * paresthesias: portend serious consequences if rapidly progress, * paralysis: weakness of dorsiflexion of the foot or toe (peroneal nerve distribution), • *other*— * collapsed superficial veins, * cold skin |
| differential features of embolization versus thrombosis | • **atrial fibrillation**—consider embolization, • **Hx of claudication**—consider thrombosis, • **physical findings**— * proximal and contralateral limb pulses are usually normal in embolization, * proximal or contralateral limb pulses are diminished to absent in thrombosis, • *pain*—abrupt onset of pain: consider embolization, • *arteriography*— * embolization: sharp cut-off, minimal atherosclerosis, few collaterals, * thrombosis: irregular cut-off, well-developed collaterals, diffuse atherosclerosis |

*Table continued on following page*

**Table 5–2. VASCULAR DISORDERS OF SURGICAL IMPORTANCE** *Continued*

| Most Common... | Answer and Explanation |
|---|---|
| cause of the "blue toe" syndrome | **microembolization of atheromatous plaque material to the distal extremity—** * artery–artery embolization: e.g., aortic aneurysm with an ulcerated atheromatous plaque, * pulses are intact but the skin is cyanotic |
| methods for Dx of acute arterial ischemia | • **arteriography,** • *Doppler ultrasound,* • *plethysmography* |
| Rx of acute arterial ischemia | • **surgery**—embolectomy, • *anticoagulation*—heparin, • *thrombolytic therapy*—select cases |
| complications associated with Rx of acute arterial ischemia | • **trauma related to catheter embolectomy**—* perforation, * dissection, * false aneurysm, • **reperfusion injury**—due to superoxide FRs, • **compartment syndrome**—particularly in pretibial area, • **byproducts of ischemic muscle**— * myoglobinuria: danger of ARF, * hyperkalemia, * lactic acidosis, * increased serum CK |
| S/S of chronic lower extremity ischemia | • **intermittent claudication**—see Table 5–1, • *Leriche syndrome*—see below, • *rest pain*—see below, • *decreased pulse amplitude*— * a bruit is often present, * obstruction is proximal to the bruit, • *cool skin temperature*—skin temperature is a measure of blood flow rate, • *pallor upon elevation of the extremity*—see below, • *muscle atrophy,* • *skin changes*— * loss of digital hair, * thickening of toe nails, * skin thin/shiny, * dermal atrophy: round, depressed areas due to superficial infarctions, * skin necrosis: punched-out, cool, ischemic ulcers on the tips of the toes, malleoli, heels, • *diminished capillary refill postcompression of the toe nail*—normally refills in <2 sec, • *gangrene*— * dry gangrene: no infection, * wet gangrene: ♦ implies an infection with anaerobes, ♦ osteomyelitis is commonly present (x-ray extremity) |
| pain site for occlusive disease of the aorta | **midabdomen** |

### Table 5–2. VASCULAR DISORDERS OF SURGICAL
### IMPORTANCE Continued

| Most Common... | Answer and Explanation |
|---|---|
| pain site for occlusive disease of the common iliac artery | **buttocks** |
| pain site for occlusive disease of the common femoral artery | **thigh** |
| pain site for occlusive disease of the superficial femoral artery | **knee** |
| pain site for occlusive disease of the popliteal artery | **calf** |
| pain site for occlusive disease of the tibial artery | **foot** |
| clinical findings in Leriche syndrome | • **site of occlusion**—aortoiliac atherosclerosis, • **S/S**— * claudication, * impotence: hypogastric arteries are involved, * calf muscle atrophy, * diminished/absent femoral artery pulse |
| clinical significance of rest pain in the lower extremity | • **far-advanced atherosclerotic disease**, • *S/S*— * severe burning pain distal to the metatarsals, * pain aggravated by elevating foot, * patient hangs the affected leg over the side of bed to relieve pain: foot swells |
| clinical significance of pallor of the lower extremity when elevated | • **indicates far-advanced atherosclerotic disease**— * elevating the extremity evaluates the arterial blood flow against gravity, * pallor indicates a poor arterial blood flow, * cool skin temperature, • *return of the extremity to the dependent position produces a violaceous color*—this indicates a loss of venomotor tone from tissue hypoxia that causes venule dilatation and pooling of blood |
| artery in lower extremity that best correlates with arterial insufficiency | **amplitude of posterior tibial artery** |

*Table continued on following page*

**Table 5–2. VASCULAR DISORDERS OF SURGICAL IMPORTANCE** *Continued*

| Most Common... | Answer and Explanation |
|---|---|
| diagnostic method to evaluate chronic ischemia of lower extremity | • **Doppler ultrasound with calculation of the ankle/brachial index (ABI)**— * Doppler measures the systolic pressure of the dorsalis pedis + posterior tibial artery and compares it with the systolic pressure of the brachial artery, * a normal ABI is 1, * intermittent claudication is associated with an ABI of 0.6–0.9, * resting pain is associated with an ABI of <0.5, • *arteriography,* • *digital subtraction angiography* |
| medical Rx of ischemic disease of the lower extremity | • **reduce risk factors**— * quit smoking, * control HTN, * glycemic control if the patient is diabetic, * Rx hyperlipidemia, • *increase exercise*—stimulate collateral circulation, • *aspirin,* • *pentoxifylline*—hemorrheologic agent that reduces blood viscosity, • *vasodilators*—e.g., * nifedipine: used in upper extremity vasospasm (Raynaud's), * papaverine |
| surgical Rx of ischemic disease of lower extremity | • **bypass operations,** • *endarterectomy*—localized disease in the distal aorta/common iliac vessels, • *percutaneous transluminal angioplasty,* • *amputation* |
| systemic disease causing atherosclerosis of the radial/brachial arteries | **DM** |
| cause of a falsely elevated ABI | **DM**—brachial artery disease decreases the denominator of the ratio |
| upper extremity artery involved in ischemic disease | **left subclavian artery** |
| site of obstruction in the subclavian steal syndrome | **proximal obstruction of the first portion of the subclavian artery**— * this may produce reversal of blood flow in the vertebral artery in order to supply blood to the arm, * reduced vertebral blood flow leads to cerebral ischemia |
| mechanism of the thoracic outlet syndrome | **compression of the arteries, veins, or nerves in the neck** |

## Table 5–2. VASCULAR DISORDERS OF SURGICAL
## IMPORTANCE *Continued*

| Most Common... | Answer and Explanation |
|---|---|
| causes of the thoracic outlet syndrome | • **positional changes in neck/arms,** • *cervical rib,* • *spastic scalenus anticus muscle* [**Note:** this is a common disorder in weight lifters.] |
| S/S of thoracic outlet syndrome | • **pain, paresthesias, or numbness in the distribution of the ulnar nerve,** • *muscular atrophy in the hand,* • *upper extremity claudication with exercise,* • *thrombosis of the subclavian vein*—see dilatation of the superficial veins, • *patient complains of the arm "falling asleep at night"* |
| screening test to document thoracic outlet syndrome | **demonstrating weakening of the radial pulse with arm abduction and head turned to the side of the lesion (Adson's test)**— * a bruit is frequently heard over the subclavian artery, * percussion over the brachial plexus may reproduce the symptoms: Tinel's test |
| confirmatory test for thoracic outlet syndrome | **arteriography** |
| Rx of thoracic outlet syndrome | • **postural correction,** • *physical therapy,* • *surgery*— * remove the cervical rib, * resect the scalenus anticus muscle |
| screening test of volar arch arteries | **Allen's test**— * examiner compresses radial and ulnar artery with each thumb, * patient opens/closes hand three times, * release thumb over radial artery to evaluate return of color, * repeat test and release thumb over ulnar artery to evaluate return of color |
| categories of cerebrovascular disease | • **transient ischemic attack** (TIA)—focal neurologic dysfunction for a few minutes that resolves completely within 24 hrs, • *stroke in evolution*—repeated neurologic dysfunction without complete recovery of deficits between attacks, • *reversible ischemic neurologic deficit* (RIND)—similar to TIA but reverses in >24 hrs with complete resolution in a few days, • *complete (acute) stroke*—stable neurologic deficit that may improve with time |

*Table continued on following page*

**Table 5–2. VASCULAR DISORDERS OF SURGICAL IMPORTANCE** *Continued*

| Most Common... | Answer and Explanation |
|---|---|
| mechanisms of ischemic CVA | • **thrombosis over atherosclerotic plaque at the carotid artery bifurcation**— * the facial vein is the landmark of the carotid bifurcation, * 90% of patients with symptomatic lesions have atherosclerosis at the bifurcation, • **embolus from the extracranial carotid artery to the MCA,** • *embolus from the heart*—particularly in the presence of atrial fibrillation, • *dissecting aortic aneurysm involving the carotid or vertebrobasilar system,* • *vessel thrombosis from a hypercoagulable state/blood dyscrasia*—e.g., PRV, • *illicit drugs*—e.g., * cocaine, * vegetation from the heart in IVDU [**Note:** bruits over the carotid bifurcation are not reliable indicators of the degree of stenosis.] |
| risk factors for ischemic CVA | • **age**— * >45 yrs in men, * >55 yrs in women, • *family Hx of CAD or stroke,* • *smoking,* • *LDL ≥160 mg/dL,* • *HDL ≤40 mg/dL,* • *DM,* • *HTN,* • *oral contraceptives,* • *atrial fibrillation,* • *CHF,* • *anterior AMI with mural thrombus* |
| modifiable risk factors to prevent ischemic CVA | • **control HTN,** • *glycemic control,* • *stop smoking,* • *lose weight,* • *lower serum CH,* • *limit alcohol intake,* • *aspirin,* • *anticoagulation for atrial fibrillation* |
| tests used to evaluate carotid artery disease | • **duplex scanning**— * the best initial screen, * determines degree of carotid stenosis, • *carotid angiography,* • *intravenous digital subtraction angiography*—helps define occlusive disease |
| cause of a TIA | **embolism of particles of atherosclerotic plaque located on the ICA** |

## Table 5–2. VASCULAR DISORDERS OF SURGICAL
## IMPORTANCE *Continued*

| Most Common... | Answer and Explanation |
|---|---|
| clinical manifestations of a TIA | • **neurologic deficits usually last <15 min,** • **~90% resolve in 24 hrs,** • **one-third progress to a stroke**—usually in the same distribution as the TIA, • 30–40% have underlying CAD, • **one-third have at least one more TIA,** • **one-third have no further problems,** • **amaurosis fugax is a classic symptom of carotid TIA**— * sudden, painless loss of vision with resolution, * atherosclerotic plaque in the retinal vessel is called a Hollenhorst plaque, * described as a curtain coming down and then going up |
| type of stroke | **atherosclerotic** |
| steps in the initial management of a cerebral infarction | • **CT scan to determine whether it is a pale or hemorrhagic infarction,** • **recombinant tPA is used if the onset of symptoms <3 hrs and it is a pale infarct**— * there is a 30% chance of escaping significant neurologic deficits, * 10 times greater risk for developing intracerebral hemorrhage, • **extended cardiac monitoring**—30–40% prevalence of CAD in patients with ischemic strokes, • **noninvasive assessment of carotid arteries** |
| recommendation for asymptomatic or symptomatic ICA stenosis > 60% | **carotid endarterectomy** |
| recommendation for symptomatic ICA stenosis 30–60% | **role of carotid endarterectomy is under investigation** |
| recommendation for ICA stenosis <30% | • **aspirin**—3% decrease in strokes over 3 yrs, • *ticlopidine if allergic to aspirin*— * 6% decrease in strokes over 3 yrs, * superior to aspirin, particularly in the first year; however, it is more expensive, * it inhibits platelet function without blocking cyclooxygenase, * problem with neutropenia requires WBC count, * Clopidogrel does not have the neutropenia effects, • dipyridamole—may be useful in patients with previous Hx of TIA or stroke |

*Table continued on following page*

### Table 5–2. VASCULAR DISORDERS OF SURGICAL IMPORTANCE *Continued*

| Most Common... | Answer and Explanation |
| --- | --- |
| sign of small vessel vasculitis | **palpable purpura (e.g., HSP)**— * palpable purpura is due to immunocomplex deposition (type III hypersensitivity) in the wall of postcapillary venules, * ICs activate the complement system: C5a is produced and is chemotactic to neutrophils, which destroy the vessel |
| clinical presentation for vasculitis involving muscular arteries | **vessel thrombosis with infarction**—e.g., PAN |
| clinical presentation for vasculitis involving the elastic arteries | • **lack of a pulse**—e.g., Takayasu's giant cell arteritis involving the subclavian artery, • *stroke,* • *blindness* |
| vasculitis in adults | **giant cell arteritis (temporal arteritis)**—a granulomatous vasculitis involving the temporal artery and extracranial vessels |
| presentation of giant cell arteritis | • **headache/tenderness in the distribution of the temporal artery,** • *jaw claudication,* • *polymyalgia rheumatica*— * 40–50%, * associated with pain and morning stiffness, * normal serum CK: polymyositis has an increase in serum CK, • *blindness*—arteritis may involve branches of the ophthalmic or posterior ciliary arteries, leading to ischemic optic neuritis |
| lab test used to screen for temporal arteritis | **ESR**— * inflammation invariably increases the ESR, * a positive clinical Hx and an increased ESR are sufficient evidence to begin Rx with corticosteroids to prevent permanent blindness, * a temporal artery Bx confirms the Dx |
| vasculitis associated with HBV | **polyarteritis nodosa (PAN)**— * PAN is a male dominant IC vasculitis involving the muscular arteries, * vascular lesions are in different stages: acute or chronic, * "nodosa" refers to focal aneurysm formation: may be palpable |

## Table 5–2. VASCULAR DISORDERS OF SURGICAL
IMPORTANCE *Continued*

| Most Common... | Answer and Explanation |
|---|---|
| S/S of PAN | • **fever with multisystem disease,** • *kidneys—* * involved in 85% of cases, * vasculitis/GN, * hematuria, * RBC casts, • *coronary vessels—* * involved in 75% of cases, * thrombosis, * aneurysms, • *liver—* * involved in 65% of cases, * calcification of the cystic duct artery: pathognomonic for PAN, • *GI tract—* * involved in 50% of cases, * bowel infarction, • *skin—* * involved in >25% of cases, * painful nodules with ulceration, * livedo reticularis, • *peripheral neuropathy* [**Note:** the lungs are usually spared in PAN.] |
| clinical associations of PAN | • **HBV—** * ~30–40% of patients with PAN have a positive HBsAg, * in the serum sickness syndrome associated with HBV in 5–10% of cases, the vasculitis and glomerulonephritis are due to PAN, • *cryoglobulinemia,* • *RA,* • *Sjögren's syndrome* |
| lab findings in PAN | • **p-ANCA—** * ~90%, * p refers to perinuclear staining, * these antibodies contribute to the inflammation, because they destroy neutrophils causing the release of their enzymes into the tissue, • *neutrophilic leukocytosis,* • *eosinophilia,* • *HBsAg,* • *thrombocytosis* |
| confirmatory tests for PAN | • **angiography,** • *tissue Bx—* * peripheral nerve, * testicle, * muscle |
| Rx of PAN | **corticosteroids**—often combined with antimetabolites or cytotoxic drugs |
| COD in PAN | • **renal failure,** • *bowel infarction* |
| vasculitis associated with young male smokers | **thromboangiitis obliterans (TAO, Buerger's disease)**—the inflammation involves the entire neurovascular compartment of digits in the upper/lower extremities |

*Table continued on following page*

### Table 5–2. VASCULAR DISORDERS OF SURGICAL
### IMPORTANCE *Continued*

| Most Common... | Answer and Explanation |
|---|---|
| S/S of TAO | • **claudication involving the instep of the foot,** • *loss of digits*—fingers and/or toes: due to thrombosis and ischemic necrosis, • *Raynaud's phenomenon*— ∗ the pulse is absent owing to vessel thrombosis, ∗ the pulse is present in Raynaud's phenomenon that is due to vasospasm |
| Rx of TAO | **stop smoking** |
| cause of pulseless disease | **Takayasu's arteritis**— ∗ granulomatous vasculitis (similar to giant cell arteritis) involving the aortic arch vessels, ∗ aneurysms may develop, ∗ other sites: ♦ AV, ♦ coronary ostia, ♦ renal arteries, ♦ pulmonary vessels, ∗ affects Asian women <50 yrs old |
| S/S of Takayasu's arteritis | • **upper extremity claudication,** • *unequal BP between the upper/lower extremity*—opposite findings to those present in coarctation of the aorta, • *blindness,* • *strokes* |
| Rx of Takayasu's arteritis | **corticosteroids** |
| COD in Takayasu's arteritis | • **CHF,** • *CVA* |
| cause of phlebothrombosis | **stasis of blood flow**—see Table 2–13 for a full discussion |
| mechanism of thrombophlebitis | **obstructive clot**— ∗ a clot may precede inflammation, ∗ inflammation may cause thrombosis, ∗ see Table 2–13 for risk factors |
| types of thrombophlebitis | • **superficial,** • *deep*—e.g., ∗ axillary vein, ∗ portal vein |
| causes of superficial thrombophlebitis | • **IV infusions into catheters,** • *IV catheters,* • *IVDU,* • *trauma,* • *varicose veins,* • *neighboring infection* |
| S/S of superficial thrombophlebitis | **fever, pain, tenderness, erythema, heat along course of vein**— ∗ palpable cord, ∗ swelling is not usually evident |
| Rx of superficial thrombophlebitis | • **anti-inflammatory agents,** • *elastic compression bandages,* • *heat,* • antibiotics if septic |

## Table 5–2. VASCULAR DISORDERS OF SURGICAL
## IMPORTANCE *Continued*

| Most Common... | Answer and Explanation |
|---|---|
| cause of phlegmasia alba dolens | **sudden thrombophlebitis and partial occlusive thrombosis of the femoral vein** |
| S/S of phlegmasia alba dolens | • **sudden onset of pain**— * confused with embolization except pallor is less intense and more cyanosis is present, * tender femoral vein, • **massive pitting edema of extremity**— due to almost complete obstruction of the femoral vein, • **pallor from arterial vasospasm**— * mild cyanosis, * Doppler identifies the reduced arterial blood flow |
| cause of phlegmasia cerulea dolens | **thrombosis blocking the entire venous return of extremity** |
| S/S of phlegmasia cerulea dolens | • **deep cyanosis of the entire limb**, • **extreme pain**, • **massive pitting edema**, • **arterial pulses may be obliterated**, • **gangrene may occur** |
| causes of axillary vein thrombosis | **overexercising upper extremity**— * called "effort" vein thrombosis, * commonly occurs in jackhammer operators |
| S/S of axillary vein thrombosis | **abrupt pain, cyanosis, and swelling of the upper extremity** |
| large superficial veins of the lower extremity | • **great saphenous vein**— * begins anterior to the medial malleolus and drains into the femoral vein in the femoral canal, * communicating (penetrating) veins drain into the deep femoral vein in the thigh and deep venous system (particularly the posterior tibial vein) in the lower leg, • **lesser saphenous vein**— * it begins on the lateral side of the foot and drains into the popliteal vein in the popliteal fossa, * perforators connect with the deep venous system [**Note:** valves keep blood moving from the superficial (greater/lesser saphenous veins) to the deep venous system (e.g., deep femoral vein in the thigh, posterior tibial vein in the lower leg). Penetrating branches are ~5 cm from each other.] |

*Table continued on following page*

Table 5–2. VASCULAR DISORDERS OF SURGICAL
IMPORTANCE *Continued*

| Most Common... | Answer and Explanation |
|---|---|
| factors responsible for drainage of blood from the lower extremities | • **competent valves in the veins**—there are more valves in the deep than in the superficial system, • *patent venous lumens,* • *voluntary muscle contractions*—muscles compress veins and aid the pumping of blood back to the right heart |
| cause of primary varicose veins in the legs | **congenital absence of the sentinel valve in the common femoral vein**— * there is usually a positive family Hx of venous incompetence, * pregnancy is a common precipitating event |
| causes of secondary varicose veins | • **vessel obstruction**—e.g., DVT, • *vessel damage*—e.g., thrombophlebitis leading to dysfunctional penetrating branches between the superficial and deep venous system: particularly the penetrators connecting the greater saphenous vein with the posterior tibial vein |
| complications of varicose veins | • **swelling of the leg,** • *thrombosis,* • *thrombophlebitis,* • *stasis dermatitis* |
| tests for evaluating the competency of the greater saphenous vein and the penetrators draining into the deep femoral vein | • **Duplex scanning**— * this is the most sensitive test, * see Table 2–13, • *venography*—see Table 2–13, • *Brodie-Trendelenburg test–* * the lower extremity is elevated to a vertical position to drain the venous blood from the leg → a tourniquet is applied to the midthigh to occlude the great saphenous vein → the patient stands up with the tourniquet in place and the time for venous filling to occur below the tourniquet is noted: normally, arterial blood flow from below the tourniquet should slowly fill the veins in ~35 seconds → the tourniquet is released in 1 min: no further filling of the veins should occur if the venous system is competent, * if slow filling occurs with the tourniquet in place and no further filling when it is released the test is negative, which indicates that the great saphenous and penetrating branches are competent |

## Table 5–2. VASCULAR DISORDERS OF SURGICAL
### IMPORTANCE *Continued*

| Most Common... | Answer and Explanation |
|---|---|
| findings in Brodie-Trendelenburg test that indicate incompetency of the great saphenous vein | • **tourniquet applied**—slow filling indicates competent penetrators, • **tourniquet released**— * quick filling from above occurs in 1–10 sec, * this is a positive test for incompetency of the great saphenous vein |
| findings in Brodie-Trendelenburg test that indicate incompetency of both the great saphenous vein and the penetrating veins | • **tourniquet applied**—rapid filling (<30 seconds) indicates incompetent penetrators, • **tourniquet released**— * further filling of the veins with blood: incompetent great saphenous vein, * this is called a double-positive test |
| test for obstruction of the deep veins in the lower extremity | **Perthes' test**— * inspect the patient's superficial varicosities after a walk around, * apply a tourniquet to the midthigh with the patient standing: when the varicosities are filled with blood, have the patient walk around for 5 min, * in a normal test, the varicose veins collapse (diminish) below the tourniquet: this indicates patency of the deep veins and competency of the penetrators |
| findings in Perthes' test if the superficial saphenous veins and penetrators are incompetent | **the varicose veins remain unchanged**—competent saphenous veins and penetrators would have directed blood into the deep system after muscular activity |
| findings in Perthes' test if the deep veins are occluded | **increase in prominence of the varicosities of the superficial saphenous veins plus pain**—sign of deep vein occlusion and incompetent penetrators |
| Rx of varicose veins | • **nonoperative**— * adequate elastic hose support, * leg elevation, * encourage walking, * discourage prolonged sitting/standing, • **operative**— * compression sclerotherapy, * venous stripping |
| cause of stasis dermatitis (postphlebitic syndrome) | **DVT in the proximal venous system**— * blood flows from the deep to superficial venous system around the ankles, * a proximal DVT increases the pressure in the penetrating vessels around the ankles |

*Table continued on following page*

### Table 5–2. VASCULAR DISORDERS OF SURGICAL IMPORTANCE *Continued*

| Most Common... | Answer and Explanation |
|---|---|
| S/S of stasis dermatitis | • **ankle edema**— * this is the first sign, * due to increased hydrostatic pressure imposed on the penetrating branches by the more proximal DVT, • *hemorrhage*—hemosiderin deposition occurs in subcutaneous tissue owing to extravasation of RBCs into the tissue, • *ulceration*—due to tissue hypoxia from stagnant venous blood, • *secondary varicose veins in the superficial saphenous veins*—increased blood is redirected from the deep to the superficial system, • *danger of squamous cell carcinoma in long-standing ulcers* |
| Rx of stasis dermatitis | • **nonoperative**—topical antibiotics and corticosteroids, • ***operative***— * skin grafting of large ulcers, * ligation of incompetent perforators |
| cause of the superior vena caval (SVC) syndrome | **obstruction of the SVC by a primary small cell carcinoma of the lung**—male predominance |
| S/S of SVC syndrome | • **face, neck, and shoulders are puffy and cyanotic,** • *distended jugular vein,* • *CNS*— * dizziness, * visual disturbances, * possibility of a stroke |
| Rx of SVC syndrome | • **prompt radiation,** • *drugs*—diuretics to reduce tissue swelling |
| causes of IVC obstruction | • **extension of a pelvic/femoral vein thrombosis into the IVC,** • *extension of a renal adenocarcinoma into the renal vein and into the IVC* |
| pathologic causes of an arteriovenous fistula | • **penetrating injury**—usually a knife wound in an extremity, • *congenital*—Klippel-Trenaunay syndrome: large hemangioma on extremity, which results in hemihypertrophy of bone and soft tissue, • *Paget's disease of bone*—the soft bone is highly vascular and contains numerous arteriovenous fistulas |

**Table 5–2. VASCULAR DISORDERS OF SURGICAL IMPORTANCE** *Continued*

| Most Common... | Answer and Explanation |
|---|---|
| S/S of arteriovenous fistulas | • **venous abnormalities**— * increased pressure, * edema, * varicose veins, * ulceration, hyperpigmentation, • *high output failure*—direct communication of arteries with veins bypasses microcirculation and increases venous return to heart, • *pain*—thrombosis, • *thrill/bruit*, • *Branham's sign*—compression of fistula to decrease blood flow causes sinus bradycardia and increased systolic/diastolic BP |
| Rx of arteriovenous fistulas | **surgery** |
| mechanisms of lymphedema | • **aplasia**—never developed, • **hypoplasia**—incomplete development, • **hyperplasia of lymphatic vessels** |
| types of primary lymphedema | • **praecox**— * presents in adolescence, * female dominant, * usually involves the legs, • *congenital*— * present at birth, * hereditary type is called Milroy's disease, * lymphedema of the hands/feet in Turner's syndrome, • *tarda*— * presents >35 yrs of age, * men/women equally involved |
| causes of secondary lymphedema in United States | • **radiation postradical mastectomy,** • *inflammatory carcinoma of the breast*—plugs of tumor block the dermal lymphatics, producing peau d'orange (orange peel) appearance, • *lymphogranuloma venereum*—scrotal/vulvar lymphedema [**Note:** parasitic diseases are the MCC of lymphedema worldwide (e.g., filariasis).] |
| S/S of lymphedema | • **painless swelling of an extremity**— * initially it produces a pitting edema relieved by elevation of the extremity, * it becomes nonpitting when it persists (chronic lymphedema): ♦ swelling is not relieved with elevation, ♦ skin is thickened, • *cellulitis,* • *lymphangiosarcoma*—a potential complication in long-standing cases |
| Rx of lymphedema | • **nonoperative**— * extremity elevation, * sequential pneumatic compression device, * elastic hose, * drainage with a large-bore needle and suction, • **operative**— * excision with grafting, * lymphatic reconstruction |

*Table continued on following page*

### Table 5-2. VASCULAR DISORDERS OF SURGICAL IMPORTANCE *Continued*

| Most Common... | Answer and Explanation |
|---|---|
| causes of a chylous effusion in the pleural cavity | • **surgical mishap during thoracic surgery**—tear in the thoracic duct, • *malignant lymphoma,* • *central venous catheter placement,* • *blunt/penetrating chest trauma* |
| lab findings in chylous effusion | • **mature lymphocytes,** • **supranate composed of chylomicrons containing TG** |
| Rx of chylothorax | • **nonoperative**— * parenteral hyperalimentation, * oral medium-chain FAs: these are directly absorbed into the blood rather than into the lymphatics, * repeated thoracentesis with drainage, • **operative**— * pleurodesis, * ligation of the thoracic duct, * pleuroperitoneal shunt |

**Question:** Which of the following are most often associated with atherosclerosis? **SELECT 4**

    (A) Arteriovenous fistula
    (B) Stroke
    (C) Leriche syndrome
    (D) Thoracic outlet syndrome
    (E) Stasis dermatitis
    (F) Sudden-onset pain and pallor in lower extremity
    (G) Pulseless disease
    (H) Dissecting aortic aneurysm
    (I) Abdominal aortic aneurysm
    (J) Berry aneurysm
    (K) Popliteal artery aneurysm

**Answers: (B), (C), (I), (K).** Arteriovenous fistulas are most often related to penetrating injury of an extremity **(choice A is incorrect).** Strokes are most often secondary to atherosclerosis at the bifurcation of the carotid artery **(choice B is correct).** Leriche syndrome is due to atherosclerosis of the aortoiliac vessel with subsequent claudication and impotence **(choice C is correct).** The thoracic outlet syndrome is due to compression of the subclavian artery and brachial plexus by positional changes, cervical rib, or tight scalenus anticus muscles **(choice D is incorrect).** Stasis dermatitis is a complication of deep venous thrombosis **(choice E is incorrect).** A sudden onset of pain and pallor in the lower extremity is most often due to embolization of thrombus material from the left side of the heart in a patient with atrial fibrillation **(choice F is incorrect).** Pulseless disease is due to a granulomatous vasculitis involving the aortic arch vessels (Takayasu's arteritis, **choice G is incorrect).** A dissecting aortic aneurysm is most often related to cystic medial degeneration and elastic tissue fragmentation **(choice H is incorrect).** Abdominal aortic aneurysms and popliteal artery aneurysms are most often secondary to atherosclerosis **(choices I and K are correct).** Berry aneurysms are most often congenital **(choice J is incorrect).**

ABI = ankle/brachial index, ACA = anterior cerebral artery, AMI = acute myocardial infarction, ARDS = adult respiratory distress syndrome, ARF = acute renal failure, AV = aortic valve, AVM = arteriovenous malformation, BP = blood pressure, Bx = biopsy, CAD = coronary artery disease, CBD = common bile duct, CH = cholesterol, CHF = congestive heart failure, CK = creatine kinase, CN = cranial nerve, COD = cause of death, CVA = cerebrovascular accident, DM = diabetes mellitus, DVT = deep venous thrombosis, ESR = erythrocyte sedimentation rate, FAs = fatty acids, FN = false-negative, FRs = free radicals, GN = glomerulonephritis, HBsAg = hepatitis B surface antigen, HBV = hepatitis B virus, HDL = high-density lipoprotein, HSP = Henoch-Schönlein purpura, HTN = hypertension, ICs = immunocomplexes, ICA = internal carotid artery, IVC = inferior vena cava, IVDU = intravenous drug user, LDL = low-density lipoprotein, MC = most common, MCA = middle cerebral artery, MCC = most common cause, MVA = motor vehicle accident, N/V = nausea/vomiting, PAN = polyarteritis nodosa, p-ANCA = perinuclear antineutrophil cytoplasmic antibody, PH = portal hypertension, PRV = polycythemia rubra vera, RA = rheumatoid arthritis, RIND = reversible ischemic neurologic defect, SiADH = syndrome of inappropriate antidiuretic hormone, SMA = superior mesenteric artery, S/S = signs/symptoms, SVC = superior vena cava, TAO = thromboangiitis obliterans, TG = triacylglycerol, TIA = transient ischemic attack, tPA = tissue plasminogen activator, $TXA_2$ = thromboxane $A_2$.

### Table 5–3. SURGICALLY CORRECTABLE CAUSES OF HYPERTENSION, ADULT CONGENITAL HEART DISEASE

| Most Common... | Answer and Explanation |
|---|---|
| cause of secondary HTN in men | **unilateral renovascular HTN—** * secondary to atherosclerosis occluding the proximal orifice of the renal artery, * activation of the renin-angiotensin-aldosterone system |
| cause of renovascular HTN in women | **fibromuscular hyperplasia**—reduced renal blood flow is due to multifocal areas of smooth muscle cell hyperplasia in the media of the renal artery |
| surgically correctable cause of secondary HTN in young individuals | **coarctation of the aorta** |

*Table continued on following page*

**Table 5–3. SURGICALLY CORRECTABLE CAUSES OF
HYPERTENSION, ADULT CONGENITAL HEART DISEASE**
*Continued*

| Most Common... | Answer and Explanation |
|---|---|
| renal tumors associated with secondary HTN | • **renal adenocarcinoma**—secrete renin, • *Wilm's tumor*—secrete renin |
| adrenal tumors associated with secondary HTN | • **primary aldosteronism,** • *pheochromo– cytoma*—most commonly occurs in adults, • *neuroblastoma*—most commonly occurs in children, • *adrenal Cushing's syndrome*— adrenal adenoma/carcinoma |
| neurogenic disorder associated with secondary HTN | **increase in intracranial pressure**—e.g., brain tumor |
| parathyroid disorder associated with secondary HTN | **primary HPTH**—it is most often due to a parathyroid adenoma involving one of the inferior parathyroid glands |
| thyroid disorders associated with HTN | • **primary hypothyroidism**—diastolic HTN due to an increase in blood volume, • *Graves' disease*—systolic HTN due to an increase in SV |
| S/S of renovascular HTN | • **abrupt onset of severe, uncontrolled HTN**—usually resistant to standard medical therapy, * most commonly occurs in men with severe atherosclerotic disease, • *epigastric bruit*—due to blood flow through the stenotic opening of the renal artery |
| noninvasive screening test for renovascular HTN | **renal radionuclide scan followed by captopril (ACE inhibitor)**— * the initial scan reveals a small kidney with decreased uptake and clearance of the radiotracer postadministration of captopril, * captopril stimulation increases PRA over the baseline values, owing to the loss of the inhibitory effect of AT II on renin release |

## Table 5–3. SURGICALLY CORRECTABLE CAUSES OF
## HYPERTENSION, ADULT CONGENITAL HEART DISEASE
*Continued*

| Most Common... | Answer and Explanation |
|---|---|
| confirmatory test for renovascular HTN | **renal arteriography and evaluation of the PRA in renal veins draining the ipsilateral and contralateral kidney**— * arteriography reveals significant atherosclerotic stenosis (>70%) in the proximal renal artery, * a "string-of-beads" effect is noted in FMH, * the ipsilateral renal vein PRA is increased: it is usually 1.5 times greater than the contralateral side, * the contralateral renal vein PRA is suppressed: ♦ increased AT II suppresses renin release in the normal kidney, ♦ lack of suppression of renin indicates parenchymal disease in the contralateral kidney, most often secondary to the sustained HTN |
| Rx of unilateral RAS | • **aortorenal bypass**—Rx of choice for atherosclerotic occlusive disease, • **angioplasty**— * Rx of choice for FMH, * Rx of choice for significant bilateral RAS |
| PRA concentration in patients with bilateral RAS | **returns to near normal**—due to the inhibitory effect of AT II suppressing the renin release from both kidneys |
| cause of primary aldosteronism (Conn's syndrome) | **unilateral adrenal adenoma involving zona glomerulosa**— * adenomas are the cause in ~60–75% of cases, * primary adrenal hyperplasia is the cause in the remainder of cases |
| S/S suggesting primary aldosteronism | • **severe muscle weakness/paralysis due to hypokalemia**—hypokalemia is due to augmented exchange of $K^+$ for $Na^+$ in the aldosterone-enhanced $Na^+/K^+$ pump in the late distal/collecting ducts, • *diastolic HTN,* • *tetany*—alkalosis increases the binding of ionized $Ca^{++}$ to albumin, • *polyuria*—hypokalemic nephropathy renders the collecting ducts refractory to ADH: nephrogenic DI, • *absence of pitting edema*—the increase in plasma volume inhibits proximal tubule reabsorption of $Na^+$, which offsets the enhanced distal reabsorption of $Na^+$ by aldosterone |

*Table continued on following page*

## Table 5–3. SURGICALLY CORRECTABLE CAUSES OF HYPERTENSION, ADULT CONGENITAL HEART DISEASE
*Continued*

| Most Common... | Answer and Explanation |
|---|---|
| screening tests for primary aldosteronism | • **plasma aldosterone/PRA ratio >20–25 after 4 hrs of standing upright**— * standing upright normally stimulates renin release, * in primary hyperplasia, there is an increase in PRA and plasma aldosterone, * in adenomas, there is suppression of PRA and little change in plasma aldosterone, • *PRA < 5 µg/dL and urine aldosterone > 20 µg in a 24-hr urine,* • *24-hr urine K⁺ > 30 mEq/day* |
| confirmatory tests for primary aldosteronism | • **failure to suppress plasma aldosterone after an isotonic saline infusion or after administration of captopril or fludrocortisone**—failure to suppress aldosterone confirms the autonomous nature of the hyperplasia/adenoma, • *CT scan*—identifies adenomas, • *elective venous sampling*—this is the most sensitive test for localizing adenomas or defining primary hyperplasia, • *measure precursor mineralocorticoids*—18-hydroxycorticosterone is more likely to be elevated in an adenoma rather than in hyperplasia |
| lab findings in primary aldosteronism | • **hypokalemia,** • *normal to slightly increased serum Na⁺,* • *marked kaluresis*—leads to hypokalemia, • *metabolic alkalosis*—increased reclaiming and regeneration of bicarbonate |
| Rx of primary aldosteronism | • **adenomas**—surgically removed, • **primary hyperplasia**—spironolactone: aldosterone blocker |
| S/S of a pheochromocytoma | • **triad of sustained hypertension in a patient with excessive sweating, anxiety, and headaches,** • *palpitations,* • *orthostatic hypotension*—a reduced plasma volume due to constriction of arterioles/venules, • *ileus*—catecholamines inhibit peristalsis, • *chest pain*—subendocardial ischemia, • *association with MEN IIa/IIb syndromes,* • *association with von Hippel-Lindau disease*—pheochromocytomas are often bilateral, • *association with neurofibromatosis* [**Note:** most pheochromocytomas are benign, most are unilateral in the adrenal medulla, and most are present in adults rather than in children.] |

**Table 5–3. SURGICALLY CORRECTABLE CAUSES OF
HYPERTENSION, ADULT CONGENITAL HEART DISEASE**
*Continued*

| Most Common... | Answer and Explanation |
|---|---|
| ancillary lab findings in pheochromocytoma | • **neutrophilic leukocytosis**—catecholamines decrease adhesion molecule synthesis, • *hyperglycemia*—increased glycogenolysis, • *polycythemia*—due to contraction of the plasma volume |
| screening tests for pheochromocytoma | **24-hr urine for metanephrine (most sensitive test) and vanillylmandelic acid (VMA)** |
| confirmatory tests for pheochromocytoma | • **lack of suppression of catecholamines after administration of clonidine,** • *CT scan*—most useful in localizing the tumor |
| Rx of pheochromocytoma | **surgical removal**— * preoperative preparation: ♦ α-adrenergic blocker (phenoxybenzamine) to control HTN and restore plasma volume, ♦ β-blockers to control tachycardias |
| Rx of hypertensive crisis during surgery | • **nitroprusside,** • *phentolamine* |
| additional screening tests that should be done in patients with a known pheochromocytoma | • **screen for MEN IIa and IIb**—screen family members for the presence of the RET proto-oncogene, • **screen for von Hippel–Lindau disease**—DNA testing is available that localizes the abnormal suppressor gene on chromosome 3 |
| differences between adult and childhood CHD | **adults have less complex and less cyanotic CHD**—~90% of children born with CHD survive until adulthood |
| adult CHDs | • **congenital bicuspid AV,** • *ostium secundum type of ASD*— * increased incidence in women, * often discovered in pregnancy due to increased plasma volume, • *pulmonic stenosis,* • *coarctation of the aorta,* • *PDA,* • *tetralogy of Fallot* |

*Table continued on following page*

## Table 5–3. SURGICALLY CORRECTABLE CAUSES OF
## HYPERTENSION, ADULT CONGENITAL HEART DISEASE
*Continued*

| Most Common... | Answer and Explanation |
|---|---|
| adult cyanotic CHD | **tetralogy of Fallot**— * adults usually have a mild degree of infravalvular pulmonic stenosis, which reduces the incidence of cyanosis: blood enters the PA for oxygenation in the lung rather than crossing the VSD into the LV causing cyanosis, * most adult patients have mild cyanosis and a systolic murmur, * echocardiography with color flow imaging and Doppler interrogation studies are diagnostic |
| problems associated with a congenital bicuspid AV | • **calcific AS/isolated AV regurgitation,** • *coarctation of the aorta*—25% of patients, • *infective endocarditis,* • **macroangiopathic hemolytic anemia**—intravascular hemolysis with schistocytes in peripheral blood: secondary iron deficiency from loss of iron in the urine is common |
| clinical findings in adult ASD | • **supraventricular atrial arrhythmias**—AF is the most common type, • *PH secondary to left to right shunting of blood*—overloading of the right heart and PA leads to PH with RVH and reversal of the shunt: this is called Eisenmenger's complex, • *cyanosis with exercise,* • *hemoptysis,* • *RHF,* • *potential for paradoxical embolism when the shunt reverses* |
| cardiac findings in an ASD | • **fixed splitting of S$_2$**—left to right shunting of blood causes even further delay in closure of the PV, • *midsystolic pulmonary flow murmur*—due to increased blood flow across the PV, • *left axis deviation,* • *accentuation of P$_2$*—sign of PH, • *step-up of oxygen in the RA, RV, and PA* |
| late complication of left to right shunts | **Eisenmenger's complex**— * refers to reversal of a left to right shunt into a right to left shunt leading to cyanosis, * due to PH from volume overload of the right heart, with subsequent development of RVH leading to reversal of the shunt and cyanosis |

### Table 5–3. SURGICALLY CORRECTABLE CAUSES OF HYPERTENSION, ADULT CONGENITAL HEART DISEASE
*Continued*

| Most Common... | Answer and Explanation |
| --- | --- |
| cardiac findings in pulmonic stenosis | • **systolic ejection murmur in the second left ICS**—intensity of the murmur increases with inspiration, • *systolic ejection click,* • *fixed splitting of $A_2$,* • *diminished $P_2$ heart sound,* • *right-sided $S_4$ heart sound*— * increased intensity with inspiration, * $S_4$ is due to RVH, • *parasternal heave*—sign of RVH, *cannon a wave*— * the a wave is normally due to contraction of the RA in late diastole to expel the remainder of blood into the RV: there is some mild reflux of blood back into the jugular vein causing the a wave, * atrial contraction against increased resistance to blood flow into the RV produces a giant a wave: resistance is due to RVH secondary to pulmonic stenosis, • *poststenotic dilation of PA* [**Note:** the majority of cases of pulmonic stenosis are mild to moderate. Many patients have a normal life expectancy.] |
| mechanism of a postductal coarctation | **defect in the media of the aorta**— * in adults, the area of narrowing in the aorta is distal to the ligamentum arteriosum, * in children, the area of narrowing is preductal: often associated with Turner's syndrome, * adult coarctations are 5 times more common in men than women, * adult coarctations usually develop after the third or fourth decade |
| S/S of a postductal coarctation | • **HTN in the upper extremities**—lower blood pressure in the lower extremities, • *greater muscular development in upper rather than lower extremities,* • *harsh systolic murmur*—heard best at the angle of the left scapula, • *leg claudication with exercise*—due to ischemia, • *diastolic HTN*—due to reduced renal blood flow, which activates the RAA system |

*Table continued on following page*

### Table 5–3. SURGICALLY CORRECTABLE CAUSES OF HYPERTENSION, ADULT CONGENITAL HEART DISEASE
*Continued*

| Most Common... | Answer and Explanation |
|---|---|
| complications/ associations of a postductal coarctation | • **increased incidence of congenital bicuspid AV**—20–25%, • *dissecting aortic aneurysm*—occurs in the proximally dilated aorta that is under increased tension, • *increased incidence of berry aneurysms*— * due to increased blood flow into the cerebral vessels, * there is a potential for a subarachnoid hemorrhage, • *infective endocarditis* |
| chest x-ray findings in a postductal coarctation | • **rib notching**—due to erosion of bone by dilated collateral intercostal arteries, • *figure "3" sign*—due to pre- and poststenotic dilatation of the aorta |
| murmur associated with an adult PDA | **machinery murmur**—chest x-ray may reveal calcification of the ductus in older adults |
| complications of cyanotic CHD | • **secondary polycythemia**—due to right to left shunting of blood and the stimulus for EPO release by hypoxemia, • *infective endocarditis,* • *multiple cerebral abscesses*—the potential exists for embolism of infected vegetations into the systemic circulation, • *clubbing*—increased collagen formation beneath the nailbed due to excessive release of PDGF from platelets shunted into the systemic circulation through the cardiac defect, • *cholelithiasis*—increased production of UCB by macrophages occurs owing to the excess number of RBCs |
| CHD that is least likely to develop IE | **ASD**— * patients with uncomplicated ASD are not placed on prophylactic antibiotics: amoxicillin, * all other CHDs are at increased risk for IE, * ASDs have an increased risk if there is a Hx of previous surgical correction of the ASD |
| congenital malformation of the coronary artery | **coronary arteriovenous fistula**—this is most often recognized by the presence of an atypical continuous murmur |

**Table 5–3. SURGICALLY CORRECTABLE CAUSES OF
HYPERTENSION, ADULT CONGENITAL HEART DISEASE**
*Continued*

**Question:** Which of the following organs are adversely affected by
hypertension? **SELECT 3**
- (A) Heart
- (B) Brain
- (C) Adrenals
- (D) Thyroid
- (E) Kidneys

**Answers: (A), (B), (E).** The heart is most affected in HTN **(choice A is
correct).** Cardiac problems include AMI, CHF, and LVH. Intracerebral
bleeds may occur in hypertension **(choice B is correct).** They are most
commonly due to rupture of Charcot-Bouchard microaneurysms of the
lenticulostriate vessels, producing a hematoma in the area of the
putamen, globus pallidus, and internal capsule. The adrenal glands
and thyroid gland have disorders that produce HTN; however, HTN
is not the direct cause of any disorders in these organs **(choices C and
D are incorrect).** The kidneys are affected by HTN **(choice E is correct).**
If HTN is due to HTN. Benign nephrosclerosis is the kidney disease of
hyaline arteriolosclerosis of cortical vessels leading to atrophy and
fibrosis of tubules and glomeruli. Proteinuria and renal failure are
potential outcomes of nephrosclerosis.

ACE = angiotensin-converting enzyme, ADH = antidiuretic hormone,
AF = atrial fibrillation, AMI = acute myocardial infarction, AS = aortic
stenosis, ASD = atrial septal defect, AT II = angiotensin II, AV = aortic
valve, BNS = benign nephrosclerosis, CHD = congenital heart disease,
CHG = congestive heart failure, DI = diabetes insipidus, EPO = erythropoietin, FMH = fibromuscular hyperplasia, HPTH = hyperparathyroidism, HTN = hypertension, ICS = intercostal space, IE = infective endocarditis, LA = left atrium, LV = left ventricle, LVH = left ventricular
hypertrophy, MC = most common, MEN = multiple endocrine neoplasia,
PA = pulmonary artery, PDA = patent ductus arteriosus, PDGF = platelet-derived growth factor, PH = pulmonary hypertension, PRA = plasma
renin activity, PV = pulmonic valve, RA = right atrium, RAA = renin-
angiotensin-aldosterone (system), RAS = renal artery stenosis, RHF =
right heart failure, RV = right ventricle, RVH = right ventricular hypertrophy, $S_2$ = second heart sound, S/S = signs and symptoms, SV =
stroke volume, TV = tricuspid valve, UCB = unconjugated bilirubin,
VMA = vanillylmandelic acid, VSD = ventricular septal defect.

Table 5–4. ISCHEMIC HEART DISEASE (IHD),
VALVULAR HEART DISEASE, MYOCARDIAL
AND PERICARDIAL DISORDERS

| Most Common... | Answer and Explanation |
|---|---|
| COD in the United States | **CAD**— * CAD accounts for ~25% of all deaths in the United States, * CAD is 4 times more common in men than women |
| coronary artery causing an acute myocardial infarction | **left anterior descending coronary artery** [**Note:** the LAD coronary artery supplies the anterior wall of the LV and anterior two-thirds of the IVS.] |
| AMI complications associated with LAD coronary artery thrombosis | • **LV mural thrombosis,** • *second/third degree AV nodal blocks requiring a permanent pacemaker*—due to location of the bundles in the anterior third of IVS, which is supplied by the LAD coronary artery, • *ventricular aneurysm,* • *myocardial rupture*—usually involves the free wall of the LV |
| coronary artery involved with an atypical presentation of chest pain with an acute myocardial infarction | **right coronary artery (RCA)**—because the RCA supplies the posterior and inferior wall of the LV, epigastric pain stimulating gastroesophageal reflux disease may occur [**Note:** the RCA supplies the posteroinferior part of the LV, the entire RV, the posterior one-third of the IVS, and 90% of the blood supply to the atrioventricular node. In ~90%, the RCA terminates with a posterior descending artery branch indicating right coronary artery dominance.] |
| AMI complications associated with RCA thrombosis | • **sinus bradycardia**—RCA supplies atrioventricular node, • **papillary muscle dysfunction/rupture**—RCA supplies the posteromedial papillary muscle, • **right ventricular infarction** |
| ECG manifestation of transmural ischemia | **ST elevation** |
| symptom of myocardial ischemia | **chest pain (angina)**—occurs when ventricular $O_2$ demand is greater than $O_2$ supply |
| cause of myocardial ischemia | • **atherosclerosis of the coronary arteries,** • *vasospasm*—e.g., Prinzmetal's angina, • *vasculitis*—e.g., * polyarteritis nodosa, * Kawasaki's disease, • *embolization,* • *dissecting aortic aneurysm* |

### Table 5–4. ISCHEMIC HEART DISEASE (IHD), VALVULAR HEART DISEASE, MYOCARDIAL AND PERICARDIAL DISORDERS *Continued*

| Most Common... | Answer and Explanation |
| --- | --- |
| clinical presentations of IHD | • **angina pectoris,** • *AMI,* • *sudden cardiac death* (SCD)—death within 1 hr of chest pain, • *chronic IHD*—severe fixed CAD with ischemic damage to the myocardium and replacement by fibrous tissue, • *cardiac arrhythmias* |
| type of angina | **exertional angina**— * associated with fixed atherosclerotic CAD, * precipitated by exercise and relieved by rest and/or nitroglycerin, * stress ECG reveals ST segment depression |
| type of angina associated with vasospasm | **Prinzmetal's angina**— * primarily occurs in women <50 yrs old, * a resting angina: usually occurs in the early AM, * a stress ECG reveals ST elevation: transmural ischemia, * coronary angiograms exhibit a mild degree of atherosclerotic CAD, * vasospasm may be due to platelet release of TXA₂ from small platelet thrombi |
| type of angina associated with rest | **unstable angina**— * usually arises out of a pre-existing exertional type of angina, * >50% patients have multivessel disease, * coronary angiograms reveal: ♦ eccentric/irregular lumens, ♦ rupture/fissuring of plaques, ♦ nonocclusive thrombi, * ~20% progress to an AMI in 3 mos, • *angiography is recommended*—patients are hospitalized |
| chest pain characteristics of angina | • **precipitating events**— * exertion, * during meals, * stress/excitement, • **relieved by**— * rest: exertional type, * nitroglycerin, • **pain characteristics**— * tightness, * squeezing, * burning, * aching, • **pain location/ radiation**— * retrosternal: 90%, * radiation to jaw, neck, left shoulder, inner aspect of arm, • **duration**— * usually <3 min, * rarely >20 min |
| ECG findings in angina | • **downsloping depression of the ST segment**—rarely ST segment elevation is present, • *T wave peaking or inversion* |

*Table continued on following page*

### Table 5–4. ISCHEMIC HEART DISEASE (IHD), VALVULAR HEART DISEASE, MYOCARDIAL AND PERICARDIAL DISORDERS *Continued*

| Most Common... | Answer and Explanation |
|---|---|
| screening test for angina | **stress ECG**— * a positive test is a 1-mm horizontal or downsloping ST segment depression at 0.08 sec after the J point, * radionuclide studies are used in equivocal cases: see **Table 5–1** |
| Rx of an acute attack of angina | **sublingual nitroglycerin**—nitrate functions include: ♦ reduce preload (venodilation), ♦ reduce afterload (arteriole vasodilatation), ♦ vasodilate coronary arteries, ♦ reduce $O_2$ demand in the heart |
| drugs that prevent angina | • **β-adrenergic blockers**— * initial drug of choice, * decreases: ♦ HR, ♦ BP, ♦ contractility, ♦ myocardial $O_2$ demands, • *isosorbides*—long-acting nitrates, • *calcium channel blockers*— * direct coronary artery vasodilator: excellent for preventing vasospasm, • *aspirin*— * prevents thrombosis/strokes,* increases survival in unstable angina, • *Rx hyperlipidemias*, • *heparin*— * mainly used for unstable angina for ~2 days, * combined with aspirin |
| advantages of PTCA over CABG for Rx of occlusive CAD | • **less mortality,** • *less post-AMI,* • *procedure of choice for 1-to-2-vessel disease*—the exception to the above is stenosis of the left main coronary artery |
| disadvantages of PTCA over CABG for Rx of occlusive CAD | • **higher rate of recurrence,** • *may require emergency CABG*—4–5%, • *risk of AMI*—4–5% |
| causes of occlusion of coronary artery post-PTCA | • **dissection,** • *thrombosis* |
| vessels used in CABG procedure | • **internal mammary artery**— * graft patency is 97% after 1 yr, * ~95% patency after 10 yrs, • **saphenous veins**— * graft patency ~90% after 1 yr, * 40–50% patency after 10 yrs: "arterialization" of the saphenous vein occurs, with subsequent fibrosis and occlusion |

**Table 5–4. ISCHEMIC HEART DISEASE (IHD),
VALVULAR HEART DISEASE, MYOCARDIAL
AND PERICARDIAL DISORDERS** *Continued*

| Most Common... | Answer and Explanation |
|---|---|
| advantages of CABG procedure over PTCA | • **greater rate of symptomatic relief from angina**—longevity is increased most notably with a CABG of the left main stem artery, • **procedure of choice with 2-vessel disease involving proximal LAD coronary artery and with 3-vessel disease,** • **lower number of recurrences**—longer graft patency than PTCA: 30–50% restenosis in 3–6 mos, • **diabetics have better outcomes with a CABG procedure** [Note: excellent presumptive evidence exists that CABG procedures prolong survival.] |
| features of a Q wave AMI | • **usually transmural**— * ST segment elevation, * large size, • *occlusive coronary artery thrombosis—>90%,* • *increased early mortality* |
| features of a non-Q wave AMI | • **usually subendocardial**— * ST depression, * small size, * difficult to distinguish from unstable angina, • *occlusive thrombosis in ~30%,* • *increased risk of SCD within several months post-AMI* |
| S/S with a high predictive value for an AMI | • **character of pain**— * crushing retrosternal chest pain lasting > 30–45 min, * pain not relieved by nitroglycerin, • **radiation of pain**—down the ulnar aspect of left arm, into the left shoulder, or jaw, • **pain associations**— * diaphoresis, * dyspnea/tachypnea: signs of pulmonary congestion, * orthopnea: sign of LHF |
| type of AMI associated with epigastric pain simulating GERD | **inferior wall AMI**—usually RCA thrombosis |

*Table continued on following page*

## Table 5–4. ISCHEMIC HEART DISEASE (IHD), VALVULAR HEART DISEASE, MYOCARDIAL AND PERICARDIAL DISORDERS *Continued*

| Most Common... | Answer and Explanation |
|---|---|
| indications for PTCA in an AMI | • **AMI < 4 hrs old**— * catheterize and decide whether a PTCA or CABG should be performed, * patient can be given intracoronary thrombolytic agents: better result than with systemic thrombolytic Rx, * CABG must be performed within 4–6 hrs of an AMI: if thrombolytic Rx is given first, the CABG is performed ~1 wk later, • **contraindication for thrombolytic agent,** • **reperfusion failure with thrombolytic agents,** • **cardiogenic shock** [Note: aspirin and heparin are given during and after the procedure.] |
| complications in an AMI | • **arrhythmias**—ventricular premature beat leading to VT and then to VF, • *LHF,* • *cardiogenic shock,* • *cardiac rupture* |
| time frame for cardiogenic shock and LHF in AMI | **first 24 hrs**—particularly if > 40% of the LV is infarcted |
| cause of cardiac tamponade in an AMI | **rupture of anterior free wall of LV**— * this usually occurs during 2nd to 7th day, * accounts for ~10% of deaths |
| clinical findings in a rupture of the IVS in an AMI | • **pansystolic heart murmur,** • **hypotension/shock,** • **step-up of $O_2$ in the RV** [Note: an IVS rupture is most common with an LAD thrombosis.] |
| causes of a mitral regurgitation murmur in an AMI | • **LHF**—volume overload of the LV dilates the MV ring, • *posteromedial papillary muscle dysfunction/rupture*—usually due to an RCA thrombosis involving the posteroinferior part of the heart |
| late complication of an AMI | **ventricular aneurysm**— * occurs in 10–20% of AMIs, * begins developing after 1–2 wks, * clinically recognized between 2–4 wks |
| clinical/lab findings of ventricular aneurysm | • **precordial bulge during systole,** • **echocardiogram**—dyskinetic movement of the involved portion of LV, • **ECG**—persistence of ST segment elevation |

### Table 5–4. ISCHEMIC HEART DISEASE (IHD), VALVULAR HEART DISEASE, MYOCARDIAL AND PERICARDIAL DISORDERS *Continued*

| Most Common... | Answer and Explanation |
|---|---|
| complications associated with a ventricular aneurysm | • **LHF**—correlates with loss of contractile muscle in the left ventricle, • *thromboembolization,* • *angina,* • arrhythmias [**Note:** rupture rarely occurs because the aneurysm is composed of scar tissue.] |
| indications for surgery of ventricular aneurysms | • **recurrent CHF,** • *angina,* • *recurrent embolization* [**Note:** scar tissue is excised and viable myocardial tissue is apposed to ensure contractility.] |
| LV assist device | **intra-aortic balloon**— * the balloon inflates during diastole right after the AV closes: this ensures proper filling of the coronary arteries, * it deflates during systole: this reduces LV afterload |
| indications for an intra-aortic balloon | • **cardiogenic shock in an AMI,** • **stabilization during MV surgery,** • **post-AMI ventricular irritability resistant to medical Rx,** • **LV failure following cardiopulmonary bypass,** • **myocardial ischemia refractory to medical Rx** |
| CK isoenzyme in cardiac tissue | **CK-MM**— * ~85%, * CK-MB accounts for 10–15% |
| time sequence of CK-MB elevation in an AMI | • **initial**—4–6 hrs, • **peak**—24 hrs, • **normal**—1.5–3 days: reappearance of CK-MB after 3 days indicates reinfarction |
| time sequence of troponin-I elevation in an AMI | • **initial**—2–12 hrs, • **peak**—24–48 hrs, • **normal**—5–14 days [**Note:** since it appears earlier and lasts longer than CK-MB, it will likely replace LDH isoenzymes. It probably will not replace the CK-MB isoenzyme because it would not detect reinfarction.] |
| factor determining the prognosis in an AMI | **degree of LV dysfunction**—LV dysfunction is evaluated, with measurement of the EF by echocardiography or radionuclide techniques |

*Table continued on following page*

### Table 5–4. ISCHEMIC HEART DISEASE (IHD), VALVULAR HEART DISEASE, MYOCARDIAL AND PERICARDIAL DISORDERS *Continued*

| Most Common... | Answer and Explanation |
|---|---|
| immune-mediated valvular heart disease | **rheumatic heart disease (RHD)**— * damage to the heart is due to cross-reactivity of antibodies directed against group A streptococci with antigens in the heart, * the initiating infection is usually a pharyngitis, * peak age is 5–15 yrs old |
| valves involved in RHD | • **MV**— * 75–80%, * nonembolic vegetations occur along the line of closure of the MV leading to MV regurgitation, * recurrent RHD results in MS, • *AV*—involved in 30%, • *TV*—uncommon, • *PV*—rare |
| chronic valvular diseases in RHD | • **MS**— * recurrent attacks lead to thickening/interadherence/calcification of valve leaflets and shortening of chordae tendineae, * usually symptomatic within 10 yrs of the initial attack, • *AV regurgitation,* • *mitral regurgitation* |
| cardiac signs in MS | • **accentuation of S$_1$**—this occurs early in the disease when the valve is still pliable, • OS—see **Table 5–1,** • **mid-diastolic rumble,** • **increased P$_2$**—indicates PH due to pulmonary venous hypertension, • **parasternal heave**—sign of RVH due to PH, • **Graham Steell murmur**—occurs in early diastole from PV regurgitation secondary to PH |
| S/S of MS | • **dyspnea on exertion,** • *AF*— * occurs in 50–80% of cases, * AF is due to LA dilatation, * danger of clot formation/embolization, * long-term anticoagulation is required, • *target organ effects of systemic embolization*—e.g., embolic stroke, • *pulmonary edema*—chronic congestion leads to malar flush, • *RHF,* • *PH,* • *hemoptysis*— * secondary to pulmonary venous HTN, * anastomoses occur between the pulmonary veins and bronchial veins, leading to formation of submucosal bronchial varices, • *dysphagia for solids*—due to LA enlargement pressing on the esophagus |
| surgical Rx of MS | • **transfemoral/transatrial MV balloon dilation,** • **closed mitral commissurotomy,** • **open commissurotomy,** • **MV replacement** |

### Table 5–4. ISCHEMIC HEART DISEASE (IHD), VALVULAR HEART DISEASE, MYOCARDIAL AND PERICARDIAL DISORDERS *Continued*

| Most Common... | Answer and Explanation |
|---|---|
| valvular diseases associated with IE | • **MVP with regurgitation**—due to its high incidence in the United States, • *degenerative disease involving AV and MV,* • *congenital heart disease,* • *RHD—30%,* • *prosthetic heart valves* |
| organisms producing infective endocarditis (IE) | • ***Streptococcus viridans***—50–75%, • *Staphylococcus aureus*—25%, • enterococci [**Note:** blood cultures are positive in >95% of cases of IE. Three cultures are commonly drawn ~3 hrs apart.] |
| organism involved with IE secondary to prosthetic heart valves | ***Staphylococcus epidermidis*** (**coagulase-negative**)—prosthetic heart valves are the MC predisposing cardiac lesion for nosocomial IE |
| source of bacteremia producing nosocomial IE | **intravenous catheters**— * *Staphylococcus aureus* is the MC organism associated with intravenous catheters, * indwelling urinary catheters are a common source of gram-negative IE due to *E. coli* |
| organism producing IE in a patient with colon cancer/IBD | ***Streptococcus bovis*** |
| procedures predisposing to bacteremia and IE | • **dental procedures inducing mucosal bleeding,** • **cystoscopy,** • **GB surgery,** • **vaginal hysterectomy,** • **urologic surgery** |
| organism producing IE after dental or upper respiratory procedures | ***Streptococcus viridans***—amoxicillin is prescribed 1 hr before dental procedures (e.g., dental extraction) or respiratory tract procedures (e.g., bronchoscopy with a rigid scope) |
| organism producing IE after a GI/GU procedure | ***Enterococcus***—amoxicillin is usually administered 1 hr before a GI/GU procedures |
| cause of a culture-negative IE | **inadequate Rx of a prior IE** |
| investigative test used to diagnose and follow IE | **echocardiography**—including transthoracic and transesophageal echocardiography |

*Table continued on following page*

### Table 5–4. ISCHEMIC HEART DISEASE (IHD), VALVULAR HEART DISEASE, MYOCARDIAL AND PERICARDIAL DISORDERS *Continued*

| Most Common... | Answer and Explanation |
| --- | --- |
| valve involved in IE | **MV** |
| organism producing IE in an IVDA | ***Staphylococcus aureus*** |
| valves involved with IE in IVDA in descending order | • **TV**— * 44%, * usually an isolated lesion, * produces tricuspid regurgitation, • *MV*—43%, • *AV*—40%, • *two valves are involved in 16% of cases* |
| S/S of IE | • **fever,** • *heart murmurs*—changing murmurs are uncommon, • *CHF,* • *signs related to systemic embolization*—e.g., * hematuria, * embolic stroke, * splenic friction rub, • *splenomegaly,* • *IC-induced vasculitis findings*— * Roth's spot in retina, * splinter hemorrhages of nails, * Osler's nodes: painful nodules on the hands/feet, * Janeway's lesions: painless lesions on hands/feet, * GN |
| complication of IE | **CHF**—most commonly occurs with left-sided valvular lesions |
| IE pathogens with highest mortality | • **IE due to fungi and aerobic gram-negative enteric organisms,** • S. aureus |
| IE valvular disease with highest mortality | **AV** |
| initial Rx for *Staphylococcus aureus* IE | **oxacillin + an aminoglycoside (gentamicin or tobramycin)** |
| initial Rx for *Streptococcus viridans* IE | **penicillin G**—vancomycin is used in penicillin allergic patients |
| initial Rx for *Staphylococcus epidermidis* | **vancomycin** |
| gold standard for diagnosing acquired valvular disease | **catheterization** |

### Table 5–4. ISCHEMIC HEART DISEASE (IHD), VALVULAR HEART DISEASE, MYOCARDIAL AND PERICARDIAL DISORDERS *Continued*

| Most Common... | Answer and Explanation |
|---|---|
| valvular heart disease | **mitral valve prolapse (MVP)—** \* ~5–10% of patients, \* typical profile is tall, thin women |
| cause of MVP | **myxomatous degeneration—** \* leads to redundancy of the MV leaflets, \* posterior leaflet is MC involved, \* AD inheritance pattern in some cases |
| genetic diseases associated with MVP | • **Marfan's syndrome,** • *Ehlers-Danlos syndrome,* • *fragile X syndrome,* • *APKD* |
| cause of SCD in Marfan's syndrome | **MVP** |
| S/S of MVP | • **most cases are asymptomatic,** • **chest pain**—MC symptomatic presentation, • *postural hypotension,* • *palpitations,* • *fatigue* |
| cardiac signs in MVP | **midsystolic ejection click followed by a mid- to late systolic murmur of mitral regurgitation** |
| complications associated with MVP | • **isolated MV regurgitation,** • *rupture of chordae*—acute MV regurgitation, • *SCD*—decreased parasympathetic/increased α-adrenergic tone leads to VT, • *IE* |
| MVP findings on echocardiography | **movement of MV leaflet(s) into LA** |
| Rx for symptomatic MVP | • **β-blockers,** • *calcium channel blockers* [**Note:** these drugs have a negative inotropic effect. This reduces stress on the chordae.] |
| causes of mitral valve regurgitation | • **MVP,** • *RHD,* • IE, • *calcification of MV annulus*—common cause of MV regurgitation in the elderly, • *papillary muscle dysfunction/rupture*—e.g., RCA thrombosis in AMI, • *CHF*—increase in LVEDV stretches MV annulus |
| cardiac findings in MV regurgitation | • **apical pansystolic murmur radiating into the axilla and left parasternal border,** • *AF*— \* 75%, \* due to LA dilatation |

*Table continued on following page*

**Table 5–4. ISCHEMIC HEART DISEASE (IHD), VALVULAR HEART DISEASE, MYOCARDIAL AND PERICARDIAL DISORDERS** *Continued*

| Most Common... | Answer and Explanation |
|---|---|
| causes of AS | • **congenital bicuspid AV,** • *degenerative AV disease*—MCC of AS in * patients > 70 yrs old, * smokers, * HTN, • *RHD* |
| valvular lesion associated with syncope with exercise and angina | **AS—** * syncope is due to: ♦ reduced cardiac output, ♦ ventricular arrhythmias, ♦ hypotension, ♦ death within 3 yrs without Rx of AS, * angina due to: ♦ increased $O_2$ demand of hypertrophied LV, ♦ less coronary artery filling in diastole (decreased cardiac output), ♦ death within 5 yrs without Rx of AS, * CHF commonly occurs: death within 2 yrs without Rx of AS |
| valvular lesion associated with macroangiopathic hemolytic anemia | **AS—** * RBCs hitting the dystrophically calcified valve are damaged, * see **Table 2–6** |
| cardiac findings in AS | • **harsh systolic ejection-type murmur heard best at the upper right or left sternal border,** • *radiation into carotid arteries,* • *delay in upstroke of peripheral pulse,* • *narrow pulse pressure,* • *normal-sized heart on chest x-ray* * concentric hypertrophy does not enlarge the heart, * increased heart size and $S_3$ indicate heart failure with volume overload, • *calcification of AV on chest x-ray*—usually evident by 40–45 yrs of age, • *see Table 5–1 for differentiation of AS from aortic sclerosis* |
| Rx of AS | **AV replacement** |
| causes of AV regurgitation | • **long-standing HTN,** • *aortic root/annulus disease*— * from annular aortic ectasia: some authors consider this the most common cause of AV regurgitation, * ankylosing spondylitis, • *bicuspid AV,* • *IE,* • *dissecting aortic aneurysm*—AV regurgitation is the most common valvular lesion in a dissection, • *coarctation of aorta*—due to stretching of AV annulus from proximal aorta dilatation |

### Table 5–4. ISCHEMIC HEART DISEASE (IHD), VALVULAR HEART DISEASE, MYOCARDIAL AND PERICARDIAL DISORDERS *Continued*

| Most Common... | Answer and Explanation |
|---|---|
| cause of acute AV regurgitation | **infective IE in IVDA** |
| cause of an Austin-Flint murmur | **AV regurgitation**— * this murmur is a rumbling diastolic murmur secondary to blood dripping onto the anterior MV leaflet, * a marker of severe regurgitant AV disease requiring surgery |
| cardiac findings in AV regurgitation | • **high-pitched blowing murmur after $S_2$,** • *wide pulse pressure,* • *bisferiens pulse*—see **Table 5–1,** • *Corrigan's water hammer pulse*—see **Table 5–1** |
| Rx of AV regurgitation | **valve replacement** |
| cause of tricuspid stenosis | **chronic RHD**—usually occurs in association with MS |
| causes of TV regurgitation | • **RHF owing to stretching of the ring from RV dilatation**—most often secondary to left heart failure, • *carcinoid syndrome,* • *IE in IVDA* |
| cardiac findings in TV regurgitation | • **pansystolic murmur**—increases with inspiration, • *giant c-v wave in JVP,* • *pulsatile liver* |
| valve abnormalities in carcinoid heart disease | • **TV regurgitation,** • **PV stenosis** [Note: the right side of the heart is flooded with serotonin coming from metastatic carcinoid tumor in the liver. Since serotonin is fibrogenic, the right-sided heart valves are most affected.] |
| types of prosthetic heart valves | • **mechanical valves,** • **biosynthetic**— * porcine valve, * pericardial valve treated with glutaraldehyde |
| indications for porcine valves | • **older patients**—durability of valve ~10 yrs, • **patients with contraindications for life-long anticoagulation**—porcine valves have a low risk for thromboembolism |

*Table continued on following page*

**Table 5–4. ISCHEMIC HEART DISEASE (IHD),
VALVULAR HEART DISEASE, MYOCARDIAL
AND PERICARDIAL DISORDERS** *Continued*

| Most Common... | Answer and Explanation |
|---|---|
| indications for mechanical valves | **younger person**— * longer durability than porcine valves, * require life-long anticoagulation due to high thromboembolism risk |
| cause of restrictive cardiomyopathy | **post-open heart surgery** |
| cardiac tumor in adults | **cardiac myxoma**— * 80% arise in LA |
| valvular lesion mimicked by cardiac myxomas | **MS**—myxomas frequently obstruct MV orifice: * mid-diastolic rumble, * syncope, * SCD, * left-sided heart failure |
| S/S of cardiac myxomas | • **constitutional signs**— * fever, * fatigue, * weight loss, * elevated ESR, • **embolization**— * ~50%, * sites: ♦ CNS, ♦ coronary arteries, ♦ peripheral organs/viscera |
| method of diagnosing cardiac myxomas | **transesophageal ultrasound** |
| Rx of cardiac myxoma | **surgery** |
| cause of pericarditis | **viral infection**—most commonly secondary to coxsackievirus B |
| causes of bacterial pericarditis | • **Streptococci spp,** • *Staphylococci spp,* • *gram-negative rods* |
| causes of metabolic pericarditis | • **uremia**— * pericarditis occurs in ~one-third of cases, * due to: ♦ nondialyzable chemicals, ♦ autoimmune disease, ♦ infection, • *myxedema,* • *amyloidosis* |
| collagen vascular diseases associated with pericarditis | • **SLE**— * pericarditis is the most common cardiac manifestation of SLE, * it may also occur in drug-induced lupus erythematosus, • *rheumatoid arthritis*—occurs in one-third of cases |
| S/S of pericarditis | • **precordial chest pain**— * aggravated by lying down, * relieved by sitting up, * pain is often referred to the shoulders from diaphragmatic irritation, • *friction rub*—see **Table 5–1,** • *pericardial effusion* |

### Table 5–4. ISCHEMIC HEART DISEASE (IHD), VALVULAR HEART DISEASE, MYOCARDIAL AND PERICARDIAL DISORDERS *Continued*

| Most Common... | Answer and Explanation |
|---|---|
| ECG findings in pericarditis | • **diffuse ST segment elevation with an upward concavity,** • *inversion of T waves* |
| causes of constrictive pericarditis | • **tuberculosis**— * MCC worldwide of constrictive pericarditis, * arises from hematogenous spread of primary TB, • **idiopathic**—MCC in United States, • *prior open heart surgery,* • *mediastinal radiation,* • *neoplastic disease,* • *previous pericarditis* |
| S/S of constrictive pericarditis | • **dyspnea,** • *JVP distention,* • *pericardial knock*—see **Table 5–1,** • *ascites,* • *hepatosplenomegaly,* • *pitting edema,* • *calcifications noted on x-rays* |
| S/S of a pericardial effusion | • **Beck's triad**— * hypotension, * elevated JVP, * muffled heart sounds, • *other signs*—Kussmaul's sign: see **Table 5–1,** * pulsus paradoxus: see **Table 5–1** |
| first step in Dx and Rx of a pericardial effusion | • **Dx**—echocardiogram, • **Rx**—pericardial paracentesis |
| causes of cardiac tamponade | • **idiopathic,** • *viral*—previous pericarditis/myocarditis, • *neoplastic disease* [**Note:** tamponade is characterized by an elevated intrapericardial pressure >15 mmHg and equal elevation of atrial and pericardial pressures. 100–250 mL of fluid in the pericardial sac compromises cardiac filling in diastole.] |
| S/S of cardiac tamponade | • **shock**— * patient is cool and diaphoretic, * sinus tachycardia with weak, thready pulse, • *muffled heart sounds,* • *jugular vein distention*—important sign of tamponade, • *pulsus paradoxus* |
| Rx of cardiac tamponade | **pericardiocentesis** |

*Table continued on following page*

## Table 5–4. ISCHEMIC HEART DISEASE (IHD), VALVULAR HEART DISEASE, MYOCARDIAL AND PERICARDIAL DISORDERS *Continued*

**Question:** The aortic valve is the most frequently involved valve in which of the following disorders? **SELECT 3**

(A) Prolapse
(B) Regurgitation murmurs
(C) Infective endocarditis in IVDA
(D) Rheumatic heart disease
(E) Systolic ejection click
(F) Wide pulse pressure
(G) Stenosis murmurs
(H) Syncope with exercise
(I) Tetralogy of Fallot
(J) Carcinoid heart disease

**Answers: (F), (G), (H).** Prolapse, regurgitation murmurs, rheumatic heart disease, and systolic ejection clicks (noted in MVP) most often involve the MV **(choices A, B, D, and E are incorrect)**. Carcinoid heart disease involves the TV **(choice J is incorrect)**. Infective endocarditis in IVDA most often involves the TV **(choice C is incorrect)**. A wide pulse pressure is most often noted in AV regurgitation **(choice F is correct)**. Stenosis of the AV is the most common stenosis murmur **(choice G is correct)**. Syncope with exercise due to a valvular lesion is most often due to AS **(choice H is correct)**. Tetralogy of Fallot most commonly has infravalvular pulmonic stenosis **(choice I is incorrect)**.

AD = autosomal dominant, AF = atrial fibrillation, AMI = acute myocardial infarction, APKD = adult polycystic kidney disease, AS = aortic stenosis, AV = aortic valve, BP = blood pressure, CABG = coronary artery bypass graft, CAD = coronary artery disease, CHF = congestive heart failure, CK = creatine kinase, CNS = central nervous system, COD = cause of death, EF = ejection fraction, ESR = erythrocyte sedimentation rate, GB = gallbladder, GERD = gastroesophageal reflux disease, GN = glomerulonephritis, HR = heart rate, HTN = hypertension, IBD = inflammatory bowel disease, IC = immunocomplex, IE = infective endocarditis, IHD = ischemic heart disease, IVDA = intravenous drug abuse, IVS = interventricular septum, JVP = jugular venous pulse, LA = left atrium, LAD = left anterior descending, LCA = left circumflex coronary artery, LDH = lactate dehydrogenase, LHF = left heart failure, LV = left ventricle, LVEDV = left ventricular end-diastolic volume, MC = most common, MCC = most common cause, MS = mitral stenosis, MV = mitral valve, MVP = mitral valve prolapse, OS = opening snap, PAN = polyarteritis nodosa, PH = pulmonary hypertension, PTCA = percutaneous transluminal coronary angioplasty, PV = pulmonic valve, RCA = right coronary artery, RHD = rheumatic heart disease, RHF = right heart failure, RV = right ventricle, RVH = right ventricular hypertrophy, SCD = sudden cardiac death, SLE = systemic lupus erythematosus, S/S = signs/symptoms, TV = tricuspid valve, $TXA_2$ = thromboxane $A_2$, VF = ventricular fibrillation, VT = ventricular tachycardia.

# CHAPTER

**6**

# THORACIC SURGERY

## CONTENTS

### Table 6–1. SIGNS/SYMPTOMS OF RESPIRATORY DISEASE AND LABORATORY TESTING

| Most Common... | Answer and Explanation |
|---|---|
| symptom of respiratory disease | **dyspnea**—see **Table 5–1** |
| causes of dyspnea | • **parenchymal lung disease**— * interstitial fibrosis, * CHF, * atelectasis, * pneumonia, * pneumothorax, * PE, • *upper/lower airway obstruction*— * asthma, * tumor, • *chest bellows disease*—e.g., obesity |
| tests for evaluation of dyspnea | • **chest x-ray**—e.g., R/O airway obstruction, • *bronchoscopy*—R/O suspected airway obstruction |
| causes of cough | • **postnasal discharge**—usually secondary to sinusitis, • *acute inflammation*— * viral URI, * atypical pneumonia: *Mycoplasma pneumoniae*, * pneumonia, • *chronic inflammation*— * CB, * bronchiectasis, * asthma, • *cancer*— * laryngeal, * bronchogenic, • *GERD*—MCC of nocturnal cough, • *diaphragmatic irritation*— * pneumonia, * tumor invasion, • *mediastinal mass*, • *drugs*—see below |
| infectious cause of nonproductive cough | **atypical pneumonia due to *Mycoplasma pneumoniae*** |

*Table continued on following page*

Table 6–1. SIGNS/SYMPTOMS OF RESPIRATORY
DISEASE AND LABORATORY TESTING *Continued*

| Most Common... | Answer and Explanation |
|---|---|
| drugs causing cough | • **ACE inhibitors**—bradykinin effect: 20% of cases, • *aspirin*—triad asthma consisting of— ♦ aspirin, ♦ nasal polyps, ♦ asthma |
| cause of persistent cough | **bronchial asthma**—persistent cough often precedes wheezing |
| tests for chronic cough | • **chest x-ray**—R/O anatomic cause for cough, • *sputum for cytology, culture, Gram stain, acid-fast stain*— * R/O infection, * cancer, • *bronchoscopy*—suspected airway abnormality, • *sinus radiographs*—suspected sinusitis, • *esophageal pH monitoring*—suspected GERD [**Note:** the cause of cough is ascertained in 95% of cases.] |
| mechanism of hemoptysis | • **parenchymal necrosis**, • *vessel damage*— bronchial or pulmonary |
| causes of hemoptysis | • **CB**, • *cancer*, • **pneumonia**, • *TB*, • *bronchiectasis*, • *fungus ball*—see below, • cardiovascular— * MS, * CHF, * aortic aneurysm, • *PE* |
| upper respiratory cause of hemoptysis | **epistaxis** |
| causes of massive hemoptysis | • **TB**, *bronchiectasis*, • *cancer*, • *aspergilloma* [**Note:** massive hemoptysis is coughing up > 250 mL/24 hr] |
| problem associated with massive hemoptysis | **asphyxiation from blood in the airway** |
| tests for evaluating hemoptysis | • **chest x-ray**, • *sputum cytology*, • Gram stain, *acid-fast stain/culture*, • **ABGs**, • *UA*—R/O Goodpasture's, • *bronchoscopy*—first step in management to R/O cancer, if risk factors are present |
| Rx of life-threatening hemoptysis | • **surgical resection when feasible**, • *bronchial artery embolization*— * 95% of massive hemoptysis originates from this source, * 85% success rate, * late rebleeding in 25% [**Note:** 5–10% require an exploratory thoracotomy to find the source of bleeding.] |

## Table 6–1. SIGNS/SYMPTOMS OF RESPIRATORY DISEASE AND LABORATORY TESTING *Continued*

| Most Common... | Answer and Explanation |
|---|---|
| causes of chest pain of respiratory origin | • **pleuritis secondary to pneumonia**, • *pleuritis due to a pulmonary infarction* [**Note:** pleuritis is a sharp, inspiratory pain that increases in magnitude with breathing.] |
| types of cyanosis | • **peripheral cyanosis**— * due to redistribution of blood from the skin to internal organs, * skin dusky but normal mucous membranes, * examples: ♦ cold temperature, ♦ hypovolemic shock, • *central cyanosis*— * decrease in $SaO_2$: <85% in fair-skinned people or <75% in dark-skinned people, * dusky skin + mucous membranes |
| causes of central cyanosis | • **lung disorders**— * V/Q defects: COPD, * alveolar hypoventilation, * *diffusion defects*—interstitial fibrosis, • *cardiac disorders*—CHD, • *Hgb disorders*—metHgb ≥ 1.5 g/dL, • *hypoxemia ≤ 60 mmHg* |
| causes of inspiratory stridor | **upper airway obstruction**— * food: cafe coronary, * laryngotracheobronchitis, * epiglottitis [**Note:** stridor is a high-pitched inspiratory sound associated with upper airway obstruction.] |
| cause of inspiratory/ expiratory stridor | **fixed upper airway obstruction**—e.g., cancer |
| cause of wheezing | • **bronchial asthma**, • *pulmonary edema*—peribronchiolar edema, • *bronchiolitis*—RSV, • *PE with infarction*—$TXA_2$ (bronchoconstrictor) released from platelets |
| cause of moist coarse rales (rhonchi) | **airflow through large bronchi encountering liquids of different viscosities**— * pulmonary edema, * bronchitis, * bacterial pneumonia |
| cause of moist, fine rales | **alveolar fluid**— * pulmonary edema, * pneumonia |
| cause of dry rales | **movements of thick exudates**—bacterial pneumonia |
| signs of lung consolidation | • **decreased percussion**, • **increased tactile fremitus**—increased vibration of chest wall, • **egophony**—*e* sounds like *a* |

*Table continued on following page*

### Table 6–1. SIGNS/SYMPTOMS OF RESPIRATORY DISEASE AND LABORATORY TESTING *Continued*

| Most Common... | Answer and Explanation |
|---|---|
| signs of a pleural effusion | • **decreased percussion,** • **absence of other consolidation signs,** • **bronchial breath sounds heard above and through the fluid** |
| causes of hyperresonance to percussion | • **increased AP diameter**—e.g., emphysema, • *pneumothorax*—lung collapse |
| causes of clubbing | • **pulmonary disease**— * bronchiectasis, * cystic fibrosis, • *cyanotic CHD,* • *GI disease*—IBD [Note: clubbing is a bulbous enlargement of the ends of the fingers and/or toes. Loss of the normal angle (≤160°) between the skin and nail (≥180°) occurs.] |
| method of measuring lung volumes/ capacities | **spirometry**—see **Table 1–1** for complete discussion |
| formula used to calculate A–a gradient | **PAO$_2$ = % O$_2$ (713) − PaCO$_2$/0.8—see Table 3–1** for a full discussion of A–a gradient and its use in acute respiratory failure |
| uses of a chest radiograph | • **detects parenchyma, vascular, and pleural space abnormalities**—e.g., * pneumonia, * pleural effusions, • *defines rib cage and diaphragmatic abnormalities*—e.g., * lytic rib lesions, * diaphragmatic hernia, • *evaluates cardiac size and chamber contours* |
| uses of CT | • **fine definition of pulmonary lesions**—e.g., calcification in solitary nodules, • *detect pleural effusions/thickening,* • *staging primary lung cancer*—identification of hilar and mediastinal lymph nodes, • *sinus films in chronic sinusitis* |
| use of echocardiography | **detecting PH**— * estimates PA pressure, * right-sided heart catheterization measures pressure and resistance |
| types of pulmonary cytology | • **sputum,** • *bronchoalveolar lavage,* • *bronchial washings,* • *fine needle aspiration* |
| use of cytology | **gold standard screening test in Dx of primary lung cancer**— * cytology is most sensitive in centrally located cancers: sensitivity ~65%, * sensitivity ~60% in Dx of malignant pleural effusions |

## Table 6–1. SIGNS/SYMPTOMS OF RESPIRATORY DISEASE AND LABORATORY TESTING *Continued*

| Most Common... | Answer and Explanation |
|---|---|
| use of a Gram stain of sputum | • **work-up of pneumonia**—chest x-ray is the gold standard for the Dx of pneumonia, • *determine adequacy of a sample for detecting bacterial pathogens* |
| criteria used to determine adequacy of a sputum sample | **satisfactory sputum**—25 or more PMNs and <10 epithelial cells per LPF |
| use of bronchoscopy | • **evaluation of airways,** • *Dx and staging of cancer,* • *work-up of hemoptysis,* • *obtain material for culture/cytology*—bronchoalveolar lavage, • *remove foreign bodies* [**Note:** flexible and rigid bronchoscopes are available, the former most often used for diagnostic studies.] |
| acid-base disorders | • **respiratory acidosis**—$PaCO_2 > 45$ mmHg, • *respiratory alkalosis*—$PaCO_2 < 33$ mmHg, • *metabolic acidosis*—$HCO_3^- < 22$ mEq/L, • *metabolic alkalosis*—$HCO_3^- > 28$ mEq/L [**Note:** see Table 1–2 for a complete discussion of acid-base.] |

**Question:** Which of the following are expected clinical findings in extensive postoperative atelectasis? **SELECT 3**

(A) Hypoxemia
(B) Normal A–a gradient
(C) Decreased tactile fremitus
(D) Ipsilateral elevation of diaphragm
(E) Normal percussion
(F) Dyspnea
(G) Normal temperature

**Answers: (A), (D), (F).** Hypoxemia (low $PaO_2$) is expected in atelectasis due to a ventilation defect (**choice A is correct**). The calculated A–a gradient should be increased owing to intrapulmonary shunting from collapse of the alveoli (**choice B is incorrect**). Tactile fremitus is increased in atelectasis, because it produces lung consolidation (**choice C is incorrect**). The ipsilateral diaphragm is elevated, because the lung mass is reduced by atelectasis (**choice D is correct**). The trachea deviates to the ipsilateral side and inspiratory lag is also noted. There is dullness to percussion with any lung consolidation (**choice E is incorrect**). Fever is present and does not relate to infection (**choice C is incorrect**). Dyspnea is invariably present (**choice F is correct**). (**choice G is incorrect**).

A–a = Alveolar-arterial, ABGs = arterial blood gases, ACE = angiotensin-converting enzyme, CB = chronic bronchitis, CHD = congenital heart disease, CHF = congestive heart failure, COPD = chronic obstructive pulmonary disease, GERD = gastroesophageal reflux disease, $HCO_3^-$ = bicarbonate, Hgb = hemoglobin, IBD = inflammatory bowel disease, LPF = low-power field, MCC = most common cause, metHgb = methemoglobin, MS = mitral stenosis, PA = pulmonary artery, $PaCO_2$ = partial pressure of arterial carbon dioxide, $PAO_2$ = partial pressure of alveolar oxygen, $PaO_2$ = partial pressure of arterial oxygen, PE = pulmonary embolus, PH = pulmonary hypertension, PMN = polymorphonuclear neutrophil [leukocytes], R/O = rule out, RSV = respiratory syncytial virus, $SaO_2$ = oxygen saturation of arterial blood, $TXA_2$ = thromboxane $A_2$, UA = urinalysis, URI = upper respiratory infection, V/Q = ventilation/perfusion.

### Table 6–2. UPPER RESPIRATORY TRACT DISORDERS, ATELECTASIS, ASPIRATION, PNEUMOTHORAX, AND FLAIL CHEST

| Most Common... | Answer and Explanation |
|---|---|
| causes of nasal polyps in adults | • **allergic rhinitis,** • *triad asthma*—aspirin/NSAID sensitivity leading to asthma, • *cystic fibrosis*—polyps noted in children |
| causes of epistaxis | • **bleeding from Kiesselbach's plexus on the anterior nasal septum secondary to trauma**— * nose picking, * impact sports, • *allergic rhinitis/polyps,* • *thrombocytopenia*—epistaxis MC symptom, • *hemorrhagic telangiectasia* |
| causes of acute sinusitis | • **blockage of sinus ostia**—e.g., * viral URI, * deviated nasal septum, • *barotrauma,* • *smoking* |
| site for acute sinusitis in adults | **maxillary sinus**—pain over the cheeks |
| pathogens causing sinusitis | • ***Streptococcus pneumoniae,*** • *Haemophilus influenzae,* • *rhinoviruses,* • *anaerobes*—chronic sinusitis |
| method of Dx of acute sinusitis | • **CT scan**—most sensitive test, • *transillumination*—helpful in differentiating sinusitis from other causes of facial pain |
| Rx of acute sinusitis | • **amoxicillin/clavulanate**—other choices: ♦ TMP/SMX, ♦ cefuroxime, ♦ newer macrolides, • *decongestants*—topical and systemic |

**Table 6–2. UPPER RESPIRATORY TRACT DISORDERS,
ATELECTASIS, ASPIRATION, PNEUMOTHORAX,
AND FLAIL CHEST** *Continued*

| Most Common... | Answer and Explanation |
|---|---|
| causes of fungal sinus infections | • ***Aspergillus fumigatus,*** • *Candida,* • *Mucor*— * especially in DM, * invades frontal lobes and produces frontal lobe abscesses |
| clinical findings in orbital cellulitis | • **fever,** • *proptosis,* • *periorbital swelling,* • *ophthalmoplegia,* • *normal retinal exam*—papilledema is present if cavernous sinus thrombosis is the cause [**Note:** organisms include *Streptococcus pneumoniae, Haemophilus influenzae, Moraxella catarrhalis, Staphylococcus aureus.*] |
| Rx of orbital cellulitis | **IV cefuroxime** |
| nasal cavity/ paranasal sinus malignancy | **squamous cell carcinoma** |
| malignancy associated with woodworking | **adenocarcinoma of nasal cavity** |
| malignant tumor of the nasopharynx | **nasopharyngeal carcinoma**— * causal relationship with EBV, * metastasizes to the cervical lymph nodes, * nasopharynx Bx should be made if no primary cancer is found for cervical node metastasis |
| types of sleep apnea | • **obstructive sleep apnea,** • *central sleep apnea*—total absence of ventilatory effort during apnea, e.g., * Cheyne-Stokes breathing [**Note:** apnea refers to breath cessation for at least 10 seconds.] |
| causes of obstructive sleep apnea (OSA) | • **upper airway obstruction**—loss of normal pharyngeal muscle tone causes pharyngeal collapse on inspiration, • *tonsillar hypertrophy,* • *obesity* |
| S/S of OSA | • **snoring at night and inordinate daytime somnolence,** • *headaches,* • *personality changes*—irritability, • *loud snoring followed by periods of apnea with increasingly strong ventilatory efforts failing to produce adequate airflow*—loud snort is coincident with the first breath after a period of apnea |

*Table continued on following page*

**Table 6–2. UPPER RESPIRATORY TRACT DISORDERS,
ATELECTASIS, ASPIRATION, PNEUMOTHORAX,
AND FLAIL CHEST** *Continued*

| Most Common... | Answer and Explanation |
|---|---|
| lab abnormalities in OSA | • **low SaO₂/PaO₂ during apneic episode**—drop of ~4% in $SaO_2$, • *respiratory acidosis*, • *polycythemia*—hypoxemic stimulus for EPO |
| complications in OSA | • **PH**—secondary to vasoconstrictive effects of chronic hypoxemia/respiratory acidosis, • *cor pulmonale*—PH + RVH, • *secondary polycythemia*, • *cardiac arrhythmias* |
| confirmatory test for OSA | **polysomnography**—also helps in determining what level of continuous positive airway pressure (CPAP) is necessary to keep the airways open |
| Rx for OSA | • **nasal CPAP**—$O_2$ may sometimes prolong periods of apnea: loss of hypoxemic drive to breathe, • *weight loss,* • *surgery*— * correction of nasal septum deviation, * uvulopalatopharyngoplasty, * tracheostomy: last resort |
| causes of hoarseness | • **viral infection,** • *smoking,* • *allergies,* • *vocal cord nodule,* • *GERD* |
| causes of recurrent hoarseness | **smoking/allergies** |
| causes of vocal cord paralysis | • **injury to the recurrent laryngeal nerve during thyroidectomy,** • *Pancoast's tumor*—see below, • *tumors involving the vagus nerve in jugular foramen*—e.g., schwannoma |
| sign of unilateral vocal cord paralysis | **hoarseness** |
| sign of bilateral vocal cord paralysis | **stridor** |
| benign tumor of vocal cords | **squamous papillomas**— * due to HPV types 6 and 11, * contracted while neonate passes through infected birth canal |
| Rx of squamous papillomas of vocal cord | **laser therapy**— * recurrence is common, * risk for laryngeal squamous carcinoma |
| cause of true vocal cord polyps | **voice abuse** |

**Table 6–2. UPPER RESPIRATORY TRACT DISORDERS,
ATELECTASIS, ASPIRATION, PNEUMOTHORAX,
AND FLAIL CHEST** *Continued*

| Most Common... | Answer and Explanation |
|---|---|
| Rx of vocal cord polyps | • **laser,** • **resection by direct laryngoscopy** |
| causes of laryngeal cancer | • **cigarette smoking,** • *alcohol* [**Note:** the two together have a synergistic effect on increasing the risk for cancer.] |
| symptom of laryngeal cancer | **hoarseness** |
| site for laryngeal squamous carcinoma | **supraglottic area above the false vocal cords**—most proximal location directly impacted upon by carcinogens in cigarette smoke |
| Rx for laryngeal carcinoma | • **lesions <2 mm—radiation,** • **lesions >2 mm**—radiation + surgery |
| indications for tracheostomy | • **respiratory failure requiring prolonged mechanical ventilation,** • *airway obstruction at or above laryngeal level* |
| causes of atelectasis | • **24-hr postoperative**—due to small airway obstruction by mucous plugs with resorption of alveolar air through the pores of Kohn: atelectasis is collapse of lung tissue, * see **Table 4–3,** • *lung compression*—e.g., pleural effusion, • *lack of surfactant*—ARDS, • *luminal obstruction*—cancer |
| S/S of atelectasis | • **fever**—not related to infection, • *cyanosis*—if widespread, • *dyspnea,* • *ipsilateral elevation of diaphragm*—loss of lung mass, • *inspiratory lag on affected side,* • *increased tactile fremitus*—sign of consolidation |
| method of preventing postoperative atelectasis | • **cough/deep breaths,** • *humidification,* • *incentive spirometry* |
| cause of the right middle lobe syndrome | **atelectasis**—the syndrome is due to recurrent or persistent atelectasis of the right middle lobe |
| cause of persistent atelectasis | **bronchial obstruction**— * enlarged hilar lymph nodes, * foreign body, * cancer |

*Table continued on following page*

Table 6–2. UPPER RESPIRATORY TRACT DISORDERS,
ATELECTASIS, ASPIRATION, PNEUMOTHORAX,
AND FLAIL CHEST *Continued*

| Most Common... | Answer and Explanation |
|---|---|
| pulmonary segments for aspiration | • **posterior segment of RUL and superior segment of RLL,** • *posterobasal segment of RLL* |
| body position for aspiration into the posterobasal segment of RLL | **sitting or standing** |
| body position for aspiration into superior segment of RLL | **lying down on the back** |
| body position for aspiration into right middle lobe and/or posterior segment of RUL | **lying down on the right side** |
| body position for aspiration into the lingula | **lying down on the left side** |
| cause of endogenous lipoid pneumonia | **obstruction of an airway by tumor**—foamy alveolar macrophages with ingested CH give the lung parenchyma a golden color |
| complication of lung transplantation | **bronchiolitis obliterans** |
| causes of cor pulmonale | • **COPD**— * cor pulmonale specifically refers to PH + RVH, * PH either primary PA or secondary to noncardiac disease, • *CF,* • *ILD* |
| causes of spontaneous pneumothorax | • **rupture of an apical subpleural bulla**— * most patients are male smokers between 30 and 40 yrs old, * recurrence in the contralateral lung is common, * blebs are secondary to high negative intrapleural pressures, • *COPD*—MC secondary cause: particularly paraseptal type, • *penetrating chest injuries,* • *PCP,* • *ruptured pneumatocele*—these usually occur with bacterial pneumonias secondary to *Staphylococcus aureus,* • *Marfan's syndrome,* • *PEEP therapy,* • *cystic fibrosis,* • *insertion of subclavian catheter*—MC postoperative cause, • *menstruation*—catamenial pneumothorax, • *Boerhaave's syndrome* [**Note:** see Table 4–3 for S/S and Rx of a spontaneous pneumothorax.] |

**Table 6–2. UPPER RESPIRATORY TRACT DISORDERS,
ATELECTASIS, ASPIRATION, PNEUMOTHORAX,
AND FLAIL CHEST** Continued

| Most Common... | Answer and Explanation |
|---|---|
| Rx of recurrent spontaneous pneumothoraces | **pleural sclerosis**—accomplished by \* surgery, \* thoracoscopy, or \* chemical pleurodesis |
| causes of tension pneumothorax | • **sucking chest wound,** • *pulmonary laceration* [**Note:** see Table 4–3 for the S/S and Rx of a tension pneumothorax.] |
| cause of a flail chest | **trauma**— \* blunt or penetrating trauma, \* multiple segmental rib fractures produce a free-floating portion of chest wall without bony fixation, \* lung contusion(s) commonly present |
| S/S of a flail chest | • **paradoxical movement of chest wall**—segment of chest moves out with inspiration and in with expiration, • *dyspnea*—inefficient breathing associated with hypoxemia |
| Rx of flail chest | • **stabilize the free-floating segment,** • **insert chest tube,** • **positive-pressure breathing through endotracheal tube** |

**Question:** A 19-yr-old patient with a stab wound to the right chest presents with dyspnea, tachypnea, hypotension, cyanosis, elevated jugular venous pressure, and deviation of the trachea to the left. You would expect which of the following additional findings? **SELECT 2**

(A) Hypoxemia
(B) Normal arterial oxygen saturation
(C) Dullness to percussion in the right lung
(D) Decreased breath sounds in the right lung
(E) Increased tactile fremitus in the right lung
(F) Elevation of the right diaphragm

**Answers: (A), (D).** The patient has a right tension pneumothorax secondary to a laceration in the right lung. Hypoxemia is likely, owing to the presence of cardiorespiratory compromise from increased pressure in the right pleural cavity pushing the mediastinal structures to the left **(choice A is correct).** The oxygen saturation should be low owing to hypoxemia and clinical evidence of cyanosis **(choice B is incorrect).** Hyperresonance to percussion, decreased tactile fremitus, and depression of the right diaphragm are likely to be present in the right lung **(choices C, E, and F are incorrect).** Decreased breath sounds on the ipsilateral side are likely **(choice D is correct).**

ARDS = adult respiratory distress syndrome, Bx = biopsy, CF = cystic fibrosis, CH = cholesterol, COPD = chronic obstructive pulmonary disease, CPAP = continuous positive pressure airway pressure, DM = diabetes mellitus, EBV = Epstein-Barr virus, EPO = erythropoietin, GERD = gastroesophageal reflux disease, HPV = human papilloma virus, ILD = interstitial lung disease, MC = most common, NSAID = nonsteroidal anti-inflammatory drug, OSA = obstructive sleep apnea, PA = pulmonary artery, $PaO_2$ = partial pressure of arterial oxygen, PCP = *Pneumocystis carinii* pneumonia, PEEP = positive end-expiratory pressure, PH = pulmonary hypertension, RLL = right lower lobe, RUL = right upper lobe, RUQ = right upper quadrant, RVH = right ventricular hypertrophy, $SaO_2$ = arterial oxygen saturation, S/S = signs and symptoms, TMP/SMX = trimethoprim sulfamethoxazole, URI = upper respiratory infection.

### Table 6–3. RESPIRATORY TRACT INFECTIONS, INTERSTITIAL AND OBSTRUCTIVE LUNG DISEASE

| Most Common... | Answer and Explanation |
|---|---|
| S/S of a typical community-acquired pneumonia | • **sudden onset of high fever/productive cough,** • *signs of lung consolidation*—see **Table 6–1** [**Note:** there is an alveolar exudate.] |
| S/S of an atypical community-acquired pneumonia | • **insidious onset of low-grade fever and non-productive cough,** • *lack of consolidation signs in the lungs* [**Note:** there is an interstitial exudate, hence the lack of signs of consolidation and productive cough.] |
| types of typical pneumonia | • **bronchopneumonia**—bronchitis leading to patchy areas of pneumonia, • *lobar* |
| tests to Dx typical pneumonia | • **chest x-ray**—gold standard screening test, • *Gram stain of sputum*, • *sputum culture*—gold standard confirmatory test, • *CBC* |
| complications associated with a typical pneumonia | • **septicemia,** • *lung abscesses*, • *metastatic abscesses*, • *empyema*—pus in pleural cavity [**Note:** complications occur in ~10% of cases of pneumonia.] |
| causes of nosocomial pneumonia | • *Escherichia coli,* • *Pseudomonas aeruginosa*—* usually respirator patients in ICU, * greenish sputum, • *Staphylococcus aureus*—yellow sputum [**Note:** the above organisms colonize the airways in the first week and spread into the lungs.] |

## Table 6–3. RESPIRATORY TRACT INFECTIONS, INTERSTITIAL AND OBSTRUCTIVE LUNG DISEASE
*Continued*

| Most Common... | Answer and Explanation |
|---|---|
| cause of ICU pneumonia | ***Pseudomonas aeruginosa*** |
| Rx of *P. aeruginosa* pneumonia | **piperacillin or mezlocillin + gentamicin or tobramycin** |
| cause of community-acquired atypical pneumonia | • ***Mycoplasma pneumoniae***—common in crowded conditions: e.g., military, college |
| Rx of *M. pneumoniae* pneumonia | • **erythromycin,** • *tetracycline* |
| Chlamydia causing atypical pneumonia | ***Chlamydia pneumoniae***— * accounts for 5–10% of atypical pneumonias, * possible causal role in CAD |
| Rx of *Chlamydia pneumoniae* | **erythromycin** |
| cause of community-acquired typical pneumonia | ***Streptococcus pneumoniae***—gram-positive, lancet-shaped diplococcus |
| risk factors for *Streptococcus pneumoniae* pneumonia | • **old age,** • *splenectomy,* • *smoking,* • *alcoholism,* • *HIV infection*—very common COD in AIDS, • *Hgb SS disease* |
| empiric Rx of community-acquired pneumonia | • **macrolide,** • *tetracycline* |
| Rx of *S. pneumoniae* pneumonia | • **penicillin G,** • *macrolide* [**Note:** Rx penicillin-resistant strains with IV vancomycin.] |
| organism producing draining sinuses in the jaw, thorax, and abdominal cavity | ***Actinomyces israelii***— * gram-positive filamentous bacteria—best seen in sulfur granules, * produces sinus tracts extending to skin surface: ♦ jaw (MC site, postdental abscess), ♦ thorax, ♦ abdomen |
| Rx of actinomycosis | **penicillin G** |
| screening test for TB | **PPD (Mantoux) intradermal skin test**— * 5 tuberculin units, * positive test is induration, not erythema |

*Table continued on following page*

**Table 6–3. RESPIRATORY TRACT INFECTIONS,
INTERSTITIAL AND OBSTRUCTIVE LUNG DISEASE**
*Continued*

| Most Common... | Answer and Explanation |
|---|---|
| criteria for positive PPD in high-risk patient | **>5-mm induration**—high-risk patients include— * immunosuppressed patient, * HIV-positive patient, * contacts of people with active TB |
| criteria for positive PPD in moderate-risk patient | **>10-mm induration**—moderate-risk patients include: ♦ foreign immigrants, ♦ low socioeconomic groups, ♦ residents of long-term facility |
| criteria for positive PPD in low-risk patient | **>15-mm induration**—a low-risk patient is an average individual |
| method of screening for TB in the elderly | **two-step PPD testing**—owing to relative anergy to skin testing in the elderly, a two-step procedure is used to enhance the reaction |
| initial work-up when a PPD is positive | • **chest x-ray,** • **clinical evaluation for active TB** |
| cause of secondary TB (reactivation TB) | **reactivation of a previous primary TB site** |
| sites for reactivation TB | • **apical or posterior segment of the upper lobe**—may be one or both lungs, • *RML or superior segment of RLL* in older people [**Note:** cavitation frequently accompanies reactivation TB.] |
| S/S of TB | • **fever,** • *drenching night sweats,* • *weight loss,* • *hemoptysis*—<25% |
| extrapulmonary sites for TB | • **kidneys**— * sterile pyuria, * hematuria, • *CNS*— * meningitis, * tuberculoma, • *epididymis,* • *pericardium*—constrictive pericarditis, • *adrenals*—Addison's disease, • *vertebral column*—Pott's disease |
| complications of pulmonary TB | • **miliary spread in lungs**—invasion into the bronchus or PA, • *systemic miliary spread*—invasion of pulmonary vein, • *empyema*—may result in a bronchopleural fistula, • *scar carcinoma*—usually an adenocarcinoma, • *massive hemoptysis*—usually the result of erosion into a pulmonary artery within a cavitary lesion or as a complication of bronchiectasis, • *bronchiectasis*—TB is MCC worldwide, • *cavity may be the site for a fungus ball* |

## Table 6–3. RESPIRATORY TRACT INFECTIONS,
## INTERSTITIAL AND OBSTRUCTIVE LUNG DISEASE
*Continued*

| Most Common... | Answer and Explanation |
|---|---|
| diagnostic methods for TB | • **fluorochrome and acid-fast stains**—presumptive evidence, • *gastric aspirate*—for patients who cannot cough: elderly, children, • *culture*—definitive Dx, • *radiometric color systems*—reduces the time for obtaining positive cultures, • *DNA probes* |
| first-line antituberculous agents | • **INH**, • *rifampin*, • *ethambutol*, • *pyrazinamide*, • *streptomycin* |
| criteria indicating nontransmissibility of TB | **3 consecutive sputum smears negative for acid-fast bacilli on separate days** |
| indications for surgical Rx in TB | • **removal of residual infection resistant to medical Rx**, • *bronchiectasis*, • *massive hemorrhage or hemoptysis* |
| systemic fungal infection involving the lungs | *Histoplasma capsulatum*— * geographic sites: Ohio/Mississippi valley states, * transmission: ♦ starlings, ♦ chickens, ♦ bats, ♦ inhalation of the spores |
| clinical findings of histoplasmosis | • **similar to TB**— * consolidations, * coin lesions, * miliary spread, • *striking dystrophic calcification in lungs and extrapulmonary sites*, • *erythema nodosum*—painful subcutaneous nodules on the lower extremities |
| methods to Dx histoplasmosis | • **culture**, • *direct visualization*—yeast forms in macrophages, • *skin tests*, • *serologic tests* |
| Rx of histoplasmosis | • **itraconazole**—moderate disease, • *amphotericin B*—severe disease |
| systemic fungal infection in the Southwest | *Coccidioides immitis*— * transmitted by inhalation of arthrospores in dust: increased with earthquakes, * called "valley fever" |
| clinical findings in coccidioidomycosis | • **flulike syndrome with a dry, nonproductive cough**, • *erythema nodosum*, • *lung*— * localized "eggshell" cavity in the lower lobes, * miliary spread, * solitary coin lesion |

*Table continued on following page*

**Table 6–3. RESPIRATORY TRACT INFECTIONS,
INTERSTITIAL AND OBSTRUCTIVE LUNG DISEASE**
*Continued*

| Most Common... | Answer and Explanation |
|---|---|
| methods to Dx coccidioidomycosis | • **culture,** • *direct visualization of spherules with endospores,* • *skin tests,* • *serologic tests* |
| Rx of coccidioidomycosis | **fluconazole** |
| fungus associated with hemoptysis, pneumonia, and asthma | ***Aspergillus fumigatus*—** * colonizes abandoned TB cavities: ♦ fungus ball, ♦ cause of massive hemoptysis, * hemorrhagic pneumonia with infarctions: invades blood vessels, * asthma: type I hypersensitivity reaction |
| methods to Dx aspergillosis | • **culture,** • *direct visualization*—fruiting bodies |
| Rx of aspergillosis | • **aspergillomas**—surgery, • **invasive disease**—amphotericin B |
| causes of a pulmonary abscess | • **aspiration of infected oropharyngeal material/infected teeth,** • *aspiration of foreign body,* • *lobar pneumonia*— * *Staphylococcus aureus,* * *Klebsiella pneumoniae,* • *bronchial obstruction from tumor,* • *hematogenous spread*— * sepsis, * infected thromboembolic material |
| sites for aspiration-induced lung abscess | **posterior segment RUL and superior segment RLL**— * most aspirations occur at night during sleep, * those to the posterior segment occur while lying down on the right side, * those to the superior segment occur while lying down [**Note:** other sites of aspiration include right posterobasal segment of the RLL (standing or sitting), right middle lobe (lying on right side), lingula (lying on left side).] |
| S/S of lung abscess | • **fever,** • *pleuritic chest pain,* • *productive cough*—often foul smelling in aspiration types owing to the presence of anaerobes |
| microbial pathogens in aspiration-induced lung abscess | **mixed population of anaerobes and aerobes**—e.g., * *Prevotella* (formerly *Bacteroides*) *melanogenicus,* * *Fusobacterium nucleatum,* * *anaerobic Peptostreptococcus* |

### Table 6–3. RESPIRATORY TRACT INFECTIONS, INTERSTITIAL AND OBSTRUCTIVE LUNG DISEASE
*Continued*

| Most Common... | Answer and Explanation |
|---|---|
| work-up of lung abscess | • **Gram stain/culture**—material obtained from protected bronchoscopy, • *chest x-ray*—note cavitation and air/fluid level |
| Rx of lung abscesses | • **drainage**— * postural, * chest percussion, * bronchoscopy if necessary, • *antibiotics*—clindamycin, • *surgical resection if residual abscess* |
| causes of ILD | • **pneumoconioses**—dust diseases, • *sarcoidosis*, • *drugs*, • *radiation*, • *infections*, • *lymphangitic spread of tumor*, • *hypersensitivity reactions*, • *pneumonitis*, • *collagen vascular disease*, • *Goodpasture's syndrome* |
| pathophysiologic abnormalities in ILD | • **functional loss of alveolar/capillary units,** • *increase in interstitial fibrosis as a reaction to injury* |
| symptoms of ILD | • **dry cough,** • *exertional dyspnea* |
| signs of ILD | • **late inspiratory crackles in lower lungs,** • *digital clubbing*, • *accentuated* $P_2$—sign of PH |
| lab findings of ILD | • **PFT**—see Table 1–1, • **ABG findings**– * hypoxemia, * chronic respiratory alkalosis, * increased A–a gradient |
| chest x-ray findings in ILD | • **diffuse bilateral reticular infiltrates**—"ground-glass" appearance, • *nodular infiltrates*—particularly in silicosis, • *reticulonodular infiltrates*, • *"honeycomb" lung*—Hamman-Rich lung |
| diagnostic tests used to evaluate ILD | • **fiberoptic bronchoscopy with Bx,** • **bronchoalveolar lavage**—useful in excluding PCP, • **PFTs,** • **ABGs** |
| cause of "egg shell" calcifications in centrally located hilar lymph nodes | **silicosis**— * inhalation produces nodulation in all lung fields after ~20 years of exposure, * simple and PMF types |

*Table continued on following page*

## Table 6–3. RESPIRATORY TRACT INFECTIONS, INTERSTITIAL AND OBSTRUCTIVE LUNG DISEASE
*Continued*

| Most Common... | Answer and Explanation |
|---|---|
| complications of silicosis | • **increased risk for typical/atypical TB**— * macrophages lysed by silica—no effector cell to kill TB, * no primary lung cancer risk, • *cor pulmonale*, • *Caplan's syndrome*—silicosis + large cavitating rheumatoid nodules in patients with rheumatoid arthritis |
| cause of ferruginous bodies in sputum | **inhalation of asbestos minerals**— * asbestos fibers become coated with iron, * crystalline silicate with two subfamilies: ♦ serpentines (e.g., chrysotile MC type), ♦ amphiboles (crocidolite) [**Note:** sources of asbestos include working in shipyards, working with roofing materials.] |
| lung lesions associated with asbestos | • **benign pleural plaque**—does not predispose to a mesothelioma, • *primary lung cancer*— * all types, * MC overall cancer, • *mesothelioma*, • *benign effusions*, • *laryngeal cancer* |
| complication of asbestos exposure plus smoking | **primary lung cancer**— * smoking + asbestos is synergistic, * 60- to 90-fold increase in primary lung cancer, * fivefold increase in nonsmokers |
| malignant pleural lesion associated with asbestos exposure | **mesothelioma**— * no smoking relationship, * requires 20–40 yrs to develop: most people die of lung cancer before they develop a mesothelioma, * must find asbestos fibers in lung parenchyma (none are present in pleura) to confirm its causal relationship to asbestos exposure, * malignant effusions are common, * poor prognosis |
| cause of COPD | **smoking**— * ~10–15% of smokers develop COPD, * fourth MC COD |
| types of COPD | • **CB**, • *emphysema*, • *bronchial asthma*, • *bronchiectasis*, • *CF* |
| clinical features of CB | • **productive cough for ~3 mos for 2 consecutive yrs**, • *airway obstruction due to inflammation/bronchoconstriction in terminal bronchioles*, • *segmental bronchi have increased mucus production* |

**Table 6–3. RESPIRATORY TRACT INFECTIONS,
INTERSTITIAL AND OBSTRUCTIVE LUNG DISEASE**
*Continued*

| Most Common... | Answer and Explanation |
|---|---|
| pathophysiologic abnormality in CB | **V/Q mismatch**— * site of obstruction is more proximally located than that of emphysema, * bronchiole obstruction affects a larger area of distal gas exchange |
| site of damage in emphysema | **functional respiratory unit**—respiratory unit consists of: ♦ RB, ♦ AD, ♦ alveoli |
| effects of smoking in respiratory unit | • **smoke attracts neutrophils into the lungs,** • **neutrophils release elastases that destroy tissue support in respiratory unit,** • **smoke inactivates AAT**—elastases are left unneutralized |
| types of emphysema (EMP) | • **centrilobular emphysema**— * involves the upper lobes, * associated with smoking and coal worker's pneumoconiosis, * RB is targeted for destruction, • *panacinar*— * the entire respiratory unit destroyed, * involves the lower lobes, • *paraseptal*— * targets AD and alveoli for destruction, * increased risk for pneumothorax |
| type of emphysema due to AAT deficiency | **panacinar emphysema**— * predilection for the lower lobes, * AR disease with decreased liver synthesis of AAT |
| S/S of COPD | • **persistent chronic productive cough with slowly progressive exertional dyspnea**— * EMP, * CB, • **hyperaerated lungs**—EMP, • **increased AP diameter**—EMP, • **flattened diaphragms**—EMP, • **diminished breath sounds**—EMP, • **normal/pink skin**— * EMP, * "pink puffer," • **weight loss/cachectic**—EMP, • **sibilant rhonchi/expiratory wheezing**—CB, • **cyanosis**— * CB, * "blue bloater," • **obese/stocky**—CB |
| chest x-ray findings in COPD | • **hyperlucent lung fields**—EMP, • **increased AP diameter**—EMP, • **vertical heart**—EMP, • **bullae/blebs**—EMP, • **low diaphragms**—EMP, • **large, horizontally oriented heart**—CB, • **increased bronchial markings**—CB |

*Table continued on following page*

**Table 6–3. RESPIRATORY TRACT INFECTIONS,
INTERSTITIAL AND OBSTRUCTIVE LUNG DISEASE**
*Continued*

| Most Common... | Answer and Explanation |
|---|---|
| lab findings in COPD | • **increased TLC**—EMP, • **increased lung compliance**—EMP, • **decreased DL$_{CO}$**—EMP, • **respiratory alkalosis/normal ABG**—EMP, • **polycythemia**—CB, • **hypoxemia**—CB > EMP, • **respiratory acidosis**—CB, • **right axis deviation/RVH/cor pulmonale**—CB |
| long-term Rx of COPD | • **stop smoking,** • *inhaled ipratropium bromide*—longer duration of action than β$_2$-agonists, • *oral theophylline,* • *O$_2$ Rx*—keep SaO$_2$ ~90%, • *glucocorticoids*—effective in 10–25%, • *yearly influenza vaccine,* • *pneumococcal vaccine*—every 6 yrs |
| causes of bronchiectasis in the United States | • **CF**—*Pseudomonas aeruginosa* is most responsible for damage to bronchi/bronchioles leading to dilatation, • *infections*— * TB, * MCC worldwide, * adenovirus, * *Staphylococcus aureus,* * histoplasmosis, • *bronchial obstruction*—e.g., tumor, • *B cell ID,* • *immotile cilia syndrome* (Kartagener's syndrome)— * absent dynein arm, * situs inversus |
| mechanisms causing bronchiectasis | **obstruction/infection**— * leads to weakening of the bronchial wall and dilatation, * bronchi/bronchioles fill with pus and extend to lung periphery, * MC in basal segment of LLL in non-TB infections and apex in TB |
| S/S in bronchiectasis | • **cough productive of copious sputum,** • *hemoptysis*—sometimes massive, • *fever,* • *cerebral abscess,* • *empyema,* • *lung abscess,* • *digital clubbing* |
| radiographic findings in bronchiectasis | • **crowded bronchial markings extending to the lung periphery,** • **high-resolution CT**—excellent in defining bronchiectasis |
| Rx of bronchiectasis | • **postural drainage,** • **antibiotics,** • **surgery**—for disease localized to segments or lobes |

### Table 6–3. RESPIRATORY TRACT INFECTIONS, INTERSTITIAL AND OBSTRUCTIVE LUNG DISEASE
*Continued*

**Question:** Which of the following would more likely be associated with chronic bronchitis than with sarcoidosis? **SELECT 2**
- (A) Respiratory alkalosis
- (B) Hypoxemia
- (C) Increased total lung capacity (TLC)
- (D) Decreased residual volume (RV)
- (E) Normal to increased $FEV_{1sec}/FVC$ ratio
- (F) Low $DL_{CO}$
- (G) Increased A–a gradient
- (H) Increased ventilation/perfusion mismatch
- (I) Hilar lymphadenopathy

**Answers: (C), (H).** Chronic bronchitis (CB) is an example of COPD, whereas sarcoidosis represents ILD. CB is characterized by increased compliance (easy to fill the lungs with air) and decreased elasticity (difficulty in expelling air), whereas sarcoidosis is associated with decreased compliance (difficult to expand lungs due to fibrosis) and increased elasticity (increased lung recoil from fibrosis). Respiratory alkalosis is more likely to be associated with sarcoidosis and ILD in general, whereas respiratory acidosis characterizes CB (choice A is incorrect). Hypoxemia is common to both conditions (choice B is incorrect). An increased TLC (choice C is correct) is noted in CB owing to an increase in RV from trapping of air behind the inflamed terminal bronchioles (choice D is incorrect). The $FEV_{1sec}/FVC$ is decreased in CB and normal to increased in sarcoidosis, the latter due to increased elasticity and similar $FEV_{1sec}$ and FVC results (choice E is incorrect). Both conditions have a low $DL_{CO}$ (choice F is incorrect). The A–a gradient is increased in both conditions, because both diseases have diffusion abnormalities (choice G is incorrect). CB is characterized by an increased V/Q mismatch (choice H is correct), whereas sarcoidosis is more often associated with diffusion abnormalities. Hilar adenopathy is a feature of sarcoidosis (choice I is incorrect). Noncaseating granulomas are present in the lymph nodes.

*Table continued on following page*

A–a gradient = Alveolar-arterial gradient, AAT = $\alpha_1$-antitrypsin, ABG = arterial blood gas, AD = alveolar duct, AR = autosomal recessive, Bx = biopsy, CAD = coronary artery disease, CB = chronic bronchitis, CBC = complete blood count, CF = cystic fibrosis, CNS = central nervous system, COD = cause of death, COPD = chronic obstructive pulmonary disease, $DL_{CO}$ = diffusion capacity using carbon monoxide, EMP = emphysema, $FEV_{1sec}$ = forced expiratory volume in 1 second, FVC = forced vital capacity, Hgb SS = sickle cell disease, HIV = human immunodeficiency virus, ID = immunodeficiency, ILD = interstitial lung disease, INH = isoniazid, LLL = left lower lobe, MC = most common, MCC = most common cause, PA = pulmonary artery, PCP = *Pneumocystis carinii* pneumonia, PFT = pulmonary function test, PH = pulmonary hypertension, PMF = progressive massive fibrosis, PPD = purified protein derivative, PZA = pyrazinamide, RB = respiratory bronchiole, RIF = rifampin, RLL = right lower lobe, RML = right middle lobe, RUL = right upper lobe, RV = residual volume, RVH = right ventricular hypertrophy, $SaO_2$ = arterial oxygen saturation, S/S = signs and symptoms, TLC = total lung capacity, V/Q = ventilation/perfusion.

### Table 6–4. LUNG TUMORS, MEDIASTINAL DISORDERS, AND DISEASES OF THE PLEURA AND PLEURAL CAVITY

| Most Common... | Answer and Explanation |
|---|---|
| term applied to a peripheral lung nodule <5 cm | **solitary pulmonary nodule or coin lesion** |
| causes of a solitary pulmonary nodule in descending order | • **granuloma**— * **histoplasmosis**, * TB, * coccidioidomycosis, • *malignant*— * **primary cancer**, * metastatic cancer, • *hamartoma* |
| risk factors for malignancy in a solitary pulmonary nodule | • **size of nodule**— * nodule >3 cm, * doubling time of lung cancer 15–450 days, * doubling of nodule size in this time frame is suspicious for malignancy, • *age of the patient*— * patients ≥50 yrs old have 50–60% risk of the nodule being malignant, * most are primary lung cancer, not metastasis, • *patient is a smoker*, • *eccentric or stippled calcification* |
| factors indicating a benign solitary pulmonary nodule | • **lack of size change over 2 yrs**, • *age <35 yrs*—1% risk, • *patterns of calcification*— * diffuse speckled calcification, * "popcorn" calcification: hamartoma, * concentric calcifications: granulomas |

**Table 6–4. LUNG TUMORS, MEDIASTINAL DISORDERS,
AND DISEASES OF THE PLEURA AND PLEURAL CAVITY**
*Continued*

| Most Common... | Answer and Explanation |
|---|---|
| tests used in evaluating solitary nodules | • **comparing previous chest x-rays,** • *skin testing for TB/systemic fungi,* • **FNA,** • *high-resolution CT scans,* • *bronchoscopy* |
| clinical findings in bronchial hamartomas | • **asymptomatic, peripherally located, solitary nodule,** • *"popcorn" calcifications* |
| COD due to cancer in men and women | **primary lung cancer**— * incidence is decreasing in men and increasing in women, * adenocarcinoma is the most common type |
| risk factors for primary lung cancer | • **cigarette smoking,** • *increasing age,* • *radon gas*—in uranium mining, • *asbestos,* • *chromium,* • *nickel,* • *beryllium,* • arsenic, • *cadmium* |
| types of primary lung cancer | • **nonsmall cell carcinoma (NSCC, ~80%)**— * **adenocarcinoma,** * squamous cell carcinoma, * large cell undifferentiated carcinoma, • *small cell carcinoma* (SCC, ~20%)—neurosecretory tumor, • *bronchial carcinoid* (2–5%)—neurosecretory tumor |
| primary lung cancers with greatest relationship to smoking | • **squamous cell carcinoma,** • *SCC* |
| primary site of origin of lung cancer | **reserve cells in the surface epithelium of the bronchi**—normally differentiate into ciliated cells, goblet cells, and neuroendocrine cells called Kulchitsky's cells |
| oncogenes involved in primary lung cancer | • **p53 suppressor gene**— * SCC: 80%, * NSCC: >50%, • *Rb suppressor gene*— * SCC: 80%, * NSCC: 25%, • *K-ras oncogene*— * adenocarcinoma: 25%, * large cell: 25%, * squamous cell: 5% |
| lung cancer | • **metastasis from breast cancer,** • *other common metastases*— * renal adenocarcinoma, * choriocarcinoma: both gestationally derived and testicular, * GI cancers: ♦ esophagus, ♦ stomach, ♦ pancreas, ♦ colorectal, * sarcomas in general, * malignant melanoma |

*Table continued on following page*

### Table 6–4. LUNG TUMORS, MEDIASTINAL DISORDERS, AND DISEASES OF THE PLEURA AND PLEURAL CAVITY
*Continued*

| Most Common... | Answer and Explanation |
|---|---|
| sites of metastasis in the lungs | • **parenchyma,** • *pleura/pleural space,* • *endobronchial mucosa,* • *lymphatics,* • *chest wall,* • *mediastinum* |
| centrally located primary lung cancers | • **squamous cell carcinoma,** • *SCC,* • *bronchial carcinoid* |
| peripherally located primary lung cancers | • **adenocarcinoma**— * filters in cigarettes allow smaller carcinogens in smoke to spread peripherally, * more common in women than men, • *bronchioloalveolar cell carcinoma,* • *large cell undifferentiated carcinoma*—most are poorly differentiated adenocarcinomas when subjected to EM, • *scar carcinoma*—most are adenocarcinomas |
| primary lung cancer with no smoking relationship | **bronchioloalveolar cell carcinoma**— * peripherally located cancer derived from Clara cells: nonciliated epithelium, * solitary nodule in early stages, * consolidation simulating lobar pneumonia in later stages |
| primary lung cancer in nonsmokers | **adenocarcinoma** |
| primary lung cancers that cavitate | • **squamous carcinoma,** • *large cell undifferentiated cancer* |
| primary lung cancer detected by cytologic examination of sputum | **squamous cell carcinoma**— * Pap stains reveal deeply eosinophilic staining of squamous cell cancers, * SCC is least likely detected by cytologic exam of sputum (often confused with lymphocytes) |
| S/S of primary lung cancer | • **cough that has changed in character**—75%, • *dyspnea*—60%, • *hemoptysis*—50%, • *weight loss*—40%, • *chest pain*—40%, • *hypertrophic osteoarthropathy*—subperiosteal bone reaction with clubbing of fingers, • *Eaton-Lambert syndrome*—see below, • *hoarseness*—left recurrent laryngeal nerve involved, • *syndromes*— * ectopic hormones, * SVC syndrome, * superior sulcus tumor: Pancoast's tumor |

**Table 6–4. LUNG TUMORS, MEDIASTINAL DISORDERS, AND DISEASES OF THE PLEURA AND PLEURAL CAVITY**
*Continued*

| Most Common... | Answer and Explanation |
|---|---|
| lung cancer associated with the Eaton-Lambert syndrome | **SCC**— * syndrome resembles myasthenia gravis, * unlike myasthenia: ♦ eyes are not usually involved, ♦ muscle strength increases with exercise, ♦ edrophonium (Tensilon) does not improve muscle function |
| symptom of lung metastasis | **dyspnea**—hemoptysis is uncommon |
| ectopic hormone-secreting primary lung cancers | • **SCC**— * secretes ACTH: ectopic Cushing's syndrome, *ADH:* ♦ ~50%, ♦ SiADH, • *squamous cell carcinoma*—PTH-like peptide: ♦ hypercalcemia, ♦ low serum parathormone (suppressed by hypercalcemia) |
| sites of metastasis of primary lung cancer in the chest cavity | **hilar and mediastinal lymph nodes** |
| sites of metastasis of primary lung cancer outside the lungs | • **adrenal glands**— * ~50%, * Addison's disease is uncommon, • *liver*— * 30%, * primary lung cancer is MCC of liver metastasis, • *brain*— * 20%, * SCC most commonly, • *bone*—predominantly lytic metastases |
| cause of the SVC syndrome | **primary small cell carcinoma with invasion and compression of SVC**—see **Table 5–2** |
| cause of the superior sulcus tumor | **primary squamous cell carcinoma**— * brachial plexus invasion: ♦ arm weakness, ♦ pain, * invasion of cervical sympathetic ganglion: Horner's syndrome with ♦ ipsilateral lid lag, ♦ miosis, ♦ anhidrosis |
| diagnostic tests used in working up lung cancer | • **cytologic evaluation of sputum**— * sensitivity 30% in asymptomatic patients, * 50% sensitivity if cough is present, * 70% sensitivity if hemoptysis is present, • **fiberoptic bronchoscopy**—sensitivity 85–95% when brushings, lavage, and biopsies are collected, • **FNA**—sensitivity 90–95% with CT guidance, • *examination of PF, if an effusion is present*—sensitivity 60–80%, • *chest x-ray*— * 95% of peripheral tumors and 70% of central tumors are visible, • *CT*— * tumor size, * extent: CT of chest and upper abdomen (adrenal/liver) |

*Table continued on following page*

**Table 6–4. LUNG TUMORS, MEDIASTINAL DISORDERS, AND DISEASES OF THE PLEURA AND PLEURAL CAVITY**
*Continued*

| Most Common... | Answer and Explanation |
|---|---|
| PFT/ABG findings indicating poor surgical risk | • **FEV$_{1sec}$ <1 liter,** • *PaCO$_2$ >45 mmHg* |
| staging guidelines used to determine Rx options in primary lung cancer | **cell type determines the approach to staging—** * TNM system is used for NSCC, * stages I and II are operable, * stage III is usually inoperable, * anatomic extent: e.g., ♦ distance from carina, ♦ <2 cm inoperable, ♦ nodal involvement (mediastinal lymph node sampling and extrathoracic spread reduce the prognosis) |
| Rx options of non-SCLC and SCLC | • **NSCC—** * surgery, * <30% candidates for resection, • **SCC—** * rarely resectable: 85% stage III, * multiple drug chemotherapy: great sensitivity to chemotherapy, * majority with distant metastasis die in < 1 yr, • *radiation—* * prevent/Rx CNS metastasis, * palliate local symptoms in advanced stages: e.g., ♦ SVC syndrome, ♦ bone metastasis [**Note:** overall 5-yr survival for all primary lung cancers is 15%.] |
| determinant of long-term survival in patients with resectable tumors | **presence or absence of mediastinal lymph node involvement** |
| 5-yr survival rates for primary lung cancer in descending order | • **bronchioloalveolar cell carcinoma—42%,** • *adenocarcinoma—17%,* • *squamous cell carcinoma—15%,* • *SCC—<5%* |
| primary lung tumor in children | **bronchial carcinoid** |
| primary neuroendocrine tumor of lung with a low-grade malignant potential | **bronchial carcinoid—** * mean age of 55 yrs old, * no smoking relationship, * ~20% metastasize locally |
| S/S of bronchial carcinoid | • **hemoptysis—** * very vascular, * protrude into lumen, • *cough,* • *postobstructive lipoid pneumonias,* • *carcinoid syndrome—<1%* |
| Rx of bronchial carcinoid | **surgery—90% 5-yr survival** |

### Table 6–4. LUNG TUMORS, MEDIASTINAL DISORDERS, AND DISEASES OF THE PLEURA AND PLEURAL CAVITY
*Continued*

| Most Common... | Answer and Explanation |
|---|---|
| presentations for mediastinal disease | • **asymptomatic,** • *vessel compression*—SVC syndrome, • *dysphagia,* • *nerve destruction*—hoarseness with recurrent laryngeal nerve involvement near the aorta or left main PA, • *Horner's syndrome*—see above, • *cough,* • *paraneoplastic syndrome*—ectopic hormones |
| structures in the anterior mediastinum | • **thymus,** • **lymphatic tissue** [**Note:** a lateral chest radiograph helps localize mediastinal masses to the correct compartment.] |
| structures in posterior mediastinum | • **sympathetic ganglia,** • **nerves,** • **esophagus** |
| structures in middle mediastinum | • **major bronchi,** • **lymphatic tissue,** • **pericardium** |
| tumor in the mediastinum | • **neurogenic tumors in posterior mediastinum**—include: ♦ neuroblastoma in children (malignant), * schwannomas and neurofibromas in adults (benign) |
| tumors in the anterior mediastinum | • **thymoma:** * 70% benign, * 30% malignant, • *malignant lymphoma:* * usually nodular sclerosing Hodgkin's disease in a young woman, * not amenable to surgery, • *teratoma* |
| mediastinal tumor associated with myasthenia gravis (MG) | **thymoma**— * ~50% express symptoms associated with MG, * only 10–15% of patients with MG have a thymoma |
| histologic findings in the thymus in patients with MG | **B cell hyperplasia**— * germinal follicles synthesize antibodies against acetylcholine receptors, * thymectomy is often required when medical Rx is not successful—~75% experience improvement |
| mediastinal tumor associated with pure RBC aplasia and hypogammaglobulinemia | **thymoma** |
| mediastinal site for germ cell tumors | **anterior mediastinum**—most germ cell tumors localize to the midline of the body |

*Table continued on following page*

**Table 6–4. LUNG TUMORS, MEDIASTINAL DISORDERS, AND DISEASES OF THE PLEURA AND PLEURAL CAVITY**
*Continued*

| Most Common... | Answer and Explanation |
|---|---|
| disorders in the middle mediastinum | • **pericardial cyst,** • *bronchogenic cyst,* • *lymphadenopathy*—due to: ♦ sarcoidosis, ♦ malignancy, ♦ granulomatous disease, • *aortic arch aneurysms* |
| cause of a "mediastinal crunch" | • **ruptured esophagus from endoscopy/retching,** • *pneumothorax* [**Note:** the crunch (Hamman's sign) occurs with each systole and is due to subcutaneous emphysema.] |
| cause of sclerosing mediastinitis | *Histoplasma capsulatum* |
| factors determining fluid movement in the pleural cavity | **hydrostatic pressure difference between the parietal and visceral pleura**— * net pressure in the parietal pleura is +9 cm $H_2O$: due to high hydrostatic pressure from the intercostal arteries, * net pressure in visceral pleura is −11 cm $H_2O$: low hydrostatic pressure from the pulmonary circulation, * fluid moves from parietal pleura → pleural space → visceral pleura, * oncotic pressure is roughly equal between parietal and visceral pleura and is not normally responsible for fluid movements |
| mechanisms for pleural fluid (PF) accumulation | • **hydrostatic pressure alterations**—e.g., high pulmonary vessel hydrostatic pressure reduces fluid uptake from visceral pleura in CHF, • *oncotic pressure alterations*—low plasma albumin causes a greater movement of PF into the pleural space, • *increased vessel permeability*—e.g., * pneumonia, * pulmonary infarction, • *lymphatic blockage*— * blocks PF uptake from pleural space, * e.g., lymphangitic spread of tumor in the lungs, • *leakage of ascitic fluid through openings in the diaphragm*—e.g., ascites in cirrhosis |
| PF tests that distinguish transudates from exudates | • **ratios favoring an exudate**— * PF protein/serum protein ratio >0.5, * PF LDH/serum LDH >0.6, * PF LDH >0.45 × upper limit of normal of serum LDH, * values less than the above indicate a transudate, • *PF protein*— * >3 gm/dL: exudate, * <3 gm/dL: transudate, • *cells*— * exudates have a cellular infiltrate, * transudates are hypocellular |

### Table 6–4. LUNG TUMORS, MEDIASTINAL DISORDERS, AND DISEASES OF THE PLEURA AND PLEURAL CAVITY
*Continued*

| Most Common... | Answer and Explanation |
| --- | --- |
| cause of a pleural effusion | **CHF**—transudate |
| causes of a PF exudate | • **pneumonia,** • *pulmonary infarction*—hemorrhagic exudate, • *cancer*—hemorrhagic exudate, • *pancreatitis*—contains amylase |
| causes of a PF pH <7.3 | • **malignancy**—primary or secondary, • *empyema*—e.g., *Staphylococcus aureus* pneumonia, • *TB,* • *collagen vascular disease*—e.g., * RA, * PSS, * SLE |
| role of cytology of PF | **detection of primary/metastatic disease**—cytology has a greater sensitivity (60–80%) than a pleural Bx in detecting malignancy |
| PF findings in TB | **exudate with a lymphocyte-dominant cell count**—culture of a pleural Bx has a higher yield than culture of PF in detecting TB |
| causes of increased amylase in the PF | • **acute pancreatitis**—left-sided PF effusion, • *Boerhaave's* syndrome—esophageal rupture |
| primary pleural malignancy | **mesothelioma**—see **Table 6–3** |
| PF pH cutoff for tube drainage of a parapneumonic effusion | **pH <7.0** |
| physical findings in a pleural effusion | **see Table 6–1** |
| Rx for recurrent malignant effusions | **pleurodesis with injection of an irritant into the pleural cavity**—doxycycline may be used |
| chest x-ray findings in a pleural effusion | • **blunting of costophrenic angle with a concave meniscus,** • *loss of definition of the hemidiaphragm,* • *increased density in the hemithorax* [**Note:** a minimum of 150–300 mL of fluid must be present to detect a PF effusion on a routine chest x-ray.] |
| x-ray position used to detect effusions | **lateral decubitus x-rays**— * suspected side in the dependent position, * detects smaller amounts of fluid, * generally more accurate in detecting effusions than upright films |

*Table continued on following page*

## Table 6–4. LUNG TUMORS, MEDIASTINAL DISORDERS, AND DISEASES OF THE PLEURA AND PLEURAL CAVITY
### *Continued*

**Question:** A 58-yr-old man with a 60-pack year history of smoking cigarettes presents with weight loss, headaches, and a change in the character of his cough. Blood has been present in the sputum on a few occasions. Physical exam reveals no localizing neurologic findings. Scattered sibilant rhonchi clear with coughing. A mental status exam is abnormal. A chest radiograph exhibits a large right hilar mass. A CT scan of the brain is negative for space-occupying lesions. The serum sodium is 110 mEq/L (135–147 mEq/L). What additional laboratory or clinical abnormalities would you expect in this patient? **SELECT 2**

- (A) Random UNa$^+$ > 40 mEq/L
- (B) UOsm > POsm
- (C) High serum blood urea nitrogen
- (D) Dependent pitting edema
- (E) Correction of hyponatremia with infusion of 0.9% normal saline

**Answers: (A), (B).** The patient has a primary SCC of the lung with the inappropriate ADH syndrome (SIADH). Ectopic secretion of ADH causes reabsorption of free water from the late distal and collecting tubules in the kidneys. This produces a dilutional hyponatremia and an osmotic gradient favoring movement of water into the ICF compartment, including the cells in the brain. CNS edema is responsible for the patient's headaches and mental status alterations. An increase in arterial blood volume in SIADH increases the glomerular filtration rate and decreases reabsorption of proximal tubule solutes like Na$^+$ and urea. Random UNa$^+$ > 40 mEq/L is the rule in SIADH, since the proximal tubule is unable to reabsorb any Na$^+$ owing to the high peritubular capillary hydrostatic pressure **(choice A is correct)**. The inappropriate presence of ADH leads to continual concentration of urine, which is the primary reason for UOsm being greater than POsm in SIADH **(choice B is correct)**. The serum BUN is usually low in SIADH due to a dilutional effect of excess water in serum and loss of urea in the urine **(choice C is incorrect)**. Dependent pitting edema, which is primarily due to an increase in TBNa$^+$ in the ECF, is not present in SIADH, since TBNa$^+$ is normal. An increase in TBW does not produce pitting edema **(choice D is incorrect)**. Hypertonic rather than isotonic saline is used to raise the serum Na$^+$ concentration in patients with SIADH **(choice E is incorrect)**. However, the best treatment for this patient is demeclocycline, which is a nephrotoxic agent that blocks the effect of ADH in the kidneys. Restricting water, the usual treatment for SIADH, is not usually recommended in the setting of a small cell carcinoma of the lung owing to poor patient compliance and the poor prognosis associated with SCC.

ABG = arterial blood gas, ACTH = adrenocorticotropic hormone, ADH = antidiuretic hormone, Bx = biopsy, CHF = congestive heart failure, CNS = central nervous system, COD = cause of death, ECF = extracellular fluid, EM = electron microscopy, $FEV_{1sec}$ = forced expiratory volume in 1 second, FNA = fine needle aspiration, ICF = intracellular fluid, LDH = lactate dehydrogenase, MCC = most common cause, MG = myasthenia gravis, NSCC = nonsmall cell cancer, PA = pulmonary artery, $PaCO_2$ = partial pressure of arterial carbon dioxide, PF = pleural fluid, PFT = pulmonary function test, POsm = plasma osmolality, PSS = progressive systemic sclerosis, PTH = parathormone, RA = rheumatoid arthritis, RBC = red blood cell, SCC = small cell carcinoma, SCLC = small cell lung carcinoma, SiADH = syndrome of inappropriate antidiuretic hormone, SLE = systemic lupus erythematosus, S/S = signs and symptoms, SVC = superior vena cava, $TBNa^+$ = total body sodium, TBW = total body water, TNM = tumor/nodes/metastasis, $UNa^+$ = urine sodium, UOsm = urine osmolality.

# CHAPTER

**7**

# GASTROINTESTINAL SURGERY

## CONTENTS

## Table 7–1. ORAL CAVITY, SALIVARY GLAND

| Most Common... | Answer and Explanation |
|---|---|
| causes of exudative tonsillitis | • **viruses**—e.g., EBV, coxsackievirus account for >50% of cases, • *group A Streptococcus pyogenes*—20–35%, • *Neisseria gonorrhoeae, • Chlamydia trachomatis, • Corynebacterium diphtheriae* [**Note:** clinical exam cannot distinguish bacterial from viral tonsillitis. Documentation by culture or direct antigen detection sensitivity 80–85%, specificity >90% for streptococcal infection.] |
| Rx of group A streptococcal pharyngitis | • **penicillin V potassium, 250 mg tid × 10 days, or** • **single IM injection of benzathine or procaine penicillin**—best for noncompliant patient [**Note:** Rx is recommended if the direct antigen test is positive. If negative, a culture should be made, with Rx based on the results.] |
| cause of deviation of the uvula to the contralateral side | **peritonsillar abscess**—it is also associated with odynophagia (painful swallowing) and medial deviation of the soft palate |
| causes of peritonsillar abscess | • **exudative tonsillitis,** • *pharyngitis,* • *dental infection* |

*Table continued on following page*

**Table 7–1. ORAL CAVITY, SALIVARY GLAND** *Continued*

| Most Common... | Answer and Explanation |
|---|---|
| organisms causing peritonsillar abscess | • β-*hemolytic streptococci*—usually children <12 yrs old, • *Fusobacterium, Bacteroides melanogenicus/mixed aerobic/anaerobic streptococci*—adults |
| S/S of peritonsillar abscess | • **medial displacement of tonsils**, • **bulging abscess through anterior tonsillar pillar**, • *fever/chills*, • *pain with talking*, • *dysphonia*—"hot potato voice," • *inflamed/deviated uvula*, • *foul-smelling breath* |
| Rx of peritonsillar abscess | • **surgical drainage of abscess**, • *penicillin* |
| causes of Ludwig's angina | • **dental extraction**, • *trauma to floor of mouth* [**Note:** Ludwig's angina is a cellulitis involving the submaxillary and sublingual space. It follows fascial planes and may spread into pharynx, carotid sheath, superior mediastinum.] |
| organisms causing Ludwig's angina | • **aerobic/anaerobic** *streptococci*, • *Eikenella corrodens* |
| Rx of Ludwig's angina | • **surgical drainage**, • *antibiotics*—IV penicillin G + metronidazole |
| cause of a submandibular sinus | ***Actinomyces israelii* infection**— * anaerobic, gram-positive, filamentous bacteria, * best identified in yellow sulfur granules, * usually associated with dental abscesses [**Note:** *Actinomyces* is a normal inhabitant of the tonsils.] |
| Rx of *Actinomyces israelii* infection | • **IV ampicillin followed by po amoxicillin**, or • **IV penicillin G followed by po penicillin V** |
| oral manifestation of AIDS | • **candidiasis**, • *aphthous ulcers*, • *hairy leukoplakia*, • *Kaposi's sarcoma*—hard palate is the most common location |
| cause of leukoplakia of the tongue in an HIV-positive patient | **hairy leukoplakia secondary to EBV**— * a glossitis located on the lateral side of the tongue, * predates the onset of AIDS, * is not a precursor lesion for squamous cancer |
| Rx for hairy leukoplakia | **high-dose acyclovir**—recurs when acyclovir is discontinued |

## Table 7–1. ORAL CAVITY, SALIVARY GLAND *Continued*

| Most Common... | Answer and Explanation |
|---|---|
| polyp syndrome associated with mucosal pigmentation | **Peutz-Jeghers syndrome**— * *AD* polyposis syndrome, * see **Table 7–3** |
| endocrine disorder associated with mucosal pigmentation | **Addison's disease**—hypocortisolism leads to an increase in ACTH, which has melanocyte-stimulating properties |
| AD disorder associated with mucosal neuromas | **MEN IIb syndrome** |
| clinical findings in MEN IIb syndrome | • **mucosal neuromas**— * >90%, * lips acromegaloid, * tongue enlarged, • *medullary carcinoma of the thyroid*—80%, • *pheochromocytoma*—60% |
| causes of leukoplakia | • **chronic irritation**—e.g., * dentures, * biting the cheek, • *tobacco smoking/smokeless tobacco,* • *alcohol* [**Note:** leukoplakia is a clinical term. It is a white (leukoplakia), red/white (erythroleukoplakia), or red (erythroplakia) patch.] |
| initial step in management of oral leukoplakia | **biopsy**— * leukoplakia does not rub off, * Bx is necessary to R/O squamous dysplasia/cancer: 4–10% chance, * erythroplakia has 80–90% chance of dysplasia/cancer |
| locations for leukoplakia | • **ventrolateral tongue,** • *floor of mouth,* • *lower lip* |
| cancer in the oral cavity | **SCC** |
| predisposing causes of squamous cancer | • **smoking,** • *alcohol,* • *Plummer-Vinson syndrome*—iron deficiency, • *poor-fitting dentures*—chronic irritation, • *Indian people chewing betel nuts,* • *UVB*—lower lip lesion, • *syphilis of tongue,* • *HPV*—these cancers are located in Waldeyer's ring [**Note:** smoking + alcohol have an additive effect that is greater than each risk factor alone.] |
| sites for SCC of the oral cavity | • **floor of mouth,** • *lower lip,* • *lateral border of tongue,* • *hard palate,* • *base of tongue* |

*Table continued on following page*

## Table 7–1. ORAL CAVITY, SALIVARY GLAND *Continued*

| Most Common... | Answer and Explanation |
|---|---|
| SCC cancers metastatic to the "tonsillar node" | • **posterior one-third of tongue,** • *oropharynx* [**Note:** the "tonsillar node" is the superior jugular node. Cancers of the tonsil also metastasize to this site.] |
| SCC cancers metastatic to jugular nodes | • **larynx,** • *hypopharynx* |
| SCC cancers metastatic to submaxillary nodes | • **anterior floor of mouth,** • *middle third of tongue* |
| SCC cancers metastatic to submental nodes | • **lower lip,** • *tip of tongue* |
| use of toluidine blue in oral cancer | **screen for oral cancer**—in general, cancers take up the dye whereas benign tumors do not |
| Rx of oral SCC | • **surgery,** • *radiation* |
| cancer associated with smokeless tobacco | **verrucous carcinoma**—variant of SCC |
| location for verrucous carcinoma | **mandibular sulcus**— * contact area of smokeless tobacco, * rarely metastasizes |
| cancer of the upper lip | **BCC**— * UVB-induced, * lesions of the upper lip and above are more commonly BCC, whereas those on the lower lip are SCC |
| site for salivary gland tumors | **major salivary glands (parotid glands)**—applies to both benign (70%) or malignant tumors of the major salivary glands, * greater percentage of minor salivary gland tumors are malignant |
| overall benign salivary gland tumor in both major/minor salivary glands | **pleomorphic adenoma** |
| benign tumors of parotid gland | • **pleomorphic adenoma (mixed tumor),** • *Warthin's tumor,* • *oncocytoma* |

## Table 7–1. ORAL CAVITY, SALIVARY GLAND *Continued*

| Most Common... | Answer and Explanation |
|---|---|
| clinical features of pleomorphic adenoma | • **painless, movable, smooth mass,** • *female predominance,* • *epithelial tissue intermixed with myxomatous/cartilaginous stroma,* • *incomplete capsule with tumor projections through capsule*—tendency to recur if normal parotid is not included in the resection |
| clinical features suggesting malignancy in a pleomorphic adenoma | • **facial nerve involvement,** • *rapid growth,* • *pain* |
| clinical features of Warthin's tumor (adenolymphoma) | • **MC monomorphic adenoma,** • *cystic glandular structures within benign lymphoid tissue,* • *only benign salivary gland tumor more common in men,* • *10% are bilateral* |
| clinical features of oncocytoma | • **begin in early adulthood,** • *rich in mitochondria* |
| overall malignant salivary gland tumor | **mucoepidermoid carcinoma** |
| radiation-induced salivary gland tumor | **mucoepidermoid carcinoma** |
| malignant tumor of parotid gland | **mucoepidermoid carcinoma** |
| clinical features of mucoepidermoid carcinoma | • **female predominance,** • *mixture of neoplastic squamous/mucus-secreting cells*—grade of squamous component determines prognosis, • *facial nerve involvement* |
| major salivary gland with malignant tumors | **sublingual**—>70–90% have malignant tumors |
| tumor of minor salivary glands | **pleomorphic adenoma** |
| malignant tumors of minor salivary glands | • **mucoepidermoid carcinoma,** • *adenoid cystic carcinoma,* • *malignant pleomorphic adenoma* |

*Table continued on following page*

## Table 7–1. ORAL CAVITY, SALIVARY GLAND *Continued*

| Most Common... | Answer and Explanation |
|---|---|
| clinical features of adenoid cystic carcinoma | • **tendency to infiltrate perineural space**—frequently painful, • *primarily a minor salivary gland tumor*—MC on palate, • *cribriform pattern,* • *tend to recur after surgery,* • *metastasize at late stage*—lung/bone metastasis is common |
| location for Kaposi's sarcoma in oral cavity in AIDS patients | • **hard palate,** • *gingiva,* • *buccal mucosa* |
| Rx for intraoral KS | • **local radiation,** • *intralesional vinblastine* |

**Question:** Which of the following are likely to represent either a malignant tumor or precancerous lesion? **SELECT 5**

- (A) Leukoplakia on lateral border of the tongue in a 26-yr-old HIV-positive patient
- (B) Leukoplakia on lateral border of the tongue in a 52-yr-old smoker/alcoholic
- (C) Movable mass below the angle of the jaw in a 35-yr-old woman
- (D) Movable mass below the angle of the jaw, pain, and ipsilateral Bell's palsy in a 35-yr-old woman
- (E) Crateriform lesion on the upper lip of a nonsmoker
- (F) Crateriform lesion on the lower lip of a smoker
- (G) Lip pigmentation in a 32-yr-old man with a positive stool guaiac
- (H) Wartlike lesion in the mandibular sulcus in a professional baseball player

**Answers: (B), (D), (E), (F), (H).** Leukoplakia along the lateral border of the tongue in an HIV-positive patient is most likely hairy leukoplakia due to an EBV infection of the tongue **(choice A is incorrect).** Leukoplakia along the lateral border of the tongue is most likely squamous dysplasia or cancer **(choice B is correct).** A movable mass below the angle of the jaw in a 35-yr-old woman is most likely a benign pleomorphic adenoma **(choice C is incorrect).** A movable mass below the angle of the jaw with pain and ipsilateral Bell's palsy is most likely a malignant salivary gland tumor **(choice D is correct).** A crateriform lesion on the upper lip of a nonsmoker is most likely a BCC, whereas a similar lesion on the lower lip of a smoker is most likely a SCC **(choices E and F are correct).** Lip pigmentation in a 32-yr-old man with a bleeding hamartomatous polyp **(choice G is incorrect).** A wartlike lesion in the mandibular sulcus in a professional baseball player is most likely a verrucous carcinoma associated with smokeless tobacco abuse **(choice H is correct).**

ACTH = adrenocorticotropic hormone, AD = autosomal dominant, AIDS = acquired immunodeficiency syndrome, BCC = basal cell carcinoma, Bx = biopsy, EBV = Epstein-Barr virus, HIV = human immunodeficiency virus, HPV = human papilloma virus, KS = Kaposi's sarcoma, MC = most common, MEN = multiple endocrine neoplasia, SCC = squamous cell carcinoma, S/S = signs and symptoms, UVB = ultraviolet light B.

### Table 7-2. ESOPHAGEAL DISORDERS, UPPER GASTROINTESTINAL BLEED

| Most Common... | Answer and Explanation |
|---|---|
| S/S of esophageal disease | • **heartburn (dyspepsia, pyrosis)**— * burning epigastric pain, * bloating, * early satiety, • *dysphagia for solids alone*—sign of obstruction, • *dysphagia for solids/liquid*—motility disorder, • *odynophagia*— * painful swallowing, * always a significant finding, • *regurgitation of recently ingested food*— * persistent: ♦ esophageal diverticulum, ♦ hiatal hernia, * intermittent: GERD, • *chronic pulmonary infection*—aspiration from GERD, • *substernal chest pain*—GERD |
| causes of dyspepsia | • **GERD**—usually in association with a hiatal hernia, • *nonulcer dyspepsia,* • *food intolerance* |
| cause of dysphagia for solids but not liquids | **obstructive esophageal lesions in the esophagus**—e.g., * web: Plummer-Vinson syndrome, * cancer [**Note:** an esophageal lumen <12 mm in diameter causes mechanical obstruction.] |
| cause of dysphagia for solids and liquids | **motility disorders**—e.g., * PSS/CREST syndrome, * DM/PM, * MG, * achalasia, * previous stroke [**Note:** the upper one-third of esophagus is skeletal muscle (site of oropharyngeal dysphagia), middle third is skeletal/smooth muscle, and the lower third is smooth muscle (site of lower esophageal dysphagia).] |
| causes of oropharyngeal dysphagia | • **neuromuscular disorders**—e.g., * DM/PM, * MG, * ALS, * stroke, • *structural disorders*—e.g., Zenker's diverticulum [**Note:** oropharyngeal dysphagia is a faulty transfer of food from the oral pharynx to the esophagus.] |

*Table continued on following page*

**Table 7–2. ESOPHAGEAL DISORDERS, UPPER GASTROINTESTINAL BLEED** *Continued*

| Most Common... | Answer and Explanation |
|---|---|
| S/S of oropharyngeal dysphagia | • **coughing/choking,** • *nasal regurgitation,* • *pulmonary aspiration* |
| causes of lower esophageal dysphagia | • **achalasia**—see below, • *PSS/CREST syndrome*—see below |
| cause of odynophagia | **inflammation**—e.g., * **infectious esophagitis**—e.g., *Candida* esophagitis in AIDS, * GERD |
| cause of intermittent dysphagia for solids only | **lower esophageal ring**— * junction of squamous with columnar epithelium, * usually asymptomatic |
| Rx of Schatzki's ring | **esophageal bougienage** |
| cause of progressive dysphagia for solids with associated heartburn | **peptic stricture secondary to Barrett's esophagus** |
| cause of progressive dysphagia for solids in elderly patients with weight loss | **esophageal cancer**—if hoarseness is present, invasive esophageal cancer with recurrent laryngeal nerve involvement is likely |
| cause of intermittent dysphagia for solids/ liquids associated with noncardiac chest pain | • **GERD,** • *nutcracker esophagus*—very high pressures recorded by manometry, • *diffuse esophageal spasm*—"corkscrew" esophagus on barium studies |
| Rx of esophageal disorders causing noncardiac chest pain | • **nitroglycerin,** • *calcium channel blockers,* • *anticholinergics* |
| cause of Plummer-Vinson syndrome (Patterson-Kelly syndrome) | **chronic iron deficiency** |
| clinical findings in Plummer-Vinson syndrome | • **upper esophageal web,** • *majority are elderly women,* • *intermittent dysphagia for solids,* • *koilonychia,* • *achlorhydria,* • *glossitis,* • *increased risk for SCC* (10–20%) *of upper esophagus and oral cavity* |

## Table 7–2. ESOPHAGEAL DISORDERS, UPPER GASTROINTESTINAL BLEED *Continued*

| Most Common... | Answer and Explanation |
|---|---|
| esophageal diverticulum | **Zenker's diverticulum**— * located in upper esophagus, * defect in cricopharyngeus muscle |
| S/S of a Zenker's diverticulum | • **oropharyngeal dysphagia**, • *halitosis*, • *diverticulitis*, • *regurgitation of undigested food* |
| clinical findings of traction diverticulum | • **located in midesophagus**, • *pathogenesis*— * **motor function defect**, * traction of fibrous adhesions from old tuberculous lymphadenitis, • *wide stoma*—does not trap food |
| congenital esophageal disorder | **tracheoesophageal fistula**— * the proximal esophagus ends blindly, * distal esophagus arises from the trachea |
| S/S of TE fistula | • **maternal polyhydramnios**—obstruction to reabsorption of amniotic fluid, • **abdominal distention**—air in the stomach from tracheal fistula, • **chemical pneumonia**—aspiration of milk into trachea |
| syndrome associated with a TE fistula | **VATER syndrome**— * v̲ertebral abnormalities, * a̲nal abnormalities (imperforate anus), * T̲E fistula, * r̲enal disease/r̲adius abnormality |
| systemic collagen-vascular disease involving the esophagus | **PSS**— * involves the smooth muscle in lower esophagus: 70–90%, * muscle atrophies and is replaced with fibrosis, * CREST syndrome is a PSS variant |
| clinical findings of PSS involving the esophagus | • **progressive dysphagia for solids/liquids**, • *reflux esophagitis*, • *abnormal esophagography*— * no peristalsis, * dilatation, * stricture, • *abnormal esophageal manometry*— * absent-to-low peristaltic amplitude, * low-to-absent LES pressure |
| cause of PSS and CREST syndrome | **small vessel vasculitis**—followed by excessive deposition of normal collagen in interstitial tissue |
| initial sign of PSS/CREST syndrome | **Raynaud's phenomenon**— * 90%, * color changes from digital vasospasm/fibrosis |

*Table continued on following page*

### Table 7–2. ESOPHAGEAL DISORDERS, UPPER GASTROINTESTINAL BLEED *Continued*

| Most Common... | Answer and Explanation |
|---|---|
| clinical findings in CREST syndrome | • *calcinosis cutis*—subcutaneous calcification, • *centromere antibody*, • **Raynaud's phenomenon**—MC initial presentation, • *esophageal motility dysfunction*, • *sclerodactyly*—tapered fingers, • *telangiectasia* |
| clinical findings in CREST syndrome that differ from PSS | • **anticentromere antibody-positive in 70–90% versus 10–20% in PSS,** • *skin tightening limited to hands/face*—no trunk involvement as in PSS, • *less renal involvement than PSS,* • *more likely to have cor pulmonale than PSS,* • *better prognosis,* • *anti-Scl-70 antibodies in 10% versus 25–30% in PSS* |
| small bowel finding in PSS | **wide-mouthed diverticula**—predispose to bacterial overgrowth: potential for malabsorption and $B_{12}$ deficiency |
| lab findings in PSS | • **positive serum ANA**—70–90%, • *anti-Scl-70 antibodies (antitopoisomerase antibodies)*—25–30%, • *anticentromere antibodies*—10–20% |
| Rx of PSS | D-**penicillamine** |
| COD in PSS | **respiratory failure**—secondary to interstitial fibrosis and restrictive lung disease |
| systemic collagen vascular diseases involving the upper esophagus | **dermatomyositis/polymyositis**—inflammation of striated muscle of upper esophagus occurs in ~50% of cases |
| S/S of DM/PM of the upper esophagus | • **oropharyngeal dysphagia,** • *regurgitation,* • *cough* |
| neuromuscular disorder of the esophagus | **achalasia** |
| pathogenesis of achalasia | • **absence of ganglion cells in the myenteric plexus**—also degenerative changes in the nucleus ambiguus and vagus nerve, • *loss of VIP from ganglion cells*— * normally, VIP is a vasodilator, * loss of VIP leads to: ♦ sustained LES contraction, ♦ aperistalsis, ♦ dilatation of proximal esophagus |

## Table 7–2. ESOPHAGEAL DISORDERS, UPPER
## GASTROINTESTINAL BLEED Continued

| Most Common... | Answer and Explanation |
|---|---|
| clinical findings in achalasia | • **older patient with progressive dysphagia for solids/liquids,** • *nocturnal symptoms*— * regurgitation of undigested food, * cough, • *weight loss,* • *predisposes to SCC,* • *chest x-ray showing air/fluid level in esophagus,* • *abnormal barium swallow*— * dilated, * aperistaltic esophagus: beaklike tapering at distal end, • *abnormal esophageal manometry*— * key test, * detects: ♦ aperistalsis, ♦ failure of relaxation of LES |
| test confirming achalasia | **esophageal manometry** |
| Rx of achalasia | • **pneumatic dilatation,** • *calcium channel blockers,* • *modified Heller's esophagotomy*—95% have excellent results |
| clinical findings in diffuse esophageal spasm | • **intermittent dysphagia for solids/liquids,** • *noncardiac chest pain*—closely simulates angina pectoris, • *abnormal barium study*—"corkscrew" esophagus, • *abnormal esophageal manometry*— * intermittent, simultaneous contractions, * normal peristalsis between contractions |
| Rx of diffuse esophageal spasm | • **calcium channel blockers,** • *nitrates* |
| abnormality reported on upper GI barium study | **hiatal hernia** |
| hiatal hernia | **sliding hiatal hernia**—herniation of the proximal cardia of the stomach through a widened diaphragmatic hiatus |
| S/S of a hiatal hernia | • **nocturnal epigastric distress**—GERD, • *hematemesis,* • *dysphagia/odynophagia,* • *ulceration*—possible Barrett's esophagus, • *stricture formation* |
| Rx of hiatal hernia | • **medical management**— * antacids, * H$_2$ blockers, • *surgery*—if medical management fails |

*Table continued on following page*

Table 7–2. ESOPHAGEAL DISORDERS, UPPER
GASTROINTESTINAL BLEED *Continued*

| Most Common... | Answer and Explanation |
|---|---|
| S/S of a paraesophageal hernia | • **postprandial pain and/or bloating,** • *early satiety,* • *breathlessness with meals,* • *mild dysphagia,* • *air/fluid level in posterior mediastinum on lateral radiographs* [**Note:** paraesophageal hernias are due to a focal defect in the diaphragmatic membrane on the anterolateral side of the esophagus. The greater curvature extends into the chest through the defect.] |
| cause of heartburn | **GERD—** * transient relaxation of the LES for as long as 2 hrs after a meal, * there is a reflux of acid/bile into the distal esophagus |
| pathogenesis of GERD | • **mechanically defective LES—**60%, • *abnormal gastric reservoir—* * increased gastric pressure, * delayed gastric emptying, * increased acid secretion, • *ineffective esophageal clearance of reflux material* |
| predisposing causes of GERD | • **factors lowering LES tone—**e.g., * smoking, * alcohol, * caffeine, * fatty foods, * chocolate, * β-adrenergics, • *sliding hiatal hernia,* • *PUD,* • *pyloric obstruction,* • *pregnancy* |
| S/S of GERD | • **heartburn 30–60 min after eating or after reclining—**initially relieved by antacids, • *dysphagia—*acid injury, • *noncardiac chest pain—*GERD MCC, • *nocturnal cough—*GERD MCC, • *chronic cough,* • *nocturnal asthma—*GERD MCC, • *laryngitis in AM—*acid injury of vocal cords, • *water-brash—* * acid taste in the mouth in AM, * acid injury to tooth enamel |
| complications associated with GERD | • **Barrett's esophagus—**see below, • *increased risk for adenocarcinoma—*see below, • *stricture—*~10%, • *hematemesis,* • *chronic pulmonary infections* |
| lab test to document GERD | **pH electrode left in distal esophagus overnight—** * pH <4 for acid reflux, * pH >7 for alkaline reflux |
| test to document extent/severity of GERD | **endoscopy—** * Bx areas involved: ♦ basal cell hyperplasia with elongation >50% of the thickness of epithelium, ♦ infiltration with eosinophils (key finding), and neutrophils, * R/O Barrett's esophagus |

## Table 7–2. ESOPHAGEAL DISORDERS, UPPER
## GASTROINTESTINAL BLEED *Continued*

| Most Common... | Answer and Explanation |
|---|---|
| test to define whether GERD is causing chest pain | **acid perfusion**— * Bernstein's test, * reproduction of pain indicates GERD |
| Rx of GERD | • **Step 1 Rx**— * raise head of bed, * lose weight, * stop smoking/drinking, * avoid foods/drugs that lower LES tone, * use antacids/alginic acid after meals and at bedtime, • *Step 2 Rx*— * proton blockers: most effective agents, * H$_2$ blockers, • *Step 3 Rx*—Nissen's fundoplication, if there is no response to medical Rx or complications are present |
| cause of Barrett's esophagus | **GERD** |
| diagnostic criteria for Barrett's esophagus | • **glandular metaplasia consisting of columnar cells appearing like gastric cardia/fundic cells**—must be ≥3 cm from gastroesophageal junction, or, • **intestinal metaplasia**—presence of goblet cells/Paneth's cells if distance <3 cm from gastroesophageal junction, • *esophageal ulceration* |
| complications of Barrett's esophagus | • **strictures**—30–50%, • *ulcers*—10–15%, * penetrate metaplastic mucosa, • *glandular dysplasia*—5–10%, • *adenocarcinoma*— * 50–100 × greater risk than general population, * Barrett's esophagus is most responsible for adenocarcinoma and has surpassed SCC as the MC esophageal cancer [**Note:** SCC is still the MCC of cancer in the midesophagus and cause of esophageal cancer world-wide.] |
| Rx of Barrett's esophagus | • **H$_2$ blockers**—prevents progression but does not reverse metaplasia, • *esophagectomy*—for high-grade dysplastic lesions |
| causes of corrosive esophagitis | • **ingestion of strong alkali**—e.g., * ammonia, * lye, • *ingestion of acid*—e.g., * hydrochloric acid, * sulfuric acid [**Note:** ~80% of ingestion of caustic agents occurs in young children. Vomiting should <u>not</u> be induced. Early endoscopy within 24 hrs is important to evaluate the extent of damage.] |

*Table continued on following page*

### Table 7–2. ESOPHAGEAL DISORDERS, UPPER GASTROINTESTINAL BLEED *Continued*

| Most Common... | Answer and Explanation |
|---|---|
| type of necrosis with strong alkali | **liquefactive necrosis**— * penetration more likely than with acid, * increased scar tissue |
| type of necrosis with strong acid | **coagulation necrosis**— * superficial damage, * less scar tissue |
| complications associated with corrosive esophagitis | • **stricture,** • *perforation,* • *esophageal cancer* |
| Rx of corrosive esophagitis | • **endoscopy**—evaluate extent of damage, • *fluids,* • *broad-spectrum antibiotics* |
| presentations of an upper GI bleed | • **hematemesis,** • **melena** [Note: see **Table 7–2** for the differential diagnosis of an upper GI bleed.] |
| COD due to an upper GI bleed | **ruptured esophageal varices** |
| cause of esophageal varices | **portal hypertension (PH)** |
| vessel causing the esophageal varices | **left gastric coronary vein**— * branch of the PV, * normally drains blood from the distal esophagus and proximal stomach to the PV and into the liver sinusoids, * blood flow in the PV in cirrhosis is reversed owing to sinusoidal hypertension |
| causes of PH | **PV obstruction**— * **intrahepatic:** cirrhosis, * hepatic vein: Budd-Chiari syndrome, * PV: PV thrombosis |
| initial steps in the management of an acute upper GI bleed | • **endoscopy**— * most important diagnostic test, * value in Rx of the bleed as well, • *assess/maintain intravascular volume,* • *insert NG tube for gastric aspirate/lavage*— * confirms upper GI source of bleeding, * assesses rate of bleeding * ice water lavage of no proven benefit |
| Rx for acute variceal bleed | **endoscopy with variceal ligation, banding, or sclerotherapy**—inject sodium morrhuate |

## Table 7–2. ESOPHAGEAL DISORDERS, UPPER GASTROINTESTINAL BLEED *Continued*

| Most Common... | Answer and Explanation |
|---|---|
| pharmacologic agents used to control upper GI bleed | • **IV octreotide**— * a somatostatin analogue, * decreases splanchnic blood flow and PV pressure, • *IV vasopressin + nitroglycerin*— nitroglycerin reduces cardiac afterload and coronary artery resistance induced by vasopressin, • *IV H₂ blockers*—? useful in lowering risk for rebleeding in PUD |
| Rx for variceal bleed if endoscopy/drugs are ineffective | • **transjugular intrahepatic portosystemic shunt (TIPS)**— * metal stent connects hepatic vein with PV, * reduces portal pressure, * increases risk for encephalopathy, • *balloon tamponade*—e.g.,   Sengstaken-Blakemore tube, • *caval shunting*— * PV anastomosed to IVC: side-to-side or end-to-side, * distal splenorenal shunt, • β-*blockers/nitrates*— * reduce portal pressure, * prevent rebleeding |
| complications associated with a Sengstaken-Blakemore tube | • **esophageal/gastric erosions,** • *esophageal obstruction*—danger of aspiration |
| causes of Mallory-Weiss syndrome | • **severe retching in alcoholics,** • *vomiting in bulimia nervosa* [**Note:** refers to a mucosal tear in the upper stomach and distal esophagus, causing vomiting of bright red blood.] |
| causes of Boerhaave's syndrome | • **instrument tear during endoscopy**—~**75% of cases,** • *severe vomiting/retching in an alcoholic or patient with bulimia nervosa,* • *foreign body,* • *esophageal cancer,* • *barotrauma* [**Note:** refers to a rupture of the distal esophagus on the left side.] |
| S/S of Boerhaave's syndrome | • **sudden onset of odynophagia,** • *systemic signs*— * fever, * leukocytosis, * tachycardia, * respiratory distress, * shock, • *pneumomediastinum*—air in subcutaneous tissue: Hamman's crunch, • *pleural effusion*—contains food, acid, amylase |
| benign tumor of the esophagus | **leiomyoma**—usually asymptomatic |

*Table continued on following page*

## Table 7-2. ESOPHAGEAL DISORDERS, UPPER GASTROINTESTINAL BLEED *Continued*

| Most Common... | Answer and Explanation |
|---|---|
| malignant tumors of the esophagus | • **adenocarcinoma**—distal esophagus, • *SCC*— * mid to lower esophagus, * MC esophageal cancer outside the United States |
| predisposing cause of esophageal adenocarcinoma | **Barrett's esophagus** [**Note:** adenocarcinoma has replaced SCC as the MC primary esophageal cancer only in recent years.] |
| predisposing causes for squamous cell carcinoma | • **smoking/alcohol**—have a synergistic effect, • *African-American,* • *lye strictures,* • *Plummer-Vinson syndrome,* • *achalasia,* • *Indians chewing betel nuts* [**Note:** there is a 3:1 male/female ratio; common cancer in Northern China and Iran.] |
| S/S of esophageal cancer | • **dysphagia for solids,** • *weight loss,* • *hoarseness*—involves the recurrent laryngeal nerve, • *hypercalcemia*—SCC ectopically produces a PTH-like peptide [**Note:** esophageal cancers spread locally first and then metastasize to the lungs and liver; 5-year survival is <15%.] |

**Question:** Which of the following disorders are predominantly associated with dysphagia for solids and liquids? **SELECT 3**
  (A) Myasthenia gravis
  (B) *Candida* esophagitis
  (C) Barrett's stricture
  (D) Achalasia
  (E) Esophageal carcinoma
  (F) Plummer-Vinson syndrome
  (G) Progressive systemic sclerosis
  (H) GERD

**Answers: (A), (D), (G).** Myasthenia gravis is an autoimmune disease with antibodies directed against acetylcholine receptors in striated muscle (**choice A is correct**). Motility abnormalities occur in the oropharyngeal musculature, leading to dysphagia for solids and liquids. *Candida* esophagitis produces odynophagia but is not associated with a motility disorder or obstruction (**choice B is incorrect**). Barrett's stricture is associated with dysphagia for solids but not liquids (**choice C is incorrect**). Both achalasia and progressive systemic sclerosis lead to dysphagia for solids and liquids owing to the loss of peristalsis in the esophagus (**choices D and G are correct**). Esophageal carcinoma and Plummer-Vinson syndrome produce both obstructive lesions without affecting esophageal motility (**choices E and F are incorrect**). GERD may be associated with strictures; however, it is not associated with dysphagia for liquids (**choice H is incorrect**).

AIDS = acquired immunodeficiency syndrome, ALS = amyotrophic lateral sclerosis, ANA = antinuclear antibody, Bx = biopsy, COD = cause of death; CREST = calcinosis/centromere, Raynaud's phenomenon, esophageal dysfunction, sclerodactyly, telangiectasia; DM = dermatomyositis, GE = gastroesophageal, GERD = gastroesophageal reflux disease, H₂-blocker = histamine blocker, HD = Hodgkin's disease, IVC = inferior vena cava, LES = lower esophageal sphincter, MC = most common, MCC = most common cause, MG = myasthenia gravis, NG = nasogastric, NSAIDs = nonsteroidal anti-inflammatory drugs, PH = portal hypertension, PM = polymyositis, PSS = progressive systemic sclerosis, PTH = parathormone, PUD = peptic ulcer disease, PV = portal vein, R/O = rule out, SCC = squamous cell carcinoma, S/S = signs/symptoms, TE = tracheoesophageal, TIPS = transjugular intrahepatic portosystemic shunt; VATER = vertebral abnormalities, anal abnormalities (imperforate anus), TE fistula, renal disease/radius abnormality; VIP = vasointestinal peptide.

## Table 7–3. NECK MASSES, STOMACH DISORDERS, HEMATEMESIS AND MELENA

| Most Common... | Answer and Explanation |
|---|---|
| site for a palpable neck mass | **thyroid gland**—~50% of all neck masses originate in the thyroid |
| nonthyroid neck masses in descending order | • **neoplastic**—adults > children, • *congenital*—children > adults, • *inflammatory*—children > adults |
| neoplastic neck masses in descending order | • **metastasis**— * usually in patients >50 yrs old, * >90% have a primary site above clavicle, * 10% have unknown primary site, • *primary malignant lymphoma*— * HD/non-HD, * patients <30 or >70 yrs old, • *major salivary gland tumors* |
| inflammatory neck masses | **reactive lymphadenitis**— * tonsillar infections, * scalp infections, * rubella—painful postauricular nodes [**Note:** tuberculous lymphadenitis (scrofula) used to be the MC neck mass in adults.] |
| benign developmental neck masses in children/ young adults | • **thyroglossal duct cyst**—midline, • *branchial cleft cyst*—anterolateral neck, • *cystic hygroma*— * lymphangiocele in infants/children, * association with Turner's syndrome |

*Table continued on following page*

**Table 7–3. NECK MASSES, STOMACH DISORDERS, HEMATEMESIS AND MELENA** *Continued*

| Most Common... | Answer and Explanation |
|---|---|
| malignant neck masses in children | • **malignant lymphoma**—HD and non-HD, • *neuroblastoma,* • *nasopharyngeal carcinoma,* • *malignant melanoma* |
| thyroid cancer metastatic to cervical lymph nodes | **papillary adenocarcinoma**—see **Table 9–2** |
| sites to Bx for SCC in cervical nodes with no obvious primary tumor | • **nasopharynx,** • *piriform sinus,* • *tonsillar fossa* |
| radiographic tests used to evaluate neck masses | • **chest x-ray**—PA and lateral, • *lateral neck views*—for suspected thyroid cancer, • *CT of sinuses, head, neck, larynx,* • *thyroid scan*—if a mass is noted on exam |
| confirmatory tests in the work-up of a neck mass | • **fine needle aspiration,** • *whole node excision*—for malignant lymphoma |
| location for parietal cells | **body of the stomach**—produces HCl and intrinsic factor: absorption of vitamin $B_{12}$ |
| location for gastric G cells | **antrum**—G cells secrete gastrin |
| function of vagus nerve in the stomach | • **increases gastric acid secretion and gastric motility**—the vagus nerve represents the parasympathetic innervation of the stomach and duodenum |
| function of the sympathetic nervous system in the stomach/duodenum | **inhibits secretion and motility**—sympathetic fibers are located in the celiac plexus from T5–T9 |
| digestive chemical reaction in gastroduodenal region | **hydrolysis** |

## Table 7–3. NECK MASSES, STOMACH DISORDERS, HEMATEMESIS AND MELENA *Continued*

| Most Common... | Answer and Explanation |
|---|---|
| sites of CHO digestion | • **mouth**—salivary gland amylase, • **duodenum**— * pancreatic amylase: amylases break polysaccharides down into branch-chained glucose polymers and glucose couplets, * brush border disaccharidases: hydrolyze above sugars into monosaccharides (glucose, fructose, galactose), • **jejunum**— * primary reabsorption site |
| sites of protein digestion | • **stomach**—pepsin hydrolyzes protein into polypeptides, • **duodenum**— * pancreatic endo-/exopeptidases further hydrolyze polypeptides into amino acids, * amino acids are reabsorbed in the small intestine |
| site for fat digestion | **small intestine**— * pancreatic lipases hydrolyze dietary TG into FAs + monoglycerides, * fat-soluble terminal of bile salts dissolve in fat, leaving the water-soluble terminal externally exposed: called micelle, * jejunum/ileum primary reabsorption site: villi reabsorb micelles and TG is resynthesized and packaged into chylomicrons |
| role of vagus nerve in gastric motility | **controls rate of relaxation in proximal stomach and magnitude of contraction in distal stomach**—plays dominant role in rate of gastric emptying |
| hormone-modulating GI muscle activity | **motilin**— * synthesized in duodenum/jejunum, * increases gastric emptying |
| factor reducing gastric motility | **fat entering duodenum** |
| drug-enhancing motilin activity | **erythromycin**—used to stimulate motility in gastroparesis |
| crystalloid solution used to replace gastric losses | **0.9% normal saline with KCl** |
| phases of gastric acid secretion | • **cephalic**—20% of acid output, • **gastric**—70% of acid output, • **intestinal**—10% of acid output |

*Table continued on following page*

### Table 7–3. NECK MASSES, STOMACH DISORDERS, HEMATEMESIS AND MELENA *Continued*

| Most Common... | Answer and Explanation |
|---|---|
| role of vagus nerve in the cephalic phase | • **directly stimulates parietal cells to release HCl,** • **stimulates G cells to release gastrin** |
| mediators involved in gastric phase | • **gastrin**— * antral release by luminal amino acids and gastric distention, * stimulates parietal cell release of acid, • **bombesin**— * gastrin-releasing peptide, * increases gastric/pancreatic secretions, * ? satiety agent, • **CCK** |
| mediators inhibiting gastric acid secretion | • **low gastric pH**—inhibits gastrin, • **somatostatin**— * synthesized in islet D cells, * inhibits gastrin, • **secretin**— * inhibits gastrin, • **VIP**—inhibits gastrin, • **GIP** |
| functions of gastrin | • **acid production,** • **increases antral/duodenal motility,** • **trophic effect on enterochromaffin cells in stomach** |
| functions of somatostatin | • **inhibits majority of GI hormones**—e.g., * insulin, * motilin, * glucagon, * gastrin, • **decreases GI motility,** • **decreases pancreatic exocrine secretion** [**Note:** somatostatin is stimulated by fat/protein in the gastric meal.] |
| functions of secretin | • **increases pancreatic bicarbonate secretion**—acid meal must be alkalinized for enzymes to work efficiently, • **inhibits gastrin** [**Note:** secretin is stimulated by an acid pH in the duodenum.] |
| functions of CCK | • **increases pancreatic secretion of enzymes,** • **stimulates GB contraction/decreases sphincter of Oddi tone,** • **enhances release of most GI hormones** [**Note:** CCK is stimulated by fat/protein in the gastric meal and bombesin.] |
| function of GIP | • **stimulates release and synthesis of insulin,** • **inhibits gastric acid secretion** [**Note:** GIP is stimulated by vagotomy, fatty acids, glucose, and amino acids.] |
| functions of bombesin | • **modulates release of GI hormones**—e.g., * gastrin, * motilin, * CCK, • **increases gastric/pancreatic secretions** [**Note:** the vagus nerve stimulates bombesin release.] |

## Table 7–3. NECK MASSES, STOMACH DISORDERS, HEMATEMESIS AND MELENA *Continued*

| Most Common... | Answer and Explanation |
|---|---|
| functions of VIP | • **increases intestinal/pancreatic secretions,** • **decreases gastrin/somatostatin release** [**Note:** the vagus nerve stimulates VIP release.] |
| S/S of stomach disease | • **N/V**— * nonbilious in pyloric obstruction, * bilious if obstruction is below ampulla, • *epigastric pain*—e.g., PUD, • *hematemesis*— see below, • *melenemesis*—see below, • *melena*—see below, • *early satiety*—e.g., gastroparesis, • *distention*—e.g., pyloric obstruction, • *specific signs of stomach cancer*—see below |
| complications of vomiting | • **electrolyte disorders**—e.g., * hypochloremic metabolic alkalosis, * hypokalemia, * hyponatremia, • *volume depletion,* • *tears*— Mallory-Weiss syndrome, • *rupture*—Boerhaave's syndrome, • *pulmonary aspiration* |
| causes of N/V of undigested food 4–6 hrs after eating | • **gastroparesis**—e.g., DM, • *pyloric obstruction*—e.g., duodenal ulcer |
| causes of hematemesis | • **duodenal ulcer,** • *gastric ulcer,* • *hemorrhagic gastritis,* • *esophageal varices* [**Note:** hematemesis is the vomiting of blood.] |
| causes of melenemesis | • **duodenal ulcer,** • *hemorrhagic gastritis,* • *gastric ulcer* [**Note:** melenemesis is vomiting of "coffee-ground" material.] |
| mechanism of black pigment in vomitus/ stools | **stomach acid**—acid converts Hgb into a black pigment called hematin |
| cause of bloody stools after liver trauma | **hematobilia**—blood in biliary tree |
| cause of melena | **duodenal ulcer**— * ~90% of causes of melena are proximal to the ligament of Treitz (duodenum/jejunum junction), * ~50–100 mL of blood produces melena, * slow bleeds below the ligament of Treitz may produce melena: colonic bacteria convert Hgb to hematin |

*Table continued on following page*

## Table 7–3. NECK MASSES, STOMACH DISORDERS, HEMATEMESIS AND MELENA *Continued*

| Most Common... | Answer and Explanation |
|---|---|
| causes in descending order of an upper GI bleed | • **duodenal ulcer,** • *acute hemorrhagic (erosive) gastritis,* • *gastric ulcer,* • *esophageal varices,* • *esophagitis,* • *Mallory-Weiss tear* |
| genetic cause of a GI bleed leading to chronic iron deficiency | **Osler-Weber-Rendu disease**—AD disease with telangiectasia on the skin, mucous membranes, and GI mucosa |
| causes of iron deficiency due to a GI bleed | • **duodenal ulcer,** • *colorectal cancer*—usually right-sided lesions, • *Meckel's diverticulum*—usually in neonates/children |
| lab test to identify blood in the stool | **Hemoccult slide test**— * the test uses guaiac to detect peroxidase activity in Hgb, * newer tests have antibodies directed against Hgb or detect heme: increases specificity |
| causes of a false-positive Hemoccult slide test | • **myoglobin in meat,** • *nonheme peroxidases in vegetables*—e.g., * horseradish, * cruciferous vegetables |
| pathogenesis of hiccups | • **direct phrenic nerve stimulation**—e.g., diaphragmatic irritation/trauma to phrenic nerve, • *central stimulation of phrenic nerve*—e.g., * **uremia,** * cerebral atherosclerosis |
| cause of hiccups | **aerophagia**—swallowing air when eating |
| gastric causes of hypergastrinemia | • **H$_2$ blockers**—decreased acid has a negative feedback on gastrin release, • *gastric distention,* • *PA,* • *ZE syndrome* |
| cause of an increased BAO and MAO in a gastric analysis | • **duodenal ulcer disease**— * increase in BAO: 5–15 mEq/hr, * increase in MAO: 20–60 mEq/hr, * increase in BAO:MAO ratio: 0.40–0.60:1, owing to an increase in parietal cell mass, • *Zollinger-Ellison syndrome*— * BAO >20 mEq/hr, * MAO >60 mEq/hr, BAO:MAO ratio >0.60:1 [**Note:** a BAO (normal <5 mEq/hr) is collected over a 1-hr period on an empty stomach. The MAO (normal 5–20 mEq/hr) is collected over 1 hour after pentagastrin stimulation. The BAO:MAO ratio is normally 0.20:1.] |

## Table 7–3. NECK MASSES, STOMACH DISORDERS, HEMATEMESIS AND MELENA *Continued*

| Most Common... | Answer and Explanation |
|---|---|
| cause of a normal to decreased BAO and MAO | **gastric ulcers** |
| complications of achlorhydria | • **maldigestion of protein**—acid is necessary to convert pepsinogen into pepsin, • *decreased release of $B_{12}$ from meat,* • *gastric polyps,* • *stomach adenocarcinoma* [**Note:** achlorhydria is a gastric pH that fails to fall below 6 after pentagastrin stimulation.] |
| factors regulating gastric emptying | • **neuroregulated distention of stomach**—activates a vagal reflex arc, • **hormones**—e.g., * gastrin: stimulates emptying, * secretin: inhibits emptying, * GIP: inhibits, * motilin: stimulates, • *gastric meal:* fats inhibit |
| causes of gastroparesis | • **autonomic neuropathy due to DM,** • *muscle disorders*—e.g., PSS, • *infiltrative disorders*—e.g., amyloidosis, • *anorexia nervosa*—gastric dysrhythmias, • *vagotomy,* • *metabolic*—e.g., * hyperglycemia: releases GIP, * hypokalemia, * hypo-/hypercalcemia, • *drugs*—e.g., * tricyclics, * anticholinergics, • *pyloric obstruction*—e.g., chronic duodenal ulcer |
| S/S of gastroparesis | • **early satiety,** • *bloating,* • *N/V*—undigested food, • *weight loss* |
| lab tests to confirm gastroparesis | • **ingest radiolabeled meal and measure transit time for emptying,** • *endoscopy*—R/O gastric obstruction |
| Rx of gastroparesis | • **prokinetic agents**—e.g., * cisapride, * metoclopramide, * erythromycin, • *dietary changes*—e.g., * avoid fatty foods, * high-fiber diet |
| clinical finding in nonulcer dyspepsia | • **persistent ulcer-like symptoms but no radiographic or endoscopic abnormalities**—prevalence ~20%, • *Bx*— * chronic inflammation due to *H. pylori,* * Rx for *H. pylori* does not remove symptoms |
| cause of acute hemorrhagic (erosive) gastritis | • **NSAIDs,** • *CMV*—AIDS patients, • *smoking,* • *alcohol,* • *burns*—Curling's ulcers, • *CNS injury*—Cushing's ulcers, • *uremia* |

*Table continued on following page*

Table 7–3. NECK MASSES, STOMACH DISORDERS,
HEMATEMESIS AND MELENA *Continued*

| Most Common... | Answer and Explanation |
|---|---|
| sign of acute hemorrhagic (erosive) gastritis | **upper GI bleed**—manifested as: ♦ hematemesis, ♦ melenemesis, ♦ melena |
| location for NSAID-induced erosions/ulcers | • **prepyloric area,** • *antrum* [**Note:** erosions/ulcers are dose-dependent.] |
| Rx of NSAID-induced erosions/ulcers | • **reduce NSAID dose,** • *D/C NSAID/replace with acetaminophen,* • *misoprostol*— * synthetic prostaglandin, * expensive, * causes diarrhea [**Note:** $H_2$-blockers and sucralfate are ineffective in preventing NSAID-induced ulcers.] |
| cause of type A body/fundus chronic gastritis | **PA**—autoimmune destruction of parietal cells in the body/fundus |
| antibodies associated with type A chronic gastritis | • **antiparietal antibodies**—90%, • *anti-IF antibodies*— * 50%, * less sensitive but more specific for PA |
| complications associated with type A chronic gastritis | • **chronic atrophic gastritis,** • *achlorhydria,* • *hypergastrinemia,* • *G cell hyperplasia*—potential for a gastric carcinoid, • *gastric polyps,* • *increased adenocarcinoma risk,* • *macrocytic anemia* |
| cause of type B antral chronic gastritis | ***Helicobacter pylori***— * a gram-negative, curved rod, * produces urease and mucolytic proteases, * prevalence of 40–50%, * transmitted by fecal-oral/oral-oral route, * colonizes mucus layer lining the antrum |
| ulcerogenic mechanisms due to *H. pylori* | • **urease converts urea into ammonia**—ammonia destroys the bicarbonate-rich mucus layer leading to gastritis and PUD, • *mucolytic proteases* |
| tests to identify *H. pylori* | • **CLO-test**— * detects urease in a gastric Bx, * 95% sensitivity/specificity, • *serologic tests*— * most cost-effective test, * 95% sensitivity, * 90–95% specificity, * remain positive over time: limits usefulness for follow-up/detection of recurrences, • *radiolabeled urea breath test*— * too expensive, * 95–98% sensitivity/specificity |

### Table 7–3. NECK MASSES, STOMACH DISORDERS, HEMATEMESIS AND MELENA *Continued*

| Most Common... | Answer and Explanation |
|---|---|
| diseases caused by *H. pylori* | • **duodenal ulcer**— * 90–95%, * usually in association with *gastric metaplasia*, • *gastric ulcer—~80%*, • *type B chronic atrophic gastritis*, • *gastric adenocarcinoma*, • *low-grade B cell malignant lymphoma* |
| cause of PUD | *H. pylori*—see above discussion |
| artery responsible for bleeds in gastric/duodenal ulcers | • **gastric ulcer**—left gastric artery, • **duodenal ulcer**—gastroduodenal artery |
| features distinguishing duodenal from gastric ulcers | • **most common PUD**, • **greater *H. pylori* association**, • **greater male to female ratio**, • **greater tendency to bleed/perforate**, • **most often located on the anterior portion of the first part of the duodenum**, • **blood group O association**, • **greater BAO and MAO**, • **MEN I relationship**, • **never malignant**—reason why they are not biopsied, • **more likely to awaken patient late at night** |
| features distinguishing gastric from duodenal ulcers | • **located on lesser curvature of the antrum**—type B chronic atrophic gastritis, • **1–3% chance of representing cancer**—see below, • **pain after eating that is aggravated by food but improved with antacids**, • **BAO and MAO levels normal to decreased**, • **blood group A relationship** |
| reason for Bx of a gastric ulcer | **R/O malignancy**—cannot grossly distinguish a benign from a malignant ulcer |
| aggravating factors for gastric ulcers | • **bile reflux**, • **COPD**, • **renal failure** [Note: smoking decreases chances of ulcer healing but does not cause ulcers.] |
| aggravating factors for duodenal ulcers | • **COPD**, • **renal failure**, • **cirrhosis** |
| complications of PUD | • **bleeding**—duodenal > gastric, • *perforation*—duodenal (anterior wall) > gastric, • *gastric outlet obstruction*— * duodenal > gastric, * aspiration of > 300 mL of fluid is diagnostic, • *pancreatitis*—duodenal (posterior ulcer) > gastric |

*Table continued on following page*

### Table 7–3. NECK MASSES, STOMACH DISORDERS, HEMATEMESIS AND MELENA *Continued*

| Most Common... | Answer and Explanation |
|---|---|
| S/S of perforated PUD | • **sudden onset of epigastric pain,** • *pain radiates to left shoulder*—plain, upright film reveals air under the diaphragm in 85% [**Note:** perforation occurs in 5–10% of duodenal ulcers. Mortality is 5–15%.] |
| Rx of *H. pylori* | **triple therapy with**— * tetracycline or amoxicillin, * metronidazole, * bismuth subsalicylate, * 90% eradication [**Note:** the goal of Rx is to heal the ulcer and eradicate the bacteria. This Rx is prescribed for 2 wks.] |
| medical Rx of PUD | • **Rx *H. pylori***—see above, • *antacids*—documented role in healing duodenal > gastric ulcers, • *H₂-blockers*—e.g., cimetidine/ranitidine are effective in both gastric/duodenal ulcers in reducing acid secretion, pain, and recurrences, • *hydrogen pump inhibitors*—e.g., omeprazole/lansoprazole are the fastest in relieving pain and in healing ulcers: duodenal > gastric, • *coating agents*—e.g., sucralfate: ♦ binds to the ulcer bed, ♦ neutralizes pepsin, ♦ stimulates $PGE_2$ production |
| indications for surgery in PUD | • **persistent bleeding**— * ~20% develop persistent bleeding, * see below, • *perforation*—see below, • *obstruction*— * usually duodenal ulcer, * consider malignancy if gastric ulcer is the cause, • *intractable pain*—consider malignancy if gastric ulcer is the cause |
| poor prognostic indicators of bleeding ulcers | • **advanced age,** • *hypovolemic shock,* • *systolic BP <90 mmHg,* • *hematemesis,* • *hematochezia,* • *RBC transfusion requirement >8–10 units* |
| types of vagotomy | • **truncal vagotomy**— * abolishes cephalic and gastric phases of digestion, * gastric stasis and diarrhea occur, • *highly selective parietal cell vagotomy*—denervates parietal cells in the proximal stomach without affecting antrum and pylorus |
| surgical recommendation for duodenal ulcer with intractable pain | **parietal cell vagotomy** |

## Table 7–3. NECK MASSES, STOMACH DISORDERS, HEMATEMESIS AND MELENA *Continued*

| Most Common... | Answer and Explanation |
|---|---|
| surgery for duodenal ulcer with obstruction | **vagotomy + antrectomy** |
| surgery for duodenal ulcer with bleeding | **suture ligation of bleeding vessel + vagotomy and drainage, or vagotomy and antrectomy** |
| surgery for duodenal ulcer with perforation | • **omental patch**—close perforation, • **ulcer operation**— * truncal vagotomy and drainage, or * superselective parietal cell vagotomy, • **antibiotics** |
| surgery for gastric ulcer | **hemigastrectomy** |
| postgastrectomy syndromes | • **delayed gastric emptying**—early satiety, epigastric pain, • *dumping*—see below, • *alkaline reflux gastritis*—see below, * 5–10% post-Billroth II, • *diarrhea*—see below, • *malabsorption*—see below, • *$B_{12}$ deficiency*—see below, • *iron deficiency*—see below, • *loop syndromes*—see below, • *recurrent marginal ulcer*—see below, • *Roux-en-Y syndrome*—see below |
| surgery causing the dumping syndrome | **Billroth II gastrojejunostomy**—occurs in 5–10% of patients |
| S/S of early dumping syndrome | **10–30 min after eating**— * diarrhea, * vasomotor symptoms: ♦ weakness, ♦ dizziness, ♦ flushing, ♦ palpitations |
| mechanism for early dumping | **rapid exit of a hyperosmolar meal into the small intestine with release of vasoactive hormones** |
| S/S of late dumping | **2–4 hrs after eating, only vasomotor symptoms**—hypoglycemia is due to increased glucose reabsorption and excessive release of insulin |
| S/S of alkaline reflux gastritis | • **epigastric pain unrelieved by antacids**—due to reflux of intestinal bile acids postresection or bypass of pylorus: e.g., Billroth type II, • **vomiting of bilious material** |

*Table continued on following page*

Table 7–3. NECK MASSES, STOMACH DISORDERS,
HEMATEMESIS AND MELENA *Continued*

| Most Common... | Answer and Explanation |
|---|---|
| Rx of alkaline gastritis | • **bile acid-binding drugs,** • *surgery*— * ensure complete vagotomy, * Roux-en-Y gastrojejunostomy |
| causes of postvagotomy diarrhea | • **bile salt deconjugation,** • **altered gastric emptying/motility,** • **dumping**—see above [**Note:** diarrhea occurs in 20% of truncal vagotomies and 4% of highly selective vagotomies.] |
| Rx of postvagotomy diarrhea | • **drugs**— * bile acid binders, * anticholinergics, • *reduce fluid intake* |
| causes of postgastrectomy malabsorption | • **bacterial overgrowth in jejunum,** • **decreased absorption time,** • **poor mixing of fats with bile salts** |
| causes of $B_{12}$ deficiency postgastrectomy | • **bacterial destruction of $B_{12}$/IF,** • **insufficient acid to break down food to release $B_{12}$** |
| causes of iron deficiency postgastrectomy | • **decreased absorption in Billroth II**— bypasses duodenum, • **achlorhydria**— acid is necessary to break down food to release iron [**Note:** iron deficiency occurs in 30% of patients 5 yrs postgastrectomy.] |
| causes of afferent loop syndrome | • **narrowing of junction of stomach with the duodenal side of a Billroth II,** • *kinking of duodenum* [**Note:** the afferent limb is the duodenum in a Billroth II procedure.] |
| S/S of afferent loop syndrome | • **postprandial epigastric fullness,** • *fullness with vomiting of bilious fluid without food,* * bilious vomiting occurs with partial obstruction, * nonbilious vomiting occurs if obstruction is complete |
| causes of efferent loop syndrome | **obstruction of jejunum** |
| S/S of efferent loop syndrome | • **postprandial epigastric fullness/pain,** • *pain relieved by vomiting of bilious material and food* |

### Table 7–3. NECK MASSES, STOMACH DISORDERS, HEMATEMESIS AND MELENA Continued

| Most Common... | Answer and Explanation |
|---|---|
| cause of marginal ulcers postgastrectomy | **incomplete vagotomy**—ulcer located at the junction of the anastomosis on the intestinal side: e.g., duodenum in type I Billroth, jejunum in type II Billroth |
| Rx of marginal ulcers | **same Rx as for duodenal ulcers** |
| indications for a Roux-en-Y procedure | • **intractable vomiting of bile**—complication of previous type I/II Billroth, • *surgical Rx of obesity,* • *bypassing stomach because of obstruction* [**Note:** a gastric remnant empties into an isolated segment of jejunum that is proximally closed with sutures. The distal stomach with attached duodenum is anastomosed to a more distal segment of jejunum. The distal stomach is no longer in the food pathway. The procedure delays gastric emptying, leading to an increase in ulcer formation.] |
| S/S of Roux-en-Y syndrome | **postprandial epigastric pain/vomiting**—due to delayed gastric emptying from jejunal atony |
| Rx of Roux-en-Y syndrome | • **drugs**—promotility agents, • *surgery*—near-total gastrectomy with the gastric remnant anastomosed to a 40-cm Roux limb |
| cause of ZE syndrome | **pancreatic islet cell tumor secreting excessive gastrin**— * 60–70% are malignant, * 85% are located in the pancreas and 15% in the duodenum, * >50% have liver metastasis when discovered |
| S/S of ZE syndrome | • **pentad of**— * epigastric pain, * weight loss, * peptic ulceration: most are solitary duodenal ulcers rather than multiple ulcers, * acid hypersecretion, * diarrhea, • *MEN I association*—20–30% |
| screening tests for ZE syndrome | • **BAO > 20 mEq/hr, MAO > 60 mEq/hr, BAO:MAO ratio > 0.60,** • *serum gastrin > 1000 pg/mL in a patient with PUD is diagnostic* |

*Table continued on following page*

**Table 7–3. NECK MASSES, STOMACH DISORDERS, HEMATEMESIS AND MELENA** *Continued*

| Most Common... | Answer and Explanation |
|---|---|
| confirmatory test for ZE syndrome | **IV secretin test**—paradoxical increase (>200 pg/mL) in an already high serum gastrin level |
| method of localizing gastrinomas | • US/CT, • *scintiscanning after injection of indium-DTPA-octreotide,* • *secretin angiography* |
| Rx of ZE syndrome | • **surgical removal**— * ~20–25% can be completely removed, * total gastrectomy is rarely indicated, • *parietal cell vagotomy,* • *high doses of H₂-blockers or proton blockers*—most effective medical Rx, • *chemotherapy for metastatic disease*— * streptozocin, * 5-fluorouracil |
| gastric cause of protein loss | **Ménétrier's disease (hypertrophic gastropathy)**— * adult type is due to overexpression of transforming growth factor-α, * childhood form is due to CMV, * characterized by giant rugal folds, * glands secrete an excessive amount of protein-rich mucus |
| clinical findings of hypertrophic gastropathy | • **peripheral pitting edema,** • *more common in men than women,* • *postprandial pain relieved by antacids,* • *precancerous* |
| gastric polyps | • **hyperplastic polyp**— * hamartomas, * no malignant potential, • *adenomatous polyp*— * neoplastic, * usually sessile, * potential for malignant transformation if > 2 cm, * >30% have foci of invasive cancer, • *Peutz-Jeghers polyp*— * AD disorder, * hamartomas, * rarely malignant |
| benign soft tissue tumor | **leiomyoma**— * stomach is the MC location for leiomyomas, * may ulcerate or bleed, * no malignant potential |
| malignancy | • **intestinal type of adenocarcinoma**— * *H. pylori* relationship, * decreasing incidence, • *diffuse type*— * not *H. pylori*-related, * "linitis plastica" or "leather bottle stomach": increasing incidence [**Note:** advanced cancers are usually polypoid or ulcerating and are less commonly diffuse.] |

## Table 7–3. NECK MASSES, STOMACH DISORDERS, HEMATEMESIS AND MELENA Continued

| Most Common... | Answer and Explanation |
|---|---|
| causes of gastric adenocarcinoma | • **H. pylori chronic atrophic gastritis,** • *adenomatous polyps,* • *nitrosamines,* • *diets lacking vitamin C,* • *smoked/pickled foods,* • *blood group A,* • *PA*—chronic atrophic gastritis of body/fundus, • *smoking,* • *alcohol,* • *Ménétrier's disease,* • *previous gastric surgery,* • *hereditary nonpolyposis colorectal cancer syndrome* [**Note:** Japan has the highest mortality due to gastric cancer. Incidence decreases when Japanese emigrate to the United States and Canada.] |
| locations of gastric adenocarcinoma | • **lesser curvature of pyloroantrum**— * 50%, * same site as gastric ulcers, • *cardia*— * 25%, * rapidly increasing at this site, • *body/fundus*—25% |
| S/S of gastric cancer | • **weight loss,** • *epigastric pain,* • *early satiety,* • *vomiting,* • *epigastric mass*—30% |
| specific signs of stomach cancer | • **Virchow's node**—left supraclavicular node metastasis, • *Irish's node*—left axillary node metastasis, • *Sister Mary Joseph sign*— metastasis to umbilicus, • *acanthosis nigricans*—pigmented skin lesion, • *Leser-Trelat sign*—outcroppings of seborrheic keratosis, • *bilaterally enlarged ovaries*— Krukenberg's tumors |
| sites of metastasis of gastric cancer | • **regional lymph nodes,** • *liver,* • *lung,* • *ovaries*—Krukenberg's tumor: bilateral |
| Rx of gastric adenocarcinoma | • **surgery**—total gastrectomy with Billroth II if confined to the stomach and regional lymph nodes, • *chemotherapy*—not generally useful, • *postoperative radiation*—may decrease local recurrence, • *prognosis*— * 19% overall 5-yr survival, * best survival with early gastric cancer: lesion confined to mucosa/submucosa |
| extranodal site for malignant lymphoma | **stomach**— * usually low-grade B cell lymphomas are *H. pylori*–related: MALToma (**mu**cosa-**a**ssociated **l**ymphoid **t**issue), * high-grade lymphomas are usually B cell immunoblastic lymphomas, * secondary involvement of stomach occurs in 20% of those with non-HD lymphomas |

*Table continued on following page*

### Table 7–3. NECK MASSES, STOMACH DISORDERS, HEMATEMESIS AND MELENA *Continued*

| Most Common... | Answer and Explanation |
|---|---|
| Rx for gastric lymphoma | • **surgery**—if localized, • *adjuvant radiotherapy*—for residual disease, • *adjuvant chemotherapy*—for cases with a high probability of recurrence, • *prognosis*—50–60% overall 5-yr survival |

**Question:** Which of the following characterizes a gastric rather than a duodenal ulcer? **SELECT 4**
- (A) MEN I relationship
- (B) Hematemesis
- (C) Greater association with *H. pylori*
- (D) Greater association with ZE syndrome
- (E) Pain aggravated by eating
- (F) Blood group A relationship
- (G) Greater malignant potential
- (H) Greater association with NSAIDs
- (I) Perforation

**Answers:** (E), (F), (G), (H). Duodenal ulcers are more likely to have a MEN I relationship, a greater association with *H. pylori*, a greater association with ZE syndrome, and a greater chance for perforation (choices A, C, D, and I are incorrect). Both gastric and duodenal ulcers are associated with hematemesis (choice B is incorrect). Gastric ulcers are more likely to be aggravated by food, have a blood group A relationship, be malignant, and be associated with NSAID-induced ulcers (choices E, F, G, H are correct).

AD = autosomal dominant, BAO = basal acid output, BP = blood pressure, Bx = biopsy, CCK = cholecystokinin, CHO = carbohydrate, CMV = cytomegalovirus, CNS = central nervous system, COPD = chronic obstructive pulmonary disease, D/C = discontinue, DM = diabetes mellitus, FAs = fatty acids, GB = gallbladder, GIP = gastric inhibitory peptide, H₂-blocker = histamine blocker, HD = Hodgkin's disease, Hgb = hemoglobin, IF = intrinsic factor, MAO = maximal acid output, MC = most common, MEN = multiple endocrine neoplasia, NSAIDs = nonsteroidal anti-inflammatory drugs, N/V = nausea/vomiting, PA = pernicious anemia, PSS = progressive systemic sclerosis, PUD = peptic ulcer disease, SCC = squamous cell carcinoma, S/S = signs/symptoms, TG = triglyceride, VIP = vasointestinal peptide, ZE = Zollinger-Ellison.

## Table 7–4. ABDOMINAL PAIN AND MISCELLANEOUS BOWEL SIGNS/SYMPTOMS

| Most Common... | Answer and Explanation |
|---|---|
| order to follow in evaluating the abdomen | • **inspection,** • *auscultation,* • *percussion,* • *palpation* [**Note:** location, mode of onset, progression, and character of pain are also important.] |
| causes of pain in hollow viscera | • **stretch or distention,** • *inflammation,* • *ischemia,* • *forceful contractions* |
| causes of pain in solid viscera | • **stretching of the capsule,** • **capsule inflammation**—e.g., hepatomegaly |
| types of pain | • **visceral,** • *parietal*—somatic, • *referred* |
| nerve fibers responsible for visceral pain | **unmyelinated afferent C fibers**—dull pain slow in onset |
| characteristics of visceral afferent fibers | • **stimuli**— * distention, * inflammation, * traction of bowel, • **insidious onset,** • **"crampy,"** • **localizes to midline closest to viscera** |
| structures referring visceral pain to the epigastrium | • **stomach,** • **duodenum,** • **liver,** • **GB** |
| structures referring visceral pain to the umbilical area | • **appendix,** • **jejunum/ileum,** • **cecum,** • **right colon** |
| structures referring visceral pain to the hypogastric/ suprapubic area | • **colon,** • **internal reproductive organs** |
| S/S of visceral pain | • **vomiting/crampy pain**— * pain/vomiting due to sudden stretch of viscera, * vomiting does not relieve pain, * vomiting is not accompanied by nausea, • *colicky pain*—sign of mechanical obstruction of a viscus with peristalsis, • *small bowel pain*— * corresponds to periodic contractions against resistance, * pain of peristaltic contractions coincides with bowel sounds, • *colon pain*— visceral pain occurs late in colonic obstruction due to lack of peristalsis in the colon, • *pain precedes systemic signs*—e.g., pain is followed by fever, leukocytosis, anorexia, • *absence of peritoneal signs*—e.g., absence of rebound tenderness |

*Table continued on following page*

Table 7–4. ABDOMINAL PAIN AND MISCELLANEOUS
BOWEL SIGNS/SYMPTOMS *Continued*

| Most Common... | Answer and Explanation |
|---|---|
| nerve fibers responsible for parietal (somatic) pain | **C fibers and myelinated Aδ fibers** |
| characteristics of parietal afferent fibers | • **stimuli**— * sudden pressure: surgical incision, * temperature or pH changes, * inflammation, • **acute onset**, • **sharp, constant pain**, • **refers to the exact location of peritoneal irritation** |
| secretions causing parietal pain | • **blood**—e.g., * ectopic pregnancy, * mittelschmerz, • *pus,* • *bile,* • *pancreatic secretions,* • *cyst fluid*—e.g., ruptured follicular cyst |
| S/S of parietal pain | • **rebound tenderness,** • *pain with coughing or movement,* • *guarding or rigidity*—involuntary contraction of abdominal muscles indicates peritonitis, • *ileus*—absent bowel sounds due to reflex intestinal inhibition of peristalsis, • *patient avoids movement* |
| sequence of pain/N/V in a surgical abdomen | **pain occurs first and is then followed by N/V**—N/V followed by pain is a nonsurgical abdomen: e.g., gastritis |
| causes of acute RUQ pain | • **acute cholecystitis,** • *cholelithiasis,* • *acute hepatitis,* • *right ureteral colic*—radiates to the ipsilateral groin, • *right-sided pleurisy*— * pneumonia, * PE, • *right-sided pyelonephritis*—urinary signs are present, • *subphrenic abscess* |
| cause of Murphy's sign | **acute cholecystitis**—RUQ palpation causes inspiratory arrest secondary to pain |
| findings in Charcot's triad | • **RUQ pain,** • **fever,** • **jaundice** |
| disorder associated with Charcot's triad | **acute cholangitis** |
| causes of acute LUQ pain | • **gastroenteritis,** • *IBS,* • *splenic infarction*—friction rub/pleural effusion are usually present, • *acute pancreatitis,* • *left ureteral colic*—radiates into the left groin, • *left pyelonephritis* |

**Table 7–4. ABDOMINAL PAIN AND MISCELLANEOUS
BOWEL SIGNS/SYMPTOMS** *Continued*

| Most Common... | Answer and Explanation |
|---|---|
| cause of Kehr's sign | **splenic rupture/infarction**—Kehr's sign is radiation of pain to the left shoulder from diaphragm irritation |
| causes of acute RLQ pain | • **acute appendicitis with perforation,** • *Meckel's diverticulitis*—simulates appendicitis in young children, • *typhlitis*—cecal inflammation, • *CD*—ileitis, • *perforated duodenal ulcer*—gastric contents settle in RLQ |
| route of pain migration in acute appendicitis | • **initially, periumbilical**— * due to irritation of C fibers, * inflamed/distended appendix, • **McBurney's point in RLQ**— * due to irritation of Aδ fibers, * localized peritonitis |
| cause of acute LLQ pain | **colonic diverticulitis**—"left-sided" appendicitis |
| mechanism of referred pain at a distant site from its source | **distant site shares similar neuronal pathways as the involved organ** |
| cause of referred pain to the right shoulder/scapular area | **acute cholecystitis**—GB receives a small afferent branch from the right phrenic nerve (C3–5) |
| cause of referred pain to the left shoulder | **perforated anterior duodenal ulcer**—pain is due to air under the diaphragm, with irritation of the phrenic nerve |
| cause of referred pain into the back or flank | **acute pancreatitis**—retroperitoneal structures refer pain into the back |
| cause of referred pain into the ipsilateral groin | **ureteral colic**—usually due to a ureteral stone |
| mechanism of colicky pain | **obstruction of a viscus that has peristalsis**—e.g., * colicky pain is pain followed by a pain-free interval: intervals vary from a few minutes to hours, e.g., * obstruction due to small bowel adhesions |

*Table continued on following page*

Table 7–4. ABDOMINAL PAIN AND MISCELLANEOUS
BOWEL SIGNS/SYMPTOMS *Continued*

| Most Common... | Answer and Explanation |
|---|---|
| causes of explosive (immediate) onset of abdominal pain | • **perforated peptic ulcer,** • *biliary "colic,"* • *ureteral colic,* • *ruptured aortic aneurysm,* • *dissecting aortic aneurysm,* • *bowel strangulation* [**Note:** biliary "colic" is a misnomer. The pain is usually constant or crampy owing to the weak contractile qualities of smooth muscle in the bile ducts.] |
| causes of rapid onset (few minutes) of severe, steady abdominal pain | • **acute pancreatitis**— * described as: ♦ "knifelike," ♦ "stabbing," ♦ "breath-taking," * radiates into the back, • *mesenteric thrombosis*—pain is out of proportion to the physical findings, • *strangulated bowel*—e.g., volvulus, • *ruptured ectopic pregnancy* |
| causes of gradual onset (over a few hours) of steady pain | • **acute appendicitis,** • *acute diverticulitis,* • *acute cholecystitis,* • *acute hepatitis,* • *acute salpingitis* [**Note:** infection is more likely to present with a gradual onset of pain.] |
| causes of intermittent colicky pain (over a few hours) | • **mechanical small bowel obstruction,** • *CD,* • *early phase of acute appendicitis*—colicky pain at first but becomes constant when localized peritonitis occurs |
| causes of early postprandial pain | • **gastric ulcer,** • *acute gastritis* |
| cause of pain at night with recumbency | • **GERD,** • *duodenal ulcer*—usually occurs around midnight to 1 AM |
| disorder in which pain is relieved following the ingestion of food | **duodenal ulcer** |
| disorder associated with late (several hours after eating) postprandial pain | **gastric outlet obstruction** |
| cause of steady, midepigastric or RUQ pain that begins in the evening | **biliary colic** |

### Table 7–4. ABDOMINAL PAIN AND MISCELLANEOUS BOWEL SIGNS/SYMPTOMS *Continued*

| Most Common... | Answer and Explanation |
|---|---|
| cause of bile-stained vomitus | **proximal small bowel obstruction** |
| cause of feculent material in vomitus | **proximal small bowel obstruction** |
| signs of a perforated viscus | • **scaphoid abdomen**, • **tense abdomen**, • **diminished bowel sounds**—late finding, • **loss of liver dullness**, • **guarding or rigidity** |
| signs of peritonitis | • **patient lies motionless**, • **absent bowel sounds**—late finding, • **rebound tenderness**, • **pain with coughing**, • **guarding or rigidity** |
| signs of intestinal obstruction | • **abdominal distention**, • *hyperperistalsis*—early finding, • *visible peristalsis*—late finding, • *diffuse pain without rebound tenderness*, • *absent bowel sounds*—late finding, • *history of previous abdominal surgery* [**Note:** colicky pain and obstipation (constipation + inability to pass gas) are common symptoms.] |
| signs of paralytic ileus | • **abdominal distention**, • *minimal bowel sounds*, • *no localized tenderness* |
| signs of ischemic or strangulated bowel | • **severe pain out of proportion to physical findings**, • *variable bowel sounds*, • *bloody diarrhea*, • *abdominal distention*—late finding |
| signs of acute cholecystitis | • **epigastric pain 15–30 min after eating**, • *vomiting does not relieve pain*, • *Murphy's sign*—see above, • *GB may be palpable*, • *right shoulder/scapula referred pain* |
| time-frame for abdominal pain in PID | **early in menstrual cycle** |
| time-frame for mittelschmerz | **midcycle**—due to rupture of the follicle at midcycle and peritoneal irritation from blood |
| cause of chronic pain throughout menses | **endometriosis**—implants of endometrial mucosa bleed during menses |
| cause of multiple quadrant abdominal pain | **generalized peritonitis** |

*Table continued on following page*

Table 7–4. ABDOMINAL PAIN AND MISCELLANEOUS
BOWEL SIGNS/SYMPTOMS *Continued*

| Most Common... | Answer and Explanation |
|---|---|
| cause of acute abdominal pain + history of chronic diarrhea | **IBD** |
| S/S of duodenal disease | • **pain**—e.g., duodenal ulcer, • *N/V*—e.g., obstruction, • *hematemesis*—e.g., duodenal ulcer, • *diarrhea*—malabsorption from: ♦ bacterial overgrowth, ♦ celiac disease, • *afferent loop syndrome*—vomiting of bilious material without food in a patient with a Billroth II procedure, • *sentinel loop*—localized ileus due to acute pancreatitis |
| S/S of jejunal/ileal disease | • **diarrhea**—e.g., gastroenteritis, • *flushing and diarrhea*—carcinoid syndrome, • *pain with distention*—e.g., * obstruction, * intussusception, • *megaloblastic anemia*—e.g., folate/$B_{12}$ deficiency from malabsorption, • *pain simulating acute appendicitis*—e.g., Meckel's diverticulitis in child, • *bloody diarrhea*—e.g., infarction, • *iron deficiency*—bleeding Meckel's diverticulum in neonate/child |
| S/S of colon disease | • **diarrhea**—e.g., infection, • *constipation*—e.g., low-fiber diet, • *pain*—e.g., ischemic colitis/ulcerative colitis, • *distention*—e.g., * obstruction, * infarction, • *anemia*—e.g., iron deficiency: colorectal cancer, • *bloody diarrhea*—e.g., * ischemic colitis, * UC, • *hematochezia*—bright red blood in stool: ♦ diverticulosis, • angiodysplasia, • *mass*—e.g., cancer, • *ileus*—e.g., obstruction: late sign, • *hyperperistalsis*—e.g., early obstruction, • *rebound tenderness*—e.g., peritonitis, • *weight loss*—cancer, • *nephrotic syndrome*—membranous GN in colorectal cancer |
| S/S of anorectal disease | • **bleeding**—e.g., internal hemorrhoids: painless, • *pain*—e.g., anal fissure, • *tenesmus*—* pain with urge to defecate, e.g., * UC, • *pruritus*—e.g., pinworm, • *ulceration*—e.g., STDs, • *mass*—e.g., anal carcinoma, • *anal fistula*—e.g., CD, • *hematochezia*—e.g., rectal cancer |

**Table 7–4. ABDOMINAL PAIN AND MISCELLANEOUS BOWEL SIGNS/SYMPTOMS** *Continued*

| Most Common... | Answer and Explanation |
|---|---|
| S/S of functional GI disease | • **absence of fever/weight loss,** • *alternating diarrhea/constipation*—e.g., IBS, • *daytime diarrhea*— * nocturnal: neoplastic, * day/night: organic cause, • *normal Hgb/Hct,* • *negative stool guaiac* |
| mechanisms of constipation | • **low-fiber diet,** • *colon motility disorder,* • *anorectal dysfunction* [**Note:** constipation is defecation <3 times/wk.] |
| life-long cause of constipation | **Hirschsprung's disease**—see **Table 7–4** |
| pathologic cause of constipation of recent onset | **obstructive lesion**—e.g., * colon cancer, * ischemic stricture |
| causes of disturbed colonic motility leading to constipation | • **drugs**—e.g., * opiates, * anticholinergics, * aluminum antacids, • *IBS,* • *pregnancy*—progesterone effect, • *metabolic conditions*—e.g., * hypokalemia, * hypercalcemia, * hypothyroidism, * DM, * pheochromocytoma: increased sympathetic stimulation decreases colonic motility, • *Hirschsprung's disease*—destruction of myenteric plexus, • *systemic disease*—e.g., PSS |
| Rx of constipation | • **increasing fiber,** • *osmotic laxatives*—e.g., * magnesium hydroxide, * lactulose, • *emollient laxatives*— * penetrate stool, e.g., * docusate, • *stimulant laxatives*—increase peristalsis: ◆ cascara, ◆ senna [**Note:** always Rx the underlying disease.] |
| cause of obstipation | **complete bowel obstruction**— * obstipation is the absence of stooling and flatus, * obstruction produces both constipation and obstipation |
| causes of hyperperistalsis | • **diarrhea,** • *early obstruction* [**Note:** hyperperistalsis refers to increased bowel sounds.] |
| cause of adynamic ileus | **intestinal obstruction due to inhibition of bowel motility**—e.g., peritonitis [**Note:** ileus refers to absent bowel sounds.] |

*Table continued on following page*

Table 7–4. ABDOMINAL PAIN AND MISCELLANEOUS
BOWEL SIGNS/SYMPTOMS *Continued*

| Most Common... | Answer and Explanation |
|---|---|
| cause of dynamic ileus | **mechanical intestinal obstruction**—e.g., postsurgical adhesions leading to absent bowel sounds |
| causes of tenesmus | • **IBS,** • **UC,** • *solitary rectal ulcer syndrome* [**Note:** tenesmus is an unproductive, often painful urge to defecate. It suggests a problem in the anal sphincter.] |
| cause of Rovsing's sign | **acute appendicitis**—palpation of LLQ results in pain in RLQ from tension on the inflamed peritoneum |
| cause of psoas sign | **acute appendicitis**—pain in RLQ on extension of right thigh |
| cause of obturator sign | **acute appendicitis**—RLQ pain on internal rotation of right thigh |
| cause of Blumberg's sign | **acute appendicitis**—rebound tenderness in RLQ |
| cause of Dance's sign | **intussusception of terminal ileum into cecum**—oblong mass palpated in epigastrium |
| cause of abdominal asymmetry in a child with hypertension | **Wilms' tumor of the kidney** |
| cause of a pulsatile mass in the abdomen | **abdominal aortic aneurysm** |
| calcified abdominal masses | • **abdominal aortic aneurysm,** • *chronic pancreatitis,* • *gallstones,* • *urinary tract stones,* • *GB*—called "porcelain GB," • *spleen*—calcified granulomas in histoplasmosis, • *liver*—echinococcal cysts, • *adrenal gland*—neuroblastoma, • *ovary*— * **cystic teratoma,** * gonadoblastoma, * ovarian fibroma |
| cause of hematuria, flank pain, flank mass in an adult | **renal adenocarcinoma** |
| cause of a palpable GB in an adult with painless jaundice | **carcinoma of head of pancreas**—a palpable GB in this setting is called Courvoisier's sign |

## Table 7–4. ABDOMINAL PAIN AND MISCELLANEOUS
## BOWEL SIGNS/SYMPTOMS *Continued*

| Most Common... | Answer and Explanation |
|---|---|
| cause of a palpable cystic mass in pancreatitis | **pancreatic pseudocyst** |
| cause of a palpable abdominal mass in a neonate or child | **hydronephrosis**—secondary to cystic disease of the kidney |
| palpable intra-abdominal adrenal tumor in young children | **neuroblastoma** |
| pelvic mass in women > 30 yrs old | **leiomyoma of uterus** |
| hematologic causes of splenomegaly | • **infectious mononucleosis,** • **MPD**—e.g., * PRV, * AMM, • **leukemia**—all types of acute and chronic leukemia, • **congenital spherocytosis,** • **AIHA**—common in SLE, • **metastasis malignant lymphoma** |
| cause of splenomegaly in cirrhosis | **portal hypertension**—produces congestive splenomegaly |
| adult lysosomal disease associated with splenomegaly | **Gaucher's disease** |
| initial diagnostic test for abdominal masses | **abdominal and pelvic CT scan** |
| use of US in abdominal masses | • **GB disease**— * stones, * hydrops, • *pelvic masses*— * solid vs. cystic mass, * Dx follicular cyst, * Dx ectopic pregnancy, * Dx appendicitis, * follow natural history of a pancreatic pseudocyst |
| cause of anterior displacement of ureters in an IVP | **retroperitoneal mass** |

*Table continued on following page*

## Table 7–4. ABDOMINAL PAIN AND MISCELLANEOUS BOWEL SIGNS/SYMPTOMS *Continued*

| Most Common... | Answer and Explanation |
| --- | --- |
| role of angiography in evaluating abdominal masses | • identify organ of origin of mass, • identify visceral artery aneurysms—e.g., splenic artery aneurysm, • **vascular vs. avascular masses**— * vascular masses imply malignancy, * avascular masses may be cystic, • **planning operative approach of a mass lesion** |

**Question:** Which of the following abdominal disorders are associated with referred pain? **SELECT 4**

(A) Diverticulitis
(B) Acute pancreatitis
(C) Acute hepatitis
(D) Acute cholecystitis
(E) Ureteral stone
(F) Gastric ulcer
(G) Perforated duodenal ulcer

**Answers: (B), (D), (E), (G).** Diverticulitis, acute hepatitis, and gastric ulcers have localized pain in the LLQ, RUQ-epigastrium, and epigastrium, respectively **(choices A, C, F are incorrect)**. Acute pancreatitis refers pain into the back **(choice B is correct)**. Acute cholecystitis refers pain into the right shoulder/scapula region **(choice D is correct)**. A ureteral stone refers pain to the ipsilateral groin **(choice E is correct)**. A perforated duodenal ulcer refers pain to the left shoulder owing to air under the diaphragm **(choice G is correct)**.

AIHA = autoimmune hemolytic anemia, AMM = agnogenic myeloid metaplasia, CD = Crohn's disease, DM = diabetes mellitus, GB = gallbladder, GERD = gastroesophageal reflux disease, GN = glomerulonephritis, Hgb/Hct = hemoglobin/hematocrit, IBD = inflammatory bowel disease, IBS = irritable bowel syndrome, IVP = intravenous pyelogram, LLQ = left lower quadrant, LUQ = left upper quadrant, MPD = myeloproliferative disease, N/V = nausea/vomiting, PE = pulmonary embolus, PID = pelvic inflammatory disease, PRV = polycythemia rubra vera, PSS = progressive systemic sclerosis, RLQ = right lower quadrant, RUQ = right upper quadrant, SLE = systemic lupus erythematosus, S/S = signs and symptoms, STDs = sexually transmitted diseases, UC = ulcerative colitis, US = ultrasound.

## Table 7–5. DIARRHEA AND INFECTIOUS DISEASE OF SMALL AND LARGE BOWEL

| Most Common... | Answer and Explanation |
|---|---|
| sites for nutrient absorption | • **duodenum**— * iron, * calcium, * water-soluble vitamins, * monosaccharides, • **jejunum**— * folate, * FAs, * AAs, * monosaccharides, * water-soluble vitamins, • **ileum**— * $B_{12}$, * conjugated bile acids, * fat-soluble vitamins, * monosaccharides, * FAs, * AAs [**Note:** the proximal small bowel is unable to reabsorb conjugated bile acids and $B_{12}$. The terminal ileum can adapt to absorbing all nutrients.] |
| site for water reabsorption | **small bowel** |
| functions of large bowel | **produces mucin and forms stool** |
| definition of diarrhea | **>250 g stool per day** |
| time distinction between acute and chronic diarrhea | • **acute diarrhea <3 wks**— * generally due to microbial pathogens, * subdivided into noninflammatory and inflammatory types, • **chronic diarrhea >4 wks** |
| mechanisms of infectious diarrhea | • **toxigenic**—toxin-induced stimulation of cAMP, • **invasive**—mucosal penetration |
| cause of acute infectious diarrhea | **viral gastroenteritis**—e.g., * Norwalk: adult, * rotavirus: child |
| tests used to evaluate infectious diarrheas | • **fecal smear for leukocytes**—presence of leukocytes indicates an invasive diarrhea: e.g., shigellosis versus an osmotic or secretory type of diarrhea, • *stool cultures,* • *stools for O/P,* • *stool guaiac*— * blood + leukocytes indicate invasive bacteria, * exceptions: ♦ UC, ♦ ischemic colitis, • *toxin assay of stool*—R/O pseudomembranous colitis due to *Clostridium difficile,* • *proctosigmoidoscopy*—R/O: ♦ pseudomembranous colitis, ♦ UC, ♦ cancer |
| causes of acute bloody diarrhea | • **invasive diarrhea**—the term *dysentery* is applied to infectious diarrheas with blood and leukocytes, • *ischemic colitis,* • *IBD* |

*Table continued on following page*

Table 7–5. **DIARRHEA AND INFECTIOUS DISEASE OF SMALL AND LARGE BOWEL** *Continued*

| Most Common... | Answer and Explanation |
|---|---|
| cause of food poisoning in the United States | *Salmonella enteritidis*—see below |
| types of food poisoning due to ingestion of preformed toxins | • **Staphylococcus aureus,** • *Bacillus cereus*—gram-positive rods • *adult Clostridium botulinum* |
| clinical findings associated with enterotoxigenic *E. coli* (traveler's diarrhea) | • toxin present in water and salads, • toxin activates c-AMP in the small intestinal cells, • secretory-type diarrhea—see below, • incubation 24–72 hrs, • +/− fever, • usually self-limited in 24–36 hrs, • Rx with TMP/SMX or quinolones if severe |
| clinical findings associated with *Clostridium difficile* | • fever, crampy abdominal pain, watery diarrhea with mucus and blood 1–6 weeks postantibiotics— * ampicillin is the MC offending drug, * vancomycin does not cause pseudomembranous colitis but resistant strains of *C. difficile* are occurring with its use, • gold standard test is a toxin assay of stool, • Rx with metronidazole—less expensive than oral vancomycin |
| clinical findings associated with *Yersinia enterocolitica* | • Gram stain—gram-negative rod, • transmission— * contaminated food, * milk products, * tofu, * water, • clinical— * dysentery with absolute neutrophilic leukocytosis, * RLQ pain simulating acute appendicitis and Crohn's disease, * mesenteric lymphadenitis, * pharyngitis in adults/children, * iron-overloaded patients susceptible to septicemia, • complications— * Reiter's syndrome, * HLA-B27 + ankylosing spondylitis, * autoimmune diseases—Graves'/Hashimoto's thyroiditis, * MC contaminant in blood transfusions, • Rx—ciprofloxacin |

### Table 7–5. DIARRHEA AND INFECTIOUS DISEASE OF SMALL AND LARGE BOWEL *Continued*

| Most Common... | Answer and Explanation |
| --- | --- |
| clinical findings associated with *Entamoeba histolytica* | • **most common parasite-induced dysentery in the United States,** • **transmission**— * ingestion of cysts in water/food, * unprotected anal intercourse, * cysts resistant to gastric acid in water/food, * excysts in alkaline environment of small bowel, * trophozoites burrow into mucosa of cecum, sigmoid colon, and rectum: "flask-shaped" ulcers, • **clinical**—* bloody diarrhea, * absence of fever, • **complications**— * hepatic abscess: "anchovy paste" abscess, * penetration through diaphragm into right pleural cavity, * dissemination, • **Dx**—stool for O/P: identify cysts/trophozoites, * indirect hemagglutination titer—80–90% sensitivity, • **Rx**—metronidazole |
| causes of acute infectious diarrhea associated with bloody stools | • *Campylobacter jejuni,* • *Shigella sonnei,* • *Entamoeba histolytica,* • *Vibrio parahaemolyticus,* • *Balantidium coli* |
| causes of chronic diarrhea | • **osmotic**—e.g., **lactase deficiency: MCC,** • *secretory*—e.g., laxatives, • *inflammatory*—e.g., IBD, • *malabsorption*—e.g., celiac disease, • *motility dysfunction*—e.g., IBS, • *chronic infections*—e.g., diarrhea in AIDS |
| tests used to document osmotic diarrhea secondary to lactase deficiency | • **hydrogen breath test**—gold standard for lactase deficiency, • *fasting*—diarrhea stops with fasting, • *stool osmotic gap*—stool osmotic gap = 300 mOsm/kg − 2 × [stool $Na^+$ + stool $K^+$], * osmotic gap in lactase deficiency is > 100 mOsm/kg, • *stool pH < 7*—due to the production of fatty acids from fermentation of lactose |
| Rx of lactase deficiency | • **avoid dairy products,** • **take lactase tablets prior to eating dairy products** |

*Table continued on following page*

Table 7–5. DIARRHEA AND INFECTIOUS DISEASE OF
SMALL AND LARGE BOWEL *Continued*

| Most Common... | Answer and Explanation |
|---|---|
| causes of secretory diarrheas | • **laxatives**— * phenolphthalein, * anthraquinones, * senna, * castor oil, * bisacodyl, • *enterotoxin-induced*— * enterotoxins stimulate cAMP enterotoxigenic: *E. coli*, * types of invasive diarrhea with mucosal injury increase permeability with a loss of isotonic fluid: e.g., ♦ *C. jejuni*, ♦ *Y. enterocolitica*, ♦ *S. sonnei*, • *pancreatic cholera*—non-β cell, malignant islet cell tumor secreting vasointestinal peptide, • *carcinoid syndrome*— * secretion of serotonin, * secretion of substance P, • *ZE syndrome*—gastrin effect, • *bile acid diarrhea*—see below, • *microscopic collagenous colitis*— * normal gross appearance, * intraepithelial lymphocytes, * subepithelial collagen band |
| tests used to document secretory diarrheas | • **stool osmotic gap**— * see above, * <50 mOsm/kg difference, • **fasting**—diarrhea continues, • **culture**—R/O invasive types of diarrhea, • *alkalinize stool with sodium hydroxide*—pink color indicates phenolphthalein ingestion, • *proctoscopy*—may reveal melanosis coli from anthracene derivatives—senna, cascara, aloe, • *barium enema*—"cathartic colon": hypomotile, dilated bowel with absent haustra, • *urine for 5-HIAA*—R/O carcinoid syndrome |
| protozoal cause of chronic diarrhea in the United States | *Giardia lamblia*— * ingestion of cysts in contaminated water, * excystation occurs in acid pH of stomach, * trophozoites attach to small bowel mucosa and may extend into the biliary tree |
| clinical signs of giardiasis | • **diarrhea**, • *malabsorption*, • *weight loss*, • *association with IgA deficiency*, • *Dx*— * stool for O/P, * Entero-Test—see below |
| Rx for giardiasis | **metronidazole** |
| organisms detected with the Entero-Test (string test) | • ***Cryptosporidium parvum***, • ***Giardia lamblia***, • ***Strongyloides stercoralis*** [**Note:** a string with one end attached to the cheek is swallowed and allowed to remain in the duodenum for a few hours. It is retrieved and the material is examined.] |

## Table 7–5. DIARRHEA AND INFECTIOUS DISEASE OF SMALL AND LARGE BOWEL Continued

| Most Common... | Answer and Explanation |
|---|---|
| cause of melanosis coli | **laxative abuse** [**Note:** laxatives contain phenanthrene pigments, which are phagocytosed by colonic macrophages in the lamina propria, giving the mucosa a black color. Laxative bowels are often distended and hypomotile.] |
| causes of malabsorption | • **small bowel disease,** • *enzyme deficiency,* • *bile salt deficiency* |
| mechanism of malabsorption in small bowel disease | • **mucosal absorptive defect**—e.g., * celiac disease, * Crohn's disease, • *loss of absorptive surface*—e.g., Billroth II, • *lymphatic obstruction*—e.g., * Whipple's disease, * malignant lymphoma |
| mechanism of diarrhea in enzyme deficiency | • **disaccharidase deficiency**—see above discussion, • *pancreatic enzyme deficiency*— * problem with breaking down of fat, protein, carbohydrates (less of a problem), * e.g., chronic pancreatitis |
| mechanism of diarrhea in bile salt deficiency | **inability to emulsify fat and produce micelles for reabsorption** |
| S/S suggesting malabsorption | • **diarrhea,** • *greasy stools*—steatorrhea, • *weight loss with good appetite*—calorie loss, • *water-/fat-soluble vitamin deficiency S/S*—see below |
| screening test for malabsorption of fat | • **qualitative stool for fat**—Sudan black fat stains, if positive, may require 72 hrs, • *quantitative stool for fat*—gold standard |
| general tests used in evaluating malabsorption | • **serum albumin**—R/O protein-losing enteropathy, particularly if globulins are decreased, • **serum calcium**—R/O vitamin D deficiency, • **CBC**—R/O anemia, • **serum carotenes**—R/O vitamin A deficiency, • **serum electrolytes**— * R/O hypokalemia, * normal AG metabolic acidosis, • **serum folate/$B_{12}$**— * R/O megaloblastic anemia, * Schilling's test is used to localize cause of $B_{12}$ deficiency, • **serum iron**—R/O iron deficiency, • **serum magnesium**— * common cause of hypocalcemia: interferes with PTH release and function, • **serum PT**—R/O vitamin K deficiency |

*Table continued on following page*

Table 7–5. DIARRHEA AND INFECTIOUS DISEASE OF
SMALL AND LARGE BOWEL *Continued*

| Most Common... | Answer and Explanation |
|---|---|
| small bowel disease causing malabsorption | **celiac disease**— * more common in women than men, * primarily involves the duodenum and jejunum |
| pathogenic factors producing celiac disease | • **autoimmune disease with antibodies against gliadin**— * gliadin is an alcohol extract of gluten in wheat, * gluten is directly toxic to the intestinal mucosa, • *HLA-B8, DrW3 associations*—60–90% |
| screening tests for celiac disease | • **antigliadin antibodies**— * >90% sensitivity, * IgG antibodies against gliadin are more sensitive, * IgA antibodies are more specific, * combined specificity of the two antibodies when both are present is >95%, • *antiendomysial antibodies*— * 70–90% sensitivity, * IgG antibodies are more sensitive and IgA antibodies are more specific for celiac disease, • *D-xylose*— * 5-carbon sugar that does not require pancreatic amylases for absorption, * a 25-g oral dose is given and urine is collected for 5 hrs: normal is ≥ 5 g, * levels < 5 g indicate small bowel disease and bacterial overgrowth, • *reappearance of normal villi after a gluten-free diet*—gold standard test for confirming celiac disease |
| serious complication of celiac disease | **small bowel T cell malignant lymphoma**— * 8–10%, * may occur 10–15 yrs into the disease |
| Rx of celiac disease | **gluten-free diet**— * ~80% respond to a gluten-free diet, * refractory cases may respond to glucocorticoids |
| clinical findings of malabsorption due to chronic pancreatitis | • **weight loss**— * anorexia from pain, * malabsorption of nutrients, • *steatorrhea*— * 40% of cases after 5–10 yrs, • $B_{12}$ *deficiency*— cannot cleave R factor off $B_{12}$ |

## Table 7–5. DIARRHEA AND INFECTIOUS DISEASE OF SMALL AND LARGE BOWEL *Continued*

| Most Common... | Answer and Explanation |
|---|---|
| mechanisms of malabsorption in chronic pancreatitis | • **maldigestion of fats**— * occurs when >90% of exocrine function is destroyed, * diminished lipase and colipase activity, * undigested neutral fats and fat droplets are noted in the stool, • *maldigestion of proteins*— * >90% of exocrine function destroyed, * diminished trypsinogen, chymotrypsinogen, proelastase, procarboxypeptidases A/B in the secretions, * undigested meat fibers are present in the stool, • *maldigestion of CHO does not occur*—salivary gland amylase is still present |
| screening tests for pancreatic insufficiency | • **CT scan of the pancreas**—look for dystrophic calcifications, • *bentiromide test*— * checks the ability of chymotrypsin to cleave off PABA from bentiromide, * PABA is reabsorbed and converted in the liver into arylamines, which are excreted in the urine, • *ERCP*— * enzyme measurements, * radiography, • *IV secretin test*—gold standard confirmatory test of pancreatic insufficiency |
| Rx of pancreatic maldigestion | • **low-fat diet**, • **oral enteric-coated pancreatic enzyme supplements**, • **vitamin supplements**—particularly fat-soluble, • **B$_{12}$ injections**, • **medium-chain TG**—directly reabsorbed |
| causes of bile salt deficiency | • **chronic liver disease**—synthetic site, • *cholestasis*—prevents delivery of bile acids to the duodenum, • *bacterial overgrowth in small bowel*—destruction of bile salts, • *cholestyramine*—binding of bile salts, • *terminal ileal disease*—interferes with the reabsorption of bile salts |
| mechanisms of diarrhea in ileal resection | • **<100-cm resection**— * mild steatorrhea, * malabsorbed bile salts enter colon and impair water/electrolyte reabsorption → diarrhea, * total bile acid pool mildly reduced, • **>100-cm resection**— * total bile acid pool significantly reduced, * free long-chain fatty acids are malabsorbed → secretory-type diarrhea and more significant steatorrhea |

*Table continued on following page*

Table 7–5. DIARRHEA AND INFECTIOUS DISEASE OF
SMALL AND LARGE BOWEL *Continued*

| Most Common... | Answer and Explanation |
|---|---|
| screening test for bile salt deficiency | **radioactive bile breath test**— * the presence of bacterial overgrowth causes the release of radioactive $CO_2$, which is reabsorbed and measured in the breath, * terminal ileal disease also produces a positive test: colonic bacteria will degrade the radioactive substrate and release radioactive $CO_2$ |
| Rx of bile salt–induced diarrhea | **low-fat diet**— * <50 g/day, * using cholestyramine further aggravates steatorrhea and decreases the bile acid pool |
| causes of bacterial overgrowth leading to malabsorption | • **intestinal stasis**—e.g., * diverticula, * motility disorders: gastroparesis, * Billroth II with blind afferent duodenal loop, • *fistulas*— * gastrocolic, * jejunocolic, • *achlorhydria*— * PA, * prolonged use of $H_2$-blockers, * gastric resection |
| screening tests for bacterial overgrowth | • **¹⁴C-xylose**— * most sensitive/specific test, * measures $^{14}CO_2$ in the breath, • *¹⁴C-glycocholate*—measures $^{14}CO_2$ in the breath, • *lactulose-$H_2$*—measures $H_2$ in the breath |
| clinical findings associated with bacterial overgrowth | • **steatorrhea,** • *bile salt deficiency,* • $B_{12}$ *deficiency* |
| Rx of bacterial overgrowth | • **surgery, if anatomic cause,** • **antibiotics**—cephalosporin + metronidazole, • **octreotide**—increases bowel motility in motility disorders, • **nutritional Rx**— * medium chain TG: directly reabsorbed, * $B_{12}$/folate, * calcium/magnesium, * iron, * vitamins |
| intrinsic colonic motility disorder producing diarrhea | **irritable bowel syndrome (IBS)**— * female dominant disease, * commonly precipitated by stress or consumption of high-fat meals |
| S/S of IBS | • **alternating bouts of diarrhea and constipation**—may be constipation- or diarrhea-dominant rather than cyclic, • *abdominal pain relieved by defecation,* • *abdominal bloating*—must R/O lactase deficiency, • *excessive mucus in the stool,* • *spastic bowel*— * urgency, * tenesmus, in some patients, • *normal flexible sigmoidoscopy* |

## Table 7–5. DIARRHEA AND INFECTIOUS DISEASE OF SMALL AND LARGE BOWEL Continued

| Most Common... | Answer and Explanation |
| --- | --- |
| Rx of IBS | • stress reduction, • high-fiber diet, • anticholinergics to relieve spasm |

**Question:** Which of the following are characteristic findings in an invasive diarrhea? **SELECT 2**
- (A) Fecal leukocytes
- (B) High-volume diarrhea
- (C) Bloody diarrhea
- (D) Stool osmotic gap >100
- (E) Acid stool pH
- (F) Steatorrhea

**Answers: (A), (C).** A positive stool for fecal leukocytes is highly predictive of an invasive diarrhea **(choice A is correct)**. Osmotic and secretory diarrheas are high-volume diarrheas, whereas invasive diarrheas are low volume **(choice B is incorrect)**. Bloody diarrhea is characteristically found in invasive diarrheas, particularly those due to *C. jejuni* and *Shigella species* **(choice C is correct)**. A stool osmotic gap >100 and an acid pH stool are findings associated with lactase deficiency, which is an osmotic diarrhea **(choices D and E are incorrect)**. Steatorrhea is the gold standard abnormality in malabsorptive states **(choice F is incorrect)**.

AAs = amino acids, AG = anion gap, AIDS = acquired immunodeficiency syndrome, BAO = basal acid output, cAMP = cyclic adenosine monophosphate, CF = cystic fibrosis, CHO = carbohydrate, CMV = cytomegalovirus, CNS = central nervous system, COD = cause of death, CPE = cytopathic effect, ERCP = endoscopic retrograde cholecystopancreatography, FAs = fatty acids, 5-HIAA = 5-hydroxyindoleacetic acid, HLA = human leukocyte antigen, IBD = inflammatory bowel disease, IBS = irritable bowel syndrome, MC = most common, MCC = most common cause, O/P = ova/parasites, PA = pernicious anemia, PABA = para-aminobenzoic acid, PT = prothrombin time, PTH = parathormone, RLQ = right lower quadrant, R/O = rule out, S/S = signs/symptoms, TG = triglyceride, TMP/SMX = trimethoprim-sulfamethoxazole, UC = ulcerative colitis, VIP = vasointestinal peptide, ZE = Zollinger-Ellison.

### Table 7–6. SMALL AND LARGE BOWEL
### DISEASE, DISORDERS OF THE APPENDIX,
### PERITONEAL DISORDERS

| Most Common... | Answer and Explanation |
| --- | --- |
| GI location for hematochezia | **below the ligament of Treitz**— * hematochezia refers to massive bleeding per rectum, * bleeding stops spontaneously in 75% of cases |
| method for identifying bleeding site in hematochezia | **inferior mesenteric artery angiography**— flexible sigmoidoscopy and colonoscopy are not generally useful in the work-up owing to blood obscuring visualization |
| causes of hematochezia | • **diverticulosis**—diverticulitis does not produce bleeding owing to scarring of the subjacent vessels, • *angiodysplasia* |
| causes of chronic lower GI bleeding | • **internal hemorrhoids,** • *colorectal cancer* |
| cause of "thumbprint" sign in bowel | **bowel infarction**—due to submucosal edema and hemorrhage into the bowel wall |
| cause of "string sign" | **Crohn's disease**—refers to narrow lumen in the terminal ileum |
| cause of a sentinel loop in RLQ | **retrocecal appendicitis**—localized ileus from appendicitis |
| cause of pneumoperitoneum | **ruptured anterior duodenal ulcer** |
| developmental abnormality in the GI tract | **Meckel's diverticulum**— * persistence of the vitelline (omphalomesenteric) duct, * 50% lined by intestinal mucosa and 50% by gastric mucosa, * rule of 2's: ♦ 2 inches long, ♦ 2 feet from ileocecal valve, ♦ 2% of the population, ♦ 2% symptomatic |
| mechanism of bleeding in a Meckel's diverticulum | **hemorrhage at the junction of ectopically located gastric mucosa and ileal mucosa** |
| cause of iron deficiency in neonates and children | **bleeding Meckel's diverticulum** |

## Table 7–6. SMALL AND LARGE BOWEL DISEASE, DISORDERS OF THE APPENDIX, PERITONEAL DISORDERS *Continued*

| Most Common... | Answer and Explanation |
|---|---|
| complications associated with Meckel's diverticulum | • **bleeding**— * symptomatic usually in children < 2 yrs old, * melena or bright red rectal bleeding, • *diverticulitis,* • *obstruction*—due to: ♦ intussusception, ♦ volvulus, • *perforation,* • *site for intussusception,* • *Littre's hernia*—Meckel's diverticulum causing an indirect inguinal hernia |
| test used to identify a Meckel's diverticulum | **99mTc nuclear scan**—technetium concentrates in parietal cells, which are ectopically located in the diverticulum |
| Rx of Meckel's diverticulum | **surgical removal** |
| congenital cause of megacolon | **Hirschsprung's disease**— * deficiency of ganglion cells in Meissner's submucosal plexus and Auerbach's myenteric plexus, * involves the distal sigmoid and rectum |
| acquired cause of Hirschsprung's disease | **Chagas' disease**— * due to *Trypanosoma cruzi,* * transmitted by the bite of the reduviid bug, * amastigotes destroy parasympathetic ganglia in Auerbach's myenteric plexus |
| chromosomal disorder associated with Hirschsprung's disease | **Down's syndrome** |
| clinical findings in Hirschsprung's disease | • **constipation**—failure to pass meconium at birth: empty rectal vault on rectal exam, • *complications*— * toxic megacolon proximal to functional obstruction, * enterocolitis: danger of perforation, • *lab Dx*—rectal biopsy, • *Rx*—reconstructive surgery |
| causes of small bowel obstruction in middle/late adulthood | • **adhesions from previous surgery**— * usually produces midgut obstruction, * adhesions occur in ~70% of patients postoperatively: ~5% develop obstruction, • *entrapment of small bowel in an indirect hernia sac*—second MCC, • *radiation,* • KCl—jejunal strictures, • *gallstone ileus*—see below, • *Crohn's disease*—see below • *endometriosis,* • *intussusception*—usually children |

*Table continued on following page*

Table 7–6. SMALL AND LARGE BOWEL
DISEASE, DISORDERS OF THE APPENDIX,
PERITONEAL DISORDERS *Continued*

| Most Common... | Answer and Explanation |
|---|---|
| cause of bowel obstruction in children/young adults | **incarceration of bowel in indirect inguinal hernia**—bowel trapped in hernia sac and cannot be reduced |
| S/S of small bowel obstruction | • **colicky abdominal pain,** • *vomiting,* • *constipation/absence of flatus*—obstipation, • *high-pitched, tinkling sounds,* • *no rebound tenderness*—no peritonitis, unless bowel ruptures or strangulation occurs, • *abdominal distension*— * trapping of swallowed nitrogen gas, * distention is not present in foregut obstruction: gas exits with vomiting, • *vomiting of feculent material*—mid- to hindgut obstruction |
| initial screening test in bowel obstruction | **plain radiography of abdomen** |
| radiographic findings in small bowel obstruction | • **distention of bowel,** • *air/fluid levels with a stepladder appearance,* • *absence of air distal to the obstruction* |
| causes of foregut obstruction | • **obstructing PUD,** • *cancer of stomach or head of pancreas* |
| S/S of foregut obstruction | • **pain**—colicky pain q2–5 min, • **vomiting**— * early symptom, * contains food, * bilious if obstruction is distal to the ampulla of Vater, • *bowel distention*—none, since vomiting expels the gas, • *hyperperistalsis*—none |
| cause of high midgut obstruction | **adhesions from previous surgery** |
| S/S of high midgut obstruction | • **pain**—colicky pain with intervals >10 min, • *vomiting*—early onset, sometimes feculent, • *bowel distention*—gas in small bowel proximal to obstruction, • *hyperperistalsis*— * early sign by auscultation, * visible peristalsis later |
| cause of hindgut obstruction | • **annular, obstructing cancer in left colon**—60–70%, • *volvulus,* • *diverticulitis* |

## Table 7–6. SMALL AND LARGE BOWEL DISEASE, DISORDERS OF THE APPENDIX, PERITONEAL DISORDERS *Continued*

| Most Common... | Answer and Explanation |
|---|---|
| S/S of hindgut obstruction (left colonic) | • **pain**—colicky pain with longer interval than above types, • **vomiting**— * later onset of vomiting than that present in midgut obstruction, * sometimes feculent, • **bowel distention**— * distention of proximal colon if ileocecal valve is competent, * if small bowel contains air: ♦ ileocecal valve is incompetent, ♦ could be confused with a high midgut obstruction, • *hyperperistalsis*—develops later than above types |
| causes of a strangulated and obstructed bowel | • **entrapment of small bowel in an indirect inguinal hernia**—10% incidence, • *volvulus*, • *intussusception* |
| S/S of a strangulated and obstructed bowel | • **pain**—continuous and not colicky: due to peritonitis, • *bowel sounds*—disappear due to peritonitis: present in simple obstruction, • *fever,* • **absolute neutrophilic leukocytosis, left shift**—not present in simple obstruction, • *abdominal distention*—also present in simple obstruction, • *rebound tenderness*—due to peritonitis: not usually significant in simple obstruction, • *lactic acidosis*—sign of bowel infarction, • *hypotension*—third spacing, • *vomiting*—also present in simple obstruction, • *air under the diaphragm* |
| causes of an intussusception in adults | • **polyp,** • *enlarged mesenteric lymph node,* • *Meckel's diverticulum* [**Note:** these lesions provide a site for the advancing peristaltic wave to grasp and drag the proximal part of the bowel into the distal bowel. Obstruction and compression of vessels lead to infarction and GI bleeding; called "currant jelly" stools.] |
| hernia that extends into the scrotum | **indirect inguinal hernia** |
| hernia in young adult males | **indirect inguinal hernia** |
| hernia types in adult women | **indirect and femoral hernias**—direct inguinal hernias are uncommon |

*Table continued on following page*

**Table 7–6. SMALL AND LARGE BOWEL
DISEASE, DISORDERS OF THE APPENDIX,
PERITONEAL DISORDERS** *Continued*

| Most Common... | Answer and Explanation |
|---|---|
| abdominal hernias in decreasing order | • **indirect inguinal hernia,** • *direct inguinal hernia,* • *femoral hernia* |
| mechanisms predisposing to acquired hernias | • **increased intra-abdominal pressure**—intermittent pressure (e.g., coughing) worse than constant pressure, • *weakness in abdominal wall*—insufficient elastic fibers for effective recoil after an increase in intra-abdominal pressure |
| clinical conditions predisposing to acquired hernias | • **obesity/old age,** • *malnourished patients,* • *weight lifting,* • *COPD*—coughing, • *prostate hyperplasia*—straining with urination, • *colonic obstruction*— * straining at stool, * e.g., obstructing colorectal cancer |
| pathogenesis of an indirect hernia in children | **persistence of the peritoneal connection between inguinal canal and tunica vaginalis** |
| pathogenesis of an indirect hernia in adults | **protrusion of a new peritoneal process into the inguinal canal**— * small bowel passes through internal inguinal ring: bowel directly hits the finger, extends out the external ring into the scrotal sac, * lateral to the triangle of Hesselbach: ♦ rectus abdominis is medial border, ♦ inguinal ligament the inferior border, ♦ superficial epigastric artery the lateral border, ♦ single layer of transversalis fascia is floor of triangle |
| pathogenesis of a Littre hernia | **indirect inguinal hernia sac containing Meckel's diverticulum** |
| complications of indirect inguinal hernia | • **incarceration**— * hernia that cannot be manually reduced with sedation, * 10% incidence, • *strangulated obstruction*—10% incidence, • *rupture*—rare |
| nonoperative management of indirect inguinal hernias | **manual reduction after sedation and relaxation of the patient** |
| Rx of indirect inguinal hernias in children | **high ligation of hernia sac at the level of the internal inguinal ring + tightening of the internal inguinal ring**—called Marcy repair |

## Table 7–6. SMALL AND LARGE BOWEL DISEASE, DISORDERS OF THE APPENDIX, PERITONEAL DISORDERS *Continued*

| Most Common... | Answer and Explanation |
|---|---|
| Rx of indirect inguinal hernias in young adults and elderly people | • transection or reduction of proximal hernia sac + tightening of internal inguinal ring—e.g., Bassini's repair: uses conjoined tendon, • *sutured mesh covering inguinal canal and Hesselbach's triangle*—e.g., Lichtenstein's repair |
| hernia bulging through floor of triangle of Hesselbach | **direct inguinal hernia** |
| mechanism of direct inguinal hernias | **single layer of transversalis is stretched in the floor of the triangle of Hesselbach** |
| clinical features of direct inguinal hernia | • **hernia bulge occurs in proximity to the external inguinal ring**— * bulge disappears when patient reclines, * small bowel cannot enter scrotal sac, • **medial to the superficial epigastric artery**—pulsation on lateral side of finger, • **rarely incarcerates** |
| Rx of direct inguinal hernias | • **sutured mesh covering inguinal canal and Hesselbach's triangle**—e.g., Lichtenstein's repair, • *Bassini's repair*—see above, • *McVay's repair*—transversalis fascia and conjoined tendon are sutured to Cooper's ligament |
| cause of a pantaloon hernia | **indirect + direct inguinal hernia** |
| hernia with the highest rate of incarceration | **femoral hernia**— * ~25–30% rate of incarceration—narrow femoral ring, * small bowel or omentum is commonly trapped |
| clinical features of a femoral hernia | • **bulge located below the inguinal ligament**—peritoneal outpouching extends into femoral canal—medial to femoral vein, • **most common in women**—>80% |
| Rx of a femoral hernia | **McVay's repair**—see above |
| mechanism of a Richter's hernia | **portion of small bowel trapped in a femoral hernia** |
| hernia in adults with ascites/pregnancy | umbilical hernia—increased incidence in obesity and intra-abdominal tumors as well |

*Table continued on following page*

**Table 7–6. SMALL AND LARGE BOWEL
DISEASE, DISORDERS OF THE APPENDIX,
PERITONEAL DISORDERS** *Continued*

| Most Common... | Answer and Explanation |
|---|---|
| hernia in newborn blacks | **umbilical hernia**—90% occur in blacks |
| clinical findings of umbilical hernias in children | • **pathogenesis**—peritoneal protrusion extends into a fascial defect containing remnants of umbilical cord, • *natural Hx*—majority close spontaneously: usually by second year, • *S/S*— * large hernias are more likely to be symptomatic, * incarceration is uncommon |
| indications for surgical Rx of umbilical hernias in children | • **incarceration,** • *presence beyond 5 yrs of age* |
| clinical findings of umbilical hernias in adults | • **gender**—more common in women than men, • **natural history**— * does not regress, * more likely to incarcerate, • **S/S**— * pain when coughing, * dragging sensation, • **Rx**—surgical repair ASAP |
| cause of a ventral hernia | **previous surgical excision** |
| predisposing causes of ventral hernias | • **obesity,** • *malnutrition,* • *postoperative wound with infection/coughing/surgical drain,* • *elderly patient* |
| mechanism of a spigelian hernia | **ventral hernia through linea semilunaris**—located above the level of the inferior epigastric artery and near the termination of the transversalis muscle along the lateral border of the rectus abdominis muscles |
| hernia with highest mortality | **obturator hernia**—difficult preoperative diagnosis |
| mechanism of an obturator hernia | **small bowel trapped in the obturator canal** |
| clinical findings of an obturator hernia | • **patient type**—elderly, thin woman, • **natural Hx**—incarcerates small bowel, leading to bowel obstruction, • **S/S**—Howship-Romberg sign: pain extending down medial aspect of the thigh with abduction, extension, or internal rotation of the knee, focal tenderness on rectal exam, • **Dx**—CT most useful, • **Rx**—prosthetic mesh |

## Table 7–6. SMALL AND LARGE BOWEL
## DISEASE, DISORDERS OF THE APPENDIX,
## PERITONEAL DISORDERS *Continued*

| Most Common... | Answer and Explanation |
|---|---|
| cause of air in the biliary tree | **gallstone ileus** |
| clinical findings of gallstone ileus | • **patient type**—elderly woman with chronic cholecystitis/lithiasis, • **pathogenesis**— * inflamed GB adheres to small bowel and fistula develops, * stone passes into small bowel and lodges at the ileocecal valve, leading to obstruction, • **S/S**—intermittent small bowel obstruction |
| Rx of gallstone ileus | **enterotomy**— * remove stone, * leave fistula to heal itself |
| site of a volvulus in elderly patient | **sigmoid colon**— * 80–90% of cases of volvulus, * bowel twists around the mesenteric root [**Note:** the cecum is the most common site in young adults: 25%.] |
| site of a volvulus in young adults | **cecum**—~20% of all cases of volvulus |
| cause of bowel obstruction in pregnancy | **volvulus** |
| causes of volvulus | • **chronic constipation**— * associated with laxative abuse, * bedridden elderly patients, • *drugs reducing motility,* • *adhesions,* • *pregnancy*—see above |
| clinical findings in volvulus | • **persistent abdominal pain,** • *abdominal distention,* • *vomiting,* • *radiographic findings in a sigmoid volvulus*— * concave portion of "coffee bean–shaped" dilated bowel points to the LLQ, * barium enema reveals a "bird's beak" appearance due to tapering of bowel toward the origin of the volvulus, • *radiographic findings in a cecal volvulus*—convex portion of distended kidney-shaped cecum extends into LUQ |
| Rx of a sigmoid volvulus | • **decompression**—rigid sigmoidoscopy with placement of a rectal tube, • *surgery*—if decompression is unsuccessful, remove redundant bowel |

*Table continued on following page*

Table 7–6. SMALL AND LARGE BOWEL
DISEASE, DISORDERS OF THE APPENDIX,
PERITONEAL DISORDERS *Continued*

| Most Common... | Answer and Explanation |
|---|---|
| Rx of a cecal volvulus | **right hemicolectomy** |
| cause of nontoxic megacolon | **Ogilvie's syndrome** |
| clinical findings in Ogilvie's syndrome | • **pseudo-obstruction**— * usually occurs in institutionalized or postoperative elderly patients, * massive distention of the right colon with a cutoff at the splenic flexure, • *S/S*— * abdominal distention, * no pain or tenderness, * danger of perforation if > 10–12 cm, • *lab*—normal diatrizoate (Hypaque) barium enema |
| Rx of Ogilvie's syndrome | **colonoscopy**—relieves the gas |
| cause of intramural gas in plain abdominal films | **pneumatosis cystoides intestinalis**—due to bowel infarction, gastroenteritis |
| cause of intramural cysts noted in plain abdominal films | **pneumatosis cystoides intestinalis**— * rare disease with intramural cysts, * danger of rupture with pneumoperitoneum |
| causes of pneumatosis cystoides intestinalis | • **bowel obstruction,** • *COPD,* • *mechanical ventilation,* • *mesenteric ischemia* |
| site for acquired diverticular disease in the GI tract | **sigmoid colon**— * >90%, * highest intraluminal pressure, * usually asymptomatic, * ~25% symptomatic: see below |
| site for acquired diverticula in small bowel | **duodenum**—usually wide-mouthed diverticula in patients > 50 yrs of age |
| collagen vascular disease associated with wide-mouthed diverticula of the small bowel | **PSS** |
| complications associated with acquired small bowel diverticula | • **usually asymptomatic,** • *diverticulitis,* • *bacterial overgrowth*—leads to: ♦ B$_{12}$ deficiency, ♦ bile salt deficiency, • *bleeding* |

## Table 7–6. SMALL AND LARGE BOWEL
## DISEASE, DISORDERS OF THE APPENDIX,
## PERITONEAL DISORDERS *Continued*

| Most Common... | Answer and Explanation |
|---|---|
| predisposing causes of colon diverticula | • **low-fiber diet with increased constipation,** • *Marfan's syndrome,* • *Ehlers-Danlos syndrome,* • *APKD* |
| specific site for colonic bacteria | **double row of diverticula between the mesenteric and antimesenteric taenia coli—** * mucosa/submucosa herniate where the vessels penetrate the muscularis propria, * sac is juxtaposed to penetrating vessel, leading to a potential for hematochezia |
| complications of diverticular disease | • **diverticulitis**—fecalith obstruction of the diverticular neck increases intraluminal pressure, leading to mucosal injury and bacterial invasion: *E. coli,* • *pericolic abscess*—20% of cases of diverticulitis, • *perforation,* • *fistula formation*—colovesical fistula: ♦ usually in men, ♦ pneumaturia, ♦ recurrent UTIs, • *hematochezia,* • *obstruction*—25% of cases |
| clinical presentation for diverticulitis of the colon | • **LLQ pain**—left-sided appendicitis, • *fever,* • *constipation/diarrhea,* • *palpable, tender mass,* • *neutrophilic leukocytosis* |
| method of diagnosing diverticulitis | • **CT scan**—test of choice for complicated diverticulitis, • *water-soluble barium study*—test of choice for uncomplicated disease, • *plain radiograph*—usually always ordered to R/O a perforation |
| Rx of diverticulitis | • **rest bowel,** • **low-fiber diet,** • **antibiotics: metronidazole + ciprofloxacin,** • **analgesic**—pentazocine, • **surgery indications**— * peritonitis, * recurrent diverticulitis, * massive hemorrhage present, * carcinoma is a possibility |
| causes of fistulas in the GI tract | • **diverticular disease,** • *Crohn's disease* |
| cause of abrupt onset of severe pain in a patient with diverticular disease | **perforation**— * signs of peritonitis, * air under the diaphragm |

*Table continued on following page*

Table 7–6. SMALL AND LARGE BOWEL
DISEASE, DISORDERS OF THE APPENDIX,
PERITONEAL DISORDERS *Continued*

| Most Common... | Answer and Explanation |
|---|---|
| arterial blood supply of stomach and duodenum | **celiac artery** |
| arterial blood supply of small bowel up to splenic flexure | **SMA** |
| arterial blood supply of left colon | **IMA**—retroperitoneal part of left colon has additional blood supply from retroperitoneal vessels |
| arterial blood supply of rectum | **IMA + rectal vessels from internal iliac artery** |
| GI site for acute ischemia | **small bowel**— * most of the small bowel is supplied by the SMA, * angle of the SMA off the aorta lends itself to obstruction by embolization |
| mechanisms of acute ischemia involving the small bowel | • **acute mesenteric ischemia**— * 50%, * SMA obstruction by embolus origination from the left side of the heart: most common, * SMA thrombosis over an atheromatous plaque, • *nonocclusive ischemia*— * 25%, * hypotension secondary to heart failure, * shock, * digitalis—? vasospasm of SMA, • *SMV thrombosis*— * 25%, * PH secondary to cirrhosis, * PRV, * hypercoagulable states |
| cardiac arrhythmia predisposing to small bowel infarction | **atrial fibrillation**—common finding in elderly patients with chronic ischemic heart disease |
| clinical findings in acute mesenteric ischemia due to embolism | • **elderly patient with a sudden onset of severe abdominal pain**—pain out of proportion to physical findings, • *Hx of heart disease with chronic atrial fibrillation*, • *vomiting*, • *bloody diarrhea*, • *hypotension*, • *absent bowel sounds*, • *absence of rebound tenderness*—peritonitis is a late sign |

## Table 7–6. SMALL AND LARGE BOWEL DISEASE, DISORDERS OF THE APPENDIX, PERITONEAL DISORDERS *Continued*

| Most Common... | Answer and Explanation |
|---|---|
| lab/radiographic findings noted in acute mesenteric ischemia | • **striking absolute neutrophilic leukocytosis with left shift,** • *increased serum amylase—*bowel origin, • *metabolic acidosis—*lactate, • *hyperkalemia—*released from RBCs in bowel, • *plain abdominal film—* * distention of small bowel, * air/fluid levels, * absence of intestinal gas, * thumbprinting: submucosal edema/hemorrhage noted in barium study, • *mesenteric arteriography—*gold standard for Dx |
| Rx of acute mesenteric ischemia due to embolism | **immediate surgical embolectomy—**postoperative anticoagulation |
| Rx of acute small bowel infarction | • **surgical removal of involved bowel—**must be removed within 12 hrs, • **prognosis–**60–90% mortality |
| methods of determining bowel viability | • **gross features—**e.g., * *pink color,* * **visible peristalsis**/arterial pulsations present, • *miscellaneous—* * Doppler, * dyes, * oximetry of tissue |
| site for chronic ischemic colitis | **splenic flexure** |
| clinical findings in chronic ischemic colitis | • **weight loss secondary to fear of eating from pain associated with mesenteric angina—**crampy pain begins 30–60 min after eating and abates in ~4 hrs, • *abdominal bruit,* • *radiography—*angiography showing vessel stenosis, • *pre-existing conditions—* * HTN, * DM, * atherosclerosis, * peripheral vascular disease |
| late complication of chronic ischemic colitis | **obstruction—**due to ischemic stricture from repair of infarcted bowel by fibrosis |
| Rx of chronic ischemic colitis | **revascularization of SMA orifice** |

*Table continued on following page*

### Table 7–6. SMALL AND LARGE BOWEL
### DISEASE, DISORDERS OF THE APPENDIX,
### PERITONEAL DISORDERS *Continued*

| Most Common... | Answer and Explanation |
|---|---|
| clinical findings in acute large bowel infarction | • **previous Hx of mesenteric angina,** • *sudden onset of left-sided crampy abdominal pain,* • *abdominal distention and diffuse abdominal tenderness,* • *bloody diarrhea*—bright red blood clots, • *radiography*—thumbprinting in splenic flexure, • *sigmoidoscopy/colonoscopy*— * bloody, edematous, friable mucosa, * pseudomembranes: simulate pseudomembranous colitis |
| Rx of acute large bowel infarction | • **crystalline fluids/antibiotics,** • *observation to R/O infarction*—infarction is uncommon, • *prognosis*—50% mortality |
| site of angiodysplasia in young versus older patients | • **young patients**— * stomach, * duodenum, • **elderly patients**—cecum/right colon |
| pathogenesis of angiodysplasia | • **vascular ectasias increase with age,** • **increased wall stress**— * wall stress increases with an increase in diameter, * right colon has an increased diameter, * increased wall stress dilates submucosal vessels, • **submucosal venules on the antimesenteric border of the right colon dilate**—dilatation due to intermittent obstruction of submucosal veins by muscle contraction and bowel distention |
| presentation of angiodysplasia | • **lower GI bleeding**—second MCC of hematochezia, • *iron deficiency* |
| associations with angiodysplasia | • **calcific aortic stenosis,** • *von Willebrand's disease* |
| methods of diagnosing angiodysplasia | • **initial step**—NG tube to R/O UGI bleed, • **colonoscopy**— * identifies lesions, * cautery of lesions, • **angiography**—localizes the disease |
| Rx of angiodysplasia | • **right hemicolectomy**—if this site has been documented to be the source of bleeding, • *correction of aortic stenosis*—bleeding often abates |
| inflammatory bowel diseases (IBD) | • **ulcerative colitis** (UC)—unknown etiology, • *Crohn's disease* (CD)—unknown etiology |

## Table 7–6. SMALL AND LARGE BOWEL
## DISEASE, DISORDERS OF THE APPENDIX,
## PERITONEAL DISORDERS *Continued*

| Most Common... | Answer and Explanation |
|---|---|
| pathologic features of UC | • **chronic relapsing ulceroinflammatory disease**— * primarily involves mucosa/submucosa of the rectum/left colon, * begins in the rectum (95%), • **gross**— * inflammatory pseudopolyps: areas of residual inflamed mucosa, * bloody, friable mucosa, • **microscopic**—* neutrophilic crypt abscesses in active disease, * lymphocytes and plasma cell inflammation in chronic disease, * possible areas of dysplasia/adenocarcinoma |
| pathologic features of CD | • **systemic, chronic granulomatous, ulceroconstrictive disease**, • **gross**— * transmural inflammation in: ♦ terminal ileum alone in 30%, ♦ colon alone in 20%, ♦ combined in 50%, * discontinuous spread, * narrow lumen: obstruction, * fistula formation, * anal fissures/fistulas, • *microscopic*— * noncaseating granulomas: 60%, * aphthous ulcers: earliest finding |
| S/S of UC | • **frequent bloody bowel movements with mucus**, • *LLQ cramping pain*, • *rectal bleeding*, • *tenesmus*, • *modifying factors*— improvement with cigarette smoking |
| S/S of CD | **intermittent RLQ colicky pain with diarrhea/bleeding**— * bleeding occurs with colonic/anal involvement, * signs of obstruction with terminal ileum involvement |
| extraintestinal findings in IBD | • **arthritis**—AS with HLA-B27 relationship or without HLA relationship: UC > CD, • *skin lesions*— * erythema nodosum: UC > CD, * pyoderma gangrenosum: UC > CD, • *primary sclerosing cholangitis*— * UC > CD, * elevated serum AP, • *uveitis*— * blurry vision, * UC > CD |
| clinical findings favoring CD over UC | • **fistula formation**, • **perianal disease**, • **malabsorption**—bile salt deficiency from terminal ileal disease, • **discontinuous lesions**, • **less risk for adenocarcinoma**, • **obstruction** |

*Table continued on following page*

Table 7-6. SMALL AND LARGE BOWEL
DISEASE, DISORDERS OF THE APPENDIX,
PERITONEAL DISORDERS *Continued*

| Most Common... | Answer and Explanation |
|---|---|
| clinical findings favoring UC over CD | • **toxic megacolon**— * hypotonic, distended bowel >6 cm in diameter, * see below, • **adenocarcinoma**, • **spreads in continuity**, • **rectal involvement**, • **extraintestinal manifestations**—see above |
| risk factors for adenocarcinoma in UC | **extent and duration of UC**— * duration >10 yrs increases risk, * pancolitis is a greater risk than limited disease |
| S/S of toxic megacolon | • **abdominal pain/distention**, • *hemorrhage*, • *volume depletion from diarrhea*, • *potential for gram-negative sepsis/perforation* |
| Rx of toxic megacolon | • **antibiotics for peritonitis**, • **volume repletion with crystalloids**, • **IV corticosteroids**, • **surgery**—total abdominal colectomy if nonresponsive in 48 hrs to medical Rx |
| radiologic findings in UC | • **"lead pipe" appearance**—fibrosis/rigidity of the colon • **loss of haustral markings**, • **irregular mucosal lining**—pseudopolyps/ulcers, • **short bowel**—chronic UC with fibrosis of bowel wall |
| radiologic findings in CD | • **"string sign" in terminal ileum**—luminal narrowing from transmural inflammation, • **fistulas**, • **cobblestone appearance**—longitudinal/transverse ulcerations, • **skip lesions** |
| Rx of UC | • **5-aminosalicylic acid**—ASA, • *glucocorticoids*— * enemas for rectal involvement, * systemic Rx for extensive disease, • *immunosuppressive agents*— * azathioprine, * 6-MP, * only for resistant disease, * corticosteroid sparing, • *anticholinergic/antidiarrheal drugs*— * reduce pain/diarrhea, * applies to acute, not chronic, UC, • *low-fiber diet*, • *surgery*—see below |
| mechanism of action of sulfasalazine | • **metabolized to sulfapyridine (toxic agent) and ASA (active ingredient)**, • **ASA mechanism**— * $O_2$ FR scavenger, * inhibits lipoxygenase pathway in arachidonic acid metabolism, • **mesalamine**— * 5-ASA preparation, * fewer side effects: see below |

### Table 7–6. SMALL AND LARGE BOWEL
### DISEASE, DISORDERS OF THE APPENDIX,
### PERITONEAL DISORDERS Continued

| Most Common... | Answer and Explanation |
|---|---|
| side effects of sulfasalazine | • **fever,** • **rash,** • **aplastic anemia,** • **folate deficiency,** • **hepatitis,** • **male infertility,** • **pancreatitis** |
| Rx of CD | • **sulfasalazine**—more effective for colonic than small bowel disease, • **5-ASA preparations**—for small bowel disease, • **corticosteroids**— * for acute exacerbations, * best for small bowel disease, • **6-MP**—steroid-sparing drug, • **metronidazole**— * perianal disease, * colonic disease, • **surgery**—see below, • **nutritional support**— * IM B$_{12}$, * low fat/low oxalate: reduce oxalate stone formation/high calcium diet |
| surgical indications for UC | • **active disease unresponsive to medical Rx,** • **increased risk for malignancy**—see above, • **toxic megacolon unresponsive to medical Rx,** • **bleeding unresponsive to medical Rx** |
| surgical indications for CD | • **complications**— * **obstruction:** 50%, * fistula, * abscess, * perforation, * bleeding, • *majority require surgery*— * 70–80% require surgery, * ~90% recurrence rate over time, * recurrence at anastomosis site, • *surgery complications*— * short bowel syndrome: occurs when ≤ 3 meters of small bowel remain, * nutritional abnormalities: occurs when <1 meter of small bowel remains |
| malignant tumor of small bowel | **metastasis**—primary sites include colon, rectum, or ovary |
| primary malignant tumors of small bowel | • **carcinoid tumor**—terminal ileum MC site, • *adenocarcinoma*—proximal jejunum MC site, • *malignant lymphoma*— * terminal ileum: Peyer's patches MC site, * usually B cell origin, * T cell if secondary to celiac disease |
| site for carcinoid tumor | **tip of appendix**— * bright yellow color, * neuroendocrine origin: contains neurosecretory granules |
| site for carcinoid tumor with ability to metastasize | **terminal ileum** |

*Table continued on following page*

Table 7–6. SMALL AND LARGE BOWEL
DISEASE, DISORDERS OF THE APPENDIX,
PERITONEAL DISORDERS *Continued*

| Most Common... | Answer and Explanation |
|---|---|
| factors determining metastatic potential in carcinoid tumors | • **tumor size**— * all carcinoid tumors are malignant, * tumors >2 cm metastasize in >80%: majority of terminal ileal tumors are >2 cm, • *depth of intramural invasion,* • *tumor site*— * foregut tumors: ♦ 5% carcinoid tumors, ♦ argentaffin-negative, ♦ bone metastasis, ♦ atypical carcinoid syndrome (see below), * midgut tumors: ♦ 90% carcinoid tumors (jejunum, **ileum,** appendix), ♦ argentaffin-positive, ♦ liver metastasis (greatest chance for carcinoid syndrome), * hindgut tumors: ♦ 5% carcinoid tumors, ♦ argentaffin-negative, ♦ nonsecretory, ♦ bone metastasis |
| signs of terminal ileum carcinoid | • **most are asymptomatic,** • **obstruction MC symptomatic presentation**—serotonin produced by tumor is fibrogenic, • *bleeding,* • *pain,* • *carcinoid syndrome*—10% chance with terminal ileal tumors, • *metastatic sites*— * regional lymph nodes, * bone: osteoblastic, * lung, * liver, • *multiple lesions in 40%* |
| factors most responsible for carcinoid syndrome | • **liver metastasis**—metastatic tumor nodules release serotonin, bradykinin, and other substances into hepatic vein tributaries, • *direct access of secretory products to the systemic circulation without metastasis*— * bronchial carcinoids directly empty into the systemic circulation, * atypical carcinoid syndrome: ♦ left-sided valvular lesions, ♦ telangiectasias, ♦ thick skin [**Note:** normally, the PV drains serotonin from the primary tumor site to the liver. The liver metabolizes serotonin into 5-HIAA, which is excreted in the urine.] |
| clinical findings of carcinoid syndrome | • **flushing**—vasodilatation from bradykinin and serotonin, • *diarrhea*—increased bowel motility: serotonin effect, • *right-sided valvular lesions*—fibroblastic effect of serotonin produces tricuspid insufficiency/pulmonic stenosis, • *increased 24-hr urine for 5-HIAA*—gold standard diagnostic test |

## Table 7–6. SMALL AND LARGE BOWEL DISEASE, DISORDERS OF THE APPENDIX, PERITONEAL DISORDERS *Continued*

| Most Common... | Answer and Explanation |
|---|---|
| Rx of ileal carcinoid tumors | **en bloc resection**— * metastasis already present in ~50%, * 5-yr survival with local disease is ~75%, * 20% 5-yr survival with metastasis |
| Rx of carcinoid syndrome | **octreotide**—somatostatin analogue—inhibits tumor release of serotonin and other products |
| overall GI site for polyps | **sigmoid colon** |
| GI tract polyp | **hyperplastic polyp**—hamartomatous polyp with no malignant potential |
| rectal polyp in children | **juvenile polyp**—solitary hamartomatous polyp that presents with rectal bleeding |
| complications associated with juvenile polyps | • **bleeding,** • *juvenile polyposis syndromes*—see below |
| syndromes associated with juvenile polyps | • **juvenile polyposis**— * AD or * **nonhereditary,** * small risk for malignancy, • *Cronkhite-Canada syndrome*— * nonhereditary, * polyps + nail abnormalities, * small cancer risk |
| polyposis associated with ovarian tumors | **Peutz-Jeghers polyp**— * AD disorder, * hamartomatous polyps: negligible GI cancer risk, * association with ovarian sex-cord stromal tumors with annular tubules |
| location for PJ polyps | • **small bowel**—100%, • *colon*—30%, • *stomach*—25% |
| oral manifestation of PJ syndrome | **buccal mucosa/lips**—also noted on the palms/soles |
| premalignant dysplastic polyp of colon | • **tubular adenoma**— * 60–75%, * stalked polyp, • *tubulovillous adenoma*—15–20%, • *villous adenoma*— * 10%, * sessile polyp with finger-like projections, * rectosigmoid colon |

*Table continued on following page*

**Table 7–6. SMALL AND LARGE BOWEL
DISEASE, DISORDERS OF THE APPENDIX,
PERITONEAL DISORDERS** *Continued*

| Most Common... | Answer and Explanation |
|---|---|
| risk factors for malignancy in adenomas | • **size of tubular adenoma**—>2 cm has 40% risk of malignancy: polyps <1 cm are rarely malignant, • *number of polyps*—risk increases with more polyps, • *percent villous component*— * villi look like those in the small intestine, * tubulovillous adenoma has ~20% risk for cancer, * villous adenomas have >50% risk if > 2 cm and >90% risk if > 4 cm |
| definition of invasion in a polyp | **cancer that has invaded through the muscularis mucosa** |
| clinical/lab findings of a villous adenoma | • **excessive mucus coating the stool**, • *hypoalbuminemia*, • *hypokalemia* |
| polyposis syndrome | **familial polyposis**— * AD disorder, * polyps absent at birth: begin to develop between 10 and 20 yrs of age, * >95% develop colorectal cancer |
| pathogenesis of familial polyposis | **inactivation of the APC suppressor gene on chromosome 5**—activation of a ras oncogene and inactivation of p53 suppressor gene are also operative in malignant transformation |
| extra-abdominal manifestation of familial polyposis | **congenital hypertrophy of retinal pigment epithelium** |
| polyposis syndrome with benign bone and soft tissue tumors | **Gardner's syndrome**— * AD disorder, * variant of familial polyposis, * benign osteomas: mandible, skull, long bones, * desmoid tumors: fibromatosis of abdominal sheath, * supernumerary teeth, * thyroid/adrenal tumors, * sebaceous cysts |
| polyposis syndrome with AR inheritance | **Turcot's syndrome**—probable variant of Gardner's syndrome |
| polyposis syndrome with brain tumors | **Turcot's syndrome**—brain tumors include astrocytomas and medulloblastoma |
| Rx for patients with familial polyposis syndrome | **prophylactic total colectomy**—usually between 35 and 40 yrs of age |

### Table 7–6. SMALL AND LARGE BOWEL DISEASE, DISORDERS OF THE APPENDIX, PERITONEAL DISORDERS *Continued*

| Most Common... | Answer and Explanation |
|---|---|
| sites for colorectal cancer in descending order | • **rectosigmoid**—50%, • *ascending colon*—15%, • *descending colon*—15%, • *transverse colon/cecum*—each 10% [**Note:** the incidence of right-sided colon cancers is increasing.] |
| risk factors for colorectal cancer | • **age >40 yrs,** • *low-fiber/high-saturated-fat diet,* • *smoking,* • *polyposis syndrome,* • *family Hx in first-degree relative*— * 25% of cases, * 3 times greater risk, • *hereditary nonpolyposis syndrome*— * Lynch's syndrome, * AD disease, * type I variant limited to colon: usually right-sided, * type II variant: family cancer syndrome and involves colon plus possible breast, gastric, endometrial/cervical cancer, • *past Hx of polyps in patient or family member,* • *IBD*—see above, • *past Hx of breast/genital cancer in a woman*—2 times increased risk [**Note:** colorectal cancer is the second most common cancer and cancer killer in men and women in the United States.] |
| proto-oncogene activated in colorectal cancer | **K-ras proto-oncogene** |
| change in colonic neoplasms predicting neoplastic transformation | **hypomethylation of DNA**— * produce alterations in gene expression and chromatin structure, * loss of tumor suppressor genes |
| factors that prevent colorectal cancer | • **FOBT annually at ≥50 yrs of age + flexible sigmoidoscopy at age 50 and q3–5 yrs,** • *high-fiber/low-saturated-fat diet,* • *aspirin,* • *antioxidants* |
| screening tests for colon cancer | • **average risk for cancer**— * no family Hx of colon cancer/polyps, * annual rectal exam after age 40 yrs, * FOBT annually ≥ 50 yrs old, * flexible sigmoidoscopy age 50 and q3–5 yrs, • **high risk for cancer**— * first-degree relative with colon cancer or polyps, * annual FOBT, colonoscopy age 35–40 yrs and q2–3 yrs thereafter, • **UC with pancolitis**—annual colonoscopy with multiple biopsies after 7 yrs' duration, • **Hx of polyposis syndrome**—annual colonoscopy beginning at puberty |

*Table continued on following page*

### Table 7–6. SMALL AND LARGE BOWEL
### DISEASE, DISORDERS OF THE APPENDIX,
### PERITONEAL DISORDERS *Continued*

| Most Common... | Answer and Explanation |
|---|---|
| procedures for evaluating positive FOBT | • **colonoscopy**— * gold standard: ♦ 75–95% sensitivity for detecting colorectal cancer within its reach, ♦ best test for polyps <1 cm, * evaluates entire colon + distal small bowel, • *flexible sigmoidoscopy*— * evaluates up to 60 cm (splenic flexure area), * detects ~65–75% of all polyps and 40–65% of all cancers, * good for polyps >1 cm, • *barium enema*— * 80–95% sensitivity for detecting cancer, * 90% sensitivity for polyps >1 cm |
| S/S of left-sided colorectal cancer | **obstruction**— * annular, "napkin-ring" appearance, * change in bowel habits: ♦ constipation/diarrhea, ♦ decreased stool diameter |
| S/S of right-sided colorectal cancer | **bleed**— * large diameter allows tumors to expand into lumen, * polypoid appearance, * melena: slow bleed, * iron deficiency |
| S/S of rectal cancer | • **bleeding,** • *constipation/diarrhea* |
| staging system for colorectal cancer | **Astler-Coller modified Dukes' staging system** |
| staging tests for colorectal cancer | • **abdominal CT scan**— * detects metastasis—liver, lymph nodes, * detects wall invasion, • *chest x-ray,* • *lab tests*— * CEA: increased in 70%, * LFTs: ♦ serum AP and GGT, ♦ indicates liver metastasis if they are elevated |
| prognostic indicators determining survival in colon cancer | • **depth of invasion and lymph node status**—see below, • *miscellaneous factors that reduce survival*— * ulceroinfiltrative tumors, * high preoperative levels of serum CEA, * vessel invasion, * poor differentiation, * mucin-secreting tumors: mucin pushes tumor into vessels, • *overall 5-yr survival*— ~35% |
| pathologic findings and prognosis in stage A colorectal cancer | • **microscopic**—tumor confined to the mucosa, • **prognosis**—100% 5-yr survival |

### Table 7–6. SMALL AND LARGE BOWEL DISEASE, DISORDERS OF THE APPENDIX, PERITONEAL DISORDERS Continued

| Most Common... | Answer and Explanation |
|---|---|
| pathologic findings and prognosis in stage B colorectal cancer | • **microscopic**— * $B_1$: tumor invades muscularis propria but not the serosa and no lymph nodes are involved, * $B_2$: tumor invades serosa and no lymph nodes are involved, • **prognosis**— * $B_1$: 60–67% 5-yr survival, * $B_2$: ~55% 5-yr survival |
| pathologic findings and prognosis in stage C colorectal cancer | • **microscopic**— * $C_1$: $B_1$ tumor with metastasis to regional lymph nodes, * $C_2$: $B_2$ tumor with metastasis to regional lymph nodes, • **prognosis**— * $C_1$: 30–40% 5-yr survival, * $C_2$: 20% 5-yr survival |
| pathologic findings and prognosis in stage D colorectal cancer | • **microscopic**—evidence of distant metastasis at any level of invasion with or without lymph node involvement, • **prognosis**—<10% 5-yr survival |
| site for metastasis of colon cancer | • **liver,** • *lungs,* • *bone,* • *brain* [**Note:** metastasis or recurrence causes an increase in CEA.] |
| surgical Rx of colon cancer | • **low anterior resection (LAR)**—cancers >12 cm from anal verge, • **abdominoperineal resection (APR)**—cancers within 7–8 cm of anal verge, • **APR or LAR for tumors 7–11 cm from anal verge** |
| surgical Rx of rectal cancer | • **APR for lower one-third,** • **LAR for proximal two-thirds** |
| complication of rectal cancer surgery | **impotence**—nerve injury related to the surgery |
| postoperative management of colon cancer | • **5-FU and levamisole**—reduce recurrence risk and mortality for stage C cancer, • **follow-up**— * yearly flexible sigmoidoscopy for low anterior resections (colonoscopy for AP resection) + serum CEA and LFTs q3–6 mos for 4 yrs, • **annual FOBT** [**Note:** ~90% of recurrences happen in the first 4 years.] |
| cause of a persistently elevated serum CEA after 6 wks | **incomplete removal of the cancer** |

*Table continued on following page*

### Table 7–6. SMALL AND LARGE BOWEL
### DISEASE, DISORDERS OF THE APPENDIX,
### PERITONEAL DISORDERS Continued

| Most Common... | Answer and Explanation |
|---|---|
| procedure to R/O local recurrence | **CT scan** |
| procedure to follow with a rising serum CEA titer | **abdominal CT scan + colonoscopy** |
| types of anal carcinoma | • **basaloid/epidermoid/cloacogenic carcinoma**— * located in the transitional zone above the dentate line, * majority of cancers are in women, • *SCC*— * located in the anal canal, * majority of cancers are in homosexual men: HPV relationship from unprotected anal intercourse, • *adenocarcinoma*—superior to the dentate line |
| Rx of basaloid carcinoma | **chemoradiation**—~40% 5-yr survival |
| Rx of anal SCC | **surgery**—~50% 5-yr survival |
| disorder of the appendix | **acute appendicitis** |
| cause of appendicitis in children | **lymphoid hyperplasia**— * 60%, * often secondary to a viral infection: e.g., adenovirus, measles (see Warthin-Finkeldey multinucleated giant cells in the tissue) |
| causes of appendicitis in adults | • **fecalith obstructing the proximal lumen**— * 35%, * fecalith obstruction increases intraluminal pressure, leading to mucosal injury and bacterial invasion, • *seeds*—e.g., * sunflower seeds, * eating persimmons, • *pinworm infection* [**Note:** pathogens include **E. coli**, *Bacteroides fragilis, Pseudomonas* species.] |
| S/S of acute appendicitis | • **colicky periumbilical pain** → • *nausea/ vomiting/low-grade fever,* → • *shift of pain to RLQ* — • *rebound tenderness at McBurney's point*—localized peritonitis |
| findings associated with Rovsing's sign in acute appendicitis | **pain in RLQ on palpation of LLQ**—due to stretching of inflamed peritoneum |
| findings associated with psoas sign in acute appendicitis | **RLQ pain on extension of right thigh**—due to stretching of inflamed peritoneum |

### Table 7–6. SMALL AND LARGE BOWEL DISEASE, DISORDERS OF THE APPENDIX, PERITONEAL DISORDERS *Continued*

| Most Common... | Answer and Explanation |
|---|---|
| findings associated with obturator sign in acute appendicitis | **RLQ pain on internal rotation of right thigh**—due to stretching of inflamed peritoneum |
| clinical findings in retrocecal appendicitis | • **diarrhea**—constipation is the rule with non-retrocecal appendicitis, • *increased urinary frequency*— * pyuria, * microscopic hematuria, • *RLQ with sentinel loop*—localized ileus on a radiograph |
| disorders simulating appendicitis | • **viral gastroenteritis,** • *mesenteric lymphadenitis*— * may be associated with *Yersinia enterocolitica,* * submit lymph node for culture, • *PID,* • *ruptured ovarian cyst,* • *torsion of a cystic teratoma,* • *ruptured ectopic pregnancy,* • *mittelschmerz*—peritoneal irritation from blood at ovulation, • *CD,* • *diverticulitis,* • *Meckel's diverticulitis* [**Note:** US differentiates many of the gynecologic problems. Pain precedes N/V in appendicitis and not vice versa. CT scan with oral contrast is the most accurate radiologic procedure for Dx of appendicitis.] |
| lab findings in acute appendicitis | • **absolute neutrophilic leukocytosis with left shift**— * WBC count usually >11,000 cells/μL with >10% band neutrophils present (left shift), * total count is often normal in elderly patients but is still left-shifted, • *abnormal UA*— * increased protein, * hematuria, * pyuria, • *US*— * wall thickening, * abscess, • *radiograph*—fecalith is sometimes visible |
| complications of appendicitis | • **periappendiceal abscess,** • *perforation*— * risk increases with time from onset of symptoms, * most common in children and elderly people, • *pylephlebitis*—infection of portal vein, • *subphrenic abscess,* • *pelvic abscess,* • *wound infection* |
| complication of a perforated appendix | **generalized peritonitis/abscess** |
| S/S of periappendiceal abscess | • **palpable mass in RLQ**—appendicitis is walled off, • *Hx of RLQ pain > 72 hrs,* • *no signs of peritonitis,* • *fever* |

*Table continued on following page*

**Table 7–6. SMALL AND LARGE BOWEL
DISEASE, DISORDERS OF THE APPENDIX,
PERITONEAL DISORDERS** *Continued*

| Most Common... | Answer and Explanation |
|---|---|
| Rx of periappendiceal abscess | **controversial—** * antibiotics: ♦ expect drop in temperature and WBC count, ♦ expect reduction in size of mass, * elective removal in 4–6 wks |
| S/S of subphrenic abscess associated with acute appendicitis | • **persistent fever 4–5 days postop,** • *diaphragm fixed on the right,* • *right-sided pleural effusion,* • *tenderness over lateral 7th–8th ribs,* • *redness, swelling, lower lateral right chest wall* |
| radiologic tests used to diagnose a subphrenic abscess | • **US/CT scan,** • *liver/lung scan,* • *gallium scan* |
| Rx of subphrenic abscess | • **extraperitoneal drainage,** • **antibiotics** |
| clinical findings suggesting perforation in acute appendicitis | • **high fever,** • *toxic appearance,* • *palpable mass,* • *diffuse abdominal tenderness,* • *neutrophilic leukocytosis* >20,000 cells/μL |
| S/S of pelvic abscess associated with acute appendicitis | • **recurrent fever/diarrhea after surgery,** • *pain on rectal exam* [**Note:** perforations are most responsible for pelvic abscesses.] |
| Rx of pelvic abscess | • **surgical drainage,** • **antibiotics** |
| S/S of pylephlebitis | • **high fever,** • *painful hepatomegaly*—liver abscesses, • *jaundice* |
| CT findings in pylephlebitis | **PV thrombosis with gas** |
| Rx of appendicitis | • **appendectomy**—open or laparoscopic approach, • **prophylactic antibiotics**—coverage of aerobic/anaerobic bacteria: e.g., ampicillin, gentamicin, metronidazole [**Note:** 10–20% of appendices are normal. This is an acceptable false-positive rate, since a lower rate of FPs is most likely complicated by perforation with peritonitis.] |
| complication of incidental appendectomy | **none**—applies to patients without CD with cecal involvement |

## Table 7–6. SMALL AND LARGE BOWEL DISEASE, DISORDERS OF THE APPENDIX, PERITONEAL DISORDERS *Continued*

| Most Common... | Answer and Explanation |
|---|---|
| causes of an appendiceal mucocele | • **non-neoplastic proximal chronic obstruction of appendix**—e.g., fecalith, • *benign cystadenoma,* • *malignant cystadenocarcinoma* |
| tumor of appendix | **carcinoid tumor**—see above |
| line demarcating the rectum from the anus | **dentate line** [**Note:** mucosa superior to the dentate line derives from endoderm. Transitional epithelium is immediately superior to the dentate line and merges with rectal mucosa. Mucosa above the dentate line is innervated by the autonomic nervous system, which is insensitive to pain. The mucosa inferior to the dentate line derives from ectoderm and contains squamous epithelium. It is innervated by the somatic nervous system and is sensitive to pain. The columns of Morgagni are immediately superior to the dentate line. The anal crypts, which empty the anal glands in the anterior and posterior midline, are located at the base of the columns. The anatomic anal canal is distal to the dentate line and ends at the anal verge.] |
| vessel causing internal hemorrhoids | **superior hemorrhoidal vein**— * hemorrhoids are superior to the dentate line, * internal hemorrhoids are nonpalpable [**Note:** hemorrhoids are dilated veins in the mucosa and submucosa.] |
| causes of internal hemorrhoids | • **straining at stool,** • *pregnancy,* • *PH* |
| symptom of internal hemorrhoids | • **painless bright red bleeding during or after stooling,** • *prolapse—* * prolapse with strangulation may be painful, * first degree: no prolapse, * second degree: prolapse into anal canal and spontaneously reduce, * third degree: prolapse with straining and require manual reduction, * fourth degree: continuously prolapsed, • *pruritus ani*—due to secondary discharge of mucus after prolapse |
| Rx of internal hemorrhoids | • **high-fiber diet/avoid straining,** • *rubber band ligation,* • *infrared coagulation,* • *sclerotherapy,* • *hemorrhoidectomy*—mainly for fourth-degree prolapse |

*Table continued on following page*

**Table 7–6. SMALL AND LARGE BOWEL
DISEASE, DISORDERS OF THE APPENDIX,
PERITONEAL DISORDERS** *Continued*

| Most Common... | Answer and Explanation |
|---|---|
| vessel causing external hemorrhoids | **inferior hemorrhoidal vein**—external hemorrhoids are inferior to the dentate line |
| symptom of external hemorrhoids | • **painful thrombosis**—blue-colored subcutaneous nodule, • *pruritus ani* |
| Rx of external hemorrhoids | • **sitz baths/stool softeners,** • *excision after local anesthesia* |
| cause of acute anal pain in adults | **anal fissure** |
| causes of anal fissures | • **trauma from hard, large-caliber stool,** • *persistent diarrhea* |
| S/S of anal fissures | • **tearing/cutting pain associated with defecation accompanied by bright red rectal bleeding,** • *location*— * 90% posteriorly located in anal canal, * 10% anteriorly located—particularly in women, • *triad of*— * anal canal ulcer, * hypertrophied column of Morgagni proximal to ulcer, * sentinel tag/pile distal to ulcer: fibrosed external hemorrhoid |
| Rx of anal fissures | • **sitz baths/stool softeners,** • *topical hydrocortisone cream,* • *surgery*—lateral anal sphincterotomy for chronic ulcers resistant to medical Rx |
| age brackets for rectal prolapse | *children <2 yrs old and elderly people* [**Note:** rectal prolapse is the intussusception of rectum through the anus.] |
| pathogenesis of rectal prolapse | **weak rectal support mechanisms**—e.g., peritoneum, musculature |
| causes of low rectovaginal fistulas | • **childbirth,** • *CD,* • *cryptoglandular abscess,* • *penetration by foreign object* |
| causes of midrectovaginal fistulas | • **ischiorectal abscess,** • *CD,* • *radiation* |
| causes of high rectovaginal fistulas | • **diverticulitis,** • *CD,* • *radiation* |

## Table 7–6. SMALL AND LARGE BOWEL DISEASE, DISORDERS OF THE APPENDIX, PERITONEAL DISORDERS *Continued*

| Most Common... | Answer and Explanation |
|---|---|
| site for anorectal abscesses/fistulas | **abscess of anal glands that empty into the crypts at the base of the columns of Morgagni**—ducts and glands penetrate to varying degrees into the anal canal, internal anal sphincter, and intersphincteric space between external and internal anal sphincter |
| causes of anorectal abscesses/fistulas | • **trauma**— * hard stools, * excessive diarrhea, * anal intercourse, * radiation, • *CD* [**Note:** the internal opening of the fistula is located in the anal crypts at the dentate line. The external opening of the fistula is where it exits on the perineum.] |
| S/S of anorectal abscesses/fistulas | • **rectal pain with purulent perianal discharge,** • *tender rectal mass on rectal exam,* • *fever* |
| external openings of anorectal fistulas | • **opening posterior to transverse anal line drawn in a coronal plane**— * internal opening of fistula is in a posterior midline crypt, * complicated fistulas penetrate into the deep ischiorectal spaces: e.g., ischiorectal abscess, • *opening anterior to transverse anal line drawn in a coronal plane*—internal opening of fistula is located in a direct radial line to the nearest crypt [**Note:** the location of the internal opening in relation to the location of the external opening is called Goodsall's rule.] |
| Rx of anorectal abscesses/fistulas | **fistulotomy** |
| causes of pruritus ani | • **poor cleansing of perianal region,** • *dietary factors*— * caffeine products, * chocolate, * spicy foods, • *infections*— * pinworm, * fungal, • *tight clothing,* • *diarrheal states*— * IBD, * CD, * lactase deficiency, • *skin disorders*— * contact dermatitis from topical anesthetics, * antibiotics, • *systemic diseases*—DM |
| cause of a pilonidal abscess | **excess hair in a deep gluteal fold becomes traumatically buried into a sinus** |
| symptom of a pilonidal abscess | **painful sacrococcygeal mass with purulent drainage** |

*Table continued on following page*

### Table 7–6. SMALL AND LARGE BOWEL DISEASE, DISORDERS OF THE APPENDIX, PERITONEAL DISORDERS *Continued*

| Most Common... | Answer and Explanation |
| --- | --- |
| Rx of a pilonidal abscess | **incision and drainage** |

**Question:** Which of the following gastrointestinal disorders are commonly associated with obstruction? **SELECT 7**

    (A) Ulcerative colitis
    (B) Gallstone ileus
    (C) Cecal cancer
    (D) Intussusception
    (E) Volvulus
    (F) Diverticulosis
    (G) Ogilvie's syndrome
    (H) Angiodysplasia
    (I) Ileal carcinoid tumor
    (J) Direct inguinal hernia
    (K) Chronic ischemic colitis
    (L) Hirschsprung's disease
    (M) Tubular adenoma
    (N) Previous abdominal surgery

**Answers: (B), (D), (E), (I), (K), (L), (N).** Unlike the transmural inflammation associated with CD leading to obstruction in the terminal ileum, the mucosal and submucosal inflammation associated with ulcerative colitis is not associated with obstruction **(choice A is incorrect)**. Gallstone ileus is associated with obstruction at the ileocecal valve from a gallstone derived from a fistulous communication of the gallbladder with the small bowel **(choice B is correct)**. Cecal cancer rarely obstructs owing to the increased diameter of the cecum **(choice C is incorrect)**. Intussusception and volvulus both cause obstruction and strangulation of bowel **(choice D and E are correct)**. Diverticulosis, per se, does not produce obstruction; however, diverticulitis may cause obstruction **(choice F is incorrect)**. Ogilvie's syndrome is a painless pseudo-obstruction of the colon seen in bedridden elderly patients **(choice G is incorrect)**. Angiodysplasia is a vascular ectasia of the cecum and right colon and does not obstruct **(choice H is incorrect)**. Carcinoid tumors of the ileum commonly kink the bowel owing to fibrosis in the intestinal wall secondary to serotonin **(choice I is correct)**. Direct inguinal hernias, unlike indirect inguinal hernias, rarely incarcerate the bowel leading to obstruction **(choice J is incorrect)**. Chronic ischemic colitis commonly leads to stricture formation at the splenic flexure **(choice K is correct)**. Hirschsprung's disease produces a functional obstruction in the rectum owing to absence of ganglion cells and aperistalsis **(choice L is correct)**. Tubular adenomas, the most common neoplastic polyp in the GI tract, do not cause obstruction **(choice M is incorrect)**. Adhesions secondary to previous abdominal surgery are the most common cause of obstruction in the small bowel **(choice N is correct)**.

AD = autosomal dominant, AP = alkaline phosphatase, APC = adenomatous polyposis coli, APKD = adult polycystic kidney disease, APR = abdominoperineal resection, AR = autosomal recessive, AS = ankylosing spondylitis, ASA = aminosalicylic acid, ASAP = as soon as possible, CD = Crohn's disease, CEA = carcinoembryonic antigen, COPD = chronic obstructive pulmonary disease, DM = diabetes mellitus, FOBT = fecal occult blood testing, FP = false-positive, FR = free radical, FU = fluorouracil, GB = gallbladder, GGT = gamma glutamyl transferase, G/M = gross and microscopic, 5-HIAA = 5-hydroxyindoleacetic acid, HLA = human leukocyte antigen, HPV = human papilloma virus, HTN = hypertension, IBD = inflammatory bowel disease, IMA = inferior mesenteric artery, LAR = low anterior resection, LFTs = liver function tests, LLQ = left lower quadrant, LUQ = left upper quadrant, MC = most common, MCC = most common cause, MP = mercaptopurine, NG = nasogastric, N/V = nausea/vomiting, PH = portal hypertension, PID = pelvic inflammatory disease, PJ = Peutz-Jeghers, PRV = polycythemia rubra vera, PSC = primary sclerosing cholangitis, PSS = progressive systemic sclerosis, PUD = peptic ulcer disease, PV = portal vein, RLQ = right lower quadrant, R/O = rule out, SCC = squamous cell carcinoma, SMA = superior mesenteric artery, SMV = superior mesenteric vein, S/S = signs and symptoms, UA = urinalysis, UC = ulcerative colitis, UGI = upper gastrointestinal tract, UTI = urinary tract infection.

# CHAPTER

8

# HEPATOBILIARY/PANCREATIC SURGERY

## CONTENTS

### Table 8–1. LABORATORY TESTS IN LIVER DISEASE

| Most Common... | Answer and Explanation |
|---|---|
| indices of hepatocellular injury | **transaminases**— * *AST,* * *ALT* [**Note:** ALT is more specific for liver disease than AST since it is localized to the liver. In acute hepatitis, transaminases range from 500–5000 U/L. In chronic hepatitis, transaminases are <500 U/L, because the amount of liver parenchyma is reduced.] |
| transaminase pattern in viral hepatitis | **ALT is higher than AST**— * ALT is the last transaminase to return to normal, * transaminases increase early in hepatitis and then decrease as bilirubin increases |
| transaminase pattern in alcohol-related liver disease | **AST is higher than ALT**— * alcohol is a mitochondrial poison, * AST is located in mitochondria, hence its preferential increase over ALT, which locates in the cytosol |
| types of cholestasis | • **extrahepatic**—e.g., * CBD stone, * carcinoma of head of pancreas, • *intrahepatic*—e.g., * **hepatitis,** * drugs |
| indices of cholestasis or infiltrative liver disease | • **ALP,** • *GGT* [**Note:** both enzymes are synthesized by bile duct epithelium in the presence of increased local levels of bile acids related to obstruction. Liver infiltration by amyloid raises the ALP. Metastatic tumor or granulomas also raise the ALP.] |
| sources of ALP | • **liver**— * 65%, * heat-stable enzyme, • *bone*— * heat-labile enzyme, * only increased during osteoblastic activity, • *intestine,* • *placenta* |

*Table continued on following page*

## Table 8–1. LABORATORY TESTS IN LIVER DISEASE
*Continued*

| Most Common... | Answer and Explanation |
|---|---|
| liver enzyme increased by drugs enhancing the microsomal system | **GGT**—e.g., * **alcohol,** * barbiturates [**Note:** enhancing the microsomal system increases the metabolism of drugs.] |
| method of determining the origin of ALP (e.g., liver versus bone) | **measurement of GGT**— * if both ALP and GGT are increased, ALP is most likely of liver origin, * if GGT is normal, ALP is most likely from another source: e.g., bone, placenta |
| index of liver excretion | **total bilirubin with fractionation into CB and UCB**—fractionation is expressed as CB%: CB = CB/TB × 100) |
| source of UCB | **destruction of senescent RBCs by BM macrophages** [**Note:** UCB is the end-product of Hgb breakdown. When released from the macrophage, UCB binds with albumin in the blood. Since it is lipid-soluble and bound to albumin, UCB cannot enter the urine. UCB is taken up by the hepatocytes and conjugated into CB (water-soluble). CB is secreted into bile canaliculi, enters the CBD, and is stored and concentrated in the GB. In the terminal ileum and colon, CB is converted into UCB. UCB is further reduced to UBG (colorless) and then oxidized to urobilin, which is responsible for the stool color. ~20% of UBG is reabsorbed into the circulation, the majority of which is recycled to the liver (90%), and the remainder enters the urine. Urobilin produces the normal color of urine.] |
| initial site of visible jaundice | **sclera**— * sclera has increased elastic tissue, which has an increased affinity for UCB or CB, * visible scleral icterus is present when TB is ≥2.0 mg/dL |
| cause of jaundice in the United States | **HAV** |
| bilirubin patterns for jaundice | • **CB < 20%**— * primarily UCB, * examples: ♦ **extravascular hemolysis,** ♦ decreased uptake or conjugation of UCB, • **CB 20–50%**— * mixed UCB and CB, * examples: ♦ hepatitis, ♦ cirrhosis, • **CB > 50%**— * intra- and extrahepatic cholestasis, * e.g., CBD stone |

## Table 8–1. LABORATORY TESTS IN LIVER DISEASE
*Continued*

| Most Common... | Answer and Explanation |
|---|---|
| urine bilirubin (UB) and urobilinogen (UBG) findings in jaundice | <table><tr><td></td><td>**UB**</td><td>**Urine UBG**</td><td>**Cause**</td></tr><tr><td>*Normal*:</td><td>negative</td><td>slight increase</td><td>—</td></tr><tr><td>*CB < 20%*:</td><td>negative</td><td>increased</td><td>EHA\*</td></tr><tr><td>*CB 20–50%*:</td><td>increased</td><td>increased</td><td>viral hepatitis</td></tr><tr><td>*CB > 50%*:</td><td>increased</td><td>absent</td><td>cholestasis</td></tr></table> <br> \*EHA = extravascular hemolytic anemia |
| cause of overproduction of UCB (CB% < 20%) | **extravascular hemolysis**—e.g., \* congenital spherocytosis, \* sickle cell anemia, \* severe thalassemia, \* folate/B$_{12}$ deficiency, \* AIHA |
| genetic cause of an increase in UCB (CB% < 20%) | **Gilbert's disease**— \* AD disease occurring in ~7% of the population, \* MCC of nonhemolytic increase in UCB, \* second MCC of jaundice in the United States |
| defects in Gilbert's disease | • **problem with uptake and conjugation of UCB**—CB < 20%, • *minor element of RBC hemolysis,* • *liver Bx is unnecessary*—normal |
| test used to Dx Gilbert's disease | **have the patient fast and note doubling of the TB over the baseline value**—Gilbert's disease has no clinical significance |
| adult causes of impaired conjugation of UCB | • **viral hepatitis,** • *cirrhosis* |
| genetic causes of a defect in the canalicular transport system (CB% > 50%) | • **Dubin-Johnson syndrome**— \* AR disease, \* black liver–nonmelanin pigment, \* nonvisualization of GB with OCG, • *Rotor's syndrome*— \* AR disease, \* normal-colored liver, \* normal OCG [**Note:** both disorders have an excellent prognosis.] |
| acquired causes of a CB% 20–50% | • **viral hepatitis,** • *alcoholic hepatitis* |
| acquired cause of a CB% > 50% | • **extrahepatic cholestasis**—e.g., \* **stone in CBD,** \* carcinoma of the head of pancreas, \* PSC, • *intrahepatic cholestasis*—e.g., \* drugs, \* pregnancy |

*Table continued on following page*

### Table 8–1. LABORATORY TESTS IN LIVER DISEASE
*Continued*

| Most Common... | Answer and Explanation |
|---|---|
| cause of a dark urine in viral hepatitis | **increase in UBG and CB** [**Note:** an inflamed liver has problems with uptake/conjugation of UCB. Liver cell necrosis with disruption of bile canaliculi occurs (release of CB into the blood → urine).] |
| cause of a dark urine in extravascular hemolysis | **increased UBG** [**Note:** increased production of UBG occurs, owing to increased production of UCB secondary to macrophage destruction of RBCs. When recycled, proportionately more UBG enters the urine.] |
| cause of a dark urine in cholestasis | **CB** [**Note:** both intra- and extrahepatic cholestasis lead to a backflow of CB into the hepatocytes, with leakage into the blood. UBG is absent in the urine as it is in the stool (clay-colored stool).] |
| initial step in the evaluation of jaundice | **US**— * detects dilated intrahepatic (normally <4 mm) and extrahepatic bile ducts (normally <10 mm), * detects GB stones |
| radiologic test to identify the cause and location of extrahepatic obstruction | **CT scan** |
| radiologic tests used for direct visualization of the biliary tree | • **PTC**— * excellent for proximal lesions causing obstruction, * better success in identifying site of obstruction if the ducts are dilated, • *ERCP*— * excellent for distal lesions causing obstruction, * excellent for localizing obstruction whether or not ducts dilated |
| indices of severity of liver disease | • **PT,** • *serum albumin* [**Note:** the PT is increased owing to decreased synthesis of coagulation factors; the best index of severity. Albumin is decreased owing to reduced synthesis. It contributes to ascites (decreased oncotic pressure) and peripheral pitting edema.] |
| cause of a drop in transaminases and increase in duration of PT | **fulminant liver failure** |

*Table continued on following page*

## Table 8–1. LABORATORY TESTS IN LIVER DISEASE
*Continued*

| Most Common... | Answer and Explanation |
|---|---|
| autoantibodies in liver disease | • **antimitochondrial**—PBC, • *antismooth muscle*—AH type I, • *antinuclear antibodies*—AH type I, • *antiliver/kidney/muscle*—AH type II |
| tumor markers | • **AFP**—marker for HCC, • *AAT*—marker for HCC |
| cause of an increase in lipoprotein X | **cholestatic jaundice**—lipoprotein X is high in free (unesterified) CH owing to reduced synthesis of lecithin-cholesterol acyltransferase (LCAT) |
| cause of a β–γ bridge on SPE | **alcoholic cirrhosis** [Note: both IgG and IgA increase in alcoholic cirrhosis. IgA migrates to the junction of the β and γ-globulin region of the SPE. Hence, when IgA is increased, it fills in the normal demarcation separating the two peaks.] |
| lab findings in extravascular hemolytic anemia | • **normal ALT,** • ↑ ↑ **AST**—present in RBCs, • **normal ALP,** • **normal GGT,** • ↑ **TB,** • **CB% < 20%,** • ↑ ↑ **urine UBG**—more UBG is synthesized in the colon due to more CB from metabolism of excess UCB, • **no urine bilirubin** [Note: TB is rarely >5 mg/dL in extravascular hemolysis.] |
| lab findings in viral hepatitis (arrows indicate magnitude) | • ↑ ↑ ↑ **ALT,** • ↑ ↑ **AST,** • ↑ **ALP,** • ↑ **GGT,** • ↑ **TB,** • **CB% 20–50%,** • ↑ ↑ **urine UBG,** • ↑ ↑ **urine bilirubin**—bile ducts in the liver are disrupted and CB has contact with the sinusoidal blood |
| lab findings in obstructive jaundice | • ↑ ↑ **ALT,** • ↑ **AST,** • ↑ ↑ ↑ **ALP,** • ↑ ↑ ↑ **GGT,** • ↑ ↑ **TB,** • **CB% > 50%,** • **absent urine UBG,** • ↑ ↑ **urine bilirubin**— * CB in bile backs up into the hepatocytes and out into the blood, * stool is clay-colored |
| lab findings in alcoholic hepatitis | • ↑ ↑ **AST,** • ↑ **ALT,** • ↑ ↑ **ALP,** • ↑ ↑ ↑ **GGT,** • ↑ **TB,** • **CB% 20–50%,** • ↑ **urine UBG,** • ↑ **urine bilirubin** |

*Table continued on following page*

## Table 8–1. LABORATORY TESTS IN LIVER DISEASE
*Continued*

| Most Common... | Answer and Explanation |
|---|---|
| lab findings in focal metastatic disease to liver | • **normal ALT,** • **normal AST,** • ↑ **ALP,** • ↑ **GGT,** • ↑ ↑ **LDH,** • **normal TB** [Note: focal liver disease does not produce enough necrosis to elevate transaminases or bile duct compression to produce cholestasis. LDH is a nonspecific tumor marker. In benign disease (e.g., granulomas), the LDH is normal.] |

**Question:** You would expect a patient with a complete obstruction of the common bile duct by a stone to produce which of the following laboratory abnormalities? **SELECT 3**
  (A) Dark stools
  (B) UBG in the urine
  (C) palpable GB
  (D) CB% > 50%
  (E) Hypertriglyceridemia
  (F) ALP proportionately greater than ALT
  (G) AST > ALT
  (H) CB in the urine

**Answers: (D), (F), (H).** Complete obstruction of the CBD causes bile containing CH and CB to back up into the liver and into the blood **(choice D is correct)**. Hence, CB% is > 50%, and hypercholesterolemia occurs **(choice E is incorrect)**. There is usually no enlargement of the GB, since most stones derive from chronically inflamed gallbladders. Hence, increased CBD pressure is unlikely to distend the thickened GB wall **(choice C is incorrect)**. Complete CBD obstruction also leads to clay-colored stools owing to a lack of UBG in the stool and urine **(choices A and B are incorrect)**. There is proportionately greater increase in ALP than ALT **(choice F is correct)**. Serum ALT is greater than AST **(choice G is incorrect)**. CB in the blood also enters the urine **(choice H is correct)**.

AAT = α₁-antitrypsin, AD = autosomal dominant, AFP = α-fetoprotein, AH = autoimmune hepatitis, AIHA = autoimmune hemolytic anemia, ALP = alkaline phosphatase, ALT = alanine transaminase, AR = autosomal recessive, AST = aspartate transaminase, BM = bone marrow, Bx = biopsy, CB = conjugated bilirubin, CBD = common bile duct, CH = cholesterol, EHA = extravascular hemolytic anemia, ERCP = endoscopic retrograde cholecystopancreatography, GB = gallbladder, GGT = γ-glutamyltransferase, HAV = hepatitis A virus, HCC = hepatocellular carcinoma, LCAT = lecithin-cholesterol acyltransferase, LDH = lactate dehydrogenase, MCC = most common cause, OCG = oral cholecystogram, PBC = primary biliary cirrhosis, PSC = primary sclerosing cholangitis, PT = prothrombin time, PTC = percutaneous transhepatic cholangiography, SPE = serum protein electrophoresis, TB = total bilirubin, UB = urine bilirubin, UBG = urobilinogen, UCB = unconjugated bilirubin.

## Table 8–2. LIVER DISORDERS

| Most Common... | Answer and Explanation |
|---|---|
| cause of hematobilia | **trauma to the liver**—hematobilia refers to blood in the bile |
| cause of segmental dilatation of intrahepatic bile ducts | **Caroli's disease**— * AR disease, * commonly associated with portal tract fibrosis, * associated with both AR and AD polycystic kidney disease, * increased incidence of cholangiocarcinoma |
| complications of Caroli's disease | • **intrahepatic cholelithiasis,** • *cholangitis,* • *hepatic abscesses,* • *PH* |
| cystic disease of the liver | **polycystic liver disease**— * AD disease, * associated with AD adult polycystic kidney disease, * abdominal pain |
| types of hepatitis that can recur in transplanted livers | • **HBV,** • **HDV** |
| types of viral hepatitis with the greatest risk for chronic disease | • **HCV**— * 70–90%, * risk increases in alcoholics, * more likely to become chronic if secondary to blood transfusion, • *HBV*— * 5–10%, * risk increases with alcohol |
| types of hepatitis associated with HCC | • **HBV,** • *HCV*—antibodies found in 40–60% of patients with HCC |
| type of viral hepatitis presenting without jaundice | **HCV** |
| types of viral hepatitis with a serum sickness–like prodrome | • **HBV,** • *HCV* [**Note:** patients may present with urticaria, vasculitis (PAN relationship), polyarthritis, or glomerulonephritis. It is a type III immunocomplex disease.] |
| types of chronic hepatitis that progress to cirrhosis | • **HBV**—~40%, • *HCV*—~30% |
| type of chronic hepatitis with fluctuation of ALT levels | **HCV** |
| cause of post-transfusion hepatitis | **HCV**—1:3300 risk per unit [**Note:** HBV has a 1:200,000 risk per unit.] |

*Table continued on following page*

Table 8–2. LIVER DISORDERS *Continued*

| Most Common... | Answer and Explanation |
|---|---|
| infection transmitted by an accidental needle stick | **HBV**—HBV has a greater viral burden in blood than other types of hepatitis have |
| beneficial effects of HBV immunization | **prevents • HBV, • HDV,** • *HCC secondary to HBV-related postnecrotic cirrhosis* |
| clinical phases of viral hepatitis | • **prodromal phase,** • **icteric phase,** • **recovery phase** |
| S/S of prodromal phase | • **fatigue,** • *"flulike" symptoms,* • *serum sickness–like symptoms*—see above, • *RUQ pain/ tenderness,* • *low-grade fever*—particularly HAV, • *transaminases progressively increase*—peak just before jaundice appears and then begin declining as jaundice declines, • *bilirubinuria before jaundice appears*—due to lower renal threshold for bilirubin, • *neutropenia with atypical lymphocytosis* |
| S/S of icteric phase | • **jaundice**— * most types of hepatitis are anicteric, * jaundice, if present, persists for 1–4 wks, • *pruritus*— * 50%, * due to deposition of bile salts in the skin, • *dark urine*—bilirubinuria, • *light stools*— * mild cholestasis occurs initially in viral hepatitis, * reduced bile flow decreases production of UBG, • *WBC count begins returning to normal,* • *constitutional symptoms lessen* |
| S/S of recovery phase | • **return of appetite,** • **decreased jaundice,** • **bile disappears from urine,** • **decreased abdominal pain,** • **decreased fatigue** |
| lab findings in viral hepatitis | • **leukopenia in prodromal phase with atypical lymphocytosis,** • **bilirubinuria before jaundice,** • **acholic stools with jaundice,** • **increased ALT/AST**—see above, • **slight increase in ALP/GGT**—particularly in HAV, • **hypoglycemia**— * 50%, * decreased glycogen stores |
| markers of active HBV, HCV | • **HBsAg,** • **anti-HCV,** respectively |
| markers of infectivity in HBV | • **HBV–DNA,** • **HBe-Ag** |

**Table 8–2. LIVER DISORDERS** *Continued*

| Most Common... | Answer and Explanation |
|---|---|
| sequence of antigens and antibodies in HBV | **HBsAg:** not infective, → HBeAg and HBV-DNA: * infective, → anti-HBc-IgM: indicator of viral replication → loss of HBeAg and HBV-DNA → loss of HBsAg: * not infective, * occurs in 90%, → persistence of anti-HBc-IgM in the window period when anti-HBs is not present: called the serologic gap → anti-HBs: protective antibody, → anti-HBc-IgG: marker of patient who has recovered from HBV, → anti-HBe: reflects low infectivity |
| definition for chronic HBV | **persistence of HBsAg >6 mos** |
| serologic marker of someone who has received recombinant HBV vaccine | **anti-HBs** |
| cause of a positive HBsAg, positive HBeAg/HBV-DNA, positive anti-HBc-IgM | **acute HBV**—high infectivity |
| cause of a negative HBsAg, HBeAg/HBV-DNA, positive anti-HBc-IgM, negative anti-HBs | **patient recovering from HBV who is in the serologic gap**—patient is not infective, since HBeAg and HBV-DNA are absent |
| serologic markers in a patient who has recovered from HBV | • **anti-HBs,** • **anti-HBc-IgG** |
| cause of a positive HBsAg, negative HBeAg, positive anti-HBc-IgG/IgM, positive anti-HBe | **chronic HBV with low infectivity** |
| cause of a positive HBsAg, positive HBeAg, positive anti-HBc-IgG/IgM, negative anti-HBe | **chronic HBV with high infectivity** |

*Table continued on following page*

Table 8–2. **LIVER DISORDERS** *Continued*

| Most Common... | Answer and Explanation |
|---|---|
| lab tests in HCV | • **screen**— * second-generation ELISA test, * positive in 2–6 wks, * ~40% sensitivity, * high FP rate in low-prevalence areas, * presence of antibody indicates infection, • **confirm**—positive ELISA is confirmed with * **RIBA:** more specific but less sensitive than ELISA, * HCV-RNA by PCR: gold standard for Dx of HCV |
| Rx of acute hepatitis | • **supportive,** • **no need to isolate,** • **handwashing precautions,** • **enteric precautions with HAV,** • **no recapping of needles** |
| prevention modalities for HBV | • **HBV recombinant vaccine**— * all children, * sexually active adolescents not previously immunized, * adults in high-risk groups: ♦ homosexuals, ♦ health care workers, ♦ travelers to high-risk countries, ♦ household contacts of HBV carriers, • *HBIG*— * intimate contacts of patients who are positive for HBsAg or those with needle stick exposure, * mucous membrane exposure of blood from HBsAg-positive patients |
| prevention modalities for exposure to HCV | **? ISG** |
| pathogenesis of ascending cholangitis | **infection (usually *E. coli*) ascends from an obstructed CBD (stone or stricture) into the portal triads** |
| S/S of ascending cholangitis | **Charcot's triad of fever, jaundice, RUQ pain** [**Note:** Reynold's pentad is the above plus shock and mental confusion.] |
| Rx of ascending cholangitis | • **decompression of bilary tract—ERCP** or placement of drainage catheter, • **antibiotics**—aminoglycosides should be avoided in jaundiced patients owing to a greater chance for nephrotoxicity |
| causes of a liver abscess in the United States | • **ascending cholangitis,** • *intra-abdominal infection*—e.g., spread via the portal vein, * diverticulitis, * bowel perforation, • *direct extension*—e.g., * empyema of GB, * subphrenic abscess, • *hematogenous spread*—e.g., bacterial endocarditis [**Note:** most liver abscesses are solitary (50%). An amebic abscess is the most common cause world-wide.] |

**Table 8–2. LIVER DISORDERS** *Continued*

| Most Common... | Answer and Explanation |
|---|---|
| organisms isolated in liver abscesses | • **gram-negative aerobes**—e.g., *E. coli,* • *anaerobes*—e.g., *Bacteroides fragilis,* • *gram-positive aerobes*—e.g., *Streptococcus fecalis* [**Note:** most liver abscesses are located in the right lobe.] |
| S/S of liver abscess | • **spiking, intermittent fever,** • *RUQ or right CVA pain* [**Note:** jaundice is uncommon in liver abscesses.] |
| initial lab test in the work-up of a liver abscess | **US**—less expensive and better for distinguishing cystic from solid masses in the liver than CT |
| Rx of pyogenic liver abscess | • **percutaneous drainage,** • **antibiotics**—e.g., * metronidazole—covers anaerobes, also covers the possibility of amebic abscess, * ampicillin: covers enterococcus, * aminoglycoside with anti-pseudomonal coverage: covers gram-negative aerobes |
| site for an intra-abdominal abscess | **below the diaphragm** |
| causes of a subdiaphragmatic abscess | • **perforated appendicitis,** • *acute cholecystitis,* • *perforated PUD,* • *acute pancreatitis* |
| diagnostic test to detect an intra-abdominal abscess | • **CT scan**—95% sensitivity, • *US*—80% sensitivity, • *plain x-rays*— * ~50% sensitivity, * raised hemidiaphragm, • *radionuclide scan*—80% sensitivity |
| world-wide cause of a hepatic abscess | ***Entamoeba histolytica***—see discussion in Table 7–4 |
| cause of "sheep herder's" disease | ***Echinococcus granulosis* or *multilocularis* (cestode tapeworm)** |
| pathogenesis of echinococcosis | • dog ingests larvae in the meat of an infected sheep (sheep intermediate host) → • larvae develop into adults and lay eggs (dog definitive host) → • eggs are unintentionally transmitted to the sheep herder → eggs develop into larvae, which penetrate the bowel wall and enter the liver (sheep herder intermediate host) → produce hydatid cysts (single or multiple) containing scolices (called hydatid sand) [**Note:** rupture of a cyst can produce anaphylactic shock.] |

*Table continued on following page*

**Table 8–2. LIVER DISORDERS** *Continued*

| Most Common... | Answer and Explanation |
|---|---|
| method to Dx echinococcosis | • **calcified cysts on x-ray,** • **serology,** • **stool for O/P** |
| Rx for echinococcosis | • **albendazole,** • **surgery** |
| parasitic cause of cholangiocarcinoma | *Clonorchis sinensis* **(Chinese liver fluke)** |
| causes of hepatic vein thrombosis (Budd-Chiari syndrome) | • **polycythemia rubra vera,** • *oral contraceptives,* • *hypercoagulable states*—e.g., * AT III deficiency, * protein C and S deficiency |
| S/S of Budd-Chiari syndrome | • **rapid onset of ascites**—>90%, • *painful hepatomegaly,* • *splenomegaly* |
| method of Dx of Budd-Chiari syndrome | • **screen with Doppler US**— * 75% sensitivity in detecting thrombosis, * hypertrophy of caudate lobe, • **hepatic vein catheterization/ angiography**—gold standard |
| Rx of Budd-Chiari syndrome | • **surgical decompression**—side-to-side porto-systemic shunt: decompresses the hepatic limb of the PV, • **fibrinolytic Rx**—variable results, • **liver transplantation with post-transplant anticoagulation** [Note: high mortality.] |
| causes of portal vein thrombosis in adults | • **pylephlebitis**—e.g., * acute appendicitis, * diverticulitis, • *postliver transplant*—fulminant liver failure, • *cirrhosis,* • *HCC*—tumor invasion, • *PRV*—hypercoagulability, • *pancreatitis*—thrombosis of splenic vein with extension into portal vein |
| causes of PH | • **cirrhosis,** • *portal vein thrombosis*—prehepatic, • *Budd-Chiari syndrome*—posthepatic |
| causes of PH in cirrhosis | • **obstruction to portal vein blood flow**—intrasinusoidal obstruction by fibrosis and regenerative nodules, • **intrahepatic anastomoses between the hepatic arterial and venous systems** |

**Table 8–2. LIVER DISORDERS** *Continued*

| Most Common... | Answer and Explanation |
|---|---|
| causes of intrahepatic cholestasis | • **viral hepatitis**—early cholestatic phase, • **drugs**—e.g., oral contraceptives, • *PBC*, • *genetic*— * Dubin-Johnson, * see above, • *alcoholic hepatitis* |
| causes of extrahepatic cholestasis | • **stone in the CBD,** • *carcinoma of the head of pancreas,* • *PSC* |
| S/S of cholestasis | • **jaundice,** • *pruritus*—due to bile salt deposition in the skin, • *skin xanthomas*— * CH deposition, * CH is eliminated in bile and backs up into the blood with obstruction, • *hepatomegaly,* • *secondary biliary cirrhosis,* • *acholic stools*—absent urobilin, • *dark urine*— * CB, * no UBG |
| lab findings of cholestasis | • **marked elevation of ALP and GGT**—markers of cholestasis, • *mild to moderate increase in ALT and AST,* • *CB% > 50%,* • *hypercholesterolemia* |
| disease associated with PSC | **ulcerative colitis**—70% of cases |
| clinical findings in PSC | • **pathology**— * multifocal, obliterative fibrosis of extra-, intrahepatic bile ducts leading to: ♦ strictures (beading effect when a dye is injected into the common bile duct), ♦ obstruction, ♦ secondary biliary cirrhosis, * absence of interlobular bile ducts, • **sex predilection**—men > women, • **S/S**— * asymptomatic increase in serum ALP, * fatigue, * pruritus, * jaundice |
| confirmatory test for PSC | **ERCP** |
| Rx of PSC | • **drugs**—immunosuppressive agents: e.g., corticosteroids, • **surgery**— * relieve obstruction with stents, * bypass operations |
| morphologic types of cirrhosis | **mixed pattern**— * *micronodular:* nodules <3 mm, * *macronodular:* nodules >3 mm |
| causes of cirrhosis | • **alcohol-related liver disease,** • *postnecrotic cirrhosis*— * **HBV,** * HCV, • *hemochromatosis,* • *PBC,* • *Wilson's disease* |

*Table continued on following page*

**Table 8–2. LIVER DISORDERS** *Continued*

| Most Common... | Answer and Explanation |
|---|---|
| histologic findings in alcoholic cirrhosis | • **regenerative nodules surrounded by fibrosis**—nodules lack the normal cord-sinusoid-cord pattern of normal liver, as well as triads and THV, • **intrasinusoidal hypertension**— * overall reduction in sinusoids, * compression of existing sinusoids by regenerative nodules, • **anastomoses between venous and arterial system leading to PH** |
| coagulation defect associated with cirrhosis | **bleeding**— * decreased synthesis of coagulation factors: prolonged PT, * platelet dysfunction: decreased clearance of FDPs, * dysfibrinogenemia: abnormal fibrinogen |
| CNS abnormality in cirrhosis | **hepatic encephalopathy**— * Stage I: ♦ confusion, ♦ agitation, ♦ daytime/night-time reversal, ♦ asterixis (failure to sustain posture, flapping tremor), * Stage II: ♦ drowsiness, ♦ dysarthria, ♦ asterixis, ♦ primitive reflexes, * Stage III: ♦ somnolent but rousable, ♦ incomprehensible speech, ♦ marked confusion, ♦ hyperreflexia, ♦ myoclonus, ♦ hyperventilation, * Stage IV: ♦ coma, ♦ decerebrate, ♦ no response to stimuli |
| mechanism of mental status abnormalities in hepatic encephalopathy | • **increase in aromatic amino acids with subsequent conversion into false neurotransmitters**— * aromatic AAs include: ♦ phenylalanine, ♦ tyrosine, ♦ tryptophan, * false neurotransmitters that are synthesized include: ♦ GABA, ♦ phenylethanolamine, ♦ octopamine, • *increase in serum ammonia*, • *increase in mercaptans*, • *increase in short chain FAs* |
| factors precipitating hepatic encephalopathy | • **increased protein**— * dietary or blood in GI tract: increases bacterial conversion of urea into ammonia, • *alkalosis*—keeps ammonia in $NH_3$ state, which is easily reabsorbed into the portal vein: fewer $H^+$ ions in alkalosis is the reason for the increase in $NH_3$ over $NH_4$, • *diuretics*—produce metabolic alkalosis, • *sedatives*, • *portosystemic shunts*—shunt ammonia away from the liver, which normally metabolizes ammonia in the urea cycle |

## Table 8–2. LIVER DISORDERS *Continued*

| Most Common... | Answer and Explanation |
|---|---|
| Rx of hepatic encephalopathy | • **restrict protein intake**—reduces ammonia production by colonic bacteria, • *lactulose*— * $H^+$ ions released by colonic bacteria combine with diffusible $NH_3$ to produce nondiffusible $NH_4$ in the colon: $NH_4$ lost in the stool, * laxative effect causes loss of nitrogenous compounds, • *neomycin*—reduces colonic bacteria, • *branched-chain amino acids*—block the synthesis of false neurotransmitters, • *use aldosterone blockers for diuresis*—retains $H^+$ ions, so less $NH_3$ is formed, • *avoid sedatives/pain medications*— * oxazepam may be used in presence of agitation, * flumazenil has also been used |
| causes of ascites in cirrhosis | • **PH**— * see below, * increased hydrostatic pressure, • *hypoalbuminemia*— * decreased synthesis of albumin, * decreased oncotic pressure, • *secondary aldosteronism*— * inability to metabolize aldosterone, * RAA stimulation from decreased cardiac output |
| lab method of distinguishing ascites secondary to cirrhosis from exudates | • **serum albumin–PF albumin gradient**— * if the gradient is >1.1 g/dL, the fluid is a transudate compatible with cirrhosis, * if the gradient is <1.1, increased vessel permeability is the cause: e.g., ♦ peritonitis, ♦ malignancy, • *PF albumin*—if <2.5 g/dL: transudate, if > 2.5 g/dL: exudate |
| Rx of ascites | • **salt restriction,** • *diuretics*—spironolactone is the drug of choice: see above, • *paracentesis,* • *peritoneovenous shunt*— * redirects ascitic fluid back into the blood, * less expensive method of replacing albumin, • *transjugular intrahepatic portosystemic shunt (TIPS)*—connects hepatic vein with portal vein via a stent |
| complications of PH | • **ascites**—see above, • *esophageal varices*— * see Table 7–1, * varices are dilated left gastric vein + azygos vein, • *periumbilical varices*—caput medusae, • *hemorrhoids,* • *congestive splenomegaly*—hypersplenism leading to cytopenias |

*Table continued on following page*

Table 8–2. **LIVER DISORDERS** *Continued*

| Most Common... | Answer and Explanation |
|---|---|
| Rx of PH | **shunting—** * portacaval shunt, * mesocaval shunt: connection of SMV with PV, * spleno-renal: ♦ most physiologic shunt, ♦ reduces PH and bleeding from varices without bypassing the liver |
| types of shunts used in Rx of PH | • **total portosystemic shunts—** * end-to-side portacaval shunt: does not reduce hepatic si-nusoidal pressure, * side-to-side portacaval shunt: ♦ reduces hepatic sinusoidal pressure, ♦ Rx for Budd-Chiari syndrome, * central splenorenal shunt (Linton): end-to-side sple-norenal shunt, * mesocaval shunt: ♦ SMV anas-tomosed to IVC, ♦ good for PV thrombosis, ♦ less risk for hepatic encephalopathy than portacaval shunts, • *selective shunts*—distal splenorenal (Warren shunt): ♦ selective de-compression of esophageal varices via shunt connections with the short gastric veins and splenic parenchyma, ♦ most physiologic of the shunts, ♦ least risk for hepatic encepha-lopathy, • *TIPS*— * metal stent connects he-patic vein with PV, * reduces portal pressure, * increases risk for encephalopathy, * Rx of acute esophageal bleeds, * Rx for patients awaiting liver transplantation |
| complication of portacaval-type shunts | **hepatic encephalopathy**—bypassing drainage of PV blood into the liver leaves ammonia from the bowel unmetabolized by the liver |
| criteria used to establish perioperative risk in cirrhosis with PH | **Child's classification** |
| components of Child's classification | • **serum albumin**, • **ascites**, • **serum bilirubin**, • **encephalopathy**, • **nutritional status** |
| criteria for minimal surgical risk using Child's classification | • **serum albumin**—>3.5 g/dL, • **ascites**—none, • **serum bilirubin**—<2.0 mg/dL, • **encephalopathy**—none, • **nutritional status**—excellent |

### Table 8–2. LIVER DISORDERS *Continued*

| Most Common... | Answer and Explanation |
|---|---|
| criteria for moderate surgical risk using Child's classification | • **serum albumin**—3.0–3.5 g/dL, • ascites—some present that is easily controlled, • **serum bilirubin**—2.0–3.0 mg/dL, • **encephalopathy**—minimal, • **nutritional status**—good |
| criteria for poor surgical risk using Child's classification | • **serum albumin**—<3.0 g/dL, • **ascites**—poorly controlled, • **serum bilirubin**—>3.0 mg/dL, • **encephalopathy**—coma, • **nutritional status**—poor: e.g., muscle wasting |
| cause of hepatorenal syndrome in cirrhosis | **prerenal hypoperfusion secondary to vasoconstriction**— * ? role of increased endothelin: vasoconstrictor, * functional renal failure with preservation of tubular function: renal concentration intact, * occurs in 40–50% of patients with terminal cirrhosis associated with jaundice, ascites, and PH |
| lab findings in HRS | • **oliguria**, • **random UNa+ <10 mEq/L**—indicates intact tubular function, • **UOsm > 500 mOsm/kg**—indicates intact renal concentration, • **UCr/PCr ratio >30:1**, • **normal urine sediment exam**—absence of renal tubular casts, • **clinical recovery in 10%** [Note: renal transplantation reverses renal function to normal.] |
| causes of hyperestrinism in cirrhosis | • **increased aromatization of androstenedione (17-KS) into estrone in the adipose tissue**, • *decreased metabolism of estrogen* |
| signs of hyperestrinism in a man with cirrhosis | • **unilateral/bilateral gynecomastia**—breast tissue has different sensitivity to estrogen, • *female secondary sex characteristics*— * female distribution of pubic hair, * soft skin, • *palmar erythema*, • *spider angiomas*— * arteriovenous fistulas, * create a lot of shunting of blood, particularly in the lungs, • *testicular atrophy/impotence*— * increased estrogen, increases synthesis of SHBG, * SHBG has an increased affinity for free testosterone |

*Table continued on following page*

Table 8–2. **LIVER DISORDERS** Continued

| Most Common... | Answer and Explanation |
|---|---|
| acid-base abnormalities in cirrhosis | • **chronic respiratory alkalosis**—toxic products overstimulate the respiratory center, • **lactic acidosis**—liver cannot metabolize lactic acid, • **hypokalemia**—due to secondary aldosteronism |
| lab findings in cirrhosis | • **low BUN/high ammonia**—dysfunctional urea cycle, • **hypoglycemia**— * defective gluconeogenesis, * low glycogen stores, • *low UNa⁺*— * decreased EABV, * secondary aldosteronism, • **mixed ABG disorders**—chronic respiratory alkalosis + metabolic acidosis (lactic), • **increased PT**—decreased coagulation factor synthesis, • **hypoalbuminemia**—decreased synthesis, • *hypocalcemia*— * hypoalbuminemia, * vitamin D deficiency from decreased first hydroxylation |
| tumor-like condition in the liver | **focal nodular hyperplasia (FNH)** [Note: there is a 2:1 female/male ratio. Etiology is unknown. FNH has no clinical significance.] |
| clinical features of FNH | • **pathogenesis**— * non-neoplastic, * probable reaction to injury, • **2:1 female/male ratio**, • **gross**—nodular mass with a central stellate scar with wagon-wheel radiations of fibrous tissue out to the periphery, • **S/S**—usually incidental finding, • **CT**—hypervascular with AV connections, • **Rx**—leave alone unless associated with pain |
| benign tumor of the liver | **cavernous hemangioma**—best diagnosed with enhanced CT |
| benign tumor of liver associated with intraperitoneal hemorrhage | **liver cell adenoma** [Note: may rupture during pregnancy. Liver cell adenomas also occur in von Gierke's glycogenosis. Adenomas are hypovascular on liver scans.] |
| clinical features of liver cell adenomas | • **pathogenesis**— * **oral contraceptives**, * **anabolic steroids**, * von Gierke's glycogenosis, • **female > male**, • **gross**—unencapsulated, smooth-surfaced mass, • **S/S**— * intraperitoneal hemorrhage while taking above medications or in pregnancy, * palpable hepatic mass, • **Rx**— * commonly regress when above drugs are discontinued, * resect if symptomatic |

## Table 8–2. LIVER DISORDERS *Continued*

| Most Common... | Answer and Explanation |
|---|---|
| liver malignancy | **metastasis**—primary sites include: * **lung,** * colorectal, * pancreas, * stomach, * breast |
| primary liver malignancy | **HCC** |
| causes of HCC | • **postnecrotic cirrhosis secondary to HBV**—enhanced risk with aflatoxins: food spoilage molds, • *postnecrotic cirrhosis secondary to HCV,* • *hemochromatosis,* • *alcoholic cirrhosis,* • *birth control pills,* • *Wilson's disease,* • *AAT deficiency,* • *hereditary tyrosinemia*—highest overall chance for HCC though a rare inborn error of metabolism [**Note:** the majority develop in a background of cirrhosis.] |
| G/M features of HCC | • **gross**—soft, hemorrhagic mass(es) with central necrosis and vessel invasion: ♦ unifocal, ♦ multifocal, ♦ diffusely infiltrative, • **microscopic**— * tumor cells with bile, * tumor giant cells |
| S/S of HCC | • **abdominal pain,** • *abdominal mass,* • *fever/ weight loss/fatigue,* • *bloody ascites*—due to: ♦ tumor invasion of the hepatic/portal vein, ♦ hemorrhage from tumor, • *paraneoplastic syndromes*— * polycythemia: EPO, * hypoglycemia: insulin-like factor, * gynecomastia, * hypercalcemia: PTH-like peptide |
| lab findings in HCC | • **increased AFP**— * tumor marker, * 30–50%: higher sensitivity in African, Far Eastern HCC, * >500 ng/mL, • *increased serum AAT*—tumor marker, • *sudden increase in serum ALP/GGT*—very characteristic, • *ectopic hormones*—see above |
| radiographic findings in HCC | • **CT/US**—localizes HCC, • *angiography*—pooling and increased vascularity |
| Rx of HCC | • **surgery**—<20% are surgical candidates, • *liver transplantation,* • *radiation*—not useful, • *chemotherapy*—not useful, • *prognosis*—majority die within 6 mos of Dx |

*Table continued on following page*

## Table 8–2. LIVER DISORDERS *Continued*

| Most Common... | Answer and Explanation |
|---|---|
| clinical features of fibrolamellar type of HCC | • **age/gender**—young men/women between 20 and 40 yrs, • **pathogenesis**—no relationship to cirrhosis or HBV, • **microscopic**—dense collagen bundles, • **prognosis**—better than usual type of HCC: 60% 5-yr survival |
| causes of cholangiocarcinoma | • **PSC,** • *Clonorchis sinensis,* • *Caroli's disease,* • *Hx of choledochal cyst* [**Note:** cirrhosis is not a prerequisite for cholangiocarcinoma, an adenocarcinoma of the bile ducts.] |
| locations for cholangiocarcinoma | • **ampulla/common bile duct**—associated with painless jaundice and Courvoisier's sign, • *junction of right/left hepatic duct*— * called Klatskin's tumor, * poorest prognosis owing to proximal location, • *intrahepatic* |
| S/S of cholangiocarcinoma | • **obstructive jaundice,** • *hepatomegaly,* • *Courvoisier's sign*—proximal to mid-CBD tumors |
| Rx of cholangiocarcinoma | **surgical resection**—distal and mid-CBD tumors are more often resectable than are proximally located cancers |
| causes of angiosarcoma | • **polyvinyl chloride,** • *arsenic,* • *Thorotrast* |
| causes of acute peritonitis | • **ruptured viscus**—e.g., * duodenal ulcer, * diverticula, * appendix, • *ruptured cyst*—e.g., benign follicular cyst, • *ischemic bowel,* • *spontaneous*— * ascites in alcoholic cirrhosis: *E. coli,* * ascites in a child with nephrotic syndrome: *S. pneumoniae* |
| S/S of spontaneous bacterial peritonitis in adults | • **fever,** • **abdominal pain,** • **abdominal tenderness** [**Note:** SBP occurs in 10–20% of cirrhotics with ascites.] |
| lab findings in SBP | • **PF leukocytes >250 cells/μL,** • *positive Gram stain*— * *E. coli:* fat gram-negative rod, * *Streptococcus pneumoniae:* gram-positive diplococcus |

## Table 8–2. LIVER DISORDERS *Continued*

**Question:** Which of the following conditions are associated with a conjugated bilirubin >50% of the total bilirubin? **SELECT 3**
- (A) Budd-Chiari syndrome
- (B) Klatskin's tumor
- (C) Primary sclerosing cholangitis
- (D) Liver cell adenoma
- (E) Alcoholic cirrhosis
- (F) Hepatocellular carcinoma
- (G) Metastatic liver disease
- (H) Gilbert's disease
- (I) Ascending cholangitis
- (J) Focal nodular hyperplasia

**Answers: (B), (C), (I).** The Budd-Chiari syndrome is not usually associated with jaundice (choice A is incorrect). Klatskin's tumor is a cholangiocarcinoma at the junction of the right and left hepatic ducts (choice B is correct). PSC is associated with fibrosis and strictures of the bile ducts leading to obstructive jaundice (choice C is correct). A liver cell adenoma is a benign tumor that is not associated with jaundice (choice D is incorrect). It has a tendency for rupturing and producing intraperitoneal hemorrhage. Alcoholic cirrhosis is usually associated with a mixed type of jaundice, with a CB% between 20 and 50% (choice E is incorrect). HCC is not usually associated with jaundice; however, the tumor cells characteristically secrete bilirubin (choice F is incorrect). Metastatic liver disease is rarely associated with jaundice because metastatic nodules do not produce diffuse liver cell injury (choice G is incorrect). Gilbert's disease is an AD disorder with a defect in the uptake and conjugation of UCB, hence CB% is < 20 (choice H is incorrect). Ascending cholangitis is most often due to infection emanating from a stone blocking the CBD, hence an obstructive type of jaundice is usually present (choice I is correct). FNH is not associated with jaundice (choice J is incorrect).

AA = amino acids, AAT = $\alpha_1$-antitrypsin, ABG = arterial blood gas, AD = autosomal dominant, AFP = $\alpha$-fetoprotein, AG = anion gap, ALP = alkaline phosphatase, ALT = alanine transaminase, ANA = antinuclear antibodies, anti-HBc = antihepatitis B core antibody, anti-HBe = antihepatitis B e antibody, anti-HBs = antihepatitis B surface antibody, AR = autosomal recessive, AST = aspartate transaminase, AT III = antithrombin III, AV = arteriovenous, BUN = blood urea nitrogen, CB = conjugated bilirubin, CBD = common bile duct, CH = cholesterol, CNS = central nervous system, CVA = costovertebral angle, DM = diabetes mellitus, EABV = effective arterial blood volume, ELISA = enzyme-linked immunosorbent assay, EPO = erythropoietin, ERCP = endoscopic retrograde cholangiopancreatography, FAs = fatty acids, FDPs = fibrin degradation products, FNH = focal nodular hyperplasia, FP = false-positive, GABA = gamma-aminobutyric acid, GB = gallbladder, GGT = γ-glutamyl transferase, G/M = gross and microscopic, GN = glomerulonephritis, HAV = hepatitis A virus, HBe-Ag = hepatitis B e antigen, HBIG = hepatitis B immune globulin, HBsAg = hepatitis B surface antigen, HBV = hepatitis B virus; HBV-DNA = hepatitis B virus DNA; HCC = hepatocellular carcinoma, HCV = hepatitis C virus, HDV = hepatitis D virus, HRS = hepatorenal syndrome, ISG = immune serum globulin, IVC = inferior vena cava, 17-KS = 17-ketosteroids, LDH = lactate dehydrogenase, LE = lupus erythematosus, O/P = ova and parasites, PAN = polyarteritis nodosa, PBC = primary biliary cirrhosis, PCr = plasma creatinine, PCR = polymerase chain reaction, PF = peritoneal fluid, PH = portal hypertension, PRV = polycythemia rubra vera, PSC = primary sclerosing cholangitis, PT = prothrombin time, PTH = parathormone, PUD = peptic ulcer disease, PV = portal vein, RAA = renin-angiotensin-aldosterone, RIBA = radioimmunoblot assay, RUQ = right upper quadrant, SBP = spontaneous bacterial peritonitis, SHBG = sex hormone–binding globulin, SMV = superior mesenteric vein, S/S = signs and symptoms, TB = total bilirubin, THV = terminal hepatic venule, TIPS = transjugular intrahepatic portosystemic shunt, UBG = urobilinogen, UCB = unconjugated bilirubin, UCr = urine creatinine, UNa⁺ = urine sodium, UOsm = urine osmolality, VLDL = very low density lipoprotein, WBC = white blood cell.

### Table 8–3. GALLBLADDER AND PANCREATIC DISORDERS

| Most Common... | Answer and Explanation |
|---|---|
| cause of air in the biliary tree | **gallstone ileus**— * fistula develops between small bowel and chronically inflamed GB: usually elderly woman, * gallstone causes obstruction at ileocecal valve |
| cystic disease of the biliary tract in children | **choledochal cyst**—most often occurs in children <10 yrs old |
| S/S of choledochal cysts | • **abdominal pain with persistent jaundice**—primarily noted in infants, • **abdominal pain with intermittent jaundice**—primarily noted in adolescents and adults, • **associations**— * cholelithiasis, * cholangiocarcinoma, * cirrhosis, * cholangitis, * pancreatitis, * Caroli's disease—see Table 8–2 |

## Table 8–3. GALLBLADDER AND PANCREATIC
DISORDERS *Continued*

| Most Common... | Answer and Explanation |
|---|---|
| radiographic findings in choledochal cysts | • **US**—screening test of choice, • **ERCP/trans-hepatic cholangiography**—useful in identifying intra- and extrahepatic cysts and sites of obstruction |
| Rx of choledochal cysts | **excision of cysts** |
| components of bile | • **bile salts (~67%)**— * hepatic product of CH metabolism, * water-soluble, * detergent action renders CH soluble in bile, • *phospholipid (22%): * mainly lecithin, * hydrophobic, * solubilizes CH in bile, • protein (4.5%), • free CH (4%), • CB (0.3%), • water/electrolytes/bicarbonate* |
| cause of stone formation | • **supersaturation of bile with CH,** • *decreased bile salts,* • *supersaturation with bilirubin* [**Note:** bile is lithogenic when the ratio of lecithin and bile salts is insufficient to keep CH soluble in bile. ~10% incidence of stones in the United States.] |
| causes of CH supersaturation of bile | • **biliary hypersecretion of CH**— * increased free CH in bile is toxic to the GB, * mucosa cannot detoxify CH by esterification, • *deficiency of bile salts,* • *deficiency of lecithin* |
| causes of an increase in biliary secretion of CH | • **obesity,** • **estrogen**— * childbearing, * birth control pills, • *increasing age,* • *Northern European,* • **drugs**— * fibric acid derivatives directly stimulate CH secretion into bile, * clofibrate increases hepatic HMG CoA reductase activity and decreases conversion of CH into bile salts: blocks 7 α-hydroxylase activity |
| mechanism for estrogen increase of CH in bile | • **upregulates LDL receptor synthesis in hepatocytes,** • **increases HMG CoA reductase activity**—rate-limiting enzyme in CH synthesis |
| causes of decreased bile salts | • **CD,** • **prolonged fasting,** • **increasing age,** • **drugs**—cholestyramine binds bile acids in bowel and eliminates them in stool |

*Table continued on following page*

### Table 8–3.  GALLBLADDER AND PANCREATIC DISORDERS *Continued*

| Most Common... | Answer and Explanation |
|---|---|
| causes of both increased biliary secretion of CH and decreased bile salts | • **increasing age,** • **American Indians,** • **estrogen Rx in women,** • **leanness** |
| factors increasing the prevalence of gallstones | • **female gender**—particularly those over 40 yrs old, • **obesity,** • *ethnicity*—highest prevalence in American Indians: ♦ **Pima,** ♦ Hopi, ♦ Navajo, • *DM,* • *extravascular hemolytic anemias,* • *cirrhosis* |
| stages in the development of CH stones | • **biliary hypersecretion of CH**— * increased hepatic synthesis of CH, * increased delivery of plasma CH to bile, • *hypomotility of GB*—promotes nucleation, • *acceleration of CH nucleation in bile,* • *hypersecretion of mucus by GB traps crystals and allows them to produce stones* |
| types of stones | • **CH**— * 75%, * usually mixed stones with: ♦ CH, ♦ calcium carbonate, ♦ some bilirubin pigment, * rarely purely CH, • *pigment stones*— * 20% black, * 5% brown |
| causes of black pigment stones | • **extravascular hemolytic anemia**—e.g., * sickle cell disease, * congenital spherocytosis, • *ineffective erythropoiesis with excess UCB*— * severe β-thalassemia, * PA/folate deficiency, • *hypersplenism secondary to cirrhosis*—macrophage destruction of RBCs with increased production of UCB [**Note:** black stones are rarely associated with infections.] |
| causes of brown pigment stones | **bile stasis in GB and CBD with infection** [**Note:** brown stones commonly occur in Asians.] |
| complications associated with stones | • **cholecystitis**—acute and chronic, • *CBD obstruction,* • *GB cancer,* • *Mirizzi's syndrome*—large stone in cystic duct compresses the subjacent hepatic duct, • *acute pancreatitis* |
| nonsurgical methods for treating gallstones | • **chemical**— * ursodeoxycholic acid: reduces CH secretion into bile, * may require up to 2 yrs of Rx, * recurrence commonly occurs, • *lithotripsy and dissolution*—extracorporeal shock wave Rx fragments stones, rendering them amenable to chemical dissolution |

## Table 8–3. GALLBLADDER AND PANCREATIC DISORDERS *Continued*

| Most Common... | Answer and Explanation |
|---|---|
| cause of acute cholecystitis | • **stone impacted in the cystic duct (90%),** • *AIDS*— * CMV, * *Cryptosporidium* [**Note:** *E. coli* is the most common pathogen in acute cholecystitis. The majority of cases resolve in 3–7 days when the stone falls out of the duct.] |
| pathogens in acute cholecystitis | • *E. coli*, • *enterococci*, • *Bacteroides fragilis*, • *Clostridium* sp |
| stages in the development of acute cholecystitis | • **stage 1**— * stone lodges in the cystic duct: ♦ stimulus of food causes GB contraction and stone is forced into cystic duct, * midepigastric, colicky pain occurs due to GB contraction against obstructed cystic duct, * N/V without pain relief, • **stage 2**— * stone becomes impacted in cystic duct, * mucus accumulates behind obstruction, * chemical irritation of mucosa, * bacterial overgrowth (no invasion), * pain shifts to RUQ: dull, continuous, aching pain, * pain radiation to right scapula/shoulder, • **stage 3**— * bacterial invasion of GB wall, * localized peritonitis with rebound tenderness, * positive Murphy's sign: see below, * neutrophilic leukocytosis, * attack subsides if the stone falls out of the cystic duct (90% subside over 3–7 days) or, if not, it perforates (next stage), • **stage 4**—perforation: wall tension from GB distention compresses lumens of intramural vessels → gangrenous necrosis |
| S/S of acute cholecystitis | • **fever,** • **RUQ constant, dull pain 15–30 min after eating,** • **vomiting—75%,** • **radiation of pain to the right scapula/shoulder,** • **Murphy's sign**—pain when the GB hits the examiner's finger on patient inspiration, • **jaundice**— * 25%, * usually indicates CBD stone, • **palpable GB—15%** |
| test used to identify stones in the cystic duct | **HIDA radionuclide scan** |
| test used to identify stones in the GB | • **US**— * gold standard test with >98% sensitivity, * detects stones >1–2 mm in diameter, * detects sludge, * evaluates GB wall thickness, * not effective in CBD stones: <30% sensitivity, • *plain film*—only 15% are radiopaque, • *CT*—too expensive |

*Table continued on following page*

Table 8–3. **GALLBLADDER AND PANCREATIC DISORDERS** Continued

| Most Common... | Answer and Explanation |
|---|---|
| lab findings in acute cholecystitis | • **absolute neutrophilic leukocytosis with left shift**—WBC counts >12,000 cells/μL with left shift, • *increased serum AST/ALP,* • *increased serum amylase*—suggests associated pancreatitis |
| pain medication used in acute cholecystitis | **meperidine**—morphine contracts the sphincter of Oddi and worsens pain |
| Rx of acute cholecystitis | • **NPO,** • **volume replacement,** • **antibiotics**—third-generation cephalosporin + metronidazole, • **surgery:** laparoscopic in most cases, within 48–72 hrs: reduces complications |
| indications for mandatory intraoperative exploration of CBD | • **jaundice,** • *CBD dilation*—>12 mm, • *filling defect in CBD noted on cholangiogram,* • *no stones in GB,* • *acute pancreatitis,* • *palpable stone in CBD* |
| causes of acute acalculous cholecystitis | **ischemic compromise of cystic artery**—cystic artery is an end-artery with no collateral circulation |
| risk factors for acute acalculous cholecystitis | • **volume depletion,** • *sepsis,* • **intravenous hyperalimentation,** • **accumulation of biliary sludge/mucus causing duct obstruction,** • **GB stasis** |
| symptomatic disorder of the gallbladder | **chronic cholecystitis** |
| cause of chronic cholecystitis | **stones in the GB with repeated attacks of minor inflammation**—chemical inflammation is more likely than infection |
| S/S of chronic cholecystitis | • **severe, persistent pain 1–2 hrs postprandially in the evening,** • *pain radiates into the right scapula,* • *recurrent epigastric distress, belching, bloating* |
| Rx of chronic cholecystitis | **laparoscopic cholecystectomy** |
| cause of cholesterolosis in the GB | **CH hypersecretion by the liver**— * CH accumulates in macrophages in the lamina propria of GB, * GB surface is studded with yellow flecks: "strawberry" GB, * no functional significance |

**Table 8–3. GALLBLADDER AND PANCREATIC
DISORDERS** *Continued*

| Most Common... | Answer and Explanation |
|---|---|
| cause of hydrops of GB | **chronic obstruction of cystic duct**— * distended GB with atrophy of the mucosa/muscle, * clear secretions |
| benign tumor of the GB | **papilloma** |
| cancer of the biliary tract | **GB cancer** |
| causes of GB cancer | • **gallstones**—>95% of cases, • *porcelain GB*— * dystrophically calcified GB, * automatic indication for elective cholecystectomy—>50% risk for cancer [**Note:** GB is a female-dominant disease.] |
| Rx of GB cancer | **surgery** [**Note:** the majority of GB cancers have already locally invaded the liver or porta hepatis when initially discovered. Poor prognosis: 5-yr survival <2%.] |
| cause of pancreas divisum | **incomplete fusion of the dorsal pancreatic bud with the ventral pancreatic bud**—ducts are not fused as well [**Note:** normally, the dorsal bud forms most of the pancreatic head and all the body and tail of the pancreas. The ventral bud is located close to the CBD and migrates posteriorly to fuse with the dorsal bud. It forms the uncinate process and inferior part of the pancreatic head. The major pancreatic duct (duct of Wirsung) derives from the entire ventral pancreatic duct plus the distal end of the dorsal pancreatic duct. In two-thirds of cases, the major duct empties directly into the CBD above the ampulla. The accessory duct of Santorini derives from persistence of the proximal dorsal pancreatic duct (usually the duct is obliterated) and enters the duodenum through a separate orifice.] |
| complication of pancreas divisum | **recurrent pancreatitis** |
| location for aberrant pancreatic tissue | • **wall of the stomach, duodenum, or jejunum**—may present as a mass or become inflamed, • *Meckel's diverticulum*—may cause peptic ulceration |

*Table continued on following page*

Table 8–3. **GALLBLADDER AND PANCREATIC DISORDERS** Continued

| Most Common... | Answer and Explanation |
|---|---|
| cause of an annular pancreas | **dorsal and ventral buds form a ring around the duodenum** |
| complication of an annular pancreas | **bowel obstruction** |
| pancreatic cyst | **pancreatic pseudocyst**— * see below, * not a true cyst |
| causes of acute pancreatitis | • **alcoholism**— * alcohol increases pancreatic duct permeability to enzymes, * alcohol thickens pancreatic secretions, * alcohol stimulates secretion of secretin, which stimulates pancreatic secretions, • *stone impacted in the distal end of the CBD*—ampullary obstruction causes reflux of bile into the major pancreatic duct, • *posterior penetration of duodenal ulcer,* • *trauma*—MCC in children, • *infection*—e.g., * mumps, * coxsackievirus, * CMV in AIDS, • *drugs*— * azathioprine, * estrogen, * pentamidine, • *hypercalcemia,* • *hypertriglyceridemia,* • *ERCP,* • *obesity*—major risk factor for severe pancreatitis |
| initiating events responsible for acute pancreatitis | **acinar cell injury due to**— * duct obstruction leads to ischemia: ♦ gallstone obstructs the major duct near the ampulla, ♦ duct obstructed by thick concretions (e.g., alcohol), * direct acinar cell injury (e.g., viruses, alcohol, drugs): intra-acinar autoactivation of trypsinogen forms trypsin, which activates other enzymes, complement, and the kinin system, * abnormal intracellular transport of proenzymes: e.g., drugs |
| S/S of acute pancreatitis | • **severe, boring midepigastric pain with radiation into the back**— * relieved by leaning forward, * worse when supine, • *fever*—low grade, • *dyspnea*— * >50%, * hypoxemia, * due to intrapulmonary shunting from atelectasis, • *N/V,* • *volume depletion*—third-space fluid losses around the pancreas, • *Grey Turner's sign*—flank hemorrhage, • *Cullen's sign*—periumbilical hemorrhage, • *tetany*—hypocalcemia from enzymatic fat necrosis, • *left shoulder pain*—pancreatic fluid may track toward left diaphragm and left pelvis |

## Table 8–3. GALLBLADDER AND PANCREATIC
DISORDERS *Continued*

| Most Common... | Answer and Explanation |
|---|---|
| lab finding in acute pancreatitis | • **elevated serum amylase**— * increased in 2–12 hrs, * returns to normal in 2–3 days: due to increased renal clearance, * sensitivity 85–90%, * FP elevation due to: ♦ bowel infarction, ♦ ruptured ectopic pregnancy, ♦ mumps, ♦ renal failure, • *increased urine amylase*— * elevated 1–14 days, * increased when serum amylase is normal, * *increased serum lipase*— * serum levels return to normal in 3–5 days, * slightly greater sensitivity/ specificity than amylase, • *amylase isoenzymes*— * S (salivary gland) and P (pancreas) bands, * presence of either band is not pathognomonic for a specific Dx, • *amylase clearance*— * urine amylase/serum amylase ÷ serum creatinine/urine creatinine, * normal 1–4% clearance, * most useful in the Dx of macroamylasemia (low value), • *neutrophilic leukocytosis,* • *hypocalcemia*— * 10–30%, • *hyperglycemia*—~30% |
| cause of an elevated serum amylase and negative urine amylase | **macroamylasemia**—immune complex of amylase with circulating antibodies |
| tumors secreting amylase | **ovarian and bronchogenic** |
| imaging findings in acute pancreatitis | • **CT scan**— * gold standard for pancreatic imaging, * not influenced by air in bowel as in US, * best test for obese patients, * identifies amount of glandular necrosis, • *US*— * pancreas is not visible in 40% of cases due to air in the bowel, * greater specificity than sensitivity, • *plain abdominal film*— * sentinel loop (localized ileus) near duodenum or transverse colon (cutoff sign), • *left-sided pleural effusion*— * 10%, * contains amylase, * diagnostic for acute pancreatis |

*Table continued on following page*

**Table 8–3. GALLBLADDER AND PANCREATIC DISORDERS** *Continued*

| Most Common... | Answer and Explanation |
| --- | --- |
| complications of acute pancreatitis | • **pancreatic necrosis**— * systemic signs occur earlier, * higher fever than usual, * sinus tachycardia, * greater degree of neutrophilic leukocytosis, * >50% chance for becoming infected, • *pseudocyst*— * ~20%, * see below, • *pancreatic abscess*—see below, • *ARDS*—destruction of surfactant by increased circulating lecithinase, • *hypovolemic shock*—third-space loss of fluids, • *DIC*—activation of prothrombin by trypsin |
| cause of persistent pain in a patient with acute pancreatitis | **pancreatic pseudocyst** |
| S/S of a pancreatic pseudocyst | • **persistent abdominal pain,** • *abdominal mass,* • *vomiting due to obstruction of gastric outlet,* • *persistence of serum amylase > 10 days,* • *radiology*—CT scan best diagnostic test [**Note:** pseudocysts are more likely to occur with chronic pancreatitis than acute pancreatitis. Must Bx the cyst wall to R/O cancer.] |
| complications of a pancreatic pseudocyst | • **infection**—produces a pancreatic abscess, • *rupture*—usually > 8 cm; • *hemorrhage*—erosion of splenic artery most commonly, • *obstruction of CBD* |
| Rx of a pancreatic pseudocyst | • **<5 cm**— * observe, * follow with CT, * most resolve without surgical intervention 2–3 mos, • *internal drainage of large or symptomatic noninfected cysts*—usually drain into the stomach |
| S/S of a pancreatic abscess | • **abdominal pain,** • *high fever*—due to sepsis: usually gram-negatives like *E. coli* or *Pseudomonas* spp., • *neutrophilic leukocytosis,* • *persistent hyperamylasemia,* • *CT*— * multiple radiolucent bubbles noted, * CT-guided aspiration of abscess identifies organisms |
| Rx of a pancreatic abscess | • **percutaneous drainage**—surgery may be necessary to debride necrotic debris (sometimes requires subtotal pancreatectomy) if external drainage is not working, • *antibiotics* |

## Table 8–3. GALLBLADDER AND PANCREATIC
### DISORDERS *Continued*

| Most Common... | Answer and Explanation |
|---|---|
| system used to determine prognosis in acute pancreatitis due to alcohol | **Ranson's criteria:** • **admission (first 24 hrs)**— * age >55, * WBC count >16,000 cells/µL, * glucose >200 mg/dL, * LDH > 350 IU/L, * AST >250 U/L, • **subsequent 48 hrs**— * Hct drop >10%, * serum BUN rise >5 mg/dL, * PaO$_2$ <60 mmHg: respiratory failure, * base deficit >4 mEq/L: metabolic acidosis, * calcium <8 mg/dL, * fluid sequestration > 6 L, • *prognosis*— * <3 signs: 0.9% mortality, * 3–4 signs: 11–16% mortality, * 5–6 signs: 33–40% mortality, * >6 signs: 100% mortality |
| system used to determine prognosis in acute pancreatitis due to biliary tract disease | **Ranson's criteria:** • **admission (first 24 hrs)**— * age >70 yrs, * WBC count >18,000 cells/µL, * glucose >220 mg/dL, * LDH > 400 IU/L, * AST >250 IU/L, • **subsequent 48 hrs**— * Hct drop >10%, * serum BUN rise >2 mg/dL, * serum calcium <8 mg/dL, * base deficit >5 mEq/L, * fluid sequestration >4 L, • *prognosis*—same as above |
| Rx of acute pancreatitis | **supportive therapy**— * NPO, * crystalloid solutions, * meperidine for pain: less sphincter of Oddi spasm, * NG suction if vomiting severe, * oxygen, * antibiotics are not indicated unless necrotizing pancreatitis |
| causes of chronic pancreatitis | • **chronic use of alcohol,** • **idiopathic,** • **CF**—MCC in children, • *hereditary,* • *protein-calorie malnutrition*—MCC in Third World countries, • *pancreas divisum* |
| mechanism of chronic pancreatitis | **repeated attacks of acute pancreatitis leading to duct obstruction**—calcified concretions occur with duct dilatation producing a "chain of lakes" appearance with radiographic dyes |
| clinical findings in chronic pancreatitis | • **severe pain**—due to duct obstruction, • *pancreatic calcifications*—CT is the best study, • *steatorrhea*— * indicates >90% exocrine destruction, * leads to weight loss, * malnutrition, • *DM*— * 70%, * usually parallels presence of pancreatic calcification, * brittle DM owing to deficiency of both glucagon and insulin |

*Table continued on following page*

Table 8–3. **GALLBLADDER AND PANCREATIC DISORDERS** *Continued*

| Most Common... | Answer and Explanation |
|---|---|
| lab findings in chronic pancreatitis | • **increased serum amylase**— * ~50%, * not reliable, • **increased urine amylase**—more reliable than serum test, • **signs of maldigestion**—meat fibers present in stool, • **low serum carotene levels**—malabsorption, • **abnormal bentiromide test**— * bentiromide is para-aminobenzoic acid + N-benzoyl tyrosine, * if chymotrypsin is present, it cleaves off PABA, which is absorbed and measured in the urine, • **abnormal stimulation tests**—IV administration of secretin/cholecystokinin and collection of pancreatic secretions, • *ERCP*— * good for evaluating ducts, * useful in distinguishing chronic pancreatitis from carcinoma |
| Rx of chronic pancreatitis | • **abstain from alcohol,** • *high-carbohydrate/ low-fat diet,* • *pancreatic enzymes,* • *fat-soluble vitamins,* • *meperidine*—addiction is common, • *? use of somatostatin analogues* |
| types of pancreatic cancer | • **adenocarcinoma,** • *islet cell tumors* |
| causes of pancreatic carcinoma | • **smoking,** • *chronic pancreatitis,* • *hereditary pancreatitis,* • *DM*—particularly in women, • *high saturated fat diet* [**Note:** point mutations of the p53 suppressor gene and ras oncogene have been strongly implicated.] |
| pancreatic sites for cancer | • **pancreatic head,** • *body,* • *tail* |
| S/S of carcinoma of the head of pancreas | • **epigastric pain,** • *painless jaundice*— * conjugated hyperbilirubinemia, * cancer in pancreatic head obstructs CBD, • *acholic stools,* • *weight loss,* • *palpable GB*— Courvoisier's sign, • *Trousseau's superficial thrombophlebitis,* • *Virchow's left supraclavicular node,* • *Sister Mary Joseph's sign*—periumbilical metastasis |
| lab findings in pancreatic cancer | • **elevated CA19-9**— * gold standard tumor marker, * other tumor markers: ♦ CEA, ♦ CA 50, • *radiologic*— * CT is best test: "C" sign, * CT guided percutaneous Bx for Dx [**Note:** enzymes are not commonly elevated.] |

### Table 8–3. GALLBLADDER AND PANCREATIC
### DISORDERS *Continued*

| Most Common... | Answer and Explanation |
|---|---|
| Rx of carcinoma of the head of the pancreas (if resectable) | **Whipple's procedure—** * en bloc resection of pancreatic head/neck (distal pancreas remains to prevent DM), * resection of part of CBD, * antrum resection with vagotomy in some cases [**Note:** radiation and chemotherapy are also used. 5-yr survival is 5–20% for resectable tumors and <1 yr with unresectable tumors.] |
| Rx of distal pancreatic cancer (if resectable) | **distal pancreatectomy with splenectomy** |
| islet cell tumor | **insulinoma—** * benign tumor in ~90%, * arises from β cells: one-third in head/body/tail, respectively, * 40- to 60-yr-old age bracket |
| clinical findings in an insulinoma | • **neuroglycopenia**—fasting hypoglycemia with mental status abnormalities, • **MEN I association in 80%**, • **Whipple's triad—** * fasting hypoglycemia, * symptoms of hypoglycemia, * symptoms reverse with glucose |
| lab findings in an insulinoma | • **fasting hypoglycemia—** * insulin normally inhibits gluconeogenesis, * 72-hr fast is the best stimulation test, • *increased serum insulin*—usually >5 μU/mL during fasting, • *increased serum C-peptide—* * excellent marker for the endogenous release of insulin, * decreased in patients taking too much insulin, • *CT scan*—useful in localizing the tumor, • *selective arteriography*—most sensitive localizing test |
| Rx of an insulinoma | • **surgery,** • *drugs—* * diazoxide, * verapamil, * octreotide: somatostatin analogue |
| islet cell tumor arising from α cells | **glucagonoma—** * 60% are malignant, * glucagon levels often >1000 pg/mL |
| S/S of a glucagonoma | • **DM—** * hyperglycemia, * osmotic diuresis, • **weight loss,** • **classic rash**—necrolytic migratory erythema, • **diarrhea,** • **venous thrombosis,** • **anemia** |
| Rx of a glucagonoma | • **surgery,** • *drugs*—octreotide |
| islet cell tumor arising from δ cells | **somatostatinoma**—majority are malignant |

*Table continued on following page*

## Table 8–3. GALLBLADDER AND PANCREATIC
## DISORDERS *Continued*

| Most Common... | Answer and Explanation |
| --- | --- |
| S/S of somatostatinoma | • **DM,** • **steatorrhea,** • **gallstones,** • **achlorhydria** |
| Rx of somatostatinoma | **surgery with cholecystectomy** |
| S/S of a VIPoma (pancreatic cholera, Verner Morrison syndrome) | • **secretory diarrhea,** • **achlorhydria,** • **muscle weakness**—due to hypokalemia, • **hypercalcemia**—70%, • **hyperglycemia**—50% [**Note:** malignant tumor of islets with excessive production of vasointestinal peptide.] |
| Rx of a VIPoma | • **surgery,** • *octreotide* |

**Question:** Gallstones are associated with which of the following clinical disorders? **SELECT 5**

    (A) Insulinoma
    (B) Small bowel obstruction
    (C) Choledochal cysts
    (D) Gallbladder cancer
    (E) Annular pancreas
    (F) Ulcerative colitis,
    (G) Congenital spherocytosis
    (H) Somatostatinoma
    (I) Chronic pancreatitis
    (J) Cholesterolosis
    (K) Pancreatic carcinoma

**Answers: (B), (C), (D), (H), (G).** Insulinomas are not associated with gallstones **(choice A is incorrect).** Small bowel obstruction may occur in patients with gallstone ileus **(choice B is correct).** Choledochal cysts have an increased incidence of gallstones **(choice C is correct).** Gallstones are the primary risk factor for gallbladder cancer **(choice D is correct).** Annular pancreas is associated with small bowel obstruction unrelated to gallstone disease **(choice E is incorrect).** Ulcerative colitis is not directly associated with GB disease **(choice F is incorrect).** In contradistinction, CD is associated with gallstones owing to bile salt deficiency related to terminal ileal disease. Congenital spherocytosis is associated with increased production of UCB owing to extravascular hemolysis of spherocytes in the spleen. Increased bilirubin in bile leads to the formation of jet black calcium bilirubinate stones **(choice G is correct).** Somatostatinomas are associated with gallstones since somatostatin has an inhibitory effect on the release of cholecystokinin **(choice H is correct).** Chronic pancreatitis is not associated with gallstones **(choice I is incorrect).** Cholesterolosis is due to hypersecretion of CH in bile and is not directly associated with gallstones **(choice J is incorrect).** Pancreatic carcinoma has no relationship to gallstones **(choice K is incorrect).**

AIDS = acquired immunodeficiency syndrome, ALT = alanine aminotransferase, ARDS = adult respiratory distress syndrome, AST = aspartate aminotransferase, BUN = blood urea nitrogen, Bx = biopsy, CB = conjugated bilirubin, CBD = common bile duct, CD = Crohn's disease, CEA = carcinoembryonic antigen, CF = cystic fibrosis, CH = cholesterol, CMV = cytomegalovirus, COD = cause of death, DIC = disseminated intravascular coagulation, DM = diabetes mellitus, ERCP = endoscopic retrograde cholangiopancreatography, FP = false-positive, GB = gallbladder, G/M = gross and microscopic, Hct = hematocrit, HIDA = technetium-99m dimethyl acetanilide imino-diacetic acid, HMG CoA = 3-hydroxy-3-methylglutaryl coenzyme A, LDH = lactate dehydrogenase, LDL = low-density lipoprotein, MCC = most common cause, MEN = multiple endocrine neoplasia, NG = nasogastric, NPO = Latin term for nothing by mouth, N/V = nausea and vomiting, PA = pernicious anemia, PABA = para-aminobenzoic acid, PaO$_2$ = partial pressure of arterial oxygen, PSC = primary sclerosing cholangitis, R/O = rule out, RUQ = right upper quadrant, S/S = signs and symptoms, TG = triglyceride, UCB = unconjugated bilirubin, VIP = vasointestinal peptide.

# CHAPTER

# 9

# ENDOCRINE SURGERY

## CONTENTS

### Table 9–1. GENERAL CONCEPTS, PITUITARY TUMORS

| Most Common... | Answer and Explanation |
|---|---|
| functional endocrine disorder | • **hypofunctioning gland**—e.g., Hashimoto's thyroiditis leading to hypothyroidism |
| causes of a hypofunctioning gland | • **autoimmune destruction**—e.g., * Addison's disease, * Hashimoto's thyroiditis, • *decreased stimulation*—e.g., secondary hypocortisolism in hypopituitarism, • *enzyme defects*—e.g., adrenogenital syndrome: 21-hydroxylase deficiency, • *neoplasms*—e.g., nonfunctioning pituitary adenoma, • *infections*—e.g., Waterhouse-Friderichsen's syndrome: secondary to *Neisseria meningitidis* sepsis, • *infarction*—e.g., Sheehan's postpartum necrosis |
| causes of a hyperfunctioning endocrine gland | • **benign adenoma**—e.g., * prolactinoma, * parathyroid adenoma, • *primary hyperplasia*—e.g., adrenal Cushing's syndrome, • *cancer*—e.g., parathyroid cancer |
| endocrine gland with a primary cancer | **thyroid** |
| type of test to evaluate hypofunctioning endocrine glands | **stimulation tests**—e.g., ACTH stimulation test in differentiating primary versus secondary hypocortisolism |

*Table continued on following page*

395

## Table 9–1. GENERAL CONCEPTS, PITUITARY TUMORS
*Continued*

| Most Common... | Answer and Explanation |
|---|---|
| type of test to evaluate hyperfunctioning endocrine glands | **suppression tests**—e.g., dexamethasone suppression test for hypercortisolism [**Note:** most hyperfunctioning glands are nonsuppressible (autonomous). Exceptions include prolactinoma and pituitary Cushing's syndrome due to a pituitary adenoma secreting ACTH.] |
| radiologic imaging study used to evaluate the pituitary gland | • **MRI**—best test for soft tissue detail of the pituitary gland: e.g., pituitary adenoma, • *CT*—best test for bony anatomy of the sella turcica |
| clinical effects of pituitary tumors | • **overactivity with hormone excess**—e.g., * **prolactinoma:** galactorrhea, * adenoma secreting excess GH: acromegaly, * pituitary Cushing's: Cushing's syndrome, • **visual disturbances (50%)**—impinge on optic chiasm, • *headache*, • *hypofunctioning endocrine glands*—see above, • *damaged pituitary stalk*— * loss of dopamine leading to galactorrhea, * central DI |
| pituitary tumors | • **prolactinoma**—40–50%, • *nonfunctioning (null) pituitary adenoma*—30–40%, • *ACTH-secreting tumors*— * 10–15%, * Cushing's disease, • *GH tumors*—10–15%, • *aldosterone-secreting tumors*, • *catecholamine-secreting tumors* |
| cause of hypopituitarism in children/young adults | **craniopharyngioma**— * derived from Rathke's pouch remnants, * Rathke's pouch is an ectodermal derivative derived from the oral cavity that forms the anterior lobe of the pituitary gland |
| clinical findings in a craniopharyngioma | • **benign tumor,** • **locations**— * **suprasellar,** * sella turcica, * stalk of the pituitary, • **gross**— * cystic, * calcifications: 75%, • **S/S**— * visual disturbances, * headache, * polyuria: central DI, * hypopituitarism: see below |
| Rx of craniopharyngiomas | **surgical removal**—radiation is used if they recur |

## Table 9–1. GENERAL CONCEPTS, PITUITARY TUMORS
*Continued*

| Most Common... | Answer and Explanation |
|---|---|
| causes of hypopituitarism in adults | • **nonfunctioning (null) pituitary adenomas,** • *removal (surgery)/ablation (radiation) for Rx of pituitary tumors,* • *pituitary apoplexy*—hemorrhage into a pituitary adenoma, • *Sheehan's postpartum necrosis*— * pituitary infarction: 90% must be destroyed to develop hypopituitarism, * sudden cessation of lactation, • *lymphocytic hypophysitis*— * autoimmune destruction of pituitary, * occurs during/after pregnancy, • *pituitary stalk disease*—head trauma, • *suprasellar craniopharyngioma* |
| sequence of tropic hormone loss in hypopituitarism due to a pituitary tumor | **FSH/LH (gonadotropins) → GH → TSH → ACTH → prolactin** |
| S/S of gonadotropin deficiency in adults | • **women**— * secondary amenorrhea, * infertility, * loss of secondary sex characteristics, * diminished libido, • **men**— * impotence: male analogue of secondary amenorrhea, * diminished libido, * loss of secondary sex characteristics, * atrophy of testes/prostate |
| S/S of GH deficiency in adults | • **decreased vigor,** • *weakness,* • *increased body fat,* • *fasting hypoglycemia* |
| S/S of TSH deficiency in adults (secondary hypothyroidism) | • **muscle weakness,** • *cold intolerance,* • *dry/brittle hair,* • *facial puffiness,* • *impaired memory,* • *constipation,* • *predisposes to mild SiADH*— * mild hyponatremia, * thyroid hormone inhibits ADH activity |
| S/S of ACTH deficiency in adults (secondary hypocortisolism) | • **fatigue/weakness,** • *propensity for adrenal crises with stress,* • *predisposes to mild SiADH*— * mild hyponatremia, * cortisol normally inhibits ADH activity: loss of cortisol negative feedback leaves ADH secretion unchecked, • *hypotension,* • *fasting hypoglycemia*—cortisol normally enhances gluconeogenesis |
| lab findings in hypogonadism (hypogonadotropic hypogonadism) | • **hypogonadism (women)**— * low FSH/LH, * low estradiol, * GnRH stimulation test: ♦ no significant increase in FSH/LH in hypopituitarism, • **hypogonadism (men)**— * low FSH/LH, * low testosterone, * low sperm count |

*Table continued on following page*

## Table 9–1. GENERAL CONCEPTS, PITUITARY TUMORS
### Continued

| Most Common... | Answer and Explanation |
|---|---|
| lab findings in GH deficiency | • **low IGF-1**— * most sensitive screening test: not adversely altered by stress and drugs, * liver-derived, • **low GH,** • **fasting hypoglycemia**— * 50%, * GH is normally gluconeogenic, • **insulin tolerance test**— * induces hypoglycemia: ♦ stimulus for GH/ACTH release, ♦ no increase in GH/IGF-1, • L-**dopa/L-arginine/sleep**—no increase in GH/IGF-1 |
| lab findings in TSH deficiency (secondary hypothyroidism) | • **low serum TSH,** • **low serum T$_4$/T$_3$,** • **hypercholesterolemia**—decreased LDL receptor synthesis, • **hyponatremia**—loss of inhibitory effect of thyroid hormone on ADH, • **TRH stimulation test**—decreased TSH response in hypopituitarism |
| lab findings in ACTH deficiency (secondary hypocortisolism) | • **decreased ACTH,** • **fasting hypoglycemia**— * decreased gluconeogenesis/glycogenolysis, * cortisol is a gluconeogenic hormone, • **hyponatremia**—loss of ADH inhibition, • **prolonged ACTH stimulation test**—eventual increase in adrenal hormones: e.g., urine for 17-hydroxycorticoids increases after 24–48 hrs of ACTH stimulation |
| Rx of pituitary adenoma | • **surgical removal,** • *glucocorticoids,* • *primary radiation*—danger of hypopituitarism |
| Rx of gonadotropin deficiency | • **conjugated estrogens with supplemental progestational agent**—if the uterus is present, • *testosterone for men* |
| Rx of GH deficiency | • **children**—GH replacement to improve impaired linear growth, • **adults**—GH is experimental in adults: increases muscle mass |
| Rx of TSH deficiency | **levothyroxine** [**Note:** glucocorticoid Rx is initiated before levothyroxine to prevent acute adrenocortical crisis. Free T$_4$ hormone levels are used to monitor Rx, since the TSH is already low.] |
| Rx of ACTH deficiency | **prednisone** |
| Rx of prolactin deficiency | **unnecessary** |

## Table 9–1. GENERAL CONCEPTS, PITUITARY TUMORS
*Continued*

| Most Common... | Answer and Explanation |
|---|---|
| types of diabetes insipidus (DI) | • **CDI**—deficiency of ADH: e.g., upper pituitary stalk trauma, • *NDI*— * end-organ defect, * e.g.: ♦ **chronic renal disease,** ♦ hypokalemia |
| S/S/lab findings of DI | • **polyuria/nocturia,** • *increased thirst* |
| lab findings in DI | • **UOsm < 100 mOsm/kg**—maximally dilute urine, • *normal to high serum Na$^+$*— * patient's access to water usually compensates for renal loss of water and may normalize the serum Na$^+$, * hypernatremia occurs when the patient does not have access to water, • *water deprivation test*— * patients with CDI have a dilute urine postwater deprivation: usually <100 mOsm/kg, * if after IM injection of vasopressin the UOsm is >50% from the baseline UOsm after water deprivation, the patient has CDI, * if after intramuscular injection of vasopressin the UOsm is <50% from the baseline UOsm after water deprivation, the patient has NDI |
| Rx of CDI | • **Rx underlying disease,** • *severe central DI*—Rx with desmopressin: ♦ nasal insufflation, ♦ spray, ♦ parenteral, • *partial CDI*— * chlorpropamide, * carbamazepine |
| Rx of nephrogenic DI | **thiazides**—thiazides produce volume contraction and increased proximal tubule reabsorption of water, which decreases polyuria |
| cause of GH excess | **GH-secreting adenoma**—hyperprolactinemia occurs in ~25% of cases [**Note:** excess GH/IGF-1 in children leads to gigantism (increased linear bone growth), because the epiphyses have not fused. In adults, an excess produces acromegaly, with increased lateral growth of bone.] |
| S/S of acromegaly | • **musculoskeletal**—acral enlargement, • *cardiovascular*— * HTN, * cardiomegaly: cardiomyopathy, * heart failure—most common COD, • *CNS*— * headache, * visual field defects |

*Table continued on following page*

### Table 9–1. GENERAL CONCEPTS, PITUITARY TUMORS
*Continued*

| Most Common... | Answer and Explanation |
| --- | --- |
| lab findings in acromegaly | • **increased IGF-1,** • *increased GH,* • *increased size of sella turcica*—majority are macroadenomas, • *hyperglycemia,* • *hyperphosphatemia,* • *OGT*—glucose does not suppress GH or IGF-1 |
| Rx of acromegaly | • **surgery**—60% successful, • *recurrent tumor*—* radiation, * drugs: ♦ bromocriptine, ♦ octreotide (somatostatin analogue) |
| S/S of a prolactinoma | • **women**— * secondary amenorrhea: prolactin inhibits GnRH, * galactorrhea, * osteoporosis: due to loss of estradiol, • **men**— * impotence, * headache, • **adolescent**—delayed puberty [**Note:** microadenomas are more common in women of reproductive age, whereas macroadenomas predominate in men and postmenopausal women.] |
| causes of galactorrhea other than prolactinoma | • **primary hypothyroidism**— * 15–30%, * low T$_4$ level increases TSH and TRH, the latter a potent prolactin stimulator: always order a TSH test in a patient with galactorrhea, • *drugs*— * estrogen: birth control pill, * cimetidine, • *pregnancy*—always R/O pregnancy, • *pituitary stalk transection/ injury*—loss of inhibitory effect of dopamine on prolactin, • *tactile stimulation of the nipple* |
| lab findings in prolactinoma | • **high serum prolactin**— * serum levels >200 ng/mL are diagnostic of a prolactinoma, * the height of prolactin correlates with tumor mass, • *low gonadotropins,* • *low estradiol,* • *low testosterone* |
| Rx of prolactinomas | • **surgery,** • *bromocriptine:* ♦ dopamine analogue, ♦ restores gonadal function in 70–80% of patients, * shrinks tumor mass in <50%, • *cabergoline*—dopamine analogue |

## Table 9–1. GENERAL CONCEPTS, PITUITARY TUMORS
*Continued*

**Question:** What laboratory tests should be ordered in a woman with secondary amenorrhea and clinical evidence of galactorrhea? **SELECT 3**

(A) Serum electrolytes
(B) Serum glucose
(C) Serum prolactin
(D) Serum TSH
(E) Serum cortisol
(F) Pregnancy test

**Answers:** (C), (D), (F). Prolactinomas, primary hypothyroidism, drug stimulation of prolactin, and pregnancy are the most common causes of galactorrhea. Prolactinomas and pregnancy are the most common causes of secondary amenorrhea + galactorrhea. Serum electrolytes, glucose, and cortisol have no value in the work-up of galactorrhea (choices A, B, and E are incorrect). Serum prolactin, serum TSH to R/O primary hypothyroidism, and a pregnancy test are always indicated in the work-up of galactorrhea (choices C, D, and F are correct).

ACTH = adrenocorticotropic hormone, ADH = antidiuretic hormone, CDI = central diabetes insipidus, CNS = central nervous system, COD = cause of death, DI = diabetes insipidus, FSH = follicle-stimulating hormone, GH = growth hormone, GnRH = gonadotropin-releasing hormone, HTN = hypertension, IGF-1 = insulin growth factor, LDL = low-density lipoprotein, LH = luteinizing hormone, MEN = multiple endocrine neoplasia, NDI = nephrogenic diabetes insipidus, OGT = oral glucose tolerance (test), SiADH = syndrome of inappropriate secretion of antidiuretic hormone, S/S = signs/symptoms, TRH = thyrotropin-releasing hormone, TSH = thyroid-stimulating hormone.

## Table 9–2. THYROID DISORDERS

| Most Common... | Answer and Explanation |
|---|---|
| steps in thyroid hormone synthesis | • **trapping of iodide**—TSH-mediated → • **oxidation of iodides to iodine**—peroxidase-mediated → • **organification**— * iodine is incorporated into tyrosine to form MIT and DIT, * TSH-mediated → • **coupling of MIT with DIT to form $T_3$ and DIT with DIT to form $T_4$** → • **hormones are bound to thyroglobulin and stored as colloid** → • **proteolysis of colloid by lysosomal proteases**—TSH-mediated → • $T_4$ **and $T_3$ bound to TBG**—one-third of binding sites → • $T_4$ **is peripherally converted to $T_3$ by an outer ring deiodinase**— * $T_3$ is the metabolically active hormone, * $T_4$ is considered a prohormone |

*Table continued on following page*

Table 9–2. **THYROID DISORDERS** *Continued*

| Most Common... | Answer and Explanation |
|---|---|
| manifestations of thyroid disease | • **mass effect**— * dysphagia for solids, * visible mass in the neck, • *hypothyroidism,* • *hyperthyroidism* |
| tests included in a thyroid profile | • **serum TSH**—best overall test • *serum T$_4$,* • *resin T$_3$ uptake* (RTU), • T$_4$ *binding ratio*—T$_4$BR = RTU/30%, • *free T$_4$-index* (FT$_4$-I)—calculated free hormone level |
| causes of an increased/decreased serum T$_4$ | • **increased/decreased free T$_4$ hormone level**—e.g., * hyperthyroidism/ * hypothyroidism, respectively, • *increase/decrease in TBG*— * an increase in TBG increases the serum T$_4$, * a decrease in TBG decreases the serum T$_4$, * the free T$_4$ and TSH are always normal when there are changes in the concentration of TBG [**Note:** the total serum T$_4$ is thyroid hormone bound to TBG (normally one-third of binding sites) and free, metabolically active T$_4$. Increasing or decreasing TBG in plasma results in an increase or decrease in the bound fraction without affecting the free hormone levels. Serum TSH is normal, since the free hormone levels are normal.] |
| causes of an increase in TBG | • **estrogen compounds**—increased hepatic synthesis of TBG, • *acute hepatitis*—increased release of TBG |
| causes of a decrease in TBG | • **androgens,** • *chronic liver disease*—decreased synthesis, • *high doses of salicylate,* • *corticosteroids,* • *nephrotic syndrome*—loss of TBG in the urine |
| use of the RTU | **indirect measurement of TBG** [**Note:** the RTU reflects the number of binding sites available on TBG. Normally, one-third of the binding sites are occupied by T$_4$. Radioactive T$_3$ (*T$_3$) is added to a tube of patient plasma. It binds to all available sites on TBG. Any residual *T$_3$ is bound by a resin and is measured and reported as a percentage. The RTU is normally 30%.] |
| effect of increased TBG on the RTU | **lowers RTU**—an increased number of available binding sites on TBG leaves less *T$_3$ to bind to the resin |
| effect of decreased TBG on the RTU | **increases RTU**—a decreased number of available binding sites on TBG leaves more leftover *T$_3$ to bind to the resin |

## Table 9–2. THYROID DISORDERS *Continued*

| Most Common... | Answer and Explanation |
|---|---|
| effect of excess free $T_4$ on the RTU | **increases RTU—** * an excess $T_4$ saturates most of the available TBG binding sites, * since there are fewer binding sites available for *$T_3$, more *$T_3$ binds to the resin, hence increasing the RTU |
| effect of a decrease in free $T_4$ on the RTU | **decreases RTU—** * less free $T_4$ leaves most of the binding sites on TBG available for binding with *$T_3$, * there is less *$T_3$ to bind to the resin, resulting in a low RTU |
| use of the $T_4BR$ | **calculate FT$_4$-index—** * free $T_4$-I = $T_4BR \times$ serum $T_4$: the free $T_4$-I is the calculated free $T_4$, * $T_4BR$ = measured RTU ÷ 30%: e.g., patient RTU = 15%, $T_4BR$ = 0.5 (15/30) |
| effect of changes in TBG on serum $T_3$ | **same as noted for serum $T_4$** |
| indication for ordering a serum $T_3$ | **R/O $T_3$ toxicosis** |
| distinction between hyperthyroidism and thyrotoxicosis | • **hyperthyroidism**—excess synthesis of thyroid hormone by the thyroid gland: e.g., ♦ Graves' disease, ♦ toxic nodular goiter, • **thyrotoxicosis**—end-organ effects of excess thyroid hormone regardless of the cause: e.g., ♦ excess ingestion of thyroid hormone, ♦ thyroiditis with release of hormone from the gland, ♦ Graves' disease, ♦ toxic nodular goiter |
| clinical uses of serum TSH | • **Dx of primary hypothyroidism—** * TSH is high in primary hypothyroidism since free $T_4$ is low, * a TSH is >20 μU/mL in most cases: normal 0.3–6.0 μU/mL, • *Dx of subclinical hypothyroidism—* * failing gland, * TSH 6–20 μU/mL, • *Dx of thyrotoxicosis*—serum TSH <0.3 μU/mL, • *follow $T_4$ therapy in patients with primary hypothyroidism—* * goal of replacement therapy is to bring the serum TSH back into normal range, * use free $T_4$ levels to monitor secondary hypothyroidism, • *identify TBG alterations versus free hormone alterations*—see above |

*Table continued on following page*

Table 9–2. **THYROID DISORDERS** *Continued*

| Most Common... | Answer and Explanation |
| --- | --- |
| clinical uses of $^{131}$I | • **Dx of primary hyperthyroidism**—e.g., Graves' disease: increased uptake of $^{131}$I, since the gland needs more iodide to synthesize thyroid hormone, • *thyrotoxicosis versus hyperthyroidism*— * increased uptake of $^{131}$I in hyperthyroidism, * decreased uptake of $^{131}$I in thyrotoxicosis due to thyroiditis or excess ingestion of thyroid hormone: ♦ in thyroiditis, inflammation in the thyroid is releasing hormone from the colloid, ♦ excess ingestion of thyroid hormone is decreasing serum TSH and causing atrophy of the thyroid gland, • *radionuclide scanning*— * distinguish "cold" nodules (nonfunctioning) from "hot" nodules (functioning), * cold nodules have no uptake of the radionuclide: the normal thyroid gland takes up the radionuclide, * hot nodules have an increase in uptake of the radionuclide: the remaining gland is suppressed by the low serum TSH from the excess free hormone and does not take up the radionuclide, • *identify metastatic thyroid cancer*—papillary and follicular thyroid cancers concentrate $^{131}$I very well, • *identify lingual thyroid*—see above, • *calculate the dose for thyroid ablation*—Rx of hyperthyroidism resistant to medical management |
| clinical uses of serum thyroglobulin | • **tumor marker for thyroid cancer recurrence**—increased in thyroid cancer, • *differentiates a silent postpartum thyroiditis from factitious thyrotoxicosis*— * increased in silent postpartum thyroiditis, * decreased in factitious thyrotoxicosis: patient taking excess thyroid hormone [**Note:** thyroglobulin does not accurately differentiate benign from malignant thyroid disease.] |
| clinical use of serum reverse $T_3$ | **diagnosis of the nonthyroidal illness syndrome** [**Note:** normally, a peripheral tissue outer ring deiodinase converts $T_4$ into metabolically active $T_3$, * in nonthyroidal illness, outer ring deiodinase is blocked and inner ring deiodinase converts $T_4$ into inactive reverse $T_3$.] |
| lab findings in the nonthyroidal illness syndrome | • **normal to decreased serum $T_4$**, • **decreased serum $T_3$**, • **normal TSH**, • **increased reverse $T_3$** |

## Table 9–2. THYROID DISORDERS *Continued*

| Most Common... | Answer and Explanation |
|---|---|
| clinical uses of thyroid-stimulating immunoglobulins (TSI) | • **immune marker for Graves' disease**— * TSI is an IgG antibody that attaches to TSH receptors and stimulates hormone synthesis, * unique to Graves' disease, • *predict remission/relapse in patients treated with thiourea drugs for Graves' disease*— * TSI decreases in remission, * TSI increases in relapse |
| antithyroid antibodies | • **antimicrosomal**—directed against peroxidase, • *antithyroglobulin* |
| clinical uses of antimicrosomal antibodies | **Dx of autoimmune thyroiditis**— * highest titers are noted in Hashimoto's thyroiditis, * moderately elevated titers in Graves' disease |
| midline vessel supplying the thyroid isthmus | **lowest thyroid artery**— * arises from the brachiocephalic trunk in ~10% of people, * danger of significant bleeding if transected during thyroid surgery |
| artery in proximity to the right recurrent laryngeal nerve | **inferior thyroid artery (ITA)**— * the right recurrent laryngeal nerve arises from the vagus nerve, * it loops inferior to the right subclavian artery, * the nerve is located between the branches of the ITA, * the nerve supplies all the intrinsic laryngeal muscles except the cricothyroid |
| nerve looping posteriorly around the ligamentum arteriosum of the aorta | **left recurrent laryngeal nerve**—the nerve can be injured with aortic arch aneurysms or an enlarged left atrium (e.g., in mitral stenosis) |
| S/S of recurrent laryngeal nerve injury | • **hoarseness,** • *true vocal cord is fixed in the midline* |
| artery in proximity to the external branch of superior laryngeal nerve | **superior thyroid artery (STA)**— * branch of the vagus nerve, * motor supply to cricothyroid muscle |
| S/S of injury to external branch of superior laryngeal nerve | **early voice fatigue**— * voice has a monotonous sound, * the cricothyroid muscle normally varies the length and tension of true vocal cord |

*Table continued on following page*

**Table 9–2. THYROID DISORDERS** *Continued*

| Most Common... | Answer and Explanation |
|---|---|
| location for the pyramidal lobe of thyroid | **extends superiorly from the isthmus**— * the pyramidal lobe occurs in 75–80% of people, * develops from remnants of the thyroglossal duct, * an isthmus may be absent |
| location for failed descent of the median thyroid anlage | **base of the tongue (foramen cecum)**—in 70%, it is the only thyroid tissue present in the patient |
| S/S of a lingual thyroid | • **dysphagia,** • *dysphonia,* • *dyspnea,* • *mass at the base of the tongue* [**Note:** a radioactive iodine uptake test with scanning should be performed to locate all thyroid tissue.] |
| Rx of a lingual thyroid | • **suppression with thyroxine**—lingual thyroids are usually hypofunctional, • *ablation with radioactive iodine,* • *surgery if obstructive* |
| cause of a cystic midline mass | **thyroglossal duct cyst**—cysts are usually in proximity to or within the body of the hyoid bone |
| S/S of a thyroglossal duct cyst | • **cystic mass in the neck,** • *ulceration through the skin of the neck,* • *papillary carcinoma*—from remnants of thyroid tissue in the cyst wall |
| Rx of thyroglossal duct cyst | **surgery**—removal of the proximal duct and hyoid bone |
| thyroid disease in the United States | **goiter**— * thyromegaly in a euthyroid patient, * thyromegaly due to excess colloid |
| types of goiter | • **endemic,** • *sporadic,* • *familial*—usually an AR enzyme deficiency: e.g., peroxidase deficiency |
| cause of an endemic goiter | **iodide deficiency** |
| causes of sporadic goiter | • **goitrogens**—e.g., * turnips, * Brussels sprouts, * lithium, • *puberty,* • *pregnancy,* • *elderly*—increasing incidence with age |

**Table 9–2.** THYROID DISORDERS *Continued*

| Most Common... | Answer and Explanation |
|---|---|
| mechanism of goiter formation | **absolute or relative deficiency of thyroid hormone**— * alternating hyperplasia (low $T_4$ increases TSH) and involution ($T_4$ increases, causing inhibition of TSH), * the thyroid gland is initially diffusely enlarged and then becomes multinodular, * danger of one or more nodule becoming autonomous and developing hyperthyroidism |
| complications associated with multinodular goiters | • **hemorrhage into a cyst**—sudden, painful, enlargement of the gland, • *hoarseness*—laryngeal nerve compression, • *dyspnea*—tracheal compression, • *compression of jugular vein*—neck congestion: Pemberton's sign, • *hypothyroidism*, • *toxic multinodular goiter*—Plummer's disease: not a variant of Graves' disease |
| test to evaluate functional status of a goiter | **serum TSH** |
| Rx of a goiter | • **thyroxine**— * reduces the size of the gland, * achieves a euthyroid state, • *surgery if compressive symptoms persist* |
| causes of thyroiditis | • **Hashimoto's thyroiditis**—see below, • *acute thyroiditis*— * bacterial: e.g., *Streptococcus pneumoniae*, * rare cause of thyrotoxicosis, • *subacute painful thyroiditis*—see below, • *subacute painless lymphocytic thyroiditis*—see below, • *Riedel's thyroiditis*—see below |
| cause of granulomatous thyroiditis | **subacute painful thyroiditis (de Quervain's thyroiditis)**— * due to a viral infection: e.g., **coxsackievirus**, * granulomatous inflammation |
| clinical findings in subacute painful thyroiditis | • **women 30–50 yrs old**, • **preceded by URI**, • **enlarged, tender gland**, • **absence of cervical adenopathy**, • **thyrotoxicosis for a few weeks**— * 50%, * due to gland destruction, • **self-limited**, • **permanent hypothyroidism is uncommon**, • **Rx**—NSAIDs |

*Table continued on following page*

Table 9–2. **THYROID DISORDERS** *Continued*

| Most Common... | Answer and Explanation |
|---|---|
| lab findings in subacute painful thyroiditis | • **high ESR,** • *antithyroid antibodies—* 10–20%, • *high serum $T_4$,* • *low serum TSH,* • *decreased $^{131}I$ uptake* |
| thyroiditis occurring in the postpartum state | **subacute painless lymphocytic thyroiditis—** * autoimmune disease, * commonly occurs 3–6 mos postpartum, * abrupt onset of thyrotoxicosis: due to gland destruction, * commonly progresses into Hashimoto's thyroiditis, with goiter or hypothyroidism * Rx transient thyrotoxicosis with β-blockers |
| thyroiditis mimicking thyroid cancer | **Riedel's thyroiditis—** * the thyroid is replaced by fibrous tissue, * fibrous tissue extends into the subjacent tissue, producing tracheal obstruction, * may produce hypothyroidism, * Rx: ♦ surgery if obstruction, ♦ tamoxifen, ♦ steroids |
| cause of hypothyroidism | **Hashimoto's thyroiditis—**symmetrically enlarged, nodular, painless gland |
| pathogenesis of Hashimoto's thyroiditis | • **autoimmune chronic thyroiditis—**increased incidence of other autoimmune diseases: e.g., ♦ Sjögren's syndrome, ♦ PA, • *antibodies—* * antimicrosomal and thyroglobulin antibodies, * IgG-blocking autoantibodies against the TSH receptor, • *cytotoxic T cells—*destroy thyroid tissue |
| S/S of hypothyroidism | • **weakness—**proximal muscle myopathy with elevated serum CK, • *periorbital puffiness—*deposition of GAGs in periorbital tissue, • *delayed recovery of Achilles reflex,* • *constipation,* • *cold intolerance,* • *mental slowing,* • *macrocytic anemia,* • *increased incidence of malignant lymphoma of the thyroid,* • *diastolic HTN,* • *dry skin/brittle hair,* • *macroglossia,* • *tightness in the throat—*from the goiter, • *menorrhagia* |
| lab findings in primary hypothyroidism | • **high serum TSH—**best test, • *low serum $T_4$,* • *low $RTU/T_4BR$,* • *low $FT_4$-I,* • *decreased uptake of $^{131}I$—*usually not a necessary test, • *high serum CH—*decreased synthesis of LDL receptors, • *high serum CK—*proximal thigh muscle myopathy, • *antimicrosomal/thyroglobulin antibodies* |

## Table 9–2. THYROID DISORDERS *Continued*

| Most Common... | Answer and Explanation |
|---|---|
| Rx of primary hypothyroidism | • **levothyroxine,** • *surgery*—for obstructive signs |
| causes of hyperthyroidism | • **Graves' disease,** • *toxic multinodular goiter*—Plummer's disease, • *toxic adenoma,* • *$T_3$ toxicosis* |
| cause of Graves' disease | **autoimmune**— * stimulatory IgG TSI antibodies are directed against the TSH receptor: type II hypersensitivity reaction, * inciting events: ♦ viral/bacterial infection, ♦ steroid withdrawal, ♦ iodide excess, ♦ lithium Rx, ♦ postpartum |
| cause of thyrotoxicosis associated with iodide excess | **Jodbasedow effect**— * common in iodide-deficient areas, * excess iodine induces hyperthyroidism: particularly in patients with toxic multinodular goiter or patients taking amiodarone (contains 37% iodine) |
| S/S unique to Graves' disease | • **exophthalmos**— * 20–40%, * infiltrative ophthalmopathy: GAGs infiltrate muscle, fat, soft tissue, * proptosis of eye, * impaired upward gaze, * periorbital edema, * extraocular muscle weakness, * conjunctival irritation, • *pretibial myxedema*—GAGs are deposited in subcutaneous tissue, • *thyroid acropachy*—defined by nail separation |
| S/S of thyrotoxicosis | • **weight loss with increased appetite,** • *heat intolerance,* • *fine tremor,* • *bruit over gland*—hypervascularity, • *gynecomastia,* • *nervousness/emotional lability,* • *diffuse enlargement of the gland,* • *diarrhea,* • *sinus tachycardia/palpitations,* • *atrial fibrillation*—common in elderly patients: always order a TSH, • *systolic HTN*— * increased systolic pressure with a wide pulse pressure, * potential for high-output cardiac failure, • *lid stare*—retraction of the upper lid due to excess sympathetic stimulation, • *osteoporosis*—increased breakdown of bone mass by osteoclasts |
| clinical findings in apathetic hyperthyroidism | • **Graves' disease of elderly patients,** • **cardiac abnormalities**— * atrial fibrillation, * CHF, • **weakness,** • **apathy,** • **weight loss due to loss of appetite,** • **thyromegaly** |

*Table continued on following page*

Table 9–2. THYROID DISORDERS *Continued*

| Most Common... | Answer and Explanation |
|---|---|
| lab findings in hyperthyroidism/ thyrotoxicosis | • **decreased serum TSH**—<0.3 μU/mL, • *increased serum $T_4$,* • *increased RTU/$T_4$BR,* • *increased F$T_4$-I,* • *increased uptake of $^{131}$I*— * Graves', * toxic multinodular goiter, • *decreased uptake $^{131}$I*— * thyroiditis, * patient taking excess hormone, • *low CH*—increased LDL receptor synthesis, • *hyperglycemia*—increased glycogenolysis/gluconeogenesis, • *lymphocytosis,* • *hypercalcemia*—increased bone turnover |
| initial Rx of Graves' disease | • **β-blockers**— * decrease catecholamine effects, * Rx for all patients, • **thionamides**— * Rx 6–9 mos and then stop, * see below [**Note:** the relapse rate is >50% after 1 yr of β-blocker and thionamide Rx.] |
| Rx if above Rx is unsuccessful | • **ablation with $^{131}$I**— * most common Rx for adults >40 yrs old, * 80–90% of patients are rendered euthyroid/hypothyroid, * all develop hypothyroidism, • *surgery*— * subtotal thyroidectomy, * primarily for Graves' disease in young patients, pregnancy |
| side effect of ablation Rx with $^{131}$I | **hypothyroidism**—70% after 10 yrs |
| antithyroid drugs used in Rx of thyrotoxicosis | • **PTU,** • *methimazole*—more potent than PTU |
| MOA of thionamides | • **inhibit organification**—see above, • *inhibit coupling*—see above, • *PTU also blocks peripheral conversion of $T_4$ to $T_3$* |
| side effects of antithyroid drugs | • **skin rash,** • *agranulocytosis*— * fever, * diarrhea, * sore throat, • *vasculitis,* • *hepatitis*—low prothrombin levels, • *teratogenic*— * PTU is used in low doses in pregnancy: greater protein binding than with methimazole and less transplacental transfer, * potential of blocking fetal thyroid: goiter with hypothyroidism, * aplasia cutis |
| drugs used to prepare patient for surgery | • **antithyroid drugs**—render euthyroid, • **iodide (Lugol's solution)**— * decreases vascularity, * inhibits organification, * inhibits proteases: decreases release of hormone from colloid |

**Table 9–2. THYROID DISORDERS** *Continued*

| Most Common... | Answer and Explanation |
|---|---|
| cause of Wolff-Chaikoff-White block | **iodine**— * inhibition of iodide trapping and synthesis of $T_3/T_4$ when plasma iodide levels are high, * useful for rapidly reducing thyroid hormone levels prior to surgery |
| causes of thyroid storm (thyrotoxic crisis) | • **inadequately treated patients with Graves' disease undergoing surgery,** • *infection,* • *trauma,* • *iodine,* • *pregnancy* |
| S/S of thyroid storm | • **tachyarrhythmias,** • *hyperpyrexia,* • *shock*—volume depletion from vomiting, • *acute metabolic encephalopathy*—coma |
| Rx of thyroid storm | • **inhibit hormone synthesis**— * PTU, * iodide, • **sympathetic blockade**—β-blockers, • **hydrocortisone,** • **IV fluids,** • **cooling blanket** |
| differences of toxic multinodular goiter versus Graves' disease | • **toxic multinodular goiter is not autoimmune**—one or more nodules are TSH independent, • **absence of antithyroid antibodies,** • **milder degree of hyperthyroidism,** • **absence of extrathyroidal signs**—e.g., exophthalmos |
| Rx of toxic multinodular goiter (Plummer's disease) | **surgery** |
| causes of a cold solitary thyroid nodule in a woman | • **multinodular goiter**—60%, • *follicular adenoma*—25%, • *cancer*—15% [**Note:** 85–90% of solitary nodules are euthyroid.] |
| cause of a hot nodule | **toxic multinodular goiter** |
| risk factors for a nodule representing cancer | • **previous Hx of radiation to the head/neck area**— * 40% chance of the nodule being malignant, * papillary cancer is the most common cancer, • *child,* • *adult male,* • *family Hx of thyroid cancer*—medullary carcinoma with a RET point mutation, • *nodule with palpable subjacent cervical lymph nodes* |

*Table continued on following page*

**Table 9–2. THYROID DISORDERS** *Continued*

| Most Common... | Answer and Explanation |
|---|---|
| diagnostic tests for evaluation of a solitary or dominant thyroid nodule | • **FNA**—sensitivity 70–98%, • *US*— * differentiates solid from cystic masses, * localizes nodules for Bx: main reason why US is sometimes performed before FNA, • *¹³¹I scans*— * useful for follicular lesions, * cannot differentiate benign vs. malignant, • *calcitonin*—if family Hx of medullary carcinoma, • *thyroid panel* |
| Rx of solitary nodules | • **FNA benign**—periodic follow-up or Rx with thyroxine for 6 mos and note any size changes, • **FNA indeterminate and nodule is "cold"/malignant/nodular mass not responding to thyroxine**—surgery |
| benign thyroid tumor | **follicular adenoma**— * an adenoma is due to somatic mutations in the TSH receptor resulting in TSH-independent cAMP production, * cold nodules |
| thyroid cancer | **papillary adenocarcinoma**— * ~80–85%, * female dominant, * mean age 35 yrs, * point mutation of RET proto-oncogene, * associations: ♦ Gardner's polyposis syndrome, ♦ radiation exposure [**Note:** presence of "benign" thyroid tissue in a lymph node is metastasis until proved otherwise. There is no such condition as a lateral aberrant thyroid.] |
| G/M findings in papillary adenocarcinoma | • **gross**— * 75% multifocal, * occult <1 cm/without local invasion, * intrathyroidal >1 cm confined to gland, * extrathyroidal with invasion of subjacent tissue, • **micro**— * papillary fronds are often intermixed with a follicular component, * empty-appearing nuclei: Orphan Annie nuclei, * psammoma bodies, * lymphatic invasion with spread to cervical lymph nodes |
| extranodal sites of papillary cancer metastasis | • **lungs**, • *bone* |

**Table 9–2. THYROID DISORDERS** *Continued*

| Most Common... | Answer and Explanation |
|---|---|
| Rx of papillary cancer | • **occult**—lobectomy with removal of isthmus, • **intra- or extrathyroidal**— * near-total (for intrathyroidal) or total (for extrathyroidal) thyroidectomy with removal of suspicious lymph nodes, * surgery followed by: ◆ suppressive $T_4$ therapy (reduces incidence of tumor recurrence) or ◆ ablative $^{131}I$ depending on the extent of tumor [**Note:** the 20-yr survival rate is ~90%. Thyroglobulin levels are useful for detecting cancer recurrence.] |
| thyroid cancer presenting as solitary cold nodule | **follicular carcinoma**— * 10%, * female dominant, * mean age 50 yrs, * high affinity for $^{131}I$ |
| G/M of follicular carcinoma | • **gross**— * encapsulated (solitary) or invasive, * metastasis to: ◆ **lung,** ◆ bone (osteoblastic, may occur 10–20 yrs after resection), ◆ liver, • **micro**— * prominent vessel invasion in >90%, * lymphatic invasion with lymph node metastasis is uncommon: <10% |
| Rx of follicular carcinoma | • **total thyroidectomy**—no lymph node resection, • **surgery followed by suppressive $T_4$ therapy (reduces incidence of tumor recurrence) or ablative $^{131}I$ depending on tumor extent** [**Note:** follicular cancers concentrate $^{131}I$ very well, since they are well differentiated. Ablation therapy is useful even with metastasis. The 10-yr survival rate is ~85%. Serum thyroglobulin levels are useful for detecting cancer recurrence.] |
| thyroid cancer with a family Hx | **medullary carcinoma**— * 5% thyroid cancers, * derives from parafollicular C cells, which synthesize calcitonin: calcitonin is the tumor marker, * neuroendocrine malignancy, * sporadic: 80%, * familial: ◆ 20%, ◆ AD MEN IIa/IIb syndromes, * tumor is commonly painful [**Note:** MEN syndromes are reviewed in Table 9–4.] |
| clinical differences between the familial and sporadic types | • **familial**— * younger age bracket: 20–40 yrs old, * premalignant C cell hyperplasia, * multicentric disease: 90% bilateral, * better 5-yr survival rate, • *sporadic*— * 50- to 60-yr-old bracket, * 75% are unilateral, * poorer prognosis than familial |

*Table continued on following page*

**Table 9–2. THYROID DISORDERS** Continued

| Most Common... | Answer and Explanation |
|---|---|
| G/M of medullary carcinoma | • **gross**— * usually located near the superior pole of the thyroid where the ultimobranchial bodies fuse with the thyroid, * unilateral: sporadic type, * multifocal: familial type, • **micro**— * sheets of tumor separated by amyloid derived from calcitonin, * lymphatic invasion with nodal involvement is common |
| hormones secreted by medullary thyroid cancer | • **calcitonin**— * produces diarrhea, * hypocalcemia rare, • *ACTH*—ectopic Cushing's syndrome, • *serotonin*—flushing |
| stimulation test to detect C cell hyperplasia | **IV infusion of pentagastrin and calcium gluconate**—in patients with C cell hyperplasia (precursor for medullary cancer), calcitonin levels increase |
| genetic testing that should be performed in familial cases | **PCR detection of DNA mutation of the RET proto-oncogene**—dominant role in MEN IIa/ IIb syndromes |
| Rx of medullary carcinoma | **total thyroidectomy with lymph node dissection**— * calcitonin/CEA levels are used to detect tumor recurrence, * 5-yr survival for sporadic cancer is ~50%, * MEN IIa 80%, * MEN IIb 50%, * positive genetic screening + C cell hyperplasia: prophylactic total thyroidectomy before age 5 yrs |
| cause of primary malignant lymphoma of the thyroid | **pre-existing Hashimoto's thyroiditis**—majority are of the diffuse, large B cell type |
| Rx of primary malignant lymphoma of the thyroid | **radiotherapy**—5-yr survival ~50% |
| clinical features of anaplastic thyroid cancers | • **elderly women**—60–80 yrs old, • **associations**— * multinodular goiter, * Hx of follicular cancer, • **rapidly aggressive**—uniformly fatal |
| complications of thyroid surgery | • **transient hypocalcemia**— * 24–48 hrs after surgery, * Rx with IV calcium gluconate, • *hemorrhage,* • *hypoparathyroidism*—see next table, • *laryngeal nerve injury*—see above |

## Table 9–2. THYROID DISORDERS *Continued*

**Question:** In which of the following thyroid disorders would you expect an elevated serum $T_4$ and suppressed TSH? **SELECT 4**
- (A) Hot nodule
- (B) Plummer's disease
- (C) Pregnancy
- (D) Nonthyroidal illness syndrome
- (E) Patient on anabolic steroids
- (F) Endemic goiter
- (G) Subacute painful thyroiditis
- (H) Follicular adenoma
- (I) Graves' disease
- (J) Medullary carcinoma of thyroid

**Answers: (A), (B), (G), (I).** Hot nodules are generally seen in toxic multinodular goiters, a cause of hyperthyroidism **(choice A is correct).** Plummer's disease is another name for a toxic multinodular goiter **(choice B is correct).** Pregnant women have an elevated $T_4$ owing to an increase in TBG, hence the serum TSH is normal **(choice C is incorrect).** In patients with nonthyroidal illness syndrome, the serum $T_4$ and TSH are usually normal **(choice D is incorrect).** Patients on anabolic steroids have a low serum $T_4$, due to a decrease in TBG and normal TSH levels **(choice E is incorrect).** Most patients with endemic goiters are euthyroid **(choice F is incorrect).** Subacute painful thyroiditis is initially associated with hyperthyroidism, due to gland destruction **(choice G is correct).** Follicular adenomas are generally nonfunctional and present as solitary cold nodules **(choice H is incorrect).** Graves' disease is the most common cause of hyperthyroidism and thyrotoxicosis **(choice I is correct).** Medullary carcinoma of the thyroid do not secrete thyroid hormone **(choice J is incorrect).**

ACTH = adrenocorticotropic hormone, AD = autosomal dominant, AR = autosomal recessive, Bx = biopsy, cAMP = cyclic adenosine monophosphate, CEA = carcinoembryonic antigen, CH = cholesterol, CHF = congestive heart failure, CK = creatine kinase, DIT = diiodothyrosine, DTRs = deep tendon reflexes, ESR = erythrocyte sedimentation rate, FNA = fine needle aspiration, $FT_4$-I = free $T_4$-index, GAGs = glycosaminoglycans, G/M = gross/microscopic, HTN = hypertension, [131]I = radioactive iodine, Ig = immunoglobulin, ITA = inferior thyroid artery, LDL = low-density lipoprotein, MEN = multiple endocrine neoplasia, MIT = monoiodotyrosine, MOA = mechanism of action, NSAIDs = nonsteroidal anti-inflammatory drugs, PA = pernicious anemia, PCR = polymerase chain reaction, PTU = propylthiouracil, R/O = rule out, RTU = resin $T_3$ uptake, SiADH = syndrome of inappropriate antidiuretic hormone, S/S = signs and symptoms, STA = superior thyroid artery, $T_3$ = triiodothyronine, $*T_3$ = radioactive $T_3$, $T_4$ = thyroxine, TBG = thyroid-binding globulin, $T_4$BR = thyroxine-binding ratio, TSH = thyroid-stimulating hormone, TSI = thyroid-stimulating immunoglobulin, URI = upper respiratory infection.

## Table 9–3. CALCIUM/PHOSPHORUS DISORDERS AND METABOLIC BONE DISEASE

| Most Common... | Answer and Explanation |
|---|---|
| origin and location of superior parathyroid glands | • **origin**—fourth branchial pouch, • **location**— * 1 cm superior to entrance of inferior thyroid artery, * level of inferior border of cricoid cartilage |
| origin and location of inferior parathyroid glands | • **origin**—third branchial pouch, • **location**— * more varied locations, * ~1 cm inferior to entrance of inferior thyroid artery, * within 2 cm of inferior pole of thyroid gland |
| functions of PTH | • **increases renal reabsorption of calcium**—proximal portion of distal tubule: ♦ same $Na^+/Cl^-$ pump blocked by thiazides, ♦ $Ca^{++}$ shares the same channel as $Na^+$ for reabsorption, • **decreases reabsorption of phosphate and reclamation of bicarbonate**—proximal tubule, • **increases synthesis of 1α-hydroxylase in proximal tubule of kidneys**—important for the second hydroxylation of vitamin D, • **increases resorption of bone to maintain the ionized calcium level** [**Note:** PTH has receptors on osteoblasts that when activated by PTH lead to release of IL-1 (OAF). IL-1 stimulates osteoclasts to remove calcium from bone. Estrogen in women and testosterone in men have an inhibitory effect on IL-1 release.] |
| functions of vitamin D | • **increases jejunal reabsorption of calcium and phosphorus**, • **activates receptors on osteoblasts to release alkaline phosphatase**—increases local phosphate concentration favorable to mineralization of bone and cartilage |
| parathyroid disorder | **primary hyperparathyroidism (HPTH)** |
| overall cause of hypercalcemia | **malignancy-induced**—see below |
| cause of hypercalcemia in the ambulatory population | **primary HPTH** |

### Table 9–3. CALCIUM/PHOSPHORUS DISORDERS AND
### METABOLIC BONE DISEASE *Continued*

| Most Common... | Answer and Explanation |
|---|---|
| cause of primary HPTH | • **benign parathyroid adenoma**— * 80–90%, * female dominant: over 50 yrs old, * right inferior gland is most often involved, * multiple adenomas in 2%, • *primary parathyroid hyperplasia*—involves all 4 glands, * wasserhelle cell (clear cell) hyperplasia variant is associated with highest calcium levels, • *parathyroid cancer*— * fibrosis, * vessel/capsule invasion |
| clinical presentation of primary HPTH | **asymptomatic patient with elevated serum calcium** |
| symptomatic presentation of primary HPTH | • **calcium stones**— * 5% of patients with a first renal stone have primary HPTH, * risk increases with recurrent calcium stones, • *polyuria*— * nephrocalcinosis leads to tubular dysfunction, * potential for CRF [**Note:** the clinical vignette that is often used to describe symptomatic primary HPTH is "stones/bones, abdominal groans, and psychic moans." These refer to renal stones, osteitis fibrosa cystica, PUD/pancreatitis, and CNS disturbances.] |
| cardiovascular findings in primary HPTH | • **diastolic HTN**—surgically correctable cause of HTN, • *short QT interval* |
| GI findings in primary HPTH | • **constipation,** • *PUD*— * ~5–15%, * usually a duodenal ulcer, * calcium stimulates gastrin release, causing hyperacidity, • *acute pancreatitis*— * ~2%, * calcium activates pancreatic enzymes |
| skeletal findings in primary HPTH | • **subperiosteal bone resorption**—occurs on the radial side of the terminal phalanges of the hand, • *bone resorption in lamina dura of tooth socket,* • *osteitis fibrosa cystica*— * late finding, * hemorrhagic cystic mass: "brown tumor," * the jaw is a common site, * pathologic fractures, * bone pain, • *"salt and pepper" appearance of the skull on x-ray,* • *increased incidence of chondrocalcinosis and pseudogout of knee* |
| sites for metastatic calcification in primary HPTH | • **kidneys**—nephrocalcinosis, • *skin*—pruritus, • *cornea*—band keratopathy [**Note:** a solubility product >40 predisposes to soft tissue calcification.] |

*Table continued on following page*

Table 9–3. CALCIUM/PHOSPHORUS DISORDERS AND
METABOLIC BONE DISEASE *Continued*

| Most Common... | Answer and Explanation |
|---|---|
| CNS finding in primary HPTH | **depression** |
| associations of primary HPTH with other disorders | • **MEN I**—see below, • *MEN IIa*—see Table 9–4 |
| lab findings in primary HPTH | • **hypercalcemia**—often requires multiple measurements, • *hypophosphatemia*—normal in ~50%, even after multiple measurements, * *high intact PTH*— * >90%, * 10% have "normal" PTH: a "normal" PTH is abnormal in the presence of hypercalcemia, • *normal anion gap metabolic acidosis*—due to a loss of $HCO_3^-$ in the urine, which is counterbalanced by a gain in $Cl^-$ ions: proximal renal tubular acidosis, • *hypercalciuria*— * amount of calcium filtered is greater than amount reabsorbed, * predisposes to stones, • *phosphaturia*, • *$Cl^-$/phosphate ratio >33*— * very high positive predictive value for HPTH * ratio <29:1 excludes primary HPTH: 100% negative predictive value |
| localizing studies performed in primary HPTH | • **noninvasive**— * CT scan, * US, * thallium-technetium subtraction scintigraphy, * technetium-labeled isotope: sestamibi scan, • **invasive**—selective venous sampling |
| Rx of primary HPTH | **surgery**— * totally excise parathyroid adenoma: ♦ Bx another gland to R/O primary hyperplasia, ♦ the second gland should show atrophy if an adenoma is present, * primary hyperplasia: remove 3.5 glands or perform a total parathyroidectomy with autotransplantation of parathyroid tissue into the forearm or neck |
| complications associated with surgery of primary HPTH | • **transient hypocalcemia,** • *hemorrhage,* • *hypoparathyroidism,* • *injury to the recurrent laryngeal nerve,* • *persistent HPTH*— * hypercalcemia is still noted postoperatively, * usually due to an improperly performed primary operation, * important to localize the parathyroid gland before reoperation, * 70–80% can be identified with neck incision, • *recurrent HPTH*— * normocalcemic for 3 mos and then hypercalcemia recurs, * must R/O familial hypocalciuric hypercalcemia: see below |

## Table 9–3. CALCIUM/PHOSPHORUS DISORDERS AND METABOLIC BONE DISEASE *Continued*

| Most Common... | Answer and Explanation |
| --- | --- |
| cause of postoperative hypoparathy-roidism | **devascularization of parathyroids**—the inferior thyroid artery supplies 80% of blood flow to the parathyroids |
| cause of hypercalcemia in a hospitalized patient | **malignancy-induced hypercalcemia**—see Table 1–3 |
| mechanisms of malignancy-induced hypercalcemia | • **metastasis to bone**—metastatic tumor releases osteoclast-activating factors (IL-1, prostaglandins), which resorb bone, • *secretion of PTH-like peptide*— * PTH-like peptide increases reabsorption of calcium from the kidneys, * tumors include: ♦ squamous cell carcinoma of the lung, ♦ renal adenocarcinoma |
| other causes of hypercalcemia other than primary HPTH and malignancy | • **metastasis to bone**—see above, • *primary HPTH,* • *ectopic secretion of PTH-like peptide,* • *hyperthyroidism,* • *sarcoidosis,* • *multiple myeloma,* • *hypervitaminosis D,* • *thiazides* |
| disorder confused with primary HPTH | **familial hypocalciuric hypercalcemia** |
| mechanism of hypercalcemia in familial hypocalciuric hypercalcemia (FHH) | **AD disease with an exaggerated reabsorption of calcium and magnesium from urine**— * hypercalcemia does not suppress PTH, which is slightly elevated, * hypermagnesemia enhances PTH activity, * renal stones develop at a young age: <10 yrs old |
| lab findings in FHH | • **hypercalcemia with a low urine calcium**—<200 mg/day, • *calcium/creatinine clearance ratio <0.01:1,* • *slight PTH elevation* |
| Rx of hypercalcemia | • **induce diuresis with isotonic saline and follow up with a loop diuretic,** • *bisphosphonates*— * drug of choice in severe hypercalcemia, * pamidronate is most often used, • *calcitonin*— * receptors are located on osteoclasts, * inhibits osteoclastic activity, * blocks renal calcium reabsorption, • *plicamycin*—inhibits osteoclast resorption, • *gallium nitrate*—inhibits osteoclast resorption, • *glucocorticoids*—mainly used for hypercalcemia due to: ♦ hypervitaminosis D (e.g., sarcoidosis), ♦ IL-1 (e.g., multiple myeloma) |

*Table continued on following page*

**Table 9-3. CALCIUM/PHOSPHORUS DISORDERS AND
METABOLIC BONE DISEASE** *Continued*

| Most Common... | Answer and Explanation |
|---|---|
| causes of secondary HPTH | • **CRF**—hypovitaminosis D causes hypocalcemia → stimulus for parathyroid gland hyperplasia, • *hypovitaminosis D from other causes*—e.g., * malabsorption, * liver disease |
| cause of tertiary HPTH | • **CRF**—autonomous secretion of PTH occurs in patients with previous secondary HPTH, • *renal transplants* |
| cause of hypocalcemia | **hypoalbuminemia**—see Table 1–3 |
| pathologic cause of hypocalcemia in a hospitalized patient | **hypomagnesemia**—see Table 1–3 |
| causes of primary hypoparathyroidism | • **previous thyroid surgery**—see above, • *autoimmune destruction*—second MCC, • *DiGeorge's syndrome*— * failure of development of the 3rd and 4th pharyngeal pouches, * combination of a pure T cell deficiency due to absent thymus + hypoparathyroidism |
| sign of hypoparathyroidism | **tetany** [Note: tetany and other causes of hypocalcemia are discussed in Table 1–3.] |
| cardiovascular finding in hypoparathyroidism | **prolonged QT interval** |
| CNS findings in hypoparathyroidism | • **basal ganglia calcification**—high serum phosphate drives calcium into this area, • **benign intracranial HTN**, • **extrapyramidal signs** |
| cutaneous/eye findings in hypoparathyroidism | • **alopecia**, • *Candida* **infections**, • **cataracts** |
| lab findings in primary hypoparathyroidism | • **hypocalcemia**—low ionized calcium, • *hyperphosphatemia*, • *low PTH* |
| causes of hyperphosphatemia | **see Table 1–3** |

**Table 9–3. CALCIUM/PHOSPHORUS DISORDERS AND METABOLIC BONE DISEASE** *Continued*

| Most Common... | Answer and Explanation |
|---|---|
| acquired causes of hypophosphatemia | **see Table 1–3** |
| metabolic bone disease | **osteoporosis—** * reduction in bone mass, * remaining bone is normally mineralized |
| mechanisms of osteoporosis | • **increased resorption of bone matrix—** * high turnover, * e.g., vertebral column in type I postmenopausal osteoporosis due to estrogen lack, • *decreased formation of bone matrix*—low turnover |
| mechanism involved in postmenopausal osteoporosis | **increased resorption of trabecular bone—** * estrogen normally dampens the release of IL-1 from osteoblasts, which enhances osteo-clastic activity, * estrogen lack allows for a greater breakdown of bone by osteoclasts than formation of bone by osteoblasts |
| mechanism involved in senile osteoporosis | **low turnover of bone or decreased formation of bone**—axial appendicular skeletal fractures predominate |
| fracture sites in postmenopausal osteoporosis | • **vertebral compression fractures,** • *Colles' fracture of distal radius* |
| fracture sites in senile osteoporosis | • **femoral neck**—danger of aseptic necrosis, • *proximal humerus,* • *tibia,* • *pelvis* |
| secondary causes of osteoporosis | • **endocrine disorders**—e.g., * Cushing's, * hyperthyroidism, * primary HPTH, * hypo-gonadism, • **drugs**—e.g., * heparin, * corti-costeroids, • **renal failure**—due to: ♦ chronic metabolic acidosis, ♦ secondary HPTH, • **immobilization,** • **malignancy**—PTH-like peptide |
| risk factors for developing osteoporosis | • **smoking,** • **sedentary life-style,** • **estrogen deficiency,** • **weight loss syndromes**—in-hibition of GnRH with reduction in FSH and LH |
| clinical findings in osteoporosis | • **pathologic fractures,** • *bone pain,* • *reduced height,* • *dowager's cervical hump* |
| radiographic finding of osteoporosis | **osteopenia—** * decreased bone density, * third metacarpal bone is a good index |

*Table continued on following page*

Table 9–3. CALCIUM/PHOSPHORUS DISORDERS AND METABOLIC BONE DISEASE *Continued*

| Most Common... | Answer and Explanation |
|---|---|
| lab test used to diagnose osteoporosis | **dual-photon absorptiometry**—noninvasive test that measures bone density at the distal radius |
| recommendations for the prevention of postmenopausal osteoporosis | • **estrogen with or without progestin**— * estrogen: ♦ inhibits bone resorption, ♦ reduces fracture risk by 50%, ♦ cardioprotective (50% reduction in CAD, maintains high HDL), * progestin protects against endometrial cancer, • *weight-bearing exercise*— * weight lifting, * walking, • *calcium*—1000–1500 mg/day, • *vitamin D*—400 U/day |
| drugs used in the Rx of established osteoporosis | • **estrogen,** • *exercise,* • *vitamin D,* • *calcium,* • *other drugs inhibiting bone resorption*— * **bisphosphonates,** * calcitonin |
| cause of osteoporosis in men | **low testosterone levels**—hip fractures are MC complication |
| benign cause of alkaline phosphatase elevation in an elderly man | **Paget's disease of bone**—osteitis deformans |
| phases of Paget's disease of bone | • **osteoclastic** → • *osteoblastic* → • *sclerotic* [**Note:** bone formed after the osteoblastic phase is structurally weak and prone to fractures.] |
| sites of predilection of Paget's disease of bone | • **pelvis,** • *skull,* • *femur,* • *tibia,* • *spine* |
| clinical findings in Paget's disease of bone | • **bone pain,** • *bone deformities*—e.g., enlarged skull, • *pathologic fractures,* • *bone tumors*—osteogenic sarcoma, • *high-output cardiac failure*—soft bone is highly vascular, leading to arteriovenous fistulas, • *deafness*—bone enlargement, • *CN palsies/vascular compression*—bone enlargement |
| radiographic studies performed in Paget's disease of bone | • **bone scan**—increased uptake, • *plain radiographs*— * ragged lytic areas, * fractures, * deformities |

## Table 9–3. CALCIUM/PHOSPHORUS DISORDERS AND METABOLIC BONE DISEASE *Continued*

| Most Common... | Answer and Explanation |
|---|---|
| lab findings in Paget's disease of bone | • **elevated alkaline phosphatase**—osteoblastic phase, • *increased urine hydroxyproline*—increased bone turnover |
| Rx of Paget's disease of bone | • **bisphosphonates**, • *calcitonin* |

**Questions 1–7:**
(A) Hypocalcemia/Low PTH  (B) Hypocalcemia/High PTH  (C) Hypercalcemia/High PTH  (D) Hypercalcemia/Low PTH  (E) Hypocalcemia/Normal PTH  (F) Normocalcemia, High PTH

For each numbered item below, select the **ONE** lettered option above that is **MOST CLOSELY** associated with it. Each lettered option may be selected once, more than once, or not at all.
1. Hypomagnesemia
2. Tetany after surgery for primary HPTH due to an adenoma
3. "Bones, abdominal groans, psychic moans"
4. Hypoalbuminemia
5. Metastatic cancer to bone
6. Chronic renal failure
7. Hyperventilation

**Answers: 1. (A), 2. (A), 3. (C), 4. (E), 5. (D), 6. (B), 7. (F).** Hypomagnesemia (1) leads to acquired hypoparathyroidism. Magnesium normally has a role in stimulating PTH synthesis and PTH release, and enhances PTH target organ activity **(choice A is correct)**. Tetany after surgery (2) may be due to devitalization of the remaining parathyroid glands leading to hypoparathyroidism **(choice A is correct)**. "Bones, abdominal groans, psychic moans" (3) is a classic description for primary HPTH **(choice C is correct)**. Bone disease (osteitis fibrosa cystica, osteoporosis), peptic ulcer disease/pancreatitis (abdominal groans), and depression (psychic moans) are findings in primary HPTH. Hypoalbuminemia (4) drops the total calcium level by decreasing the amount bound to albumin without altering the ionized calcium level, hence PTH levels are normal **(choice E is correct)**. Metastatic cancer to bone (5) causes hypercalcemia and a drop in serum PTH **(choice D is correct)**. CRF (6) leads to hypovitaminosis D with hypocalcemia and a stimulus for secondary HPTH **(choice B is correct)**. Hyperventilation (7) causes respiratory alkalosis. Alkalosis increases negative charges on albumin, leading to binding of some of the ionized calcium to albumin. This lowers the ionized calcium level (tetany), hence increasing PTH without reducing the total calcium **(choice F is correct)**.

*Table continued on following page*

AD = autosomal dominant, Bx = biopsy, cAMP = cyclic adenosine monophosphate, ATP = adenosine triphosphate, CAD = coronary artery disease, CN = cranial nerve, CNS = central nervous system, CRF = chronic renal failure, DI = diabetes insipidus, DKA = diabetic ketoacidosis, FHH = familial hypocalciuric hypercalcemia, FSH = follicle-stimulating hormone, GnRH = gonadotropin-releasing hormone, HDL = high-density lipoprotein, HPTH = hyperparathyroidism, HTN = hypertension, IL-1 = interleukin 1, LH = luteinizing hormone, MC = most common, MCC = most common cause, MEN = multiple endocrine neoplasia, OAF = osteoclast-activating factor, PFK = phosphofructokinase, PTH = parathormone, PUD = peptic ulcer disease, R/O = rule out, SD = standard deviation, S/S = signs and symptoms.

### Table 9–4. ADRENAL DISORDERS, MEN SYNDROMES, ECTOPIC HORMONE SYNDROMES

| Most Common... | Answer and Explanation |
| --- | --- |
| hormones synthesized in the zona glomerulosa | • **aldosterone**, • **weak mineralocorticoids**— * deoxycorticosterone, * corticosterone [**Note:** AT II activates the 18-OHase enzyme, which converts corticosterone into aldosterone. ACTH does not stimulate aldosterone release.] |
| hormones synthesized in the zona fasciculata/ reticularis | • **glucocorticoids**— * 11-deoxycortisol, * cortisol, • **17-ketosteroids**— * DHEA, * androstenedione, * both compounds are weak androgens, • **testosterone**—synthesized from androstenedione [**Note:** The urine for 17-hydroxycorticoids measures 11-deoxycortisol and cortisol byproducts.] |
| cause of Cushing's syndrome | **exogenous administration of glucocorticoids** |
| pathologic causes of Cushing's syndrome | • **pituitary adenoma**— * Cushing's disease, * 60% of cases, • *adrenal adenoma/cancer/ hyperplasia*— * 25%, * a functioning adenoma is the most common cause, • *ectopic Cushing's*— * 15%, * SCC of the lung is the most common cause: 50%, * endocrine tumors— ♦ 35%, ♦ thymic carcinoid, ♦ bronchial carcinoid, ♦ medullary carcinoma of the thyroid |

## Table 9–4. ADRENAL DISORDERS, MEN SYNDROMES, ECTOPIC HORMONE SYNDROMES *Continued*

| Most Common... | Answer and Explanation |
|---|---|
| S/S of cortisol excess in Cushing's syndrome | • **central obesity**— * moon facies (75%), * buffalo hump, * truncal obesity, * insulin is responsible for increased fat deposition in these areas, • *violaceous striae*— * 65%, * excess cortisol weakens collagen, leading to vessel rupture in the stretch marks, • *glucose intolerance*— * 65%, * cortisol is gluconeogenic, • *proximal muscle weakness*— * 60%, * due to muscle breakdown for gluconeogenesis, • *plethoric face*— * 60%, * due to polycythemia from stimulation of erythropoiesis, • *easy bruising*—40%, • *osteoporosis*—40% |
| S/S of weak mineralocorticoid excess in Cushing's syndrome | • **weight gain**— * 90%, * salt/water retention, • *diastolic HTN*—75%, • *dependent pitting edema*—40%, • *hypokalemic metabolic alkalosis*—15% |
| S/S of androgen excess in Cushing's syndrome | • **hirsutism**— * 65%, * increase in 17-KS, • *menstrual dysfunction*—60%, • *acne*—40% |
| type of Cushing's with hyperpigmentation | **ectopic Cushing's** |
| type of Cushing's syndrome associated with virilization | **adrenal Cushing's**— * usually a primary adrenal carcinoma, * a marked increase in DHEA-sulfate (unique to the adrenal gland) and 17-KS is seen |
| screening tests for Cushing's syndrome | • **24-hr urine for free (unbound) cortisol**—increased in >97%: represents the excess cortisol that is not bound to transcortin that is excreted in the urine, • *1-mg low-dose dexamethasone suppression test*— * dexamethasone is a cortisol analogue: there is no suppression of cortisol from pituitary, adrenal, or ectopic Cushing's, * 13–25% FP rate due to: ♦ obesity, ♦ chronic disease, ♦ depression |
| confirmatory tests for Cushing's syndrome | • **8-mg high-dose dexamethasone suppression test**— * cortisol suppression in pituitary Cushing's, * no suppression in adrenal/ectopic Cushing's, • *plasma ACTH*— * lowest in adrenal Cushing's, * highest in ectopic Cushing's, * "normal" to increased in pituitary Cushing's |

*Table continued on following page*

### Table 9–4. ADRENAL DISORDERS, MEN SYNDROMES, ECTOPIC HORMONE SYNDROMES *Continued*

| Most Common... | Answer and Explanation |
|---|---|
| localizing tests for Cushing's syndrome | **CT/MRI sella**— * if negative, then check the abdominal cavity, * >50% of pituitary Cushing's have a normal sella: indicates that the tumor is a microadenoma, * venous petrosal sinus sampling is recommended in equivocal pituitary Cushing's cases |
| Rx of pituitary Cushing's | **surgery** |
| Rx of adrenal Cushing's | • **adenoma**—unilateral adrenalectomy, • *carcinoma*—unilateral adrenalectomy + o,p'-DDD |
| Rx of ectopic Cushing's | • **surgical removal of tumor, if operable,** • *block steroid synthesis if inoperable*— * ketoconazole, * metyrapone, * somatostatin analogue |
| cause of Nelson's syndrome | **bilateral adrenalectomy in a patient with an underlying pituitary adenoma**—drop in cortisol causes further enlargement of the pituitary adenoma [**Note:** 10–15% of patients with bilateral adrenalectomy for Cushing's develop this syndrome. This underscores why adrenalectomy is not indicated as a treatment modality.] |
| S/S of Nelson's syndrome | • **headache,** • *hyperpigmentation*—due to increased ACTH |
| mineralocorticoid excess states | **see Table 5–3**—discussion of primary aldosteronism |
| adrenal medulla tumor in adults | **pheochromocytoma**—see Table 5–3 for complete discussion |
| cancer associated with hyponatremia or ectopic Cushing's syndrome | **SCC of the lung**—ectopic secretion of ADH and ACTH, respectively |
| cancer associated with hypercalcemia or secondary polycythemia | **renal adenocarcinoma**—ectopic secretion of PTH-like peptide and EPO, respectively |

## Table 9–4. ADRENAL DISORDERS, MEN SYNDROMES, ECTOPIC HORMONE SYNDROMES *Continued*

| Most Common... | Answer and Explanation |
|---|---|
| cancer associated with hypoglycemia or secondary polycythemia | **HCC**—ectopic secretion of an insulin-like factor and EPO, respectively |
| cancer associated with hypocalcemia or hypercortisolism | **medullary carcinoma of thyroid**—secretion of calcitonin and ACTH, respectively |
| cancers associated with gynecomastia | **gestationally or nongestationally derived trophoblastic tumors that secrete β-hCG**—e.g., * hydatidiform moles: benign, * choriocarcinoma: malignant, * testicular cancers with trophoblastic tissue [**Note:** Syncytiotrophoblast secretes the hormone.] |
| cancers associated with secondary polycythemia | • **renal adenocarcinoma**—alone or in association with von Hippel–Lindau disease, • *Wilms' tumor,* • *HCC* |
| cancer associated with the carcinoid syndrome | **carcinoid tumor arising from the terminal ileum**—see Table 7–6 |
| cause of acute adrenal insufficiency | • **abrupt withdrawal of glucocorticoids,** • *bilateral adrenal hemorrhage*— * **meningococcemia,** * trauma, * anticoagulation, • *Rx of primary hypopituitarism with thyroid hormone replacement before glucocorticoid replacement* |
| clinical findings of acute adrenal insufficiency | • **hypovolemic shock**—out of proportion to the intercurrent illness, • *hyponatremia,* • *hyperkalemia,* • *prerenal azotemia,* • *abdominal pain,* • *eosinophilia*—due to loss of glucocorticoids, • *hypercalcemia*—due to volume depletion, • *fasting hypoglycemia*—reduced gluconeogenesis |
| causes of chronic primary adrenal insufficiency (Addison's disease) | • **autoimmune destruction**—Addison's disease, • *infectious disease*— * **TB:** ♦ MCC in Third World countries, ♦ calcifications are very characteristic, ♦ histoplasmosis, • *AIDS*—disseminated CMV, • *adrenogenital syndrome*—MCC in children: 21-hydroxylase deficiency with loss of mineralocorticoids, • *drugs*— * ketoconazole, * aminoglutethimide, • *metastasis*—most commonly lung cancer |

*Table continued on following page*

Table 9–4. ADRENAL DISORDERS, MEN SYNDROMES,
ECTOPIC HORMONE SYNDROMES *Continued*

| Most Common... | Answer and Explanation |
|---|---|
| S/S of Addison's disease | • **weakness/weight loss**—100%, • *hyperpigmentation*— * 95%, * due to MSH activity of increased ACTH, * sites: ♦ buccal mucosa, ♦ scars, ♦ nipples, • *orthostatic hypotension*—salt loss from aldosterone deficiency |
| lab findings in Addison's disease | • **hyponatremia**—90%, • *hyperkalemia*— * 65%, * cannot excrete potassium, • *normal anion gap metabolic acidosis*—cannot excrete H⁺ ions, • *fasting hypoglycemia*—reduced gluconeogenesis, • *prerenal azotemia*—volume depletion, • *high plasma ACTH*—loss of negative feedback with cortisol, • *hypercalcemia*—volume depletion, • *antiadrenal antibodies*— ~50%, • *no cortisol response to short or prolonged ACTH stimulation,* • *hematologic abnormalities*— * eosinophilia, * lymphocytosis, * neutropenia |
| Rx of Addison's disease | • **hydrocortisone**—for glucocorticoid deficiency, • **fludrocortisone**—mineralocorticoid replacement, • **increase salt intake** |
| disorders in the MEN I syndrome (AD, Wermer's syndrome) | • **primary HPTH**— * 80%, * hypercalcemia, * bilateral parathyroid hyperplasia is more common than adenomas, • *pancreatic islet cell tumor*— * 75%, * **usually Zollinger-Ellison,** * insulinoma is the second most common tumor, • *pituitary adenoma*— * 60%, * usually nonfunctional, * occasionally functional: ♦ prolactin, ♦ GH, • *PUD* |
| disorders in the MEN IIa syndrome (Sipple's syndrome) | • **medullary carcinoma of the thyroid**— * >90%, * see Table 9–2, • *primary HPTH*— * 50%, * adenoma or hyperplasia, • *pheochromocytoma*— * 20–35%, * usually bilateral, * see Table 5–3 for screening tests |
| disorders in the MEN IIb syndrome | • **mucosal neuromas**— * >90%, * lips acromegaloid, * tongue enlarged, • *medullary carcinoma of the thyroid*—80%, • *pheochromocytoma*—60% |
| pancreatic endocrine tumors | **see Table 8–3** |

## Table 9–4. ADRENAL DISORDERS, MEN SYNDROMES, ECTOPIC HORMONE SYNDROMES *Continued*

**Question:** Which of the following laboratory findings, signs and symptoms, or gross features characterize Cushing's syndrome, primary aldosteronism, and pheochromocytoma? **SELECT 3**

(A) Hyperkalemia
(B) Hypertension
(C) MEN syndrome relationship
(D) Metabolic acidosis
(E) Adenomas
(F) Adrenal origin
(G) Nonsuppressible

**Answers: (B), (E), (F).** Hypokalemia is more likely than hyperkalemia in each of the syndromes **(choice A is incorrect)**. Hypertension is present in all the syndromes **(choice B is correct)**. A MEN IIa/IIb syndrome relationship is noted only with pheochromocytoma **(choice C is incorrect)**. Metabolic alkalosis is more likely to occur than metabolic acidosis in Cushing's and primary aldosteronism **(choice D is incorrect)**. Benign adenomas are more common than malignant tumors or primary hyperplasia for each of the syndromes **(choice E is correct)**. An adrenal location may occur for each of the syndromes. The cortex is involved in Cushing's syndrome and primary aldosteronism **(choice whereas the medulla is the usual site for a pheochromocytoma (choice F is correct)**. Pituitary Cushing's is suppressible, whereas the other syndromes are nonsuppressible **(choice G is incorrect)**.

ACTH = adrenocorticotrophic hormone, AD = autosomal dominant, ADH = antidiuretic hormone, AIDS = acquired immunodeficiency syndrome, AT II = angiotensin II, CMV = cytomegalovirus, DHEA = dehydroepiandrosterone, DIC = disseminated intravascular coagulation, DM = diabetes mellitus, EPO = erythropoietin, FP = false-positive, GH = growth hormone, HCC = hepatocellular carcinoma, HCG = human chorionic gonadotropin, HPTH = hyperparathyroidism, HTN = hypertension, 17-KS = 17-ketosteroids, MCC = most common cause, MEN = multiple endocrine neoplasia, MSH = melanocyte-stimulating hormone, OHase = hydroxylase, o,p'-DDD = mitotane, PTH = parathormone, PUD = peptic ulcer disease, SCC = small cell carcinoma, S/S = signs and symptoms.

## Table 9–5. DIABETES MELLITUS, HYPOGLYCEMIA

| Most Common... | Answer and Explanation |
|---|---|
| classification scheme for DM | • **primary DM**— * **type I: 10–20%**, * **type II: 80–90%**, * subtypes: ♦ obese (80%), ♦ nonobese, maturity-onset type, • *secondary DM*— * pancreatic disease: e.g., chronic pancreatitis, * drugs: e.g., glucocorticoids, * endocrine disease: e.g., Cushing's, * genetic disease: e.g., hemochromatosis, • *impaired glucose tolerance*, • *gestational DM* |
| pathogenesis of type I DM | **absolute insulin lack** |
| pathogenesis of type II DM | • **relative insulin deficiency**, • *insulin resistance*— * receptor deficiency—obesity down-regulates insulin receptor synthesis, * postreceptor defect: e.g., tyrosine kinase defects |
| pathologic processes in DM | • **NEG**— * refers to glucose combining with amino groups, * examples include: ♦ basement membranes of small vessels, which increases vessel permeability to protein, causing hyaline arteriolosclerosis, ♦ Hgb to produce HgbA$_{1c}$, ♦ LDL to produce oxidized LDL (more atherogenic than native LDL), • *osmotic damage*— * aldose reductase in certain cells (e.g., Schwann cells, lens, pericytes in retinal vessels) converts glucose into sorbitol, * sorbitol is osmotically active and draws water into the cells, leading to damage: e.g., ♦ peripheral neuropathy, ♦ microaneurysms, ♦ cataracts |
| disease where DM is the MCC | • **peripheral neuropathy**, • **nontraumatic amputation of leg**, • **blindness**, • **chronic renal disease** |
| clinical presentation of type I | • **abrupt-onset polyuria, polydipsia, polyphagia, unexplained weight loss**, • *nocturia*, • *volume depletion*, • *DKA*, • *coma* |
| clinical presentation of type II DM | • **insidious onset**, • *recurrent blurry vision*—alteration of lens refraction by sorbitol: constant changing of glasses, • *recurrent infections*—e.g., *Candida*, • *signs of target organ disease*—e.g., neuropathy, • *pruritus*, • *HNKC*, • *reactive hypoglycemia* |

## Table 9–5. DIABETES MELLITUS, HYPOGLYCEMIA
*Continued*

| Most Common... | Answer and Explanation |
|---|---|
| S/S of insulin-induced hypoglycemia | • **sympathetic signs**— * sweating, * tachycardia, * palpitations, • *parasympathetic signs*— * nausea, * hunger [**Note:** focal neurologic deficits, mental confusion, coma may also occur.] |
| Rx of hypoglycemia | • **candy bar**, • *glucagon injection*—patients eventually lose the glucose response to glucagon, • *infusion of 50% glucose in comatose patients* |
| precipitating causes of DKA | • **medical illness**, • *omission of insulin*, • *unknown* |
| clinical presentation of DKA | • **N/V**, • *abdominal pain*— * acute pancreatitis from increased TG, * decreased splanchnic blood flow from increased TG, • *severe volume depletion*, • *coma* |
| cause of volume depletion in DKA | **osmotic diuresis from glucosuria and loss of water, sodium, and potassium**— * ~6 L of hypotonic salt solution is lost in urine, * volume repletion with crystalloids is most important initial step in management |
| lab findings in DKA | • **hyperglycemia/hyperketonemia**—glucose ranges from 250–>1000 mg/dL, • *dilutional hyponatremia*—glucose draws water out of the ICF into the ECF, • *hyperkalemia*— * transcellular shift due to increased $H^+$ ions in the ECF, • *increased AG metabolic acidosis*— * ketoacidosis, * lactic acidosis, • *prerenal azotemia*—volume depletion |
| cause of HNKC | **type II DM**—enough insulin to prevent ketogenesis is present but not enough to prevent hyperglycemia |
| precipitating causes of HNKC | • **medical illness**—e.g., pancreatitis, • *drugs*—e.g., corticosteroids, • *surgery* |
| causes of pressure ulcers on the feet in DM | **peripheral neuropathy**—see Table 4–4 |
| urogenital findings due to autonomic neuropathy in DM | • **male impotence**— * 50%, * absent testicular sensitivity, • **female hypogonadism**— * 25%, * vaginal dryness, • **retrograde ejaculation**, • **neurogenic bladder**— * susceptible to urinary retention, * LUT/UUT infection |

*Table continued on following page*

**Table 9–5. DIABETES MELLITUS, HYPOGLYCEMIA**
*Continued*

| Most Common... | Answer and Explanation |
|---|---|
| infections noted in DM | • **cutaneous infections**— * *Staphylococcus aureus* abscesses, * skin pyodermas, • *UTIs*— * cystitis, * pyelonephritis, • *malignant external otitis—Pseudomonas aeruginosa*, • *rhinocerebral mucormycosis*—extension of *Mucor* from the sinuses through the cribriform plate into the frontal lobe to produce frontal lobe abscesses, • *emphysematous cholecystitis*—anaerobic infection (*Clostridium perfringens* >50%) with gas formation |
| lab criteria for the diagnosis of DM | • **random plasma glucose ≥ 200 mg/dL + classic symptoms of DM**— * polyuria, * polydipsia, * unexplained weight loss, • **FPG ≥ 126 mg/dL**, • **2-hr glucose post-75-g glucose challenge ≥ 200 mg/dL** [**Note:** any of these 3 criteria is consistent with a presumptive Dx of DM. To confirm DM, one of the 3 criteria must be present on a subsequent day.] |
| uses of a FPG | • **defines normal**—FPG < 110 mg/dL, • **defines impaired glucose tolerance (IGT)**—FPG ≥ 110 and < 126 mg/dL, • **provisional Dx of DM**— * FPG ≥ 126 mg/dL, * must be confirmed on subsequent day with one of the previously described 3 criteria [**Note:** fasting is defined as no caloric intake for at least 8 hrs.] |
| use of OGTT | • **defines normal**—2-hr 75-g postload glucose < 140 mg/dL, • **defines IGT**—2-hr 75-g postload glucose ≥ 140 mg/dL and < 200 mg/dL, • provisional Dx of DM— * 2-hr 75-g postload glucose ≥ 200 mg/dL, * must confirm with one of the previously described 3 criteria |
| types of insulin treatment regimens | • **split dose insulin mixtures**—split doses of regular + NPH twice daily: AM and PM, • *intensive insulin therapy*— * 3 injections including: ♦ regular + NPH in AM, ♦ regular to cover PM dinner, ♦ NPH at bedtime, * long-acting insulin for maintaining a basal level throughout the day plus insulin lispro (peaks 1–3 hrs) to cover each meal: ♦ most physiologic, ♦ labor intensive, • *insulin pump* |
| recommendation for fasting and premeal glucose | **glucose 80–120 mg/dL** |

## Table 9–5. DIABETES MELLITUS, HYPOGLYCEMIA
*Continued*

| Most Common... | Answer and Explanation |
|---|---|
| recommendation for $HbA_{1c}$ % | **$HbA_{1c}$ 6–7%**—additional action is suggested if the $HgbA_{1c}$ is > 8% |
| role of $HbA_{1c}$ in DM | **measure of glycemic control for the last 4–8 wks** |
| benefits of intensive glycemic control in DM | **50–75% reduction in risk of development or progression of (in decreasing order of benefit) retinopathy, neuropathy, and nephropathy** |
| Rx for type II DM | • **glycemic control**, • **weight reduction**, • **exercise** |
| types of oral agents used in Rx of type II DM | • **sulfonylureas**— * e.g.: ♦ glyburide, ♦ glipizide, * stimulate insulin secretion by the remaining β-islet cells, • *biguanides*—e.g., * metformin, * enhances insulin effect on liver/peripheral tissue, * reduces gluconeogenesis, • α-*glucosidase inhibitor*—e.g., * acarbose, * interferes with digestion of disaccharides and complex CHO, • *thiazolidinedione*—e.g., * troglitazone, * enhances peripheral uptake of insulin |
| method of patient monitoring of glucose | **SMBG** |
| COD in DM | • **AMI**, • *stroke*, • *renal failure* |
| complications associated with impaired glucose tolerance (IGT) | • **macrovascular complications**—e.g., * AMI, * PVD, • **~30% develop DM within 10 yrs** |
| lab findings in IGT | • **FPG ≥ 110 mg/dL but < 126 mg/dL**, • **2-hr glucose post-75-g glucose load ≥ 140 mg/dL but < 200 mg/dL** |
| types of hypoglycemia | • **fed state**, • *fasting* |
| S/S of fed state hypoglycemia | • **sweating**, • **tremor**, • **anxiety**, • **palpitations**, • **weakness**, • **hunger** [Note: symptoms are adrenergic. Symptoms usually begin 1–5 hrs after eating. β-Blockers mask these symptoms, hence they should not be used in patients with DM.] |

*Table continued on following page*

## Table 9–5. DIABETES MELLITUS, HYPOGLYCEMIA
*Continued*

| Most Common... | Answer and Explanation |
|---|---|
| S/S of fasting-state hypoglycemia | • **headache,** • **dizziness,** • **altered mentation,** • **visual disturbances,** • **motor disturbances,** • **seizures,** • **coma** [Note: symptoms are related to neuroglycopenia. The brain primarily uses glucose in the fasting state.] |
| causes of fed-state hypoglycemia | • **insulin-dependent DM,** • *alimentary hypoglycemia*—e.g., * dumping syndrome post-Billroth II operation, * postvagotomy/pyloroplasty, • *IGT,* • *idiopathic postprandial syndrome* |
| mechanism of alimentary hypoglycemia | **rapid entry of glucose load into small bowel with rapid increase in plasma glucose and inappropriately large increase in insulin release** [Note: symptomatic hypoglycemia usually develops 1–2 hrs after eating.] |
| causes of fasting hypoglycemia | • **alcohol**—decreased gluconeogenesis, • *renal failure*—kidney is a gluconeogenic site, • *sepsis,* • *malnutrition,* • *liver disease*— * decreased gluconeogenesis, * glycogen depletion, • *insulinoma*—see Table 8–3 |
| test used to document fasting hypoglycemia | **prolonged fast and satisfying Whipple's triad**— * symptoms, * hypoglycemia, * symptoms relieved by glucose |

**Question:** Which of the following are more often associated with type II DM rather than type I DM? **SELECT 4**
- (A) Age > 30 yrs
- (B) HLA association
- (C) Positive family history
- (D) Obesity
- (E) Absolute insulin deficiency
- (F) Insulin receptor deficiency
- (G) Insulin antibodies

**Answers:** (A), (C), (D), (F). Patients with type II DM are usually > 30 years old, have a positive family Hx of DM, are obese in >80%, and have insulin receptor deficiencies (choices A, C, D, and F are correct). Patients with type I DM have an HLA Dr3/Dr4 association, have absolute insulin deficiency, and commonly have anti-islet cell and insulin antibodies (choices B, E, and G are incorrect).

AG = anion gap, AMI = acute myocardial infarction, CHO = carbohydrate, COD = cause of death, DKA = diabetic ketoacidosis, DM = diabetes mellitus, ECF = extracellular fluid, FPG = fasting plasma glucose, GDM = gestational diabetes mellitus, Hgb = hemoglobin, HgbA$_{1c}$ = hemoglobin A$_{1c}$, HNKC = hyperosmotic nonketotic coma, ICF = intracellular fluid, IFG = impaired fasting glucose, IGT = impaired glucose tolerance, LDL = low-density lipoprotein, LUT = lower urinary tract, MCC = most common cause, NEG = nonenzymatic glycosylation, NPH = neutral protamine Hagedorn, N/V = nausea/vomiting, OGTT = oral glucose tolerance test, PVD = peripheral vascular disease, SMBG = self-monitoring of blood glucose, S/S = signs/symptoms, TG = triglyceride, UTIs = urinary tract infections, UUT = upper urinary tract.

# SURGICAL ONCOLOGY

## CONTENTS

### Table 10–1. TUMOR BIOLOGY

| Most Common... | Answer and Explanation |
|---|---|
| contributory factor responsible for cancer in the United States | **cigarette smoking**—cancer is the second most common COD in the United States |
| primary prevention modalities in cancer | • **life-style modification**— * stop smoking, * increase fiber/decrease dietary saturated fat, * reduce alcohol intake, * reduce weight, • *aspirin*—decreases incidence of the following cancers: ♦ esophageal, ♦ stomach, ♦ colon, ♦ rectal, • *isotretinoin (retinoic acid)*—decreases leukoplakia in the lungs and GI tract, • *tamoxifen*— * reduces risk for a second primary malignancy in the remaining breast in a woman with previous breast cancer, * may reduce the incidence of a primary malignancy in women who have a strong family Hx of breast cancer |
| name applied to malignant tumors derived from epithelium | **carcinomas**— * squamous: e.g., squamous cell carcinoma of larynx, * adenocarcinoma (gland-forming): e.g., prostate adenocarcinoma, * transitional epithelium: e.g., TCC of bladder |
| name applied to malignant tumors derived from connective tissue | **sarcomas**—e.g., * rhabdomyosarcoma: striated muscle, * liposarcoma: adipose tissue |
| adult sarcomas | • **malignant fibrous histiocytoma**, • *liposarcoma*—close second |

*Table continued on following page*

Table 10–1. TUMOR BIOLOGY *Continued*

| Most Common... | Answer and Explanation |
|---|---|
| childhood sarcoma | **embryonal rhabdomyosarcoma**—derives from skeletal muscle |
| features of APUD tumors | • **definition**—*a*mine *p*recursor *u*ptake and *de*carboxylation, • **neuroendocrine tumors**— * contain dense core neurosecretory granules, * S100 antigen-positive, * primarily develop from neural crest/neural ectoderm, • **examples**— * small cell carcinoma of lung, * carcinoid tumors, * malignant melanoma, * neuroblastoma |
| site for mixed tumors (pleomorphic adenoma) | **parotid gland** [**Note:** mixed tumors have two different morphologic patterns derived from the same germ cell layer: the MC tumor of the major and minor salivary glands.] |
| germ cell tumor | **cystic teratoma of the ovary** [**Note:** teratomas derive from all three germ cell layers. Locations include ovary, testis, anterior mediastinum, and pineal gland. They commonly have teeth and bone that are visible on x-ray.] |
| benign trophoblastic tumor | **hydatidiform mole** [**Note:** trophoblastic tumors contain syncytiotrophoblast (secretes β-hCG) and cytotrophoblast. Hydatidiform moles are benign tumors of the chorionic villus.] |
| malignant trophoblastic tumor | **choriocarcinoma** [**Note:** most derive from complete moles.] |
| location for choriocarcinomas in men | **testicle** [**Note:** they are highly aggressive cancers and do not respond well to chemotherapy as gestationally derived choriocarcinomas do.] |
| leukemia in adults and children, respectively | **CLL (adults), ALL (children)** [**Note:** leukemias are cancers derived from bone marrow stem cells. No benign bone marrow tumors exist.] |
| malignant lymphoma in adults and children, respectively | **poorly differentiated B cell follicular lymphoma (adults), Burkitt's lymphoma (children)** [**Note:** lymphomas are cancers derived from lymph nodes. The MC type is non-Hodgkin's lymphoma, followed by Hodgkin's lymphoma.] |

**Table 10–1. TUMOR BIOLOGY** *Continued*

| Most Common... | Answer and Explanation |
|---|---|
| extranodal site for a primary malignant lymphoma | • **stomach**, • *terminal ileum*—second MC site |
| non-neoplastic tumors | • **hamartoma**— * non-neoplastic lesions due to an overgrowth of tissue that is normally present in the organ, * examples: ♦ bronchial hamartoma, ♦ Peutz-Jeghers and hyperplastic polyps, • *choristoma (heterotopic rest)*— * normal tissue in a foreign location, * examples: ♦ pancreatic tissue in the wall of the stomach, ♦ gastric/pancreatic tissue in a Meckel's diverticulum |
| differentiating feature of a malignant versus a benign tumor | **metastasis** |
| malignant tumor that does not metastasize | • **BCC**— * MC skin cancer, * invades but does not metastasize, • *GBM*— * MC adult primary CNS cancer, * does not metastasize outside the CNS |
| types of metastasis | • **lymphatic**— * usual route of carcinomas, * initially localizes in regional lymph nodes, * eventually becomes hematogenous once it breaks through the lymph nodes, • *hematogenous*— * usual route for sarcomas, * lung (MC) and bone metastasis, • *seeding*— * implants of tumor that invade, * e.g., ovarian cancer seeding omentum |
| carcinomas that invade blood vessels | • **renal adenocarcinoma**, • *follicular thyroid carcinoma*, • *hepatocellular carcinoma* |
| sarcoma that invades lymphatics | **rhabdomyosarcomas** |
| sites for seeding of tumor | • **peritoneal cavity**—primary ovarian carcinoma, • *pleural cavity*— * primary lung cancer, * metastasis: e.g., ♦ breast, ♦ ovarian, • *subarachnoid space*—GBM |

*Table continued on following page*

Table 10–1. **TUMOR BIOLOGY** *Continued*

| Most Common... | Answer and Explanation |
|---|---|
| mechanisms of invasion by malignant cells | • **malignant cells have receptors for the integrin molecules laminin and fibronectin**—receptors help malignant cells adhere to the extracellular matrix, • **malignant cells contain enzymes**— * type IV collagenases: ♦ dissolve basement membranes, ♦ zinc is the metalloenzyme in collagenase, * proteases, • **malignant cells secrete TGF-α and -β**— * promote angiogenesis and collagen deposition, * TGF-α in breast cancer is blocked by tamoxifen |
| tissues resistant to invasion | **mature cartilage/elastic tissue in arteries** |
| factors influencing the growth rate of cancers | • **cell division time**—most cancers have a longer cell cycle than the parent tissue, • *percent of cells in the cell cycle*—growth fraction, • *rate of cell death* |
| relationship of tumor growth rate with doubling time | **growth rate = tumor aggressiveness/host defenses = 1/doubling time**— * a short doubling time correlates with an increased tumor growth rate, * a long doubling time correlates with a decreased tumor growth rate [**Note:** size of the tumor is a good indicator of growth rate. It requires 30 doubling times before tumors are clinically detected. This is equivalent to $10^9$ cells, 1 g of tissue, or a volume of 1 mL.] |
| DNA study abnormalities in highly aggressive malignancies | • **aneuploidy**—uneven multiple of 23 chromosomes, • *S phase fraction >5%*—measure of the number of malignant cells in the proliferating pool |
| relationship of doubling time with tumor-free interval | • **long doubling time**— * slow-growing cancers: e.g., breast cancer, * long tumor-free interval before recurrences, * 5-yr survival rates are not effective prognostic indicators: recurrence/death occurs after 5 yrs, • **short doubling time**— * fast-growing tumors: e.g., colon cancer, * short tumor-free interval before recurrences, * death comes quickly after recurrences, * 5-yr survival statistics are better prognostic indicators: recurrences are rare after 5 yrs |

**Table 10–1. TUMOR BIOLOGY** *Continued*

| Most Common... | Answer and Explanation |
|---|---|
| relationship of early metastasis to tumor size/survival | **good correlation with tumor size/survival—** * cancer is more likely to be widespread, * Rx of local recurrences or resection of metastatic lesions does not alter survival |
| relationship of late metastasis to tumor size/survival | **poor correlation with tumor size/survival—** * cancer is more likely to be localized than widespread, * Rx of local recurrences does improve survival, * resection of metastatic lesions often improves survival |
| bone sites for metastasis | • **vertebral column,** • *proximal femur—* second MC site [**Note:** the Batson vertebral venous plexus extends along the vertebral column from the cranial plexus to the pelvis. Tributaries penetrate the vertebrae, surround the spinal cord, and connect with the vena cava.] |
| symptom of bone metastasis | **pain** |
| Rx of bone metastasis | • **local radiation,** • *bisphosphonates—*inhibit bone resorption, • *ERA-positive breast cancer—*tamoxifen, • *prostate cancer—* antiandrogen drugs |
| radiographic techniques to identify bone metastases | • **radionuclide bone scans—**most sensitive screening test, • *plain radiographs—*30–50% of cortical bone must be involved to be visualized, • *CT scan—*most useful in vertebral metastasis |
| primary cancer with osteoblastic metastasis | **prostate cancer—**radiodense loci are noted on plain films |
| enzyme elevated in osteoblastic metastases | **alkaline phosphatase—**due to increased bone mineralization by osteoblasts (contain alkaline phosphatase) activated by cytokines released by the tumor |
| malignancies producing purely osteolytic metastases | **lung/kidney—**lytic metastases produce bone lucencies and predispose to pathologic fractures |
| organ metastasized to | **lymph nodes** |

*Table continued on following page*

## Table 10–1. TUMOR BIOLOGY *Continued*

| Most Common... | Answer and Explanation |
|---|---|
| malignancies of lymph nodes | • **metastasis**—e.g., carcinomas: ♦ breast, ♦ colorectal, • *primary cancer*—NHL |
| malignancies of the lungs | • **metastasis**—breast cancer, • *primary cancer*—adenocarcinoma: peripherally located |
| malignancies of the brain | • **metastasis**—lung cancer, • *primary cancer*—GBM: poorly differentiated astrocytoma |
| malignancies of the liver | • **metastasis**—lung cancer, • *primary cancer*— * HCC secondary to HBV or HCV postnecrotic cirrhosis |
| malignancy of bone | • **metastasis**—breast cancer, • *primary cancer*— * multiple myeloma: adults, * osteogenic sarcoma: children/adolescents |
| malignancy of the adrenal glands | **metastasis**—lungs |
| primary site for metastasis to Virchow's node | • **stomach adenocarcinoma,** • *pancreas adenocarcinoma* [**Note:** the left supraclavicular lymph node, or Virchow's node, drains the abdominal cavity.] |
| metastatic sites in descending order for breast cancer | • **lung,** • *bone,* • *liver* |
| metastatic sites in descending order for colorectal cancer | • **liver,** • *adrenal,* • *bone* |
| metastatic site for renal adenocarcinoma | **lungs**—metastases tend to be hemorrhagic |
| metastatic site for TCC of the bladder | **adrenal glands** |
| metastatic sites in descending order for lung cancer | • **liver,** • *bone,* • *brain/adrenal* |
| metastatic sites in descending order for malignant melanoma | • **liver/lung,** • *adrenal/brain/bone/skin* |

**Table 10–1. TUMOR BIOLOGY** *Continued*

| Most Common... | Answer and Explanation |
|---|---|
| metastatic sites in descending order for ovarian cancer | • **liver,** • *lung* |
| metastatic sites in descending order for prostate cancer | • **bone,** • *lung,* • *liver* |
| Rx for a woman with metastasis to axillary lymph nodes but no obvious primary site | **Rx as a primary breast cancer—** * ~5–10% of all metastatic carcinomas have an unknown primary, * majority are undifferentiated adenocarcinomas |
| Rx for peritoneal carcinomatosis in a woman with no obvious primary site | • **exploratory laparotomy,** • *surgical cytoreduction of tumor tissue as if the primary is ovarian* |
| steps in oncogenesis | • **initiation**—irreversible mutation→ • *promotion*—growth enhancement: due to ♦ growth factors, ♦ hormones (e.g., estrogen)→ • *tumor progression*— * subdivision of tumor cells into special functions: e.g., ♦ resist chemotherapy drugs, ♦ metastasize |
| types of genes associated with cancer | • **proto-oncogenes**— * precursors of <u>oncogenes</u>: genes that produce cancer, * proto-oncogenes are regulatory genes that code for proteins involved in normal growth/repair processes: see examples listed below, * growth factor synthesis: e.g., sis proto-oncogene, * synthesis of growth factor receptors: e.g., ♦ erbB₂/neu (HER-2), ♦ ret, * signal transduction (membrane-related guanine triphosphate–binding proteins): ras, * signal transduction (nonreceptor tyrosine kinase): abl, * nuclear transcription regulators: e.g., ♦ myc, ♦ N-myc, • **tumor suppressor genes**— * antioncogenes, * guardians of unregulated cell growth: see below |
| mechanisms of initiation | • **point mutations,** • *translocations,* • *overexpression,* • *amplification* |
| factors responsible for mutations leading to cancer | • **chemicals,** • *viruses,* • *bacteria,* • *radiation*— * UVB light, * ionizing radiation, • *physical agents*—e.g., burn scars |

*Table continued on following page*

Table 10–1. **TUMOR BIOLOGY** Continued

| Most Common... | Answer and Explanation |
|---|---|
| cancer associated with overexpression of erbB$_2$ | **invasive ductal cancers of the breast**—predicts poor survival |
| cancer associated with t9;22 translocation of abl | **chronic myelogenous leukemia**—formation of bcr-abl fusion gene on chromosome 22: called Philadelphia chromosome |
| tumors associated with a point mutation of ret | **MEN AD syndromes** |
| cancers associated with point mutation of ras | **~30% of all human cancers**— * lung, * colon, * pancreas, * acute myelogenous leukemia |
| cancer associated with a t8;14 translocation of myc | **Burkitt's lymphoma**—EBV causes polyclonal stimulation of B cells, which increases chances for the translocation to occur |
| cancer associated with amplification of N-myc | **neuroblastoma** |
| cancer associated with t14;18 translocation of B cell Ig heavy chain | **B cell follicular lymphoma**—B cell Ig heavy chain is translocated in the proximity of the bcl-2 gene on chromosome 18→overexpression of bcl-2 gene product→inactivates apoptosis gene involved in programmed cell death→B cells are immortal→B cell follicular lymphoma |
| suppressor genes associated with human cancers | • **p53 suppressor gene**— * chromosome 17, * normally codes for a protein product that inhibits activated cyclin-dependent kinase (cdk) in the cell cycle: activated cdk normally phosphorylates the Rb protein (see below) that allows a cell to pass from the G$_1$ into the S phase, • *Rb-1 gene*— * chromosome 13, * codes for Rb protein: ♦ normally prevents a cell from moving from the G$_1$ into the S phase, ♦ phosphorylation of the Rb protein by activated cdk allows the cell to move into the S phase, • *APC suppressor gene*—chromosome 5, • *NF-1 (chromosome 17) and NF-2 (chromosome 22) suppressor genes*—NF = neurofibromatosis, • *BRCA-1*—chromosome 17, • *BRCA-2*—chromosome 13, • *WT-1*— * chromosome 11, * WT = Wilms' tumor |

## Table 10–1. TUMOR BIOLOGY *Continued*

| Most Common... | Answer and Explanation |
|---|---|
| cancers associated with a point mutation of the p53 suppressor gene | • **accounts for ~25–50% of all human cancers**— * examples: ♦ colon, ♦ breast, ♦ lung, ♦ CNS, ♦ AD Li-Fraumeni multicancer syndrome (increased incidence of breast cancer, sarcomas, brain tumors, leukemia), • *oncogenesis in HPV*—gene products E6 and E7 in HPV infections inhibit the p53 suppressor gene leading to cancer: see below |
| cancers associated with inactivation of the Rb-1 suppressor gene | • **retinoblastoma**— * sporadic type requires 2 inactivations of the Rb suppressor gene on chromosome 13, * AD type requires only 1 inactivation: 1 is already inactivated at birth, • *osteogenic sarcoma,* • *breast cancer* |
| cancers associated with a point mutation of the APC suppressor gene | • **AD familial polyposis syndrome**— * APC = *a*denomatous *p*olyposis *c*oli, * AD Gardner's syndrome, • *other cancers*— * lung, * esophagus, * stomach, * pancreas |
| disorder associated with point mutation of the NF-1/NF-2 suppressor genes | • **inactivation of NF-1 suppressor gene**— * type I neurofibromatosis: ♦ café-au-lait macules, ♦ axillary freckling, ♦ Lisch's nodules (iris hamartomas), ♦ pigmented neurofibromas (benign tumors involving all peripheral nerve elements), ♦ CNS tumors (optic nerve glioma, meningiomas, unilateral acoustic neuroma [nerve deafness]), ♦ pheochromocytoma (hypertension), ♦ neurofibrosarcoma (usually involves large nerve trunks), ♦ Wilms' tumor, • **inactivation of NF-2 suppressor gene**—type 2 neurofibromatosis: ♦ bilateral acoustic neuromas, ♦ CNS tumors (meningiomas) |
| cancers associated with inactivation of the BRCA-1/BRCA-2 suppressor genes | • **inactivation of BRCA-1**— * breast cancer, * ovarian cancer, * colon cancer, * prostate cancer, • **inactivation of BRCA-2**— male/female breast cancer |
| cancer associated with inactivation of the WT-1 suppressor gene | **AD Wilms' tumor** |

*Table continued on following page*

**Table 10–1. TUMOR BIOLOGY** Continued

| Most Common... | Answer and Explanation |
|---|---|
| carcinogenic agent | **chemicals**— * 80–90% of cancers: particularly polycyclic hydrocarbons in cigarette smoke, * most are inactive in their native states: ♦ activated by enzymes in the cytochrome P-450, ♦ electron-deficient (attracted to nuclear proteins rich in electrons—e.g., DNA), * direct-acting chemical carcinogens: e.g., alkylating agents |
| chemical carcinogens inducing TCC of the bladder | • **polycyclic hydrocarbons in cigarette smoke,** • aniline dyes, • cyclophosphamide, • benzidine, • phenacetin |
| chemical carcinogens inducing liver angiosarcoma | • **vinyl chloride,** • arsenic, • Thorotrast |
| chemical carcinogens inducing primary lung cancer | • **polycyclic hydrocarbons**—cigarette smoke, • uranium—radon gas in mines, • asbestos—additive carcinogenic effect if combined with smoking, • chromium, • arsenic, • nickel, • cadmium |
| chemical carcinogens inducing HCC | • **aflatoxins**—especially in association with HBV postnecrotic cirrhosis, • oral contraceptives, • Thorotrast, • alcohol |
| chemical carcinogens inducing leukemia | • **alkylating agents**—also predispose to malignant lymphoma, • benzene, • polycyclic hydrocarbons |
| chemical carcinogens inducing SCC of oral pharynx | • **polycyclic hydrocarbons in cigarette smoke/smokeless tobacco,** • alcohol [Note: the two together are synergistic and greatly increase the risk for cancer.] |
| chemical carcinogens inducing SCC of larynx | • **polycyclic hydrocarbons in cigarette smoke/smokeless tobacco,** • alcohol |
| chemical carcinogens inducing SCC of esophagus | • **polycyclic hydrocarbons,** • alcohol, • nitrosamines |

**Table 10–1. TUMOR BIOLOGY** *Continued*

| Most Common... | Answer and Explanation |
|---|---|
| chemical carcinogens inducing stomach adenocarcinoma | • **nitrosamines,** • *polycyclic hydrocarbons* |
| chemical carcinogens that induce SCC of the skin | • **immunosuppressive agents**—MC overall cancer associated with immunosuppressive agents, • *arsenic,* • *tar/soot/oils*—"chimney sweeper" cancer |
| chemical carcinogens that induce pancreatic adenocarcinoma | • **polycyclic hydrocarbons,** • *alcohol*—associated with chronic pancreatitis |
| chemical carcinogen that induces clear cell adenocarcinoma of the vagina | **diethylstilbestrol (DES)** |
| chemical carcinogens inducing SCC of cervix | • **polycyclic hydrocarbons,** • *oral contraceptives* |
| oncogenic viruses associated with leukemia/lymphoma | • **EBV**— * primary CNS lymphoma: HIV is a cocarcinogen, * polyclonal lymphoma, * Burkitt's lymphoma, • *HTLV-1*—adult T cell leukemia, • *HTLV-2*—? hairy cell leukemia, • *HIV*—primary CNS lymphoma |
| oncogenic virus associated with nasopharyngeal carcinoma | **EBV** |
| oncogenic viruses associated with HCC | • **HBV,** • *HCV* |
| oncogenic virus associated with Kaposi's sarcoma | **herpesvirus 8** |
| oncogenic virus associated with cervical/anal squamous cell carcinoma | **HPV types 16, 18, 31** [**Note:** the anal variety is associated with unprotected anal intercourse.] |

*Table continued on following page*

### Table 10–1. TUMOR BIOLOGY *Continued*

| Most Common... | Answer and Explanation |
|---|---|
| MOA of radiation-induced cancer | • **UVB light**—formation of thymidine dimers: distort the DNA molecule, • *ionizing radiation*— * ionizing particles: ♦ α- and β-particles, ♦ γ-rays, ♦ x-rays, * hydrolyze water into free OH·radicals: mutagenic to DNA |
| UVB light–induced cancers | • **BCC,** • *SCC,* • *malignant melanoma* |
| ionizing radiation-induced cancers | • **leukemia**— * increased in radiologists, * increased in atomic bomb victims, • *papillary carcinoma thyroid,* • *lung cancer*—radon gas from uranium, • *breast cancer,* • *liver angiosarcoma*—Thorotrast, • *osteogenic sarcoma* |
| AR disease associated with skin cancers from UVB radiation | **xeroderma pigmentosum**—deficiency of DNA repair enzymes |
| bacteria associated with cancer | *Helicobacter pylori*— * gastric adenocarcinoma involving antrum, * low-grade mucosa-associated primary malignant lymphoma of the stomach |
| scar-related cancers | • **scar carcinoma in lungs**— * peripherally located scars: e.g., old TB scar, * usually adenocarcinoma, • *burn scars*—SCC, • *chronically draining sinus tracts*—SCC |
| terms applied to grading of cancer | • **low grade**—well differentiated, • **intermediate grade**—moderately well differentiated, • **high grade**— * poorly differentiated, * anaplastic [**Note:** grade is based primarily on histologic appearance of the tumor: how differentiated the tumor appears, nuclear features (e.g., chromatin pattern, mitotic activity), invasiveness.] |
| elements involved in staging cancer | • **tumor size (T),** • **lymph node status (N),** • **presence or absence of other metastatic spread (M)** [**Note:** stage is more important than grade in prognosis. M has greater prognostic significance than N. Nodal involvement indicates the need for adjuvant therapy (e.g., drugs and/or radiation).] |

**Table 10–1. TUMOR BIOLOGY** *Continued*

| Most Common... | Answer and Explanation |
|---|---|
| host defenses against cancer | • **type IV cell-mediated immunity**— * most efficient mechanism, * cytotoxic T cells, • *humoral mechanisms*— * antibodies, * complement, • *NK cells*— * direct killing, * indirect through type II hypersensitivity, * lymphokine-activated NK cells: NK cells activated by IL-2, • *macrophages*—activated by γ-interferon, • *nonspecific enhancement of immune system*— * use of BCG: infuse into bladder in TCC, * vaccinate with *Corynebacteria* species, • *tumor vaccines prepared from host tumor tissue,* • *antibodies against tumor-specific antigens (TSAs)*— * TSAs are produced by tumors, * host develops antibodies against TSAs, * virus-induced cancers produce the most antigenic TSAs, * chemical-induced cancers produce the least antigenic TSAs |
| chemical factor associated with cachexia due to cancer | **tumor necrosis factor-α**— * secreted by host macrophages and cancer cells, * tumor traps nitrogen: patients have a negative nitrogen balance, * megestrol is an appetite stimulant commonly used in treating cachexia: cachexia is usually irreversible |
| anemias associated with cancer | • **ACD,** • *iron deficiency*—e.g., right sided colon cancers, • *macrocytic anemia*—secondary to folate deficiency from rapid tumor growth, • *autoimmune hemolytic anemia*— * CLL, * HTLV-1, • *microangiopathic hemolytic anemia*— * schistocytes in peripheral blood, * RBCs damaged by tumor emboli in vessels, • *myelophthisic anemia*—metastasis to the marrow, • *bone marrow suppression*— * radiation, * chemotherapy |
| cause of a leukoerythroblastic peripheral smear | **metastasis to the bone marrow** [Note: this pushes hematopoietic elements into the peripheral blood (immature WBCs, nucleated RBCs).] |

*Table continued on following page*

## Table 10–1. TUMOR BIOLOGY *Continued*

| Most Common... | Answer and Explanation |
|---|---|
| coagulation abnormality in cancer | • **hypercoagulability,** • *DIC*—common finding in disseminated cancers [**Note:** hypercoagulability in cancer is multifactorial. Factors include increased synthesis of coagulation factors (e.g., fibrinogen, V, VIII), release of tissue thromboplastin, thrombocytosis, and decreased liver synthesis of antithrombin III and protein C.] |
| overall COD in cancer patients | **infections**—most often secondary to gram-negative sepsis |
| cause of hypercalcemia in cancer | • **metastasis to bone**—cancers secrete factors that stimulate osteoclast activity: e.g., IL-1, prostaglandins, • *secretion of a PTH-like peptide*—see Table 1–3 |
| term applied to remote effects of a cancer that are unrelated to metastasis | **paraneoplastic syndrome**— * occurs in 10–15% of tumors, * may predate the onset of metastasis in the tumor |

**Question:** In which of the following organs is malignancy most often due to a primary cancer rather than metastasis? **SELECT 4**
- (A) CNS
- (B) Thyroid
- (C) Lymph node
- (D) Lung
- (E) Liver
- (F) Skin
- (G) Kidney
- (H) Adrenal
- (I) Ovary
- (J) Bone

**Answers: (B), (F), (G), (I).** The correct answers for each of the choices are: CNS (A)—metastasis from a primary in lung; thyroid (B)—primary papillary carcinoma; lymph node (C)—metastasis from a carcinoma; lung (D)—metastasis from a primary in breast; liver (E)—metastasis from a primary in lung; skin (F)—primary BCC; small intestine (G)—primary adenocarcinoma; adrenal (H)—metastasis from a primary in lung; ovary (I)—primary serous cystadenocarcinoma; bone (J)—metastasis from a primary in breast.

ACD = anemia of chronic disease, AD = autosomal dominant, ALL = acute lymphoblastic leukemia, AML = acute myelogenous leukemia, APC = adenomatous polyposis coli, APUD = amine precursor uptake and decarboxylation, AR = autosomal recessive, BCC = basal cell carcinoma, BCG = Bacille Calmette-Guérin, BRCA = breast cancer, cdk = cyclin-dependent kinase, CLL = chronic lymphocytic leukemia, CML = chronic myelogenous leukemia, CNS = central nervous system, COD = cause of death, DES = diethylstilbestrol, DIC = disseminated intravascular coagulation, EBV = Epstein-Barr virus, ERA = estrogen receptor assay, GBM = glioblastoma multiforme, HBV = hepatitis B virus, HCC = hepatocellular carcinoma, β-hCG = beta-human chorionic gonadotropin, HCV = hepatitis C virus, HIV = human immunodeficiency virus, HPV = human papilloma virus, HTLV = human T cell lymphotropic virus, Ig = immunoglobulin, IL = interleukin, IVC = inferior vena cava, MC = most common, MEN = multiple endocrine neoplasia, MOA = mechanism of action, NF = neurofibromatosis, NHL = non-Hodgkin's lymphoma, NK = natural killer, PTH = parathormone, Rb = retinoblastoma, SCC = squamous cell carcinoma, S/S = signs and symptoms, TCC = transitional cell carcinoma, TGF = transforming growth factor, TSA = tumor-specific antigen, UVB = ultraviolet B (light), WT = Wilms' tumor.

### Table 10–2. PARANEOPLASTIC SYNDROMES, CANCER EPIDEMIOLOGY, RISK FACTORS FOR CANCER

| Most Common... | Answer and Explanation |
|---|---|
| paraneoplastic syndrome | **hypercalcemia secondary to secretion of a PTH-like peptide**—see Table 1–3 |
| cause of the Eaton-Lambert syndrome | **small cell carcinoma of the lung**— * muscle weakness resembles myasthenia gravis, * key differences from myasthenia: ♦ eye muscle weakness is not present, ♦ muscle strength increases with exercise, ♦ edrophonium chloride (Tensilon) does not improve muscle function |
| cancer associated with Sweet's syndrome | **acute leukemia**—syndrome consists of: ♦ fever, ♦ neutrophilic leukocytosis, ♦ red papular rash |
| phenotypic markers for gastric adenocarcinoma | • **acanthosis nigricans**—black, verrucoid lesion usually located in the axilla, • *Leser-Trélat sign*—multiple outcroppings of seborrheic keratoses |
| cancer associated with pulmonary osteoarthropathy | **primary lung cancer**—clubbing of the nails with an underlying periosteal reaction of bone |

*Table continued on following page*

Table 10–2. PARANEOPLASTIC SYNDROMES, CANCER
EPIDEMIOLOGY, RISK FACTORS FOR CANCER *Continued*

| Most Common... | Answer and Explanation |
|---|---|
| cancer associated with Trousseau's sign | **pancreatic adenocarcinoma**—Trousseau's sign refers to superficial migratory thrombophlebitis |
| collagen vascular disease associated with an underlying cancer | **dermatomyositis**—increased incidence of primary lung and breast cancer |
| renal disease associated with cancer | **nephrotic syndrome**— * most commonly an immunocomplex-mediated diffuse membranous glomerulonephritis, * cancers include: ♦ Hodgkin's lymphoma, ♦ colon cancer |
| cancers associated with granulocytosis (>8000 cells/μL) | • **primary lung cancer**, • *GI cancers* |
| cancer associated with subacute sensory peripheral neuropathy | **primary lung cancer**—may occur in 50% of lung cancers |
| adenocarcinomas associated with marantic vegetations | • **pancreas**, • *colon* [**Note:** marantic vegetations are sterile vegetations usually located on the mitral valve. Mucin-secreting cancers are prone to this complication.] |
| cancer associated with hyponatremia or ectopic Cushing's syndrome | **small cell carcinoma of the lung**—ectopic secretion of ADH and ACTH, respectively |
| cancer associated with hypercalcemia or secondary polycythemia | **renal adenocarcinoma**—ectopic secretion of PTH-like peptide and erythropoietin, respectively |
| cancer associated with hypoglycemia or secondary polycythemia | **HCC**—ectopic secretion of an insulin-like factor and erythropoietin, respectively |
| cancer associated with hypocalcemia or hypercortisolism | **medullary carcinoma of the thyroid** |

## Table 10–2. PARANEOPLASTIC SYNDROMES, CANCER EPIDEMIOLOGY, RISK FACTORS FOR CANCER *Continued*

| Most Common... | Answer and Explanation |
| --- | --- |
| cancers associated with gynecomastia | **gestationally or nongestationally derived tro-phoblastic tumors that secrete β-hCG—** * choriocarcinoma: malignant, * β-hCG is an LH analogue that stimulates progesterone synthesis |
| cancers associated with secondary polycythemia | • **renal adenocarcinoma**—alone or in association with von Hippel–Lindau disease, • *Wilms' tumor,* • *HCC* |
| cancer associated with flushing of the skin and diarrhea | **carcinoid tumor arising from the terminal ileum**—see Table 7–6 |
| cancers associated with secretion of AFP | • **HCC,** • *endodermal (yolk sac) sinus tumors*—most often located in the ovaries or testicles of young children [**Note:** AAT is also increased in HCCs.] |
| tumor markers ordered in the evaluation of testicular cancer | • **AFP**—derives from endodermal (yolk sac) tumors, • **β-hCG**— * derives from syncytio-trophoblast in a choriocarcinoma, * small amount secreted in a seminoma |
| tumor markers for multiple myeloma | • **Bence Jones protein**— * light chains in the urine, * best detected with urine immuno-electrophoresis, • β₂-*microglobulin* |
| tumor marker for surface-derived ovarian cancers | **CA 125** |
| tumor markers for small cell carcinoma of the lung | • **CEA,** • *neuron-specific enolase,* • *bombesin* |
| tumor marker for prostate cancer | **prostate-specific antigen (PSA)**— * more sensitive than it is specific: also elevated in prostate hyperplasia, * indicates tumor burden as well |
| tumor markers for breast cancer | • **CEA,** • **CA 15-3** |
| tumor marker for medullary carcinoma of the thyroid | **calcitonin** |

*Table continued on following page*

## Table 10–2. PARANEOPLASTIC SYNDROMES, CANCER EPIDEMIOLOGY, RISK FACTORS FOR CANCER *Continued*

| Most Common... | Answer and Explanation |
|---|---|
| tumor marker for colorectal cancer | **CEA**—primarily used to detect recurrences rather than as a primary screen for colorectal cancer |
| tumor markers for pancreatic carcinoma | • **CA 19-9**, • **CEA** |
| enzyme that is commonly elevated in malignant lymphomas | **LDN, particularly the LDH$_3$ isoenzyme fraction**—LDH is also increased in cystic teratomas, a germ cell tumor of the ovary or testes |
| cancers in children in order of decreasing frequency | • **ALL**, • *CNS tumors*— * cerebellar astrocytoma: ♦ benign tumor, ♦ MC overall CNS tumor in children, * medulloblastoma: ♦ MC primary malignant tumor of the CNS in children, ♦ located in the cerebellum, • *Burkitt's lymphoma,* • *neuroblastoma,* • *Wilms' tumor,* • *Ewing's sarcoma* [**Note:** cancer is second to accidents as the most common COD in children.] |
| cancers in decreasing order of incidence in men | • **prostate,** • *lung,* • *colorectal* |
| cancers in decreasing order of incidence in women | • **breast,** • *lung,* • *colorectal* |
| cancer mortalities in decreasing order in men | • **lung,** • *prostate,* • *colorectal* |
| cancer mortalities in decreasing order in women | • **lung,** • *breast,* • *colorectal* [**Note:** colorectal cancer is the second most common cancer and cancer killer in men and women.] |
| gynecologic cancers in decreasing order of incidence | • **endometrial,** • *ovarian,* • *cervical* |
| gynecologic cancers in decreasing order of mortality | • **ovarian,** • *cervical,* • *endometrial* |
| gynecologic cancer at ages 45, 55, 65 yrs | • **45 yrs**—cervical cancer, • **55 yrs**—endometrial cancer, • **65 yrs**—ovarian cancer |

## Table 10–2. PARANEOPLASTIC SYNDROMES, CANCER EPIDEMIOLOGY, RISK FACTORS FOR CANCER *Continued*

| Most Common... | Answer and Explanation |
|---|---|
| cancers that are decreasing in incidence in the United States | • **SCC of cervix**—due to Pap screens detecting cervical dysplasia (precursor for SCC of cervix), • *stomach adenocarcinoma,* • *endometrial adenocarcinoma* |
| cancers that are increasing in incidence in the United States | • **malignant melanoma**—most rapidly increasing cancer in the world, • *prostate*—due to detection by PSA and DRE, • *lung—* * particularly in women, * the incidence is decreasing in men, • *multiple myeloma,* • *pancreatic adenocarcinoma,* • *malignant lymphoma* |
| cancer in Southeast China | **nasopharyngeal carcinoma secondary to EBV** [Note: in Northern China, esophageal cancer is more common.] |
| cancer in Japan | **stomach adenocarcinoma**—primarily due to consumption of smoked products |
| cancer in Southeast Asia | **HCC secondary to HBV**—incidence is enhanced by aflatoxins, a mold present in food |
| malignant lymphoma in Africa | **Burkitt's lymphoma** |
| cancer prevented by immunization | **HCC**—vaccination against HBV also reduces the risk for developing HBV and HDV hepatitis |
| cancers associated with parasitic diseases | • **SCC of the bladder**—due to *Schistosoma hematobium,* • **cholangiocarcinoma**—due to *Clonorchis sinensis* |
| chromosome disorder associated with ovarian cancer | **Turner's syndrome**— * majority of patients are 45 XO: no Barr's bodies on a buccal smear, * streak gonads predispose to ovarian dysgerminomas: germ cell tumor |
| components of the MEN I/IIa/IIb syndromes | **see Table 9–4** |
| AD polyp syndrome associated with ovarian tumors | **Peutz-Jeghers syndrome**—PJ syndrome has an increased incidence of benign sex cord tumors with annular tubules |

*Table continued on following page*

**Table 10–2. PARANEOPLASTIC SYNDROMES, CANCER EPIDEMIOLOGY, RISK FACTORS FOR CANCER** *Continued*

| Most Common... | Answer and Explanation |
|---|---|
| risk factors for BCC of the skin | • **UVB light,** • *xeroderma pigmentosum* |
| risk factors for SCC of the skin | • **UVB light,** • *actinic keratosis*—precursor lesion for SCC, • *xeroderma pigmentosum,* • *arsenic,* • *immunosuppression,* • *radiation,* • *draining sinus tracts,* • *burn scars,* • *tars/soot/oils* |
| risk factors for malignant melanoma | • **UVB light**—severe sunburn at an early age is the greatest risk factor, • *dysplastic nevus syndrome,* • *xeroderma pigmentosum,* • *cellular blue nevus* |
| risk factors for nasopharyngeal carcinoma | • **EBV,** • *nickel* |
| risk factors for SCC of larynx | • **polycyclic hydrocarbons,** • *asbestos,* • *laryngeal papillomas*—HPV |
| risk factors for primary lung cancer | • **polycyclic hydrocarbons,** • *uranium*—radon gas in mines, • *asbestos*—additive carcinogenic effect if combined with smoking, • *chromium,* • *arsenic,* • *nickel,* • *cadmium* |
| risk factor for pleural mesothelioma | **asbestos exposure**— * see Table 6–4, * smoking is not a risk factor for mesothelioma |
| risk factor for SCC in the oral cavity | **polycyclic hydrocarbons**— * alone or in synergism with alcohol, * see Table 7–1 for other risk factors |
| risk factor for SCC of esophagus | • **polycyclic hydrocarbons**—see Table 7–2 for other risk factors |
| risk factor for distal adenocarcinoma of the esophagus | **Barrett's esophagus**— * MC cancer of esophagus, * see Table 7–2 |
| risk factor for gastric adenocarcinoma | • ***Helicobacter pylori*–induced chronic atrophic gastritis of antrum/pylorus**— * chronic inflammation produces intestinal metaplasia (goblet cells): precursor for adenocarcinoma, * see Table 7–3 for other risk factors |

### Table 10–2. PARANEOPLASTIC SYNDROMES, CANCER EPIDEMIOLOGY, RISK FACTORS FOR CANCER *Continued*

| Most Common... | Answer and Explanation |
|---|---|
| risk factor for low-grade gastric malignant lymphoma | ***Helicobacter pylori***—see Table 7–3 |
| risk factor for high-grade malignant lymphoma of the stomach | **immunosuppression**—see Table 7–3 |
| risk factors for primary small intestine malignant lymphoma | • **celiac disease**—high-grade T cell lymphoma, • *IgA heavy chain disease,* • *Crohn's disease* |
| risk factors for colorectal cancer | • **age >50 yrs old,** • **adenomatous polyps**—see Table 7–6 for other risk factors |
| type of inflammatory bowel disease with the greatest risk for colorectal cancer | **UC**— * risk increases most with: ♦ UC for >10 yrs, ♦ pancolitis, * see Table 7–6 |
| risk factor for SCC of anus | **HPV types 16, 18, 31**—unprotected anal intercourse |
| risk factors for HCC | **postnecrotic cirrhosis due to HBV/HCV**—see Table 8–2 for other risk factors |
| risk factor for liver angiosarcoma | **vinyl chloride**—see Table 8–2 for other risk factors |
| risk factor for cholangiocarcinoma | **primary sclerosing cholangitis**—see Table 8–2 for other risk factors |
| risk factor for gallbladder cancer | **cholelithiasis**—see Table 8–3 for other risk factors |
| risk factor for pancreatic cancer | **polycyclic hydrocarbons**—see Table 8–3 for other risk factors |
| risk factors for SCC of vulva | • **HPV types 16, 18, 31,** • *Bowen's disease,* • *immunosuppression* |
| risk factor for clear cell adenocarcinoma of the vagina | **DES exposure of the fetus during pregnancy**—vaginal adenosis is the precursor lesion for the cancer |

*Table continued on following page*

**Table 10–2. PARANEOPLASTIC SYNDROMES, CANCER
EPIDEMIOLOGY, RISK FACTORS FOR CANCER** *Continued*

| Most Common... | Answer and Explanation |
|---|---|
| risk factors for SCC of the cervix | • **HPV types 16/18**—risk for exposure to the virus increases with: ♦ early age of sexual intercourse, ♦ multiple high-risk partners, • *polycyclic hydrocarbons,* • *oral contraceptives,* • *immunosuppression* |
| risk factors for endometrial adenocarcinoma | • **excessive exposure to unopposed estrogen**—risk factors for unopposed estrogen include: ♦ early menarche/late menopause, ♦ estrogen Rx without progesterone, ♦ obesity (increased aromatization of 17-ketosteroids in adipose tissue), ♦ nulliparity, ♦ granulosa cell tumor of ovary, ♦ polycystic ovarian syndrome, • *Hx of breast cancer* |
| risk factors for ovarian cancers | • **age >50 yrs old,** • **nulliparity**—the greater the number of times ovulation has occurred, the greater the risk for ovarian cancer, • *high-fat/low-fiber diet,* • *late menopause,* • *Turner's syndrome*—see above, • *Peutz-Jeghers syndrome*—see above, • *polycyclic hydrocarbons,* • *BRCA-1* |
| risk factors for breast cancer | • **age >50 yrs old,** • **unopposed estrogen**— * atypical ductal hyperplasia is a precursor lesion for ductal cancer, * excessive exposure to estrogen includes: ♦ early menarche/late menopause, ♦ estrogen Rx without progesterone, ♦ nulliparity, ♦ high-fat/low-fiber diet, • **family Hx of breast cancer**— * particularly first-generation relatives: e.g., mother, sister, * BRCA-1/BRCA-2 suppressor genes, • *Hx of endometrial cancer,* • *radiation,* • *Li-Fraumeni multicancer syndrome* |
| risk factor for papillary adenocarcinoma of the thyroid | **radiation exposure of the head and neck**—see Table 9–2 for additional risk factors |
| risk factor for medullary carcinoma of the thyroid | **Hx of MEN IIa or IIb in the family**— * C cell hyperplasia is the precursor lesion of the cancer, * see Table 9–2 |
| risk factors for pheochromocytoma | • **MEN IIa/IIb**—see Table 9–4, • *neurofibromatosis,* • *von Hippel–Lindau disease* [**Note:** see Table 5–3 for a full discussion of pheochromocytoma.] |

**Table 10–2. PARANEOPLASTIC SYNDROMES, CANCER EPIDEMIOLOGY, RISK FACTORS FOR CANCER** *Continued*

| Most Common... | Answer and Explanation |
|---|---|
| risk factors for renal adenocarcinoma | • **polycyclic hydrocarbons,** • *von Hippel–Lindau disease*— * AD disease, * cerebellar hemangioblastoma, * >50% chance for bilateral renal adenocarcinoma |
| risk factors for TCC of the urinary bladder | • **polycyclic hydrocarbons,** • *aniline dyes,* • *phenacetin,* • *cyclophosphamide,* • *benzidine* |
| risk factors for testicular cancer | • **cryptorchid testis**— * risk extends to the cryptorchid testis and the uninvolved testis, * seminoma is the MC germ cell tumor in cryptorchidism, • *testicular feminization*—seminoma risk, • *DES exposure of the male fetus* |
| risk factors for prostate cancer | • **age >50 yrs**—an age-dependent cancer, • *family Hx of prostate cancer,* • *polycyclic hydrocarbons,* • *cadmium exposure,* • *BRCA-1 suppressor gene* |
| risk factors for SCC of the penis | • **uncircumcised state**—with poor hygiene, • *Bowen's disease,* • *erythroplasia of Queyrat,* • *balanitis xerotica obliterans* |
| risk factors for osteogenic sarcoma | • **irradiation,** • *Paget's disease of bone* |
| risk factor for chondrosarcoma | **enchondromatosis**—Ollier's disease |
| risk factors for soft tissue sarcomas | • **previous history of radiation**—malignant fibrous histiocytoma, • *neurofibromatosis*—neurofibrosarcoma, • *trauma*—malignant fibrous histiocytoma, • *herpesvirus 8*—Kaposi's sarcoma, • *chronic lymphedema*—lymphangiosarcoma |
| risk factors for astrocytoma | • **Turcot's syndrome**—AR polyposis syndrome, • **tuberous sclerosis,** • **neurofibromatosis,** • **Li-Fraumeni multicancer syndrome,** • **CNS lymphoma**—HIV/EBV: increased incidence of primary CNS lymphoma is directly related to increased incidence of AIDS |

*Table continued on following page*

**Table 10–2. PARANEOPLASTIC SYNDROMES, CANCER EPIDEMIOLOGY, RISK FACTORS FOR CANCER** *Continued*

| Most Common... | Answer and Explanation |
|---|---|
| risk factor for primary CNS lymphoma | **HIV**— * increase in AIDS parallels the increased incidence of primary CNS lymphoma, * EBV is a cocarcinogen with HIV |
| risk factor for acute leukemias | **radiation exposure**—see Table 2–8 for additional risk factors |
| risk factor for T cell leukemia/lymphoma | **HTLV-1** |
| risk factor for Burkitt's lymphoma | **EBV** |

**Question:** Smoking is a risk factor for which of the following cancers? **SELECT 9**

(A) Lung cancer
(B) Adenocarcinoma of the distal esophagus
(C) Mesothelioma
(D) Pancreatic cancer
(E) Stomach cancer
(F) Bladder cancer
(G) Embryonal rhabdomyosarcoma
(H) Gallbladder cancer
(I) Acute leukemia
(J) Colorectal cancer
(K) Squamous cell carcinoma of the anus
(L) Hepatocellular carcinoma
(M) Cervical cancer
(N) Laryngeal cancer
(O) Tongue

**Answers: (A), (D), (E), (F), (I), (J), (M), (N), (O).** Smoking is a risk factor for lung **(choice A is correct,** SCC and small cell carcinoma predominantly), pancreatic **(choice D is correct,** adenocarcinoma), stomach **(choice E is correct,** adenocarcinoma), bladder **(choice F is correct,** TCC), acute leukemia **(choice I is correct),** colorectal **(choice J is correct,** adenocarcinoma), cervical **(choice M is correct,** SCC), laryngeal **(choice N is correct,** SCC), and tongue **(choice O is correct,** SCC). Mesotheliomas have a relationship only with asbestos exposure and not smoking **(choice C is incorrect).** No sarcomas have any relationship to smoking **(choice G is incorrect).** There is no association of gallbladder cancer with smoking **(choice H is incorrect).** SCC of the anus is associated with HPV in unprotected anal intercourse **(choice K is incorrect).** HCC is not associated with smoking **(choice L is incorrect).**

AAT = α₁-antitrypsin, ACTH = adrenocorticotropic hormone, AD = autosomal dominant, ADH = antidiuretic hormone, AFP = alpha-feto-protein, AIDS = acquired immunodeficiency syndrome, ALL = acute lymphoblastic leukemia, AR = autosomal recessive, BCC = basal cell carcinoma, BRCA = breast cancer, CEA = carcinoembryonic antigen, CNS = central nervous system, COD = cause of death, DES = diethylstil-bestrol, DRE = digital rectal exam, EBV = Epstein-Barr virus, GERD = gastroesophageal reflux disease, HBV = hepatitis B virus, HCC = hepatocellular carcinoma, β-hCG = beta-human chorionic gonadotropin, HCV = hepatitis C virus, HDV = hepatitis D virus, HIV = human immunodeficiency virus, HPV = human papilloma virus, HTLV = human T cell lymphotropic virus, LDH = lactate dehydrogenase, LH = luteinizing hormone, MC = most common, MEN = multiple endocrine neoplasia, Pap = Papanicolaou, PJ = Peutz-Jeghers, PSA = prostate-specific antigen, PTH = parathormone, SCC = squamous cell carcinoma, TCC = transitional cell carcinoma, UC = ulcerative colitis, UVB = ultraviolet B (light).

### Table 10-3. CONCEPTS OF CANCER AND CANCER THERAPY IN SURGERY

| Most Common... | Answer and Explanation |
|---|---|
| cancer treatment modalities | • **surgery,** • *radiation,* • *chemotherapy* |
| benefits of surgery | • **potential cure,** • *remove tumor burden,* • *staging*—e.g., endometrial/ovarian cancers, • *complications*—e.g., * bowel adhesions secondary to previous surgery, * radiation |
| benefits of debulking operations | • **facilitate chemotherapy/radiation**—less tumor mass to kill, • *remove a potential complication related to Rx*—e.g., removal of bowel segment with infiltrating cancer to prevent perforation after adjuvant Rx begins |
| benefits of radiation | • **potential cure**—e.g., may be the sole Rx in laryngeal cancer, oral cavity, certain CNS tumors, • *adjuvant to chemotherapy,* • *Rx of complications*—e.g., * SVC syndrome, * pain due to bone metastasis [**Note:** radiation is used in the Rx of 50–60% of cancers.] |
| effect of tumor necrosis/fibrosis in tumor response to radiation | **decreases killing of tumor cells**—molecular oxygen is necessary for effective killing of tumor cell by radiation |

*Table continued on following page*

Table 10–3. CONCEPTS OF CANCER AND CANCER
THERAPY IN SURGERY *Continued*

| Most Common... | Answer and Explanation |
|---|---|
| cancers in which radiation alone is effective Rx | • **head/neck squamous carcinoma,** • **prostate,** • **anal squamous carcinoma,** • **HD** |
| complication of tumor recurrence after excision | **higher incidence of widespread metastases—** * malignant cells resistant to chemotherapy and radiation, * shorter cell cycle of malignant cells than original tumor cells prior to surgery |
| cancers with a high degree of dissemination near disease inception | • **small cell carcinoma of lung,** • *anaplastic thyroid cancer,* • *esophageal cancer,* • *pancreatic cancer,* • *Ewing's sarcoma,* • *osteogenic sarcoma* [**Note:** Rx should involve local and systemic Rx at the outset. The object is to attack cancer in the local and regional stage before dissemination.] |
| cancer utilizing lymphatic mapping | **malignant melanoma—** * using dyes and radiolabeled isotopes, regional lymph nodes (sentinel nodes) most likely to contain metastatic tumor are identified, * this method is being tried on breast cancer |
| chemotherapy agents | • **cytotoxic drugs**—e.g., alkylating agents, • *hormones*—e.g., * DES in prostate cancer, * progesterone in endometrial cancer, • *cytokines*—e.g., recombinant α-interferon in malignant melanoma, • *antihormones*—e.g., * tamoxifen: antiestrogen used in Rx of ERA-positive breast cancers, * 5-α reductase inhibitors: block DHT effect in prostate cancer, • *biologic*—e.g., intravesical BCG in bladder cancer, • *plant products*—e.g., paclitaxel from the Pacific yew tree |
| benefits of chemotherapy | • **adjuvant therapy along with surgery/radiation,** • *potential cure*—e.g., * gestationally derived choriocarcinoma, * HD, • *palliation,* • *preoperative modality to diminish tumor mass* |

### Table 10–3. CONCEPTS OF CANCER AND CANCER THERAPY IN SURGERY *Continued*

| Most Common... | Answer and Explanation |
|---|---|
| terms applied to chemotherapy | • **induction**—object: ♦ try to induce complete remission, ♦ kill all cancer cells, • **consolidation**—object: try to kill any remaining cancer cells in those that enter remission, • **maintenance**—try to prolong remissions, • **adjuvant**— * similar in concept to consolidation therapy, * most important modality to destroy micrometastases |
| routes of administration of chemotherapeutic agents | • **oral**, • *intravenous*, • *intracavitary*— * bladder, * peritoneum, • *intrathecal*—subarachnoid space: methotrexate in the Rx of ALL, • *intra-arterial*— * for administering high drug concentrations, * e.g., liver metastasis |
| causes of failure of advanced cancers to respond to chemotherapy | • **tumor heterogeneity**—cell populations resistant to chemotherapy, • *majority of neoplastic cells not in the cell cycle*—cells in the $G_0$ phase of cell cycle |
| cell cycle–specific chemotherapy agents | • **antimetabolites**, • **bleomycin**, • **plant alkaloids** [Note: cycle-specific drugs act during a specific phase of the cycle.] |
| cell cycle–nonspecific chemotherapy agents | • **alkylating agents**, • **antibiotics**, • **cisplatin**, • **nitrosourea**, • **L-asparaginase** [Note: cycle-nonspecific drugs are active throughout the cell cycle. Drugs inhibiting DNA synthesis (alkylate, intercalate) and inhibiting mitosis are in this group.] |
| antitumor MOA of antimetabolites | **blocks DNA synthesis in the S phase of the cell cycle**— * compete with normal metabolites for the regulatory site of a key enzyme, * substitute for a metabolite normally incorporated into DNA/RNA, * useful in rapidly dividing tumors |
| MOA of methotrexate (MTX) | **antimetabolite that blocks DNA synthesis**—inhibits dihydrofolate reductase in folic acid metabolism |

*Table continued on following page*

Table 10–3. **CONCEPTS OF CANCER AND CANCER THERAPY IN SURGERY** Continued

| Most Common... | Answer and Explanation |
|---|---|
| MTX complications | • **hematologic**— * megaloblastic anemia: prevent with leucovorin rescue, * BM suppression: cytopenias, • *GI*— * stomatitis, * liver fibrosis, • *lung*—interstitial fibrosis, • *GU*—crystal formation: keep urine pH alkaline |
| cancers treated with MTX | • **breast,** • *gestational choriocarcinoma,* • *testicular,* • *SCC of head/neck* |
| MOA of 5-fluorouracil (5-FU) | **antimetabolite that blocks DNA synthesis**— * pyrimidine analogue, * blocks thymidylate synthetase, * inhibits methylation of deoxyuridylic to thymidylic acid, * effective throughout cell cycle |
| 5-FU complications | • **GI**—stomatitis, • *hematologic*—BM suppression, • *CNS*—cerebellar ataxia |
| cancers treated with 5-FU | • **GI**— * colorectal, * stomach, * pancreas, • *breast,* • *ovarian* |
| MOA of antitumor antibiotics | **interfere with DNA metabolism by breaking up DNA** [Note: majority of the drugs derive from *Streptomyces*.] |
| MOA of bleomycin (BLM) | **MOA**— * antibiotic, * breaks DNA by an oxidative process involving FRs, * inhibits DNA ligase involved in DNA repair, * most effective in the $G_2$ phase in which tubulin is synthesized |
| BLM complications | • **lungs**—interstitial fibrosis, • *GI*—stomatitis |
| cancers treated with BLM | • **testicular,** • *head/neck* |
| MOA of dactinomycin (actinomycin D; antibiotic) | **interferes with DNA synthesis by intercalating between DNA base pairs, leading to the formation of FRs that break the DNA strand** [Note: it is effective in the S phase and inhibits topoisomerases (enzymes that repair single or double DNA breaks).] |
| complications associated with dactinomycin | • **severe myelosuppression,** • *stomatitis,* • *alopecia* |

## Table 10–3. CONCEPTS OF CANCER AND CANCER THERAPY IN SURGERY *Continued*

| Most Common... | Answer and Explanation |
| --- | --- |
| cancers treated with dactinomycin | • **Wilms' tumor,** • **choriocarcinoma,** • **Ewing's sarcoma** |
| complications associated with doxorubicin (antibiotic; Adriamycin) | • **marrow suppression,** • **dose-dependent cardiotoxicity,** • **alopecia,** • **red urine due to the drug** [**Note:** has a mechanism similar to that of dactinomycin.] |
| cancers treated with doxorubicin | **breast** |
| MOA of paclitaxel (antibiotic; plant alkaloid) | **antimicrotubule agent that blocks the disassembly of microtubules**—inhibits M phase of cycle [**Note:** binds to tubulin and stabilizes it so that it cannot disassemble.] |
| complications associated with paclitaxel | • **BM suppression,** • **hypersensitivity reactions**— * flushing, * angioedema, * urticaria, • *peripheral neuropathy,* • *alopecia* |
| cancers treated with paclitaxel | • **ovarian,** • **breast,** • **nonsmall cell lung cancer,** • **malignant melanoma** |
| MOA of vincristine/ vinblastine (antibiotics; plant alkaloids) | **bind to tubulin and prevent polymerization of tubulin dimers used to assemble microtubules**—inhibits the M phase of the cell cycle [**Note:** they derive from the periwinkle plant.] |
| complications associated with vincristine/ vinblastine | • **peripheral neuropathy,** • **BM suppression,** • **alopecia,** • **SiADH,** • **Raynaud's phenomenon** |
| cancers treated with vincristine/ vinblastine | • **bladder,** • **breast,** • **testicular** |
| MOA of alkylating agents | **impair cell function by alkylating DNA, RNA, and other proteins** [**Note:** alkylation primarily leads to breakage of DNA strands and cross-linking, which inhibits strand replication.] |

*Table continued on following page*

**Table 10–3. CONCEPTS OF CANCER AND CANCER THERAPY IN SURGERY** *Continued*

| Most Common... | Answer and Explanation |
|---|---|
| complications associated with cyclophosphamide (alkylating agent; Cytoxan) | • **hemorrhagic cystitis**—blocked with mesna, • *bladder cancer*, • *BM suppression*, • *SiADH* [**Note**: it is a nitrogen mustard changed by the cytochrome system into phosphoamide, which interacts with DNA.] |
| cancers treated with cyclophosphamide | • **breast**, • **small cell carcinoma**, • **ovarian**, • **Ewing's sarcoma** |
| complications associated with chlorambucil (alkylating agent; Leukeran) | • **BM suppression**, • *second malignancies*—NHL |
| cancers treated with chlorambucil | • **ovarian**, • **breast** |
| complications associated with melphalan (alkylating agent; Alkeran) | • **BM suppression**, • **interstitial pneumonitis**, • **second malignancies**—NHL |
| cancers treated with melphalan | • **ovarian**, • **breast** |
| complications associated with cisplatin (alkylating agent) | • **nephrotoxicity**— * magnesium wasting leading to hypoparathyroidism, * potentiates aminoglycoside nephrotoxicity, • *ototoxicity*, • *peripheral neuropathy* |
| cancers treated with cisplatin | • **bladder**, • **cervical**, • **ovarian**, • **testicular**, • **osteogenic sarcoma** |
| MOA of IL-2 (cytokine from $CD_4$ T helper cells) | • **increases T cell proliferation**, • **increases lymphokine-activated NK cells** |
| complications associated with IL-2 | **vascular leak syndrome** |
| cancers treated with IL-2 | • **metastatic renal adenocarcinoma**, • **malignant melanoma** |
| MOA of tamoxifen | **weak estrogen that acts as an estrogen antagonist that binds to estrogen receptors**—disrupts estrogen's effect on RNA synthesis |

## Table 10–3. CONCEPTS OF CANCER AND CANCER THERAPY IN SURGERY *Continued*

| Most Common... | Answer and Explanation |
|---|---|
| complications associated with tamoxifen | • **endometrial carcinoma**, • **hypercalcemia**, • **hot flushes** |
| cancer treated with tamoxifen | **adjuvant therapy in ERA-positive breast cancers** [Note: in addition, its weak estrogenic activity prevents osteoporosis and CAD.] |
| MOA of DES | **estrogen compound that competes with androgens for intracellular receptor sites**— blocks growth-promoting effect of estrogens |
| complications associated with DES | • **gynecomastia**, • *venous thrombosis* |
| cancer treated with DES | **prostate** |
| MOA of leuprolide | **analogue of GnRH**—when administered in a sustained fashion, it inhibits LH/FSH release and decreases synthesis of testosterone and DHT |
| complication associated with leuprolide | **hypogonadism** |
| cancer treated with leuprolide | **prostate** |

**Question:** Which of the following groups of chemotherapy agents are cell cycle-specific in their activity? **SELECT 3**
  (A) DNA alkylating agents
  (B) DNA synthesis inhibitors
  (C) Mitotic inhibitors
  (D) Bleomycin
  (E) Most DNA intercalating agents

**Answers: (B), (C), (D).** DNA synthesis inhibitors, like methotrexate and fluorouracil, are cell cycle-specific in that they block the S phase **(choice B is correct)**. Mitotic inhibitors, like paclitaxel and vincristine/ vinblastine, are cell cycle-specific since they block the mitotic phase of the cycle **(choice C is correct)**. Bleomycin is a DNA intercalating drug but its main effect is on the $G_2$ phase of the cycle **(choice D is correct)**. DNA alkylating agents and most DNA intercalating drugs act throughout the cycle **(choices A and E are incorrect)**.

*Table continued on following page*

ALL = acute lymphoblastic leukemia, BCG = Bacille Calmette-Guérin vaccine, BLM = bleomycin, BM = bone marrow, CAD = coronary artery disease, CNS = central nervous system, DES = diethylstilbestrol, DHT = dihydrotestosterone, ERA = estrogen receptor assay, FRs = free radicals, FSH = follicle-stimulating hormone, 5-FU = 5-fluorouracil, $G_0$ = resting phase of cell cycle, $G_2$ phase = gap 2, GnRH = gonadotropin-releasing hormone, HD = Hodgkin's disease, IL-2 = interleukin 2, LH = luteinizing hormone, M = mitotic phase of the cell cycle, MOA = mechanism of action, MTX = methotrexate, NHL = non-Hodgkin's lymphoma, NK = natural killer, S = synthesis of DNA phase of the cell cycle, SCC = squamous cell carcinoma, SiADH = inappropriate antidiuretic hormone syndrome, SVC = superior vena cava.

# CHAPTER

## 11

# BREAST SURGERY

## CONTENTS

### Table 11–1. BENIGN BREAST DISORDERS

| Most Common... | Answer and Explanation |
|---|---|
| causes of breast masses in order of decreasing frequency | • **fibrocystic change (FCC)**, • *no disease,* • *other types of benign disease,* • *cancer,* • *fibroadenoma* |
| locations for breast tissue | • **upper outer quadrant**—underscores why cancer is most commonly located in this quadrant, • *beneath the nipple* |
| role of estrogen in the breast | **ductal and alveolar growth** |
| role of progesterone in the breast | **alveolar differentiation** |
| hormones involved in lactational events | • **prolactin**—stimulates and maintains lacto-genesis, • *human placental lactogen*—stimulates alveolar growth and lactogenesis, • *cortisol and insulin*—support lactational development, • *oxytocin*— * released by the suckling reflex, * contracts myoepithelial cells with expulsion of milk into ducts |
| breast mass in a woman <50 yrs old | **fibrocystic change (FCC)** |
| breast mass in a woman >50 yrs old | **infiltrating ductal carcinoma**—slightly more common in the left than right breast |
| tumor in a woman <35 yrs old | **fibroadenoma** |
| cause of bloody nipple discharge in a woman <50 yrs old | **intraductal papilloma**— * confirm that it is blood with a Hemoccult test, * lactiferous duct is identified and excised [**Note:** bloody nipple discharges unrelated to papillomas occur during 2nd–3rd trimester.] |

*Table continued on following page*

## Table 11–1. BENIGN BREAST DISORDERS *Continued*

| Most Common... | Answer and Explanation |
|---|---|
| cause of a bloody nipple discharge in a woman >50 yrs old | **infiltrating ductal carcinoma** |
| physiologic cause of galactorrhea after lactation has ceased and menses resumed | **mechanical stimulation of nipple** [Note: galactorrhea refers to milk production unrelated to lactation.] |
| pathologic cause of galactorrhea | **prolactinoma** |
| nonpituitary endocrine disease causing galactorrhea | **primary hypothyroidism**—low serum thyroxine increases TSH and TRH, the latter a potent stimulator of prolactin |
| drugs associated with galactorrhea | • **birth control pills,** • *phenothiazines,* • *tricyclic antidepressants,* • *cimetidine,* • *reserpine,* • *methyldopa,* • *calcium channel blockers* |
| diseases involving the nipple/areola complex | • **Paget's disease,** • *abscess* |
| diseases involving the lactiferous duct/sinus | • **intraductal papilloma,** • *galactocele,* • *abscess,* • *mammary ectasia (plasma cell mastitis)* |
| diseases involving the large ducts | • **FCC,** • *ductal cancer* |
| disease involving the terminal duct | **tubular carcinoma** |
| diseases involving the terminal lobules | • **sclerosing adenosis,** • *lobular carcinoma* |
| diseases involving breast stroma | • **fibroadenoma,** • *phyllodes tumor (cystosarcoma phyllodes)* |
| cause of a nipple discharge | **lactation** |
| cause of a purulent nipple discharge | **subareolar abscess due to *Staphylococcus aureus*—** * usually in the setting of a lactating woman, * child does not have to be weaned during antibiotic Rx while lesion is in the cellulitis stage, * an abscess must be incised and drained |

### Table 11–1. BENIGN BREAST DISORDERS *Continued*

| Most Common... | Answer and Explanation |
|---|---|
| greenish-brown nipple discharge | **mammary duct ectasia (plasma cell mastitis)**— * chronic mastitis in multiparous women, * perimenopausal, * ectatic lactiferous ducts are filled with debris, * may simulate cancer, * not associated with smoking, * Rx patients with recurrent infections with incision/drainage and antibiotics covering aerobic/anaerobic bacteria |
| cause of a serous or clear nipple discharge | **birth control pills**—particularly common just prior to menses |
| time frame for cyclic breast pain | **midcycle and premenstrual**— * disappears with increasing age, * reduction in caffeine often helps relieve pain, * a good supporting bra is mandatory, * reduction in fat intake is useful [**Note:** pain in the breast is more often due to hormone imbalance than cancer.] |
| vitamins used in Rx of cyclic breast pain | • **vitamin E,** • *vitamin A,* • *pyridoxine* [**Note:** these have not been scientifically proved but do provide relief for some women. Other modalities of Rx include evening primrose oil, danazol, and birth control pills.] |
| Rx of noncyclic breast pain | • **evening primrose oil plus reduction in fat intake and use of a supporting bra**—evening primrose oil increases synthesis of PGE$_1$, which blocks prolactin effect in breast tissue, • *danazol,* • *lidocaine + steroid injection,* • *surgical excision*—if nothing else works [**Note:** noncyclic pain is usually in women >40 yrs old. It is usually subareolar.] |
| causes of breast pain unrelated to breast parenchymal disease | • **referred pain from gallbladder/lung disease,** • *Tietze's syndrome*—costochondritis, • *Mondor's disease*— * superficial thrombophlebitis of veins overlying breast, * palpable, painful cord, * Rx with NSAIDs |
| site of pain for Tietze's syndrome | **2nd–4th costal cartilages along parasternal border** |
| Rx of Tietze's syndrome | **NSAIDs and local heat** |
| cause of painless lump in the breast >50 yrs of age | **infiltrating ductal carcinoma** |

*Table continued on following page*

## Table 11–1. BENIGN BREAST DISORDERS *Continued*

| Most Common... | Answer and Explanation |
|---|---|
| components of FCC | • **cysts,** • **fibrosis,** • *sclerosing adenosis*—proliferation of small ductules/acini, • *ductal hyperplasia*— * benign papillary proliferation, * apocrine metaplasia, * atypical hyperplasia: precancerous [**Note:** FCC is a disorder during the reproductive period of life.] |
| variant of FCC confused with invasive cancer | **sclerosing adenosis**— * proliferative lesion in the terminal lobules has an infiltrative pattern but remains in the lobule, * it is commonly associated with microcalcifications |
| cause of acute mastitis | *Staphylococcus aureus* **in lactating woman** |
| cause of periductal, subareolar mastitis | **smoking**— * chemicals in smoke alter epithelium in lactiferous sinuses, predisposing to infection with abscess formation, * no relation to age or lactation |
| cause of fat necrosis | **breast trauma**— * undergoes fibrosis and dystrophic calcification, * calcification simulates breast cancer in a mammogram, * may retract skin and simulate cancer |
| clinical presentation of a fibroadenoma | **painless to painful freely movable mass**— * estrogen-sensitive tumor, * stromal tumor with compression of ducts, * may enlarge or infarct during pregnancy, * commonly multiple [**Note:** a mild risk for ductal cancer exists if associated with a family Hx of cancer or FCC with proliferative changes.] |
| drug associated with development of fibroadenomas | **cyclosporine**—in women who are postrenal transplant |
| Rx of fibroadenoma | **excision** |
| histologic reaction to silicone breast implants | **granulomatous reaction with foreign body giant cells and chronic inflammatory cells** [**Note:** the relationship of these implants with an increase in autoimmune disease has not been verified.] |
| disorder of the male breast | **gynecomastia** [**Note:** it refers to a benign proliferation of the glandular component of the male breast. It may be unilateral or bilateral depending on breast sensitivity to estrogen.] |

**Table 11–1. BENIGN BREAST DISORDERS** *Continued*

| Most Common... | Answer and Explanation |
|---|---|
| time frames when gynecomastia is normal | • **neonate**— * 60–90%, * transplacental passage of estrogen, • **puberty**— * unilateral or bilateral, * peaks ages 13–14 yrs, • **old age**—50–80 yrs old |
| cause of gynecomastia | **increased estrogen stimulation** |
| sources of estrogen in males | • **peripheral aromatization of androgens**— * 85%, * testosterone → estradiol, * androstenedione → estrone, • *Leydig cells*—15% |
| mechanisms of gynecomastia | • **increased free estrogen**, • *decrease in endogenous free androgens*—leaves estrogen unopposed, • *defects in androgen receptors*—leaves estrogen unopposed |
| causes of increased free estrogen | • **aromatization of 17-KS to estrogen in liver disease**, • *conversion of estrone to estradiol*— * 17-KS reductase, * estradiol is the most potent estrogen and estrone the weakest, • *decreased liver metabolism of estrogen,* • *drug displacement from SHBG*—e.g., * spironolactone, * ketoconazole, • *drugs with estrogen activity*—e.g., * DES, * digoxin, which activates estrogen receptors |
| causes of decreased free androgens | • **old age,** • *increased SHBG*—hyperestrinism increases the liver synthesis of the protein, • *drugs*—e.g., * leuprolide, * spironolactone/ketoconazole (these inhibit testosterone synthesis), • *primary hypogonadism*—refers to testicular disease, • *secondary hypogonadism*—refers to hypothalamic/pituitary dysfunction, • *genetic diseases*—e.g., Klinefelter's syndrome |
| causes of androgen receptor defects | • **drugs**—e.g., * flutamide, * spironolactone, • *genetic diseases*—e.g., testicular feminization |
| drugs of abuse causing gynecomastia | • **alcohol,** • *marijuana,* • *amphetamines,* • *heroin* |
| tests used to evaluate gynecomastia | • **serum hCG,** • **serum FSH/LH,** • **serum testosterone,** • **serum estradiol ($E_2$)** |

*Table continued on following page*

## Table 11–1. BENIGN BREAST DISORDERS *Continued*

| Most Common... | Answer and Explanation |
| --- | --- |
| cause of gynecomastia if the above studies are normal | **idiopathic gynecomastia** |
| cause of gynecomastia if hCG is high | **testicular cancer with trophoblastic component**—hCG is an LH analogue and stimulates breast tissue |
| cause of gynecomastia when LH is high and testosterone low | **primary testicular dysfunction**—e.g., Klinefelter's syndrome |
| cause of gynecomastia when FSH/LH and testosterone are low | • **secondary hypogonadism**, • *prolactinoma*, • *androgen/estrogen–producing tumor*— * testes, * adrenal |
| cause of gynecomastia when LH and testosterone are high | **androgen receptor insensitivity** |
| cause of gynecomastia when estradiol is high | **estrogen-producing tumor in testes or adrenal gland** |
| overall causes of pathologic gynecomastia in decreasing frequency | • **idiopathic**, • *drugs*, • *cirrhosis*, • *primary hypogonadism*, • *testicular tumors*, • *secondary hypogonadism*, • *hyperthyroidism*—increased breast sensitivity to estrogens, • *renal disease* |

**Question:** Which of the following breast site:breast disorder groupings are correctly matched? **SELECT 3**
- (A) Nipple:Paget's disease
- (B) Lactiferous duct:lobular carcinoma
- (C) Major duct:fibrocystic change
- (D) Terminal lobule:sclerosing adenosis
- (E) Stroma:plasma cell mastitis

**Answers: (A), (C), (D).** Paget's disease of breast is invasion of the nipple by an underlying ductal cancer, producing an eczematous-appearing nipple **(choice A is correct)**. Fibrocystic change is the most common lesion of the major duct **(choice C is correct)**. Sclerosing adenosis is a variant of FCC that involves the terminal lobules and is often confused with invasive cancer **(choice D is correct)**. It is commonly associated with microcalcifications. Lobular carcinoma is the most common cancer of the terminal lobules **(choice B is incorrect)**. Plasma cell mastitis is most commonly located in the lactiferous ducts **(choice E is incorrect)**.

DES = diethylstilbestrol, FCC = fibrocystic change, FSH = follicle-stimulating hormone, hCG = human chorionic gonadotropin, 17-KS = 17-ketosteroid, LH = luteinizing hormone, SHBG = sex hormone–binding globulin, TRH = thyrotropin-releasing hormone, TSH = thyroid-stimulating hormone.

### Table 11–2. MALIGNANT BREAST DISORDERS

| Most Common... | Answer and Explanation |
| --- | --- |
| overall cancer in women | **infiltrating ductal carcinoma** [**Note:** it is the second most common COD due to cancer. The incidence has stabilized over the last few years. One in nine women are at risk for breast cancer.] |
| risk factors for breast cancer | • **age**— * incidence 1/232 in 4th decade and 1/29 in 7th decade, * average age is 64 yrs, • *family Hx*— * 5–10% have AD disorder, * first-degree relatives (mother/sister) are at greater risk than second-degree relatives (e.g., aunts), • *excessive estrogen exposure*— * early menarche/late menopause, * nulliparity, * postmenopausal obesity: aromatization, • *Bx showing atypical ductal/lobular hyperplasia,* • *Hx of endometrial carcinoma,* • *Hx of previous breast cancer,* • *radiation*— * atomic bomb exposure, * radiation for other cancers, • *Li-Fraumeni multicancer syndrome*—AD disorder due to inactivation of p53 suppressor gene: ♦ breast cancer, ♦ sarcomas, ♦ brain tumors, ♦ leukemia, • *Cowden disease*— * AD disease, * multiple hamartoma syndrome: ♦ skin, ♦ polyposis, * 50% risk of breast cancer by 50 yrs of age |
| genetic association with breast cancer | • **BRCA1 gene,** • **BRCA2 gene** [**Note:** these genes can be identified to evaluate women for cancer risk. Less than 20% of women with a family Hx of breast cancer have these genes.] |

*Table continued on following page*

**Table 11–2. MALIGNANT BREAST DISORDERS** *Continued*

| Most Common... | Answer and Explanation |
|---|---|
| differences between BRCA1 and BRCA2 cancers | • BRCA1 is located on chromosome 17 and BRCA2 is located on chromosome 13, • breast cancer at earlier age in BRCA1 (40–50 yrs old) than BRCA2 ($\geq$50 yrs old), • breast cancer >70% by age 80 yrs in BRCA1 and >60% by age 70 yrs in BRCA2, • medullary carcinoma is more common with BRCA1 than BRCA2, • male breast cancer greater in BRCA2 than BRCA1, • greater risk for ovarian cancer by age 70 yrs in BRCA1 than BRCA2, • bladder/pancreatic cancer greater in BRCA2 than BRCA1, • colon cancer greater in BRCA1 than BRCA2 |
| differences in breast cancer in blacks versus whites | • lower incidence in blacks, • greater mortality, • higher grade, • younger age, • less likely to be ERA/PRA positive |
| oncogene relationships with breast cancer | • ras oncogene, • p53 suppressor gene, • erbB$_2$, • Rb suppressor gene |
| S/S of breast cancer | • **painless mass in upper outer quadrant,** • *skin retraction,* • *nipple retraction,* • *axillary lymphadenopathy,* • *peau d'orange*— * orange-skin appearance due to plugged up dermal lymphatics, * a sign of inflammatory carcinoma |
| uses of mammography | • **screening test for nonpalpable breast masses**— * not a diagnostic test, * sensitivity is 90% for detecting nonpalpable masses, * does not distinguish solid from cystic lesions, * cancerous lesions are usually stellate and have fuzzy borders, • *evaluate for multicentric cancer if the FNA is positive,* • *evaluate extent of a cancer,* • *identify microcalcifications* |
| primary screening modality in women <30 yrs | **ultrasonography**—breast tissue is very dense in young women, which renders mammography less useful |
| mammography pattern of microcalcification suggesting cancer | **5 or more tightly clustered microcalcifications that are punctate, microlinear, or branching** |

## Table 11–2. MALIGNANT BREAST DISORDERS *Continued*

| Most Common... | Answer and Explanation |
|---|---|
| benign breast disease with microcalcifications | **sclerosing adenosis**—proliferative variant of FCC that targets terminal lobules |
| malignant breast cancer with microcalcifications | **ductal carcinoma in situ (DCIS)** |
| screening recommendation for breast cancer | • **40–49 yrs old**—annually or every other year, • **≥50 yrs on**—annually, • **Hx of cancer in mother/sister**—begin 5–10 yrs earlier than age of cancer in mother/sister |
| initial step in work-up of a palpable breast mass | **fine needle aspiration**— * determines whether it is cystic or solid, * provides cytologic Dx, * sensitivity 90–98% [**Note:** some surgeons first use ultrasonography to distinguish a cystic from a solid mass.] |
| management step if the FNA shows the lesion is cystic and cytologically benign, and the mammogram is normal | **observe for evidence of recurrence in 1 mo**—if fluid is bloody or multiple recurrences occur, outpatient excisional Bx is recommended |
| management step if the FNA shows the lesion is cystic and cytologically benign, and the mammogram is abnormal | **outpatient excisional Bx** |
| management step if the FNA shows the lesion is solid and cytologically benign or suspicious, and the mammogram is normal or abnormal | **outpatient excisional Bx** |
| management step if the FNA is cytologically malignant, and the mammogram is normal or abnormal | **intraoperative incisional Bx with a frozen section to confirm malignancy before definitive surgery is performed** |

*Table continued on following page*

### Table 11–2. MALIGNANT BREAST DISORDERS *Continued*

| Most Common... | Answer and Explanation |
|---|---|
| use for a core Bx of a breast lesion | **large, palpable, solid masses** |
| Bx techniques for nonpalpable masses | • **needle-localized Bx**—using mammography for guidance, a needle with a hookwire is inserted at the periphery of the lesion, • *core Bx with computer-driven stereotactic unit*— * good alternative to needle localization (some use it as primary technique), * sensitivity and specificity is >95% |
| G/M appearance of infiltrating ductal carcinoma | **stellate, indurated, gray-white tumor that is gritty on cut section**— * induration is due to reactive fibroplasia secondary to a stromal reaction against the tumor, * the majority exhibit multifocality, * the grading system for breast cancer is based on: ♦ percent tubule formation, ♦ nuclear polymorphism, ♦ mitoses per 10 hpf |
| types of ductal carcinoma in situ (DCIS) | • **noncomedo type**—netlike pattern in the ducts with central necrosis, • *comedocarcinoma*— * central area of necrosis, * tends to have a poorer prognosis [**Note:** ~one-third of low-grade DCIS will eventually invade. Most high-grade DCIS will invade if left untreated.] |
| cancer with an eczematous appearance of the nipple | **Paget's disease**— * variant of DCIS, * an underlying breast cancer that extends up into the nipple and invades the skin, * usually seen in elderly women, * erbB₂ relationship, * a palpable mass is present in 50–60%, * poor prognosis |
| subtype of breast cancer associated with BRCA1 gene | **medullary carcinoma**— * bulky, soft tumor with large cells, a benign lymphocytic infiltrate, and pushing rather than infiltrating margins, * high nuclear grade, * majority are ERA/PRA-negative, * better survival rate and younger age group than with infiltrating ductal cancer |
| cancer misdiagnosed as acute mastitis | **inflammatory carcinoma**— * it is a clinical Dx, * the skin is erythematous, * plugs of tumor block the dermal lymphatics, causing lymphedema and a peau d' orange appearance: Cooper's ligaments tether the skin to the underlying breast tissue, * has the poorest prognosis of all the breast cancers |

## Table 11–2. MALIGNANT BREAST DISORDERS *Continued*

| Most Common... | Answer and Explanation |
|---|---|
| cancers with an increased incidence of bilaterality | • **lobular carcinoma in situ (LCIS)**— * 50–75% bilaterality, * contralateral tumor does not have to be a lobular carcinoma, * slow-growing cancer: 25–35% eventually invade over next 20 yrs if left untreated: risk ~1% per yr, * the majority are ERA/PRA-positive, * excellent prognosis, • *invasive lobular carcinoma*— * ~20% bilaterality, • *tubular carcinoma*— * 10–40% bilaterality, * MC cancer of the terminal duct, * majority are ERA/PRA-positive |
| subtype of invasive breast cancer with "Indian filing" | **invasive lobular carcinoma**— * neoplastic cells line up behind each other ("Indian file"), or form concentric circles like a bulls-eye, * this pattern may also be seen in invasive ductal carcinoma |
| subtype of breast cancer with the greatest propensity for CNS, ovary, uterus, and bone marrow metastasis | **invasive lobular carcinoma** |
| subtype of breast cancer found incidentally on a Bx specimen | **LCIS**— * nonpalpable, * LCIS does not produce a density on a mammogram, * LCIS does not have microcalcifications |
| invasive breast cancers with an excellent prognosis | • **tubular**, • *colloid (mucinous) carcinoma*— * neoplastic cells float in lakes of mucin, * good prognosis applies only if it is not associated with another type of invasive cancer, • *lobular*, • *medullary* |
| malignant stromal cancer | **phyllodes tumor (cystosarcoma phyllodes)**— * hypercellular stroma is malignant but the epithelial component is benign, * bulky tumor with necrosis, * microscopic study shows cystic spaces with leaflike extensions, * low-grade malignancy that does not metastasize to the axillary lymph nodes, * Rx with simple mastectomy |

*Table continued on following page*

#### Table 11–2. MALIGNANT BREAST DISORDERS *Continued*

| Most Common... | Answer and Explanation |
|---|---|
| factors affecting the prognosis in breast cancer | • **status of the axillary lymph nodes**—tumors >2 cm impose an increased risk for nodal metastasis: ~one-third have nodal metastasis at the time of presentation, • *ERA-PRA status*— * postmenopausal patients are more often positive than younger women, * positive assays indicate a better remission rate (60–80%) and a slightly better prognosis: patients are candidates for tamoxifen, • *cancer grade,* • *erbB₂ oncogene status*—poor prognosis if present, • *skin/muscle invasion*—poor prognosis, • *vascular space invasion*—poor prognosis, • *S-phase fraction*—>5% is a bad prognosis, • *DNA ploidy*—diploid (even number) is better than aneuploid (odd number) |
| lymph node groups involved in order of decreasing frequency | • **axillary nodes**— * level I nodes are inferior to the pectoralis minor muscle, * level II nodes are beneath the pectoralis minor, * level III nodes are medial and superior to the pectoralis minor, • *internal mammary nodes,* • *supraclavicular nodes* [**Note:** nonpalpable lymph nodes have metastasis in 25–30% of cases. Palpable nodes do not have metastasis in 25–30% of cases.] |
| lymph node group involved in outer quadrant cancers | **axillary lymph nodes** |
| lymph node group involved in inner quadrant cancers | **internal mammary nodes** |
| metastatic sites in descending order for breast cancer | • **lung,** • *bone,* • *liver* |
| cancers in stage 0 | **DCIS and LCIS**—5-yr survival rate is >90% |
| criteria for stage I cancers | • **invasive,** • **≤2 cm,** • **no nodal involvement,** • **no distant metastasis,** • **5-yr survival rate 80–87%** |
| criteria for stage II cancers | • **invasive,** • **<5 cm**—also includes tumors ≥5 cm without nodal involvement or distant metastasis, • **nodes involved**—must be movable, • **5-yr survival rate 65–75%** |

## Table 11–2. MALIGNANT BREAST DISORDERS *Continued*

| Most Common... | Answer and Explanation |
|---|---|
| criteria for stage III cancers | • **invasive,** • **>5 cm with nodal involvement,** • **any-sized tumor with**— * fixed axillary nodes, * ipsilateral internal mammary node involvement, * skin/chest wall/muscle involvement without distant metastasis, * clinical inflammatory carcinoma without nodal/distant metastasis, • **5-yr survival rate 40–45%** |
| criteria for stage IV cancers | • **any breast cancer with**— * distant metastasis, * ipsilateral supraclavicular nodal involvement, • **5-yr survival 10–13%** |
| preoperative screening tests for breast cancer | • **CBC,** • **biochemical profile**—including liver enzymes and calcium, • **chest x-ray** |
| indications for a preoperative radionuclide bone scan | • **symptomatic bone pain,** • **elevated serum alkaline phosphatase**—γ-glutamyl transferase should not be elevated or suspect liver metastasis, • **hypercalcemia** |
| indications for a preoperative CT scan of liver | • **hepatomegaly,** • **elevated liver function tests**— * alkaline phosphatase, * γ-glutamyl transferase, * LDH |
| surgical options for stage I and II breast cancers | • **modified radical mastectomy**— * nipple/areolar complex, * all breast tissue, * pectoralis minor, * levels I and II axillary lymph nodes in continuity, * level III nodes if levels I and II nodes are grossly involved, • **breast conservation therapy**— * lumpectomy with microscopically free margins, * removal of levels I and II axillary nodes, * breast irradiation |
| contraindications for breast conservation therapy | • **tumor >5 cm,** • **unacceptable cosmetic result based on tumor versus breast size,** • **woman is pregnant,** • **diffuse, malignant-appearing microcalcifications,** • **autoimmune disease**— * PSS, * SLE |
| cause of a winged scapula after a modified radical mastectomy | **damage to the long thoracic nerve** |

*Table continued on following page*

### Table 11–2. MALIGNANT BREAST DISORDERS *Continued*

| Most Common... | Answer and Explanation |
|---|---|
| Rx of lymphedema postmodified radical mastectomy | **pneumatic device + elevation of arm**— * complication occurs in 10–15%, * cellulitis commonly accompanies lymphedema and requires antibiotics |
| long-term complication of lymphedema | **potential for lymphangiosarcoma** |
| management of locally advanced (stage IIB, IIIA/B) breast cancer | • **modified radical mastectomy,** • **irradiation**— * chest wall, * axilla, * supraclavicular nodes, • **systemic chemotherapy**—given prior to and after surgery |
| adjuvant systemic therapy in node-positive, ERA-positive premenopausal women | **combination chemotherapy**—with or without tamoxifen |
| adjuvant systemic therapy in node-positive, ERA-negative premenopausal women | **combination chemotherapy** |
| adjuvant systemic therapy in node-positive, ERA-positive postmenopausal women | **tamoxifen**—with or without chemotherapy |
| adjuvant systemic therapy in node-negative, ERA-positive premenopausal women | **depends on the risk of recurrence**— * risk is determined by tumor size and grade, * low risk: no Rx versus tamoxifen, * good risk: tamoxifen, * high risk: chemotherapy ± tamoxifen |
| adjuvant systemic therapy in node-negative, ERA-positive postmenopausal women | **depends on the risk of recurrence**— * low risk: no Rx versus tamoxifen, * good risk: tamoxifen, * high risk: tamoxifen ± chemotherapy |

## Table 11–2. MALIGNANT BREAST DISORDERS *Continued*

| Most Common... | Answer and Explanation |
|---|---|
| adjuvant systemic therapy in node-negative, ERA-negative premenopausal women | **automatically high risk**—chemotherapy |
| adjuvant systemic therapy in node-negative, ERA-negative postmenopausal women | **automatically high risk**—chemotherapy ± tamoxifen |
| drugs used in adjuvant chemotherapy | • **CMF regimen**— * c̲yclophosphamide, * m̲ethotrexate, * 5-f̲luorouracil, • **CAF regimen for high-risk recurrence**—cyclophosphamide, A̲driamycin (doxorubicin), 5-f̲luorouracil |
| indications for postoperative radiation | • **tumor >5 cm**, • **tumor with extension into chest wall or skin**, • **perineural/lymphatic invasion**, • **fixed axillary nodes**, • **positive surgical margins**, • **≥4 positive axillary nodes**, • **adherent to pectoralis fascia** |
| Rx of LCIS | • **clinical surveillance**— * clinical breast exam every 6 mos, * yearly mammography, • *bilateral mastectomy*—prophylactic |
| Rx of bone metastasis | **radiation**—tamoxifen is often added |
| Rx of chest wall recurrence | **excision + radiation** |
| management of a breast mass during pregnancy | **FNA** |
| preoperative studies for pregnant women with breast cancer | • **CBC**, • **biochemical profile**, • *radiologic studies*— * based on the risk to the fetus, * ultrasound is satisfactory for liver evaluation |

*Table continued on following page*

## Table 11–2. MALIGNANT BREAST DISORDERS *Continued*

| Most Common... | Answer and Explanation |
|---|---|
| Rx for stages I and II breast cancer in pregnancy | **modified radical mastectomy during the pregnancy**— * breast conservation therapy is contraindicated, * no increased risk to the fetus |
| Rx for stage III breast cancer in pregnancy | **combined chemotherapy after organogenesis has occurred** |
| risk factors for breast cancer in men | • **family Hx in first-degree relative,** • *BRCA2 gene,* • *Klinefelter's syndrome,* • *exposure to ionizing radiation,* • *exposure to exogenous estrogens*—e.g., DES |
| breast cancers to occur in men | **all types except DCIS and LCIS** |

**Question:** A 58-yr-old woman with a 20-year history of smoking has a history of breast cancer in her mother. Her diet is poor in fiber and rich in saturated fats. Menarche occurred at 13 years of age and menopause began at 52 yrs of age. She has had 3 children. She had a cervical conization at 28 yrs of age for severe cervical dysplasia and has since had normal cervical Pap smears. Which of the following is her greatest risk factor for breast cancer? **SELECT 1**
- (A) Age
- (B) Family history
- (C) Smoking history
- (D) Severe cervical dysplasia
- (E) Low-fiber, high-saturated-fat diet

**Answer: (B).** The history of breast cancer in a first-degree relative overrides age as the most important risk factor for cancer in this woman **(choice A is incorrect).** Cervical dysplasia is not a risk factor for breast cancer **(choice D is incorrect).** Smoking is a minor risk factor for breast cancer **(choice C is incorrect).** A low-fiber/high-saturated-fat diet is a risk factor but does not have the same significance as family history **(choice E is incorrect).**

AD = autosomal dominant, BRCA = breast cancer, Bx = biopsy, CAF = cyclophosphamide, Adriamycin, 5-fluorouracil, CMF = cyclophosphamide, methotrexate, 5-fluorouracil, CNS = central nervous system, COD = cause of death, DCIS = ductal carcinoma in situ, ERA = estrogen receptor assay, FCC = fibrocystic change, FNA = fine needle aspiration, G/M = gross and microscopic, hpf = high-powered field, LCIS = lobular carcinoma in situ, LDH = lactate dehydrogenase, MC = most common, PRA = progesterone receptor assay, PSS = progressive systemic sclerosis, Rb = retinoblastoma, SLE = systemic lupus erythematosus, S/S = signs and symptoms.

# CHAPTER

## 12

# SELECTED ORTHOPEDIC DISORDERS

## CONTENTS

### Table 12–1. SELECTED ORTHOPEDIC DISORDERS I

| Most Common... | Answer and Explanation |
|---|---|
| symptom of a musculoskeletal disorder | **pain** |
| types of musculoskeletal pain | • **localized**—present at the site of the pathologic process, • *diffuse*—deep tissue type of pain, • *radicular*—follows the anatomic distribution of a peripheral nerve: e.g., sciatic nerve pain, • *referred*—pain is located at a site remote from the primary pathologic process: e.g., knee pain is often manifested in the hip |
| causes of shoulder pain | • **rotator cuff tear,** • **rupture of a cervical disc,** • **arthritis of the acromioclavicular joint,** • **shoulder dislocation**— * the majority are anteriorly dislocated, * often injure the axillary artery/nerve |
| components of the rotator cuff | **tendon insertions of—supraspinatus, infraspinatus, teres minor, subscapularis muscles** |
| rotator cuff injuries | • **tendinitis/bursitis**—impingement of rotator cuff on the coracoacromial ligament, • **tears**—pain/weakness with active shoulder abduction |
| diagnostic tests for rotator cuff injuries | • **arthrography,** • **MRI,** • *ultrasound* |

*Table continued on following page*

**Table 12–1. SELECTED ORTHOPEDIC DISORDERS I**
*Continued*

| Most Common... | Answer and Explanation |
|---|---|
| causes of elbow pain | • **tennis elbow**— * pain occurs in the area where the extensor muscle tendons insert near the lateral epicondyle, * pain is reproduced by extending the wrist against resistance with the elbow extended, * common in— ♦ racket sports, ♦ repetitive use of a hammer or screwdriver, • *golfer's elbow*— * pain is located where the flexor muscle tendons insert near the medial epicondyle, * pain is reproduced by resisting wrist flexion or forearm pronation, • *ulnar nerve compression*— * the ulnar nerve may be entrapped in the following areas: ♦ transverse carpal ligament, ♦ elbow ("funny bone area"), * pain and numbness of the ulnar aspect of the forearm and ring and little finger exist, plus weakness of the intrinsic muscles of the hand, • *radicular pain from cervical disc disease* |
| S/S of herniation of $C_4$–$C_5$ disc | • **pain**—$C_5$ distribution: ♦ medial scapula, ♦ lateral border of arm, • **sensory loss**—lateral border of upper arm, • **reflex loss**—biceps: musculocutaneous nerve $C_5$–$C_6$, • **motor deficit**— * deltoid, * supraspinatus, * infraspinatus, * rhomboids |
| S/S of herniation of $C_5$–$C_6$ disc | • **pain**—$C_6$ distribution: ♦ lateral forearm, ♦ thumb, ♦ index finger, • **sensory loss**— * lateral forearm, * index finger, • **reflex loss**—supinator, • **motor deficit**— * biceps, * brachioradialis, * pronators/supinators of the forearm |
| S/S of herniation of $C_6$–$C_7$ disc | • **pain**—$C_7$ distribution: ♦ posterior arm, ♦ lateral hand, ♦ midforearm, ♦ medial scapula, • **sensory loss**— * midforearm, * middle finger, • **reflex loss**—triceps: radial nerve $C_6$–$C_8$, • **motor deficit**— * latissimus dorsi, * triceps, * pectoralis major, * wrist flexors |
| causes of hand/wrist pain | • **tendinitis/synovitis,** • **carpal tunnel,** • **arthritis**—e.g., * osteoarthritis, * rheumatoid arthritis, • *ganglion cyst*—synovial cyst located on the wrist or hand |

## Table 12–1. SELECTED ORTHOPEDIC DISORDERS I
*Continued*

| Most Common... | Answer and Explanation |
|---|---|
| clinical findings of de Quervain's disease | • **definition**—chronic stenosing tenosynovitis of the first dorsal compartment of the wrist, • **pathogenesis**— * overuse of the hands and wrist: e.g., ♦ gripping and wringing clothes, ♦ use of an EZ curl bar in weight lifting, * the first dorsal compartment contains the abductor pollicis longus (APL) and the extensor pollicis brevis (EPB): excessive friction causes thickening of the tendon sheath and stenosis of the osseofibrous tunnel, • **S/S**— * pain occurs on the radial aspect of the wrist: aggravated by moving the thumb, * Finkelstein's test: ♦ the patient flexes the thumb into the palm→ the examiner pushes the base of the flexed thumb in an ulnar direction→ the patient feels pain in the region of the radial styloid process |
| cause of a bulge on the dorsum of the wrist when the wrist is flexed | **"ganglion" (synovial) cyst**— * a cyst filled with mucinous material, * communicates with synovial sheaths on the dorsum of the wrist, * enlarges with flexion of the wrist and causes pain, * sometimes called the Bible tumor since a Bible is often used to smash the cyst, * recurs unless it is surgically removed |
| S/S of a compartment syndrome | • **pain**, • *paresthesias*, • *pallor*, • *paralysis*, • *pulselessness* [**Note:** a compartment syndrome refers to an increase of pressure in a confined space. The pressure reduces perfusion, which may lead to permanent ischemic contractures of the muscle(s) in that compartment. The 5 P's listed above are the same as those listed for arterial insufficiency.] |
| causes of compartment syndromes | • **fractures**, • **injuries to arteries/soft tissue**, • **prolonged limb compression**—e.g., tight-fitting cast, • **third-degree burns** [**Note:** compartment pressures are measurable with needles inserted into the compartment. Pressures > 30 mmHg are considered dangerous.] |

*Table continued on following page*

**Table 12–1. SELECTED ORTHOPEDIC DISORDERS I**
*Continued*

| Most Common... | Answer and Explanation |
|---|---|
| compartment syndrome in the forearm | **Volkmann's ischemic contracture**— * a complication of a supracondylar fracture of the humerus, * injury to the brachial artery and median nerve occurs, * brachial artery ischemia leads to increased pressure in the closed muscle compartments of the forearm, with a subsequent decrease in venous and then arterial perfusion: this may lead to permanent ischemic contractures of the muscle, * Rx: fasciotomy to relieve pressure |
| entrapment syndrome of the median nerve | **carpal tunnel syndrome**— * the median nerve is most commonly entrapped in the transverse carpal ligament of the wrist, * may also be entrapped between the bellies of the pronator teres muscle |
| causes of the carpal tunnel syndrome | • **RA/pregnancy,** • *overuse of the hands/wrist,* • *amyloidosis,* • *hypothyroidism* |
| S/S of the carpal tunnel syndrome | • **pain, numbness, or paresthesias in the thumb; index, second, and third fingers; and radial side of fourth finger**—nocturnal pain is common, • **thenar atrophy**—"ape" hand appearance, • **physical exam**— * positive Tinel's sign: the pain is reproduced by tapping over the median nerve, * positive Phalen's sign: symptoms are reproduced with forced flexion of the wrist for 1 min |
| tests used to evaluate a carpal tunnel syndrome | • **lab tests ordered depending on the clinical suspicion include**— * uric acid: gout, * glucose: diabetes mellitus, * TSH: primary hypothyroidism, * serum ANA: collagen vascular disease, • **electrodiagnostic tests**—nerve conduction studies: ♦ must be ordered if surgery is contemplated, ♦ electromyography to R/O muscle degeneration related to the nerve compression |
| Rx of carpal tunnel syndrome | • **conservative**— * wrist splint with the wrist held in mild dorsiflexion, * NSAIDs, * osteopathic manipulation, * local corticosteroid injection, • *surgery to release the nerve* |

## Table 12–1. SELECTED ORTHOPEDIC DISORDERS I
*Continued*

| Most Common... | Answer and Explanation |
|---|---|
| Rx of a felon and paronychia | **incision and drainage**— * a felon is an abscess of the fingertip pulp: *Staphylococcus aureus* is a common pathogen, * a paronychia is an infection of the eponychial fold: *Staphylococcus aureus* and *Candida* species are common offenders |
| cause of "claw hand" | **ulnar nerve palsy**— * ulnar nerve functions include: ♦ adduction of the fingers due to innervation of the palmar and dorsal interosseus muscles, ♦ adduction of the thumb: adductor pollicis muscle, * injury may be due to: ♦ fracture of the medial epicondyle of the humerus, ♦ lead poisoning, ♦ arm wrestling, ♦ slashing of the wrist |
| cause of "wrist drop" | **radial nerve palsy**— * the radial nerve supplies the extensor muscles of the wrist and digits: wrist drop refers to a hand that is flexed at the wrist and cannot be extended, * injury may be due to: ♦ midshaft fractures of the humerus, ♦ draping the arm over a park bench (called "Saturday night palsy") |
| cause of "waiter's tip deformity" | **brachial plexus lesion (Erb-Duchenne) involving $C_5$ and $C_6$**—upper trunk injury |
| clinical findings in Erb-Duchenne palsy | • **birth injury of the brachial plexus with damage to $C_5$–$C_6$ nerves**—upper trunk injury, • **S/S**— * loss of abduction of the arm from the shoulder, * inability to rotate the arm externally, * inability to supinate the forearm, * absent biceps reflex, * asymmetric Moro reflex: no movement on the affected side |
| clinical findings in Klumpke's paralysis | • **birth injury of the brachial plexus with injury to the $C_7$–$C_8$ and $T_1$**—lower trunk injury, • **S/S**— * paralysis of the hand, * Horner's syndrome: ♦ ipsilateral ptosis of the eye, ♦ miosis, ♦ anhidrosis |
| lung disease associated with Horner's syndrome | **superior sulcus tumor with destruction of the cervical sympathetic ganglion**—usually a primary squamous cell carcinoma |

*Table continued on following page*

## Table 12–1. SELECTED ORTHOPEDIC DISORDERS I
### *Continued*

| Most Common... | Answer and Explanation |
|---|---|
| causes of axillary nerve injury (C₅–C₆) | • **fracture of the surgical neck of the humerus,** • **dislocation of the shoulder joint**— * usually anterior dislocation, * may also injure the axillary artery |
| S/S of axillary nerve injury | • **patient cannot abduct the arm to the horizontal position or hold the horizontal position when a downward force is applied to the arm**—paralysis of deltoid muscle, • **weakening of lateral rotation of the arm**—paralysis of teres minor muscle, • **sensory loss on lateral side of the upper arm** |
| arteries, nerves, tendons cut with a deep laceration of the radial side of the wrist | • **artery**—radial artery, • **nerve**—median nerve: courses along the radial artery, • **tendons**— * palmaris longus, * flexor carpi radialis |
| arteries, nerves, tendons cut with a deep laceration of the ulnar side of the wrist | • **artery**—ulnar artery, • **nerve**—ulnar nerve, • **tendon**—flexor carpi ulnaris |
| causes of lower extremity pain | • **foot pain**— * metatarsalgia: due to repetitive loading on the metatarsal heads, * plantar fasciitis: ♦ due to repetitive loading on the attachment of the plantar ligament to the calcaneus, ♦ commonly causes the formation of a heel spur, * arthritis: ♦ rheumatoid arthritis, ♦ Charcot's neuropathic joint (e.g., peripheral neuropathy due to diabetes mellitus), • **tibial pain**— * stress fractures, * compartment syndrome, • **knee pain**— * meniscal tears, * arthritis, * chondromalacia of the patella, * patellar tendinitis, • **hip pain**— * osteoarthritis of the femoral head, * Legg-Perthes disease: see Table 12–2, * trochanteric bursitis: produces lateral hip pain, * sciatica: produces posterior hip pain, • **miscellaneous**— * peripheral vascular disease: see Tables 5–1 and 5–2, * deep venous thrombosis: see Table 5–2, * radicular pain from lumbar disc herniations |

## Table 12–1. SELECTED ORTHOPEDIC DISORDERS I
*Continued*

| Most Common... | Answer and Explanation |
|---|---|
| cause of "shin splints" | **repetitive loading of the anterior compartment muscles of the tibia**— * inflammation occurs at the musculotendinous insertions: these are often called "stress fractures," * Rx with: ♦ rest, ♦ icing, ♦ NSAIDs, ♦ correction of training errors |
| site for a compartment syndrome in the leg | **anterior compartment of the tibia**—see the above discussion of compartment syndromes |
| mechanisms of low back pain | • **spasm of the paraspinal muscles**, • *ligament strains*— * anterior/posterior longitudinal ligaments, • *facet disease*—see below, • *nerve root irritation*—e.g., intervertebral disc disease with nerve root compression, • *spinal stenosis*, • *extradural compression of spinal cord*, • *diseases involving vertebral column*— * metastasis: breast cancer, * multiple myeloma, * osteoporosis: compression fractures, * osteomyelitis: Pott's disease, * Paget's disease of bone, * rheumatologic diseases: ♦ OA, ♦ RA, ♦ AS [**Note:** myofascial pain and discogenic pain are more common in patients < 50 yrs old. Paget's disease, spinal stenosis, osteoporosis, and malignancy are more common in patients > 50 yrs old.] |
| diagnostic procedures used in evaluating low back pain | • **radiographs**—should be ordered in all: ♦ trauma patients, ♦ adolescents, ♦ adults > 50 yrs old, • **bone scans**, • **CT/MRI**—usually for those in whom surgery is likely, • **miscellaneous tests**— * CBC, * rheumatoid factor (RF), * serum ANA |
| Rx of low back pain | • **conservative**— * NSAIDs, * muscle relaxants, * physical therapy modalities: ♦ ice, ♦ heat, ♦ ultrasound, * osteopathic/chiropractic manipulation, * relative rest for 1–2 days with early return to activity, * lose weight if obese, • *epidural injection of corticosteroids,* • *surgery* |

*Table continued on following page*

## Table 12–1. SELECTED ORTHOPEDIC DISORDERS I
*Continued*

| Most Common... | Answer and Explanation |
|---|---|
| cause of intervertebral disc disease | **degeneration of fibrocartilage/nucleus pulposus**— * the ruptured disc material may herniate posteriorly and compress the nerve root and/or spinal cord, * pain (sciatica) radiates from the low back to: ♦ the buttocks, ♦ down the leg, ♦ below the knee |
| disc herniation | $L_5$–$S_1$ |
| S/S of disc herniation | **radicular pain**—leg pain is aggravated by: ♦ straight leg raising, ♦ coughing, ♦ sitting, ♦ sneezing, ♦ forward flexion, • **physical exam**—straight leg raising on the affected side with the patient in the supine position: ♦ called Lasègue's test, ♦ exacerbates pain in the leg (not the back) by putting traction on the sciatic nerve, ♦ pain is further enhanced by dorsiflexing the foot, which is called Lasègue's sign |
| S/S of herniation of $L_5$–$S_1$ disc | • **pain**—$S_1$ distribution: ♦ back of thigh, ♦ back of calf, ♦ lateral foot, • **sensory loss**— * lateral and posterior calf, * plantar aspect of foot, • **reflex loss**—Achilles reflex: tibial nerve $L_4$–$S_3$, • **motor deficit**— * loss of plantar flexion, * loss of foot eversion: weakness of peroneus longus/brevis |
| S/S of herniation of $L_4$–$L_5$ disc | • **pain**—$L_5$ distribution: ♦ back of thigh, ♦ lateral calf, ♦ dorsum of foot, • **sensory loss**— * dorsum of foot, * webbed space between the great toe and first digit, • **reflex loss:** none, • **motor deficit:** loss of dorsiflexion of the big (great) toe: weakness of the extensor hallucis longus |
| S/S of herniation of $L_3$–$L_4$ disc | • **pain**—$L_4$ distribution: down to the medial malleolus, • **sensory loss**—medial leg to the malleolus, • **reflex loss**—knee jerk: femoral nerve $L_2$–$L_4$, • **motor deficit**— * quadriceps weakness: weakness of knee extension, * loss of dorsiflexion of the foot: weakness of the tibialis anterior |
| Rx of disc herniation | • **conservative**—80–90% of patients improve without surgery, • *surgery*— * laminectomy with removal of the extruded disc, * digestion with percutaneous injection of chymopapain/collagenase: select cases, * microdiscectomy: select cases |

**Table 12–1. SELECTED ORTHOPEDIC DISORDERS I**
*Continued*

| Most Common... | Answer and Explanation |
|---|---|
| S/S of the lateral recess syndrome in lumbar spine (facet syndrome) | • **radicular pain**, • **unilateral/bilateral pain/ paresthesias in $L_5$ or $S_1$**, • **pain is brought on by walking/standing and relieved by sitting**, • **negative straight leg test**—recall that a positive straight leg test indicates a ruptured intervertebral disc [**Note:** the facet syndrome is frequently due to an osteophyte involving the superior articular facet in a patient with osteoarthritis.] |
| S/S of lumbar stenosis | • **patient is usually >50 yrs old**, • **symptoms are usually bilateral**, • **pain is described as dull or aching**—involves the whole extremity, • **pain is provoked by walking and/or standing (pseudoclaudication) and is relieved by sitting and/or leaning forward**, • **feeling of deadness in the leg** [**Note:** spinal stenosis refers to narrowing of the spinal canal or neuroformina. It is best diagnosed with MRI or CT scans.] |
| causes of spinal cord compression | • **trauma**, • *epidural tumor*, • *herniated intervertebral disc*, • *epidural/subdural abscess/ hematoma*, • *AVM* |
| causes of extradural hematomas | • **trauma**, • *anticoagulants*, • *AVM*, • *hemophilia* |
| extradural spinal tumors leading to cord compression | **metastatic breast, prostate, or lung cancer**— 85% of patients also have evidence of vertebral metastasis |
| clinical findings in extradural compression on the cord | • **pain comes first**, • **second**—corticospinal tract dysfunction: ♦ weakness, ♦ spasticity, ♦ hyperreflexia, • **third**—posterior column disease: ♦ paresthesias, ♦ loss of vibration and position sense, • **bladder/bowel dysfunction if the conus medullaris or cauda equina is compressed** [**Note:** in cord compression, distal signs occur before proximal signs.] |
| Rx of spinal cord compression | • **MRI of the entire spine to identify all lesions**, • **dexamethasone**, • **radiation if the compression is due to metastatic lesions**— >80% are ambulatory after radiation, • **neurosurgical consultation** |

*Table continued on following page*

**Table 12–1. SELECTED ORTHOPEDIC DISORDERS I**
*Continued*

| Most Common... | Answer and Explanation |
|---|---|
| S/S of cauda equina syndrome | • **bowel or bladder dysfunction,** • **saddle area anesthesia** |
| S/S of low back pain in ankylosing spondylitis | **bilateral sacroiliac pain in the AM that improves with exercise** |
| cause of forward subluxation of one vertebral body on another | **spondylolisthesis**—best demonstrated by lateral and oblique radiographs of the spine |
| causes of spondylolisthesis | • **spondylosis**—defect in the vertebral lamina (pars interarticularis) with separation from the main body of the vertebra, • *congenital facet deficiency,* • *fracture of posterior elements,* • *facet deficiency due to intervertebral disc disease* |
| S/S of spondylolisthesis | **low back pain**— * hamstring tightness, * sciatica without neurologic deficits |
| causes of superior gluteal nerve injury | • **surgery,** • **poliomyelitis,** • **Duchenne's muscular dystrophy** |
| S/S of superior gluteal nerve injury | **waddling gait**— * the superior gluteal nerve supplies the gluteus medius and minimus muscles, * loss of abduction of the thigh and inability to pull the pelvis down, * positive Trendelenburg's sign: ♦ raising of the foot on the injured side causes the contralateral pelvis to fall down, ♦ a positive Trendelenburg test also occurs in patients with a hip dislocation and in those with fractures of the femoral neck |
| S/S of inferior gluteal nerve injury | **patient is unable to walk**— * the inferior gluteal nerve supplies the gluteus maximus muscle, * the patient cannot: ♦ walk, ♦ climb stairs, ♦ rise from a seated position, * the patient leans backward when the heel strikes the ground |
| site of sciatic nerve entrapment | **sciatic notch in the buttocks** |
| site of peroneal nerve entrapment | **behind the knee**— * common in people who cross their legs a lot, * the patient has a slapping gait |

## Table 12–1. SELECTED ORTHOPEDIC DISORDERS I
*Continued*

| Most Common... | Answer and Explanation |
|---|---|
| S/S of a common peroneal nerve injury (L₄–S₂) | • **motor deficits**— * loss of foot eversion: due to weakening of the peroneus longus and brevis muscles, * loss of foot dorsiflexion: ♦ due to weakening of the tibialis anterior muscle, * "slapping gait" or "high-stepping gait" like a horse, * loss of toe extension: due to weakening of the extensor digitorum longus and hallucis longus muscles, * the combined effect of all the above produces an equinovarus deformity: plantar flexion with foot drop and inversion of the foot, • **sensory deficits**—anterolateral aspect of the leg and dorsum of the foot, • **loss of the ankle jerk reflex** |
| site for lateral femoral nerve entrapment | **inguinal ligament**— * entrapment of the nerve produces meralgia paresthetica, * numbness or burning sensation over the lateral part of the thigh with walking or prolonged standing, * common in obese patients |
| signs of an obturator nerve injury (L₂–L₄) | • **motor deficit**— * the leg swings out when walking because the obturator nerve supplies muscles that are involved with hip adduction, • **sensory loss**—medial aspect of thigh, • **loss of knee reflex** |
| signs of a tibial nerve injury (L₄–S₃) | • **motor deficits**— * loss of plantar flexion of the foot due to weakening of the gastrocnemius, soleus, and plantaris muscles, * loss of flexion of the toes due to weakening of the flexor digitorum longus and hallucis longus muscles, * foot inversion due to weakening of the tibialis posterior muscle, * the above motor deficits combine to produce calcaneovalgocavus, with dorsiflexion and inversion of the foot, • **sensory loss**—sole, • **loss of ankle jerk reflex** |
| signs of femoral nerve injury (L₂–L₄) | • **motor deficits**— * the patient cannot flex the thigh due to weakening of the sartorius and iliacus muscles, * the patient cannot extend the leg due to weakening of the quadriceps muscle, • **sensory loss**— * anterior portion of the thigh, * medial side of the leg and foot, • **loss of knee jerk reflex** [**Note:** femoral nerve injuries are due to injury in the area of the femoral triangle, a common site for catheterization punctures.] |

*Table continued on following page*

**Table 12–1. SELECTED ORTHOPEDIC DISORDERS I**
*Continued*

| Most Common... | Answer and Explanation |
|---|---|
| term applied to forward displacement of the thoracic spine | **kyphosis (humpback)**— * stated another way, kyphosis is an increase in the normal posterior convexity of the thoracic spine, * forward displacement of the spine is seen: humpback * if severe, kyphosis may lead to chest restriction and respiratory acidosis |
| causes of kyphosis in adolescents | • **muscular/postural problems**— * the benign type of kyphosis that responds well to exercise, * commonly seen in tall adolescents, • *Scheuermann's disease*—due to abnormal vertebral end-plates leading to disc herniations into the vertebrae, called Schmorl's nodes |
| cause of senile kyphosis | **osteoporosis**—multiple compression fractures cause wedging of the vertebrae |
| term applied to lateral curvature of the spine | **scoliosis** |
| clinical findings in idiopathic scoliosis | • **usually affects adolescent girls between 10 and 16 yrs of age,** • **S/S**—usually a right thoracic curve: forward bending causes a paraspinous prominence on the right from a hump in the ribs due to a rotational component of the vertebra, • **Rx**— * bracing, * postural exercise, * surgical correction with rods if curvature is > 40° |
| fibromatosis | **Dupuytren's contracture**— * a fibromatosis is a non-neoplastic proliferation of connective tissue, * Dupuytren's contracture involves thickening of the palmar fascia, which causes contraction of the 4th and 5th fingers, * common in alcoholics and smokers |
| fibromatosis associated with Gardner's polyposis syndrome | **desmoid tumor**—usually occurs in the anterior abdominal wall |
| fibromatosis associated with methysergide | **retroperitoneal fibrosis**—often leads to hydronephrosis, owing to entrapment of the ureters in collagen |
| benign soft tissue tumor | **lipoma**—arises from adipose cells |

## Table 12–1. SELECTED ORTHOPEDIC DISORDERS I
*Continued*

| Most Common... | Answer and Explanation |
|---|---|
| risk factors for producing sarcomas | • **ionizing radiation**—e.g., * malignant fibrous histiocytoma, * osteogenic sarcoma, • *genetic predisposition*—e.g., neurofibrosarcoma involving the sciatic nerve in patients with neurofibromatosis |
| sarcoma in adults | • **malignant fibrous histiocytoma**, • *liposarcoma*—second MC sarcoma |
| positions the knee joint is forced into that result in injury | • **valgus position**— * valgus injury is angulation away from the midline, * knee joint is in a knockknee position: knees together, * laterally originating force is applied to the knee: e.g., clipping injury in football |

**Frontal View (Valgus Injury)**

• *varus position*—varus is angulation toward the midline: ♦ medially originating force is applied to the knee, ♦ knee has bowlegged appearance

**Frontal View (Varus Injury)**

*Table continued on following page*

**Table 12–1. SELECTED ORTHOPEDIC DISORDERS I**
*Continued*

| Most Common... | Answer and Explanation |
|---|---|
| functions of the menisci in the knees | • **evenly distribute joint fluid,** • **joint shock absorber,** • **provide rotary joint stability,** • **keep the articular surfaces of the bones from rubbing against each other**—provides a protective filler in the joint |
| meniscus injury | **medial meniscus injury**—the lateral meniscus is less frequently torn due to: ♦ smaller diameter, ♦ greater thickness, ♦ attachment to both cruciate ligaments |
| mechanism of a meniscus injury | **rotational force is applied to the flexed knee when it is moving toward an extended position** |
| tear in a medial meniscus injury | **longitudinal tear of the posterior portion of the medial meniscus** |
| test used to evaluate meniscus injuries | **McMurray's test**— \* test for the medial meniscus: patient is supine→ knee is acutely flexed→ foot is grasped and the leg is externally rotated→ knee is slowly extended while the other hand feels the posteromedial margin of the knee joint→ a click along the posteromedial margin indicates a medial meniscus tear: femur passes over the tear, \* test for a lateral meniscus injury: same procedure as above except the leg is rotated internally and extended→ a click is palpated along the posterolateral margin of the joint |
| location and function of the anterior cruciate ligament (ACL) | **ACL attaches the anterior part of the tibia to the lateral condyle of the femur**—prevents anterior movement of the tibia in relation to the femur |
| location and function of the posterior cruciate ligament (PCL) | **PCL extends from the posterior part of the tibia to the medial condyle of the femur**—prevents posterior movement of the tibia in relation to the femur |

## Table 12–1. SELECTED ORTHOPEDIC DISORDERS I
*Continued*

| Most Common... | Answer and Explanation |
|---|---|
| tests used to evaluate the cruciate ligaments in the knee | • **Lachman's test for ACL**—knee is flexed ~15–30° and the femur is stabilized by one of the examiner's hands→ other hand of the examiner is placed on the posterior aspect of the tibia→ anterior force is applied to evaluate whether the tibia moves forward or remains stabilized→ anterior movement of the tibia indicates an ACL injury, • **anterior draw test to evaluate ACL**—patient supine, hip flexed 45°, knee flexed 90°→ examiner places hand on the posterior aspect of the tibia→ anterior force is applied in neutral, external, internal direction→ positive anterior draw test is noting anterior displacement of the tibia, • **posterior draw test to evaluate PCL**—patient supine, hip flexed 45°, knee flexed 90°→ examiner places hand on the anterior aspect of proximal tibia→ posterior force is applied in neutral, external, internal direction→ positive posterior draw test is noting posterior displacement of the tibia |
| functions of the medial collateral ligament | **supports the medial side of the knee joint**— * attaches the medial epicondyle of the femur with the shaft of the tibia, * resists valgus and external rotational forces of the proximal tibia in relation to the distal femur |
| functions of the lateral collateral ligament | **supports the lateral side of the knee joint**— * attaches the lateral epicondyle of the femur to the head of the fibula, * resists varus forces and rotational forces of the proximal fibula in relation to the distal femur |
| S/S of a meniscus injury | • **pain**, • **quadriceps atrophy**—chronic injury, • **knee catches, locks, or gives way when walking**, • **swelling/popping of knee** |

*Table continued on following page*

## Table 12–1.  SELECTED ORTHOPEDIC DISORDERS I
*Continued*

| Most Common... | Answer and Explanation |
|---|---|
| clinical findings of a medial meniscus injury | • **mechanism of injury**— * MC internal derangement of knee joint, * most commonly part of a valgus injury: clipping in football, * hyperextension of the knee joint: second MC mechanism of injury, • **structures damaged**— * medial meniscus, * medial collateral ligament, * ACL, • **S/S**— * inability to extend the knee: locked, * pain, * quadriceps atrophy: chronic injury, * knee catches or gives way when walking, * swelling of the knee, * positive McMurray's test: click on posteromedial margin with the knee flexed, externally rotated, and slowly extended, • **lab studies**—double contrast arthrography is confirmatory test, • **Rx**— * conservative therapy: if longitudinal and partial tears, * arthroscopy/open surgery: ♦ partial/complete meniscectomy, ♦ suture |
| clinical findings of a lateral meniscus injury | • **mechanism of injury**— * less common than medial meniscus, * varus injury, * injury to lateral collateral ligament, • **S/S**—similar to medial meniscus injury, * positive McMurray's test: click on posterolateral margin with the knee flexed, externally rotated, and slowly extended, • **lab studies**—double-contrast arthrography is confirmatory test: 95% accuracy, • **Rx**—similar to that for medial meniscus |
| clinical findings of ACL injury | • **mechanism of injury**— * MC ligament injury, * torn most commonly in a valgus injury secondary to clipping or skiing, * hyperextension of the knee: occurs in 30% of medial meniscus injuries, * direct blow to a flexed knee: dashboard injury, • **S/S**—knee gives way or buckles when walking, * a pop is heard, * positive anterior draw sign, * positive Lachman's test: best test, • **lab studies**—MRI is the best test, • **Rx**— * conservative, * surgery |

**Table 12–1. SELECTED ORTHOPEDIC DISORDERS I**
*Continued*

| Most Common... | Answer and Explanation |
|---|---|
| clinical findings of a PCL injury | • **mechanism of injury**— * hyperextension of the knee secondary to an anterior force pushing the tibia in a posterior direction, * direct fall on a flexed knee with the foot in plantar flexion: jumping from a height, * dashboard injury with knee flexed and tibia posteriorly displaced, • **S/S**— * similar to those of ACL, * positive posterior draw test, • **lab studies**—MRI is the best test, • **Rx**— * conservative, * surgery |
| clinical findings of a medial collateral ligament injury | **torn with valgus injuries**— * more common than lateral collateral ligament tears, * patient describes a pop after receiving a lateral blow to the knee joint |
| clinical findings of a lateral collateral ligament injury | **torn with varus injuries**— * patient describes pain in the posterolateral aspect of the knee, * sensory and motor findings from possible injury to the peroneal nerve |
| cause of an ankle sprain | **sprain of lateral ankle ligaments from inversion of a plantar flexed foot**—common in basketball, volleyball, and football |
| lateral ligament that is sprained | **anterior talofibular ligament**—very important ligament in stabilization of plantar flexion in the foot |
| test used to evaluate ankle sprains | **x-rays of the ankle**— * lateral, * AP, * mortise view: evaluates injury to the deep deltoid ligament |
| Rx of ankle sprains | • **compression bandages,** • **ice,** • **elevation,** • **NSAIDs,** • **reduce weight bearing on the joint**—crutches |
| nerve injured with clavicular fractures | **ulnar nerve**—most clavicular fractures are in the middle one-third and are secondary to thoracic trauma |
| nerve injured in proximal humerus fractures | **axillary nerve**—sensory loss along lateral aspect of the deltoid muscle |

*Table continued on following page*

## Table 12–1.  SELECTED ORTHOPEDIC DISORDERS I
*Continued*

| Most Common... | Answer and Explanation |
|---|---|
| nerve injured in midshaft/distal third of humerus | **radial nerve**— * nerve travels in the spiral groove, * wrist drop |
| danger of a supracondylar fracture of the elbow | **damage to the brachial artery and/or median nerve**—vascular compromise may result in Volkmann's ischemic contracture in the forearm compartment (see above) |
| classification scheme for growth plate fractures in children | **Salter–Harris**— * epiphyseal plate is the weakest part of a child's bones, * type I: fracture through the growth plate without bony involvement, * type II: fracture through the growth plate and metaphysis, * type III: fracture through the growth plate and epiphysis into the joint, * type IV: fracture through the metaphysis, growth plate, and epiphysis into the joint, * type V: crush injury to the growth plate |
| clinical findings of the boxer's fracture | • **fracture**— * neck of fifth metacarpal, * trauma with a closed fist: ♦ hitting a wall, ♦ jaw of another individual, * danger of human bite infection, • **Rx**— * closed reduction with splinting, * percutaneous pitting if severe angulation, * if human bite: ♦ irrigation of wound, ♦ debridement, ♦ intravenous antibiotics |
| cause of pain in the elbow and inability to supinate the forearm in 1–4 yr olds | **subluxation of the head of the radius**—usually due to jerking of the hand by an impatient or abusing parent |
| clinical findings of Monteggia's fracture | **dislocation of the radial head + diaphyseal fracture of the ulna**— * sometimes called the "nightstick fracture," * Rx with ORIF of ulna and closed reduction of radial head |
| clinical findings of Galeazzi's fracture | **dislocation of the distal radioulnar joint + fracture of the diaphysis of the radius**—Rx with ORIF of radius + cast the forearm in supination to reduce distal radioulnar joint |

### Table 12–1. SELECTED ORTHOPEDIC DISORDERS I
*Continued*

| Most Common... | Answer and Explanation |
|---|---|
| fracture associated with falling on the outstretched hand | **Colles' fracture of the distal radius—** * MC fracture of the wrist, * radiologically, it produces a "dinner fork" deformity of the proximal radial fragment: ◆ displaced upward and backward, ◆ fracture of ulnar styloid process commonly occurs as well, * second most common fracture in osteoporosis in women, * Rx with closed reduction with application of a plaster splint |
| carpal bone fracture | **scaphoid—** * second MC fracture of the wrist, * majority occur at the waist of the scaphoid, * pain in the anatomic snuff box located below the radial styloid process, * high incidence of aseptic necrosis, * Rx with thumb spica cast |
| use of the Allen's test | **evaluate the radial and ulnar artery circulation in the hand—** * the patient opens and closes the hands a few times and then the examiner occludes both vessels with the patient's wrist closed, * the patient opens the hand and the examiner releases one of the vessels and notes the time interval for the return of color to the hand, * the procedure is repeated and the other vessel is released [**Note:** the ulnar artery is most responsible for the circulation of the hand.] |
| cause of a mallet finger | **avulsion fracture of the extensor tendon to the distal phalanx—** * produces a flexion deformity of the DIP joint, * Rx with splinting of the DIP joint in hyperextension |
| cause of pelvic fractures | **automobile accidents** |
| cause of pelvic fractures in patients >60 yrs old | **falls at home in patients with underlying osteoporosis—**particularly true for elderly white women |
| complications of pelvic fractures | • **severe hemorrhage,** • *disruption of the urethra/bladder*—retrograde urethrography is performed before catheterization, • *bowel perforations* [**Note:** a 40–50% mortality exists in open pelvic fractures.] |

*Table continued on following page*

**Table 12–1. SELECTED ORTHOPEDIC DISORDERS I**
*Continued*

| Most Common... | Answer and Explanation |
|---|---|
| hip dislocations | • **posterior**—usually due to a car accident when the flexed knee in an abducted position is forced into the dashboard, • *anterior,* • *central* |
| clinical findings in posterior versus anterior dislocation | • **posterior**—the lower extremity: ♦ limb is shortened, ♦ flexed, ♦ adducted, ♦ internally rotated at the hip, • **anterior**—the lower extremity: ♦ limb is shortened, ♦ abducted, ♦ externally rotated at the hip |
| complications of a posterior dislocation | • **damage to sciatic nerve,** • *osteoarthritis of femoral head* |
| complications of an anterior dislocation | • **neurovascular compromise of the femoral artery, vein, nerve,** • *aseptic necrosis of femoral head,* • *osteoarthritis* |
| clinical features of a slipped capital femoral epiphysis | • **most commonly found in obese adolescent males from 9–15 yrs of age,** • **pain is classically located on the medial aspect of the knee** |
| femoral fracture | **femoral neck fracture**— * most commonly occurs in an elderly male patient with osteoporosis, * groin or knee pain is present |
| complications of femoral neck fracture | • **aseptic necrosis of femoral head**—damage to the medial femoral circumflex artery, • *non-union,* • *fat embolism syndrome,* • *severe hemorrhage* |
| clinical findings in fat embolization | • **mechanism**—fat enters the microcirculation from the bone marrow and surrounding fat, • **S/S**— * begin within 24–72 hrs, * CNS dysfunction: mental status changes, * respiratory failure: ♦ hypoxemia, ♦ dyspnea, ♦ potential for ARDS, * thrombocytopenia: ♦ platelets stick to the fat globules in the circulation, ♦ petechiae develop in the upper half of the body, • **lab**— * increased serum lipase, * fat in urine, • **Rx**— * corticosteroids, * oxygen with PEEP |
| complication of a knee dislocation | **neurovascular compromise**— * evaluation of sensory/motor function is very important, * arteriography is necessary |

## Table 12–1. SELECTED ORTHOPEDIC DISORDERS I
*Continued*

| Most Common... | Answer and Explanation |
|---|---|
| complication associated with tibial fractures | **compartment syndrome**—see above |
| clinical finding in march fractures | **stress fracture of metatarsal bones** |
| mechanisms of ankle fractures | **supination and external rotation injury with fractures of medial and lateral malleoli** |
| foot bone(s) fractured after a fall from a height | **calcaneus**—additional areas of concern include: ♦ spinal injury, ♦ tibial plateau fractures, ♦ femoral neck fractures |
| mechanism for cervical spine fractures | **extreme cervical compression**— * e.g., diving into a shallow pool, trampoline, football, * $C_2$–$C_7$ most affected |
| mechanism for a teardrop fracture of cervical spine | **hyperflexion of the neck** |
| radiograph ordered in the initial work-up of a cervical spine injury | **lateral radiograph of the neck** |
| Rx of localized soft tissue injuries involving muscles/ ligaments | **RICE**— * rest, * ice, * compression bandage, * elevation |
| fracture associated with ecchymoses of the mastoid | **basilar skull fracture**—petrous portion of the temporal bone [**Note:** otorrhea (CSF fluid leaking out of the ear) may also occur.] |
| fracture associated with rhinorrhea (CSF leaking from the nose | **orbital fractures** [**Note:** rhinorrhea occurs after a fracture of the cribriform plate. Orbital fractures also produce raccoon eyes (periorbital hemorrhage) and ophthalmoplegia (eye muscle entrapment).] |

*Table continued on following page*

### Table 12–1. SELECTED ORTHOPEDIC DISORDERS I
*Continued*

**Question:** In which of the following disorders is the knee jerk reflex lost? **SELECT 3**
(A) $L_3$–$L_4$ disc rupture
(B) $L_4$–$L_5$ disc rupture
(C) $L_5$–$S_1$ disc rupture
(D) Femoral nerve injury
(E) Obturator nerve injury
(F) Tibial nerve injury
(G) Common peroneal nerve injury
(H) Superior gluteal nerve injury

**Answers: (A), (D), (E).** The knee jerk reflex is mediated by $L_2$–$L_4$. Therefore, a disc rupture at $L_3$–$L_4$ or injury to the femoral or obturator nerves is associated with an absent knee reflex **(choices A, D, E are correct).** The ankle jerk reflex is diminished with lesions involving $L_4$–$S_3$. Therefore, an $L_5$–$S_1$ disc rupture or injury to the common peroneal or tibial nerve causes a loss of the ankle jerk reflex **(choices C, F, G are incorrect).** No reflexes are lost with $L_4$–$L_5$ disc ruptures or injury to the superior gluteal nerve **(choices B, H are incorrect).**

ACL = anterior cruciate ligament, ANA = antinuclear antibodies, APL = abductor pollicis longus, ARDS = adult respiratory distress syndrome, AS = ankylosing spondylitis, AVM = arteriovenous malformation, CNS = central nervous system, DIP = distal interphalangeal joint, EBP = extensor pollicis brevis, MC = most common, NSAIDs = nonsteroidal anti-inflammatory drugs, OA = osteoarthritis, ORIF = open reduction and internal fixation, PCL = posterior cruciate ligament, PEEP = positive end-expiratory pressure, RA = rheumatoid arthritis, RF = rheumatoid factor, RICE—rest, ice, compression bandage, elevation, R/O = rule out, S/S = signs and symptoms, TSH = thyroid-stimulating hormone.

### Table 12–2. SELECTED ORTHOPEDIC DISORDERS II

| Most Common... | Answer and Explanation |
|---|---|
| routine SF tests | • **cell count and differential**—should be < 200 WBCs/μL, • **culture,** • **crystal analysis,** • **mucin clot test**—see below |
| monoclinic SF crystals | • **MSU,** • *CPP* [Note: monoclinic crystals are needle-shaped. Without special polarization, it is not possible to distinguish MSU from CPP monoclinic crystals.] |
| triclinic crystal | **CPP**—triclinic crystals are rhomboid shaped and are pathognomonic of CPP crystals |

## Table 12–2. SELECTED ORTHOPEDIC DISORDERS II
### Continued

| Most Common... | Answer and Explanation |
|---|---|
| appearance of MSU crystals when aligned parallel to the slow axis of the compensator | **yellow monoclinic crystal**— * by placing a red compensator in the microscope, the background of the slide with the SF becomes red and the crystals are yellow and blue, depending on their orientation, with the slow axis of the compensator located at the base of the microscope, * if the crystal is yellow when aligned parallel to the slow axis of the compensator, it represents negative birefringence, which defines MSU crystals |
| appearance of CPP crystal when aligned parallel to the slow axis of the compensator | **blue monoclinic or triclinic crystal**—if the crystal is blue when parallel to the slow axis of the compensator, it represents positive birefringence and defines CPP crystals |
| test evaluating SF viscosity | **mucin clot test**— * acid added to a tube of SF clots hyaluronic acid, which is the lubricant of the SF, * poor clot formation indicates deficient hyaluronic acid and the presence of joint inflammation |
| S/S of joint disease | • **arthralgia**—a general term for joint pain, • *arthritis*—refers to pain associated with: ◆ joint swelling, ◆ tenderness, ◆ warmth, • *morning stiffness*—e.g.,: ◆ RA, ◆ SLE, ◆ polymyalgia rheumatica, • *abnormal mobility*—indicates damage to ligaments or the joint capsule, • *swelling*—indicates increased joint fluid: e.g., ◆ exudate, ◆ blood, • *joint crepitus*—refers to a crackling feeling when moving the joint: e.g., articular degeneration in OA |
| classification of joint disorders | • **group I**—noninflammatory, • *group II*—inflammatory, • *group III*—septic, • *group IV*—hemorrhagic: e.g., ◆ trauma, ◆ hemophilia A or B, ◆ scurvy |
| noninflammatory joint diseases | • **osteoarthritis (OA),** • *neuropathic (Charcot) joint* |
| disabling joint disease | OA—OA is a female dominant disease, characterized by progressive and disabling degeneration of the articular cartilage |

*Table continued on following page*

### Table 12–2. SELECTED ORTHOPEDIC DISORDERS II
*Continued*

| Most Common... | Answer and Explanation |
|---|---|
| predisposing cause of OA | **abnormal load placed on a weight-bearing joint**—increased pressure leads to ischemia, generation of FRs, and eventual destruction of the articular cartilage |
| joints involved in OA | • **weight-bearing joints**—e.g., * hip, * knee, • *hands*— * **DIP** and PIP joints, * usually indicates a genetic predisposition, • *vertebral column*—see below |
| vertebral findings in OA | • **anterolateral spinous osteophytes** ("spurs"), • **degenerative disc disease**—see below, • **narrow joint space**, • **compression neuropathies**, • **spondylolysis**— * defect in posterior neural arch development, * bilateral spondylolysis causes subluxation of one vertebra over another: called spondylolisthesis |
| secondary causes of OA | • **trauma**—usually involves an isolated joint: e.g., ◆ OA from a chronic rotator cuff tear, ◆ OA from a meniscus tear in knee, • *Legg-Perthes*—aseptic necrosis of the femoral head in young boys: see below, • *obesity,* • *hemochromatosis*— * 50%, * chondrocalcinosis with pseudogout is common, • *Wilson's disease*— * 50%, * AR disease with a defect in secreting copper into bile |
| sites never involved by primary OA | • **shoulders**, • **MCP joints**, • **ulnar side of the wrist** |
| site for primary isolated nodal OA | **DIP joint** |
| S/S of OA | • **arthralgia**, • *joint stiffness*—<15 min, • *Heberden's node of DIP joint*—osteophyte at the margin of the joint, • *Bouchard's node of PIP joint*—osteophyte at margin of joint, • *compression neuropathies from vertebral involvement* |
| x-ray findings in OA | • **narrow joint space**—due to a wearing down of the articular cartilage, • *osteophytes*—reactive bone formation at the margins of the joint, • *subchondral bone cysts,* • *dense subchondral bone,* • *fibrillation of the articular cartilage*—perpendicular clefts in the articular cartilage that break off to form joint mice |

**Table 12–2. SELECTED ORTHOPEDIC DISORDERS II**
*Continued*

| Most Common... | Answer and Explanation |
|---|---|
| Rx of OA | • **pain relievers**—e.g., * acetaminophen, * NSAIDs, • **weight loss**, • **protect joints from overuse**, • **? glucosamine salts + chondroitin sulfate**, • **surgery** |
| causes of a neuropathic (Charcot) joint | • **DM**—targets the tarsometatarsal joint, • *syringomyelia*—involves the following joints: ◆ shoulder, ◆ elbow, ◆ wrist joint, • *tabes dorsalis*—targets the: ◆ hip, ◆ knee, ◆ ankle [**Note:** a neuropathic joint is due to a combination of insensitivity to pain (neuropathy) plus ischemia.] |
| predisposing factors for developing RA | • **HLA Dr₄**—present in 60–70%, • **infection**—e.g., * **EBV**, * rubella, * parvovirus, • **autoimmunity against immunoglobulins**, • **unknown genetic factors** [**Note:** RA occurs between 30 and 50 yrs of age and is more common in women than men.] |
| mechanism of destruction of articular cartilage in RA | **chronic synovitis with pannus formation** [**Note:** pannus refers to hyperplastic synovial tissue that grows over articular cartilage in a joint and destroys it and the underlying bone (erosions). Reactive fibrosis in the repair process causes fusion of the joint (ankylosis).] |
| antibody synthesized by synovial tissue lymphocytes in RA | **rheumatoid factor (RF)**—positive in 70% [**Note:** RF is an IgM antibody against IgG. It forms complexes with itself by binding to the Fc components of IgG. The immunocomplexes activate the complement system, producing chemotactic factors that attract neutrophils and macrophages into the joint.] |
| joints involved in RF | • **symmetric involvement of the second and third MCP joints and PIP joints**— * >85%, * leads to: ◆ ulnar deviation of the hands, ◆ morning stiffness > 1 hr, ◆ carpal tunnel syndrome, • *knees*—80%, • *ankles*—80%, • *elbows*—50%, • *hips*—50%, • *shoulders*—50% * AC joint—50%, • *cervical spine*—40%, • *TMJ*—30% |

*Table continued on following page*

**Table 12–2. SELECTED ORTHOPEDIC DISORDERS II**
*Continued*

| Most Common... | Answer and Explanation |
|---|---|
| clinical findings associated with cervical spine disease in RA | • **atlantoaxial joint instability**—subluxation occurs when the patient looks down, • *danger of vertebrobasilar insufficiency*— * ataxia, * limb weakness, * tetraplegia |
| cause of a popliteal (Baker's) cyst in RA | **outpouching of the posterior portion of the joint space due to increased intra-articular pressure** [**Note:** US is diagnostic of the cyst. It must be differentiated from a popliteal artery aneurysm.] |
| complication of a popliteal cyst | **rupture**— * rupture usually occurs into the calf muscle, * clinically resembles an acute thrombophlebitis: ♦ fever, ♦ neutrophilic leukocytosis, ♦ ecchymoses around the ankle |
| S/S of tenosynovitis in RA | • **swelling between the joints,** • **palpable grating in the flexor tendon sheaths when the digit is moved** |
| cause of paresthesias in the hand in RA | **carpal tunnel syndrome**—RA is second to pregnancy as the MCC of this compartment syndrome, * median nerve is compressed in the transverse carpal ligament |
| locations for rheumatoid nodules | • **extensor aspect of the forearm,** • *lungs,* • *heart* [**Note:** they occur in 20–35% of patients, particularly those with high titers of RF. Ulceration and infection may occur.] |
| clinical appearance of the "swan neck" deformity in RA | • **flexion of the DIP joint,** • **extension of the PIP joint** <br><br> DIP → ◣ ← PIP |
| clinical appearance of the boutonnière deformity in RA | • **hyperextension of the DIP joint,** • **flexion of the PIP joint** <br><br> ← PIP <br> DIP → |
| radiographic findings in RA | • **symmetric narrowing of joint space,** • *periarticular osteoporosis,* • *bone erosions at the joint margins* |

## Table 12–2. SELECTED ORTHOPEDIC DISORDERS II
*Continued*

| Most Common... | Answer and Explanation |
|---|---|
| initial first-line Rx of RA | **NSAIDs**—glucocorticoids may be used to preserve function |
| disease-modifying (second-line) drugs used in RA | • **methotrexate,** • *hydroxychloroquine*—danger of pigmentary retinitis, • *penicillamine,* • *sulfasalazine*—danger of: ♦ neutropenia, ♦ thrombocytopenia, • *gold salts*— * 60% response, * complications: ♦ dermatitis, ♦ proteinuria, • *azathioprine,* • *cyclophosphamide* |
| inheritance pattern noted in primary gout | **multifactorial inheritance** |
| causes of secondary gout | • **alcoholism,** • *chronic renal insufficiency,* • *lead nephropathy,* • *DM,* • *diuretics* |
| primary causes of an increase in uric acid synthesis | • **obesity**—the relationship to obesity is unknown, • *decrease in HGPRT,* • *increase in PRPP* [**Note:** uric acid is a byproduct of purine metabolism. Overproduction of UA accounts for ~10% of cases.] |
| cause of hyperuricemia in primary and secondary gout | **decreased excretion of uric acid in the kidneys**—underexcretion accounts for 90% of cases |
| secondary cause of overproduction of UA | **Rx of disseminated cancer**—excess release of purines: e.g., ♦ leukemia, ♦ malignant lymphoma |
| secondary causes of underexcretion of UA | • **alcohol**—lactate and β-OHB compete with UA for excretion in the proximal tubule, • *chronic renal insufficiency,* • *low-dose aspirin*—high-dose aspirin is uricosuric, • *diuretics* |
| clinical presentation of acute gouty arthritis | **acute onset (usually nocturnal) of inflammation in the first metatarsophalangeal joint (big toe)**— * 50%, * this is called podagra, • *fever,* • *neutrophilic leukocytosis* [**Note:** gout is more likely to occur in men than women except after menopause, when the attack rate is the same in both sexes.] |

*Table continued on following page*

### Table 12–2. SELECTED ORTHOPEDIC DISORDERS II
*Continued*

| Most Common... | Answer and Explanation |
|---|---|
| factors precipitating acute gouty arthritis | • **alcohol use,** • *trauma,* • *postoperative state,* • *postcardiac transplantation—* * 25%, due to: ♦ diuretics, ♦ cyclosporine |
| cause of joint inflammation in acute gouty arthritis | **interaction of MSU with neutrophils and release of leukocyte-derived chemotactic factor** |
| lab test used to confirm gout | **SF analysis with demonstration of negatively birefringent crystals** [Note: hyperuricemia does not define gout. UA is usually > 7.5 mg/dL; however, not all patients with gout have an elevated UA (~20%).] |
| Rx of acute gouty arthritis | • **NSAIDs**—e.g., indomethacin, • *intra-articular injection of corticosteroids,* • *colchicine—* * rarely used due to GI effects, * it blocks the release of leukocyte-derived chemotactic factor and interferes with leukocyte motility by blocking microtubules |
| clinical findings in interval gout | **usually asymptomatic**—UA crystals are confined to vacuoles within SF neutrophils |
| clinical finding in chronic gout | **tophus formation** [Note: tophi occur in deposits of MSU in tissue (multinucleated granulomatous reaction) around the joint (most common) and other sites. Tophi develop after ~10 yrs of the disease, particularly in poorly controlled patients.] |
| complications of gout | • **disabling arthritis,** • **renal disease**—urate nephropathy |
| clinical disorders associated with gout | • **HTN,** • **obesity,** • **CHD,** • **chronic renal insufficiency** |
| drugs used to lower UA during the interval period | • **uricosuric drugs**—e.g., * **probenecid,** * sulfinpyrazone, * UA levels in urine < 1000 mg/day, • *drugs that decrease UA production*—e.g., * allopurinol, which blocks xanthine oxidase, * UA levels in urine > 1000 mg/day |
| causes of CPPD disease | • **metabolic disease**—e.g., * primary HPTH, * hemochromatosis, * Wilson's disease, * ochronosis, • *idiopathic,* • *genetic,* • *trauma* |

## Table 12–2. SELECTED ORTHOPEDIC DISORDERS II
*Continued*

| Most Common... | Answer and Explanation |
|---|---|
| S/S of CPPD disease (pseudogout) | **chondrocalcinosis involving the knee**—inflammatory arthritis with CPP crystals and linear deposits of CPP in the articular cartilage [**Note:** other joints that may be affected include the wrists, elbows, intervertebral discs, and ankles.] |
| Rx of CPPD disease | • **NSAIDs,** • *IV colchicine,* • *drain joint and inject corticosteroids in resistant cases* |
| seronegative (RF = negative) spondyloarthropathy | **ankylosing spondylitis (AS)**—an inflammatory arthritis most commonly afflicting young men who are HLA B27 positive (>90%) |
| joints and other sites targeted in AS | • **sacroiliac joint,** • *vertebral column*— * "bamboo spine", * other joints: ♦ shoulder, ♦ hip, • *aorta*—aortitis with aortic insufficiency, • *uveal tract*—uveitis with blurry vision |
| S/S of AS | • **morning stiffness in the sacroiliac joints**—stiffness abates with exercise, • *fever,* • *diminished anterior flexion*—eventual restrictive lung disease, • *kyphoscoliosis,* • *aortic insufficiency,* • *visual problems,* • *Achilles tendinitis,* • *plantar fasciitis* |
| Rx of AS | • **NSAIDs**—indomethacin, • *exercise* |
| S/S of Reiter's syndrome | • **urethritis**—*Chlamydia trachomatis,* • *dysentery*— * *Shigella,* * *Campylobacter,* * *Yersinia,* • *conjunctivitis*—noninfectious, • *HLA B27–positive arthritis*— * 80% are HLA B27 positive, * "sausage" toe: fusiform swelling of the digit, * erosive arthritis, • *mucocutaneous disease*—e.g., * balanitis, * aphthous ulcers in the mouth, • *Achilles tendinitis*—x-ray reveals periostitis at the tendon insertion, • *skin disease*— * keratoderma blennorrhagicum, * similar to psoriasis, • *cardiac conduction abnormalities,* • *aortitis* |
| cell of origin of Reiter's cell in SF | **macrophage that has phagocytosed a neutrophil** |
| Rx of Reiter's syndrome | • **NSAIDs,** • *Rx underlying infectious disease if present* |

*Table continued on following page*

Table 12–2. SELECTED ORTHOPEDIC DISORDERS II
*Continued*

| Most Common... | Answer and Explanation |
|---|---|
| S/S of psoriatic arthritis | • **morning stiffness that is similar to RA**—symmetric disease, • *sausage-shaped DIP joints (finger or toe) with nail pitting and erosive joint disease*—radiographs exhibit a "pencil-in-cup" deformity, • *psoriatic spondylitis*— * HLA B27–positive in 50–75%, * involves sacroiliac joint, * AS is commonly present, • *severe skin disease*—precedes arthritis in 80%, • *hyperuricemia*—increased turnover of skin with release of purines |
| Rx of psoriatic arthritis | • **NSAIDs,** • *methotrexate,* • *gold* |
| IBD associated with HLA B27–positive arthritis | **UC**—next to anemia, HLA B27–positive arthritis (~75%) is the second MC extraintestinal manifestation of IBD |
| infections associated with aseptic (reactive) HLA B27–positive arthritis | ***Chlamydia trachomatis,*** • *Ureaplasma urealyticum,* • *Shigella flexneri,* • *Campylobacter jejuni,* • *Yersinia enterocolitica,* • *Salmonella* [**Note:** ~80% of cases are HLA B27 positive. The arthritis is self-limited and not erosive in nature.] |
| cause of episodic destruction of cartilage in the ears/nose/upper airways + arthritis | **relapsing polychondritis** |
| nongonococcal cause of septic arthritis | ***Staphylococcus aureus***— * usually spread by the hematogenous route in children, * spread most commonly by direct extension in elderly people: e.g., ♦ infection in fractures, ♦ prosthetic devices, * gram-negative organisms such as *Escherichia coli, Pseudomonas aeruginosa* are more likely in the elderly population |
| cause of septic arthritis in urban populations | ***Neisseria gonorrhoeae***— * female to male ratio is 3:1, * in women, it most commonly occurs during menses or pregnancy |

**Table 12–2. SELECTED ORTHOPEDIC DISORDERS II**
*Continued*

| Most Common... | Answer and Explanation |
|---|---|
| S/S of disseminated gonorrhea | • **tenosynovitis**— * 60%, * sites: ♦ wrists, ♦ ankles, • *septic arthritis*—knee, • *dermatitis*—pustules involving: ♦ wrists, ♦ ankles, • *fever*—<50% have fever, • *genitourinary signs*— * <25% have genitourinary symptoms, * all sites still should be cultured: ♦ urethra, ♦ cervix |
| complement deficiencies in disseminated gonococcemia | **C5–C9**—these complement components are necessary for phagocytosis of the organisms |
| lab findings in gonococcal septic arthritis | • **SF Gram stain**—positive in 25%, • **SF culture**—positive in 30–50%, • **blood culture**— * positive in 40% of those with tenosynovitis, * negative in those with suppurative arthritis, • **culture of skin lesions**—positive in 40–60% |
| Rx of gonococcal septic arthritis | **ceftriaxone** |
| cause of Lyme disease | **tick-transmitted (*Ixodes dammini* in East/ Midwest, *Ixodes pacificus* in West), *Borrelia burgdorferi* (spirochete)** [Note: the white-tailed deer is the animal reservoir for the organism.] |
| skin lesion in early Lyme disease | **erythema chronicum migrans**— * a red, expanding lesion with concentric circles emanating from the site of the tick bite, * present in 50% of patients: pathognomonic of Lyme disease |
| Rx of early Lyme disease | **doxycycline** |
| late manifestations of Lyme disease | • **arthritis**—30–50%, • *CNS disease*— * ~15%, * bilateral Bell's palsy: pathognomonic of Lyme's disease, • *cardiovascular disease*— * ~5%, * myocarditis/pericarditis |
| musculoskeletal findings in Lyme disease | • **most commonly involves the knee, • may develop popliteal cysts that rupture, • obliterative endarteritis in synovial tissue, • disabling arthritis if left untreated** |

*Table continued on following page*

## Table 12–2.  SELECTED ORTHOPEDIC DISORDERS II
*Continued*

| Most Common... | Answer and Explanation |
| --- | --- |
| lab findings in Lyme disease | • **ELISA assay**— * screening test, * many FP test results, * requires 4–6 wks to become positive, • **Western blot assay**—confirmatory test, • *culture*—60–70% sensitivity in biopsy specimens of ECM, • *silver stains of synovial biopsy*—positive in ~30% |
| Rx of late stages of Lyme disease | **ceftriaxone** |
| hereditary bone disease | **osteogenesis imperfecta**—an AD or AR disease with a defect in synthesis of type I collagen |
| S/S of osteogenesis imperfecta | • **pathologic fractures**—"brittle bone" disease, • *blue sclerae*—loss of collagen in the sclera allows bluish discoloration of the choroidal veins to show through, • *deafness* |
| metabolic bone disease | **osteoporosis**— * see Table 9–3, * osteoporosis refers to an overall reduction in mineralized bone |
| cause of osteomyelitis in young adults | ***Staphylococcus aureus***— * usually spreads by the hematogenous route, * other mechanisms include: ♦ spread to bone from a subjacent soft tissue infection, ♦ trauma |
| site in bone targeted by osteomyelitis | **metaphysis**—the metaphysis has the richest blood supply |
| complications of osteomyelitis | • **draining sinus tracts**, • **nidus for septicemia**, • *squamous cell carcinoma in the sinus tract*, • *secondary amyloidosis* |
| type of osteomyelitis in sickle cell anemia | ***Salmonella species***—over 75% of cases are due to *Salmonella* species, followed by *Staphylococcus aureus* |
| method for diagnosing osteomyelitis | • **radionuclide bone scan**—plain radiographs do not reveal the moth-eaten appearance with sclerotic margins during the first week, • *bone biopsy with culture for confirmation* |
| cause of Pott's disease | ***Mycobacterium tuberculosis***— * Pott's disease refers to a TB infection involving the vertebral column, * leads to destruction of bone and extension of inflammation along the sheath of the psoas muscle |

## Table 12–2. SELECTED ORTHOPEDIC DISORDERS II
### *Continued*

| Most Common... | Answer and Explanation |
|---|---|
| common sites for Pott's disease | • **lower thoracic vertebra,** • *lumbar vertebra* |
| infection due to puncture wounds while wearing rubber footwear | ***Pseudomonas aeruginosa* osteomyelitis** |
| site/cause of avascular (aseptic) necrosis of bone | **femoral head/femoral head fracture**—other causes of avascular necrosis of the femoral head include: ♦ corticosteroids, ♦ sickle cell disease, ♦ Legg-Perthes disease |
| osteochondritis | **Legg-Perthes disease involving the femoral head**— * osteochondritis refers to aseptic necrosis of secondary ossification centers, * Legg-Perthes is more common in boys between 3 and 10 yrs of age and presents with a painless limp, * OA is a common sequela |
| wrist bone fracture leading to aseptic necrosis | **scaphoid (navicular) fracture**— * pain in the anatomic snuff box, * MC wrist bone fracture, * MRI is excellent in detecting fracture |
| osteochondritis of the tibial tuberosity | **Osgood-Schlatter disease**— * self-limited disease that most commonly occurs in 13- to 15-yr-old children, * pain and swelling of the tibial tuberosity: ♦ fragmented appearance on x-ray, ♦ knobby knee is a common sequela |
| osteochondritis of lunate bone | **Kienbock's disease** |
| osteochondritis of vertebral bodies | **Scheuermann's disease**—see above discussion |
| osteochondritis of the tarsal navicular bone | **Kohler's disease**— * affects children between 3 and 6 yrs old, * pain/swelling in the foot: x-ray shows sclerosis of navicular bone |
| test used to identify aseptic necrosis | • **MRI**—exhibits increased density in the area of involvement, • *plain x-ray*—increased density from reactive bone formation |
| S/S of Albright's syndrome | • **polyostotic fibrous dysplasia**—benign bone disease, • *café-au-lait pigmentation,* • *precocious puberty*—usually in females: due to a midline hamartoma in the hypothalamus |

*Table continued on following page*

## Table 12–2. SELECTED ORTHOPEDIC DISORDERS II
### Continued

| Most Common... | Answer and Explanation |
|---|---|
| cancer associated with hypertrophic osteoarthropathy | **primary lung cancer**—hypertrophic osteoarthropathy refers to periosteal inflammation with new bone formation and arthritis, which may or may not be associated with clubbing of the fingers |
| benign bone tumor producing nocturnal pain relieved by aspirin | **osteoid osteoma**— * involves the cortical aspect of the proximal femur, * an x-ray reveals a radiolucent nidus surrounded by dense sclerotic bone |
| primary bone tumors in order of increasing age | • **Ewing's sarcoma**—first and second decade, • **osteogenic sarcoma**—10–25 yrs old, • **chondrosarcoma**–>30 yrs old, • **multiple myeloma**—>50 yrs old |
| primary bone tumors in descending order of frequency | • **multiple myeloma**, • **osteogenic sarcoma**, • **chondrosarcoma**, • **Ewing's sarcoma**, • **giant cell tumor of bone** |
| malignancy of bone | **metastatic breast cancer** |
| bone metastasized to | **vertebral column**—due to the Batson system: see Table 10–1 |
| benign bone tumor | **osteochondroma**— * benign cartilaginous tumor arising as an outgrowth from the metaphysis of bone, * capped by benign proliferating cartilage |
| bone tumors arising in the epiphysis of bone | • **giant cell tumor of bone**—adult, female-dominant tumor arising in the distal end of femur/proximal tibia, • *chondroblastoma*— * benign cartilaginous tumor, * "popcorn appearance" on x-ray |
| classic x-ray findings in osteogenic sarcoma | • **"sunburst appearance"**—due to calcified malignant osteoid invading the soft tissue surrounding the tumor, • *Codman's triangle*—due to lifting up of the periosteum from tumor infiltrating out of the metaphysis into the soft tissue |
| classic x-ray finding in Ewing's sarcoma | **concentric "onion skin layering" due to new bone formation around the primary tumor**—usually located in the tibia or flat bones of the pelvis |
| location of an osteogenic sarcoma | **distal femur or proximal tibia**—both these sites are around the knee |

## Table 12–2. SELECTED ORTHOPEDIC DISORDERS II
*Continued*

| Most Common... | Answer and Explanation |
|---|---|
| risk factors for an osteogenic sarcoma | • **radiation,** • *Paget's disease of bone,* • *retinoblastoma*—Rb suppressor gene relationship on chromosome 13 |
| bone tumor associated with Gardner's polyposis syndrome | **osteoma**—benign tumor most commonly located in the sinuses, jaws, and facial bones |
| primary bone tumor located in the vertebrae | **osteoblastoma**—essentially a "giant osteoid osteoma" |
| malignant cartilaginous tumor and its location | **chondrosarcoma**—most often located in the pelvis and upper end of the femur |
| risk factors for chondrosarcoma | • **multiple osteochondromas**—osteochondromatosis: AD disease, • *Ollier's disease*—multiple enchondromas that arise in the medullary cavity |
| bone tumor with multinucleated giant cells | **giant cell tumor**— * benign tumor arising in the epiphysis of bone in young/middle-aged women, * mononuclear fibroblast-like cells are the neoplastic component, whereas the multinucleated giant cells are benign |
| cause of pathologic fractures | **metastatic disease to bone**—breast cancer is the most common cause of bone metastasis |

**Question:** Which of the following bone disorders are more common in patients less than 30 years of age? **SELECT 5**
- (A) Osteochondroma
- (B) Hip fracture
- (C) Chondrosarcoma
- (D) Legg-Perthes disease
- (E) Osteoid osteoma
- (F) Ewing's sarcoma
- (G) Paget's disease
- (H) Osteogenic sarcoma

**Answers: (A), (D), (E), (F), (H).** Hip fractures, chondrosarcoma, and Paget's disease are more common in patients > 30 years of age (**choices B, C, G are incorrect**). Osteochondroma, Legg-Perthes disease, osteoid osteoma, Ewing's sarcoma, and osteogenic sarcoma are more common in a younger age-bracket (**choices A, D, E, F, H are correct**).

*Table continued on following page*

AC = acromioclavicular joint, AD = autosomal dominant, AR = autosomal recessive, AS = ankylosing spondylitis, β-OHB = beta-hydroxybutyric acid, CHD = coronary heart disease, CNS = central nervous system, CPP = calcium pyrophosphate, CPPD = calcium pyrophosphate deposition, DIP = distal interphalangeal joint, DM = diabetes mellitus, EBV = Epstein-Barr virus, ECM = erythema chronicum migrans, ELISA = enzyme-linked immunosorbent assay, FP = false-positive, FRs = free radicals, GC = gonococcus, HGPRT = hypoxanthine-guanine phosphoribosyltransferase, HLA = human leukocyte antigen, HPTH = hyperparathyroidism, HTN = hypertension, IBD = inflammatory bowel disease, MC = most common, MCC = most common cause, MCP = metacarpophalangeal (joint), MSU = monosodium urate, NSAIDs = nonsteroidal anti-inflammatory drugs, OA = osteoarthritis, β-OHB = beta-hydroxybutyric acid, PRPP = 5-phospho-α-D-ribosyl-1-pyrophosphate, PIP = proximal interphalangeal joint, RA = rheumatoid arthritis, Rb = retinoblastoma, RF = rheumatoid factor, SF = synovial fluid, SLE = systemic lupus erythematosus, S/S = signs and symptoms, TMJ = temporomandibular joint, UA = uric acid, UC = ulcerative colitis.

# CHAPTER

## 13

# SELECTED NEUROSURGICAL/ OPHTHALMOLOGY/AUDITORY DISORDERS

## CONTENTS

### Table 13–1. SELECTED NEUROSURGICAL DISORDERS

| Most Common... | Answer and Explanation |
|---|---|
| primary disturbances of arousal | • **stupor**— * psychologic unresponsiveness, * response only to vigorous external stimulation, • **coma**— * unarousable state, * eyes closed, * no evidence of awareness of inner thoughts or outer events |
| mechanisms for stupor/coma | • **supratentorial lesions involving posterior ventromedial diencephalon**— * central/uncal herniation, * invasion/destruction of posterior VMD, • **subtentorial lesions compressing/ damaging upper pontine midbrain reticular formation**—e.g., pontine/cerebellar bleed, • **metabolic/diffuse lesions**—e.g., * drugs/poisons, * myxedema coma, * liver failure, * hypo-/hypernatremia, * meningitis, * hypoglycemia |
| causes of sudden acute coma | • **self-induced drug poisoning,** • **brain trauma,** • **acute intracranial bleed,** • **hypoglycemia,** • **meningitis** |
| clinical findings of supratentorial mass lesions | • **focal cerebral signs**—e.g., * headache on side of lesion, * aphasia, * contralateral hemiparesis, • **dysfunction moves front to back**—focal motor → bilateral motor → stupor/coma, • **dysfunction localized to a single or adjacent anatomic level,** • **absence of brain stem signs unless herniation occurs**—see below |

*Table continued on following page*

## Table 13–1. SELECTED NEUROSURGICAL DISORDERS
*Continued*

| Most Common... | Answer and Explanation |
|---|---|
| clinical findings of central transtentorial herniation | • **midline diencephalon displaced caudally toward and through tentorial notch against the midbrain,** • **early decline in arousal,** • **pupils small, equal, and reactive,** • **bilateral UMN signs,** • **decerebrate early** |
| clinical findings of uncal transtentorial herniation | • **temporal fossa lesion herniates uncus over edge of ipsilateral tentorium,** • **compression of CN III—** * unilateral mydriasis: earliest finding, * ptosis, • **late decline in arousal and decerebrate state**—see below |
| cause of decerebrate state | **upper brain stem injury**—e.g., * brain stem infarction, * pontine/posterior fossa bleed, * tumor, * metabolic encephalopathy: ♦ hepatic encephalopathy, ♦ hypoglycemia, * brain stem compression secondary to increased intracranial pressure |
| clinical findings in decerebrate state | • **arms adducted/extended,** • **wrists pronated/ fingers flexed,** • **extension of both legs with plantar flexion of feet** [Note: it is an abnormal extensor response.] |
| neurologic test to establish whether the brain stem is intact | **oculocephalic test (doll's eyes)—** * performed by quickly turning the head laterally or vertically, * eyes should move conjugately in opposite direction of head movement if brain stem is intact, * absence of all eye movements indicates bilateral pontine lesion, * eye deviation toward side of hemiparesis indicates a contralateral pontine lesion, * eye deviation away from the side of hemiparesis indicates a contralateral frontal lobe lesion |
| cause of the decorticate state | **damage to one or both corticospinal tracts**—e.g., * CVA, * head injury, * brain abscess, * brain tumor |
| clinical findings in the decorticate state | • **adduction/flexion of arms up to chest,** • **wrists/fingers flexed on chest,** • **legs extended and internally rotated with plantar flexion of feet** [Note: it is an abnormal flexor response.] |

## Table 13–1. SELECTED NEUROSURGICAL DISORDERS
*Continued*

| Most Common... | Answer and Explanation |
|---|---|
| clinical findings of subtentorial lesions | • **compression of reticular activating system,** • **upper CN palsies,** • **sudden onset of coma**—brain stem dysfunction may precede coma, • **absent caloric responses,** • **pupil abnormalities**— * pinpoint: pons, * fixed: midbrain, * irregular and/or unequal: mid-brain-pontine, • **cerebellar dysfunction,** • **bilateral motor dysfunction** |
| clinical findings of metabolic/diffuse lesions | • **stupor/coma often preceded or replaced by delirium**—see below, • **commonly noted in elderly patients on multiple drugs admitted to medical/surgical units,** • **symmetric motor signs,** • **moderate hypothermia,** • **bilateral asterixis/myoclonus,** • **multiple anatomic levels involved,** • **preserved sensory function,** • **preserved pupillary function** |
| uses of Glasgow Coma Scale (GCS) | • **quantify level of consciousness,** • **quantify severity of head injury** |
| parameters in GCS | • **eye-opening response**—scale of E1 (no response) to E4 (eyes open and blinking), • **verbal response**—scale of V1 (no verbal response at all) to V5 (oriented to person, place, time, etc.), • **best motor response**— * scale of M1 (no movement at all) to M6 (obeys verbal commands, moves limbs spontaneously), * best motor score is taken from any extremity even though worse responses may be present in other extremities |
| definition of coma according to GCS | • **unable to open eyes,** • **unable to follow commands,** • **unable to utter words** |
| drugs associated with delirium | • **sedative/hypnotics,** • *NSAIDs,* • β*-blockers,* • *antipsychotic agents,* • *anticholinergic agents* |
| S/S of delirium | • **clouding of consciousness/lack of awareness of environment,** • **worse at night/early morning,** • **lack orientation to time and place**—not person, • **coarse tremor,** • **breathing alterations**—e.g., hyperpnea, • **visual hallucinations** |

*Table continued on following page*

Table 13–1. SELECTED NEUROSURGICAL DISORDERS
*Continued*

| Most Common... | Answer and Explanation |
|---|---|
| S/S of psychogenic coma | • **resists passive opening of eyelids, when eyelids raised,** • **eyelids shut abruptly when released,** • **brisk pupillary reactions,** • **normal caloric studies**—quick nystagmus, • **normal EEG,** • **no pathologic reflexes,** • **associations**— * severe depression, * catatonia of schizophrenia, * hysteria, * malingering |
| clinical findings of vegetative state | • **absent cognitive activity,** • **preservation of sleep-wake cycles,** • **primitive motor responses** |
| clinical findings of locked-in state | • **paralysis of communication and facial movements with retained consciousness**—bilateral ventral pontine lesions: e.g., ♦ pontine bleed, ♦ central pontine myelinolysis, • **quadriplegic**—damage to corticospinal tracts, • **reticular-activating system intact**—conscious, • **can communicate by blinking eyelids**—supranuclear ocular motor pathways intact |
| criteria used to define brain death | • **permanent loss of all essential brain functions**—no cerebral or brain stem function: e.g., ♦ no response to noxious stimuli, ♦ fixed pupils, ♦ apneic off ventilator, • **isoelectric EEG for 30 min,** • **known structural or irreversible systemic metabolic cause** |
| Rx of coma | • **intubate/oxygenate,** • **hyperventilate**—respiratory alkalosis vasoconstricts CNS vessels: prevents cerebral edema, • **IV thiamine**—R/O Wernicke's encephalopathy, • **IV glucose**—R/O hypoglycemic coma, • **consider naloxone**—R/O drug of abuse overdose, • **obtain emergency brain scan,** • **increase serum osmolality with mannitol,** • **Rx specific cause if known** |
| clinical findings in communicating hydrocephalus dementia (normal-pressure hydrocephalus) | • **may follow head trauma, infection, intracranial bleeds,** • **problem with absorption of CSF out of subarachnoid space,** • **shuffling, wide-based gait,** • **urinary incontinence,** • **bilateral UMN dysfunction in legs > arms**—positive Babinski's sign, • **ataxic/spastic gait,** • **dilated ventricles noted on CT/MRI,** • **normal CSF pressure in most patients** |

## Table 13–1. SELECTED NEUROSURGICAL DISORDERS
### *Continued*

| Most Common... | Answer and Explanation |
|---|---|
| mechanisms of spinal cord injury | • **dislocation with or without fracture at the atlas-axis junction,** • *fracture-dislocations with or without bony fragmentation at other spinal levels,* • *penetrating missile or stab wounds* |
| locations for dislocations of spine | • $C_7$–$T_1$ junction, • $T_{12}$–$L_1$ junction |
| hallmarks of spinal cord dysfunction | **interruption of motor, sensory, autonomic function below a level of injury** |
| spinal cord segments involved in bulbocavernous reflex | $S_1$ and $S_2$ [Note: the reflex is dependent on an intact $S_1$ and $S_2$. Stimulus to the glans penis or wall of vagina should cause a contraction of the anal sphincter around the examiner's finger. Absence of the reflex in a patient with spinal cord injury indicates that $S_1$ and $S_2$ are involved.] |
| types of shock associated with spinal injuries | • **spinal cord shock,** • **neurogenic shock** |
| clinical findings in spinal shock | • **occurs soon after either complete or partial spinal cord injuries,** • **absence of motor, sensory, autonomic function below level of injury,** • **spinal shock disappears in 1–3 days,** • **previously flaccid muscle becomes spastic, DTRs are exaggerated, and Babinski's sign is positive** |
| clinical findings in neurogenic shock | • **dysfunction of descending sympathetic pathways,** • **heart/BV do not respond to sympathetic responses**— * no compensatory tachycardia, * bradycardia present, • **vasomotor tone decreased**—pooling of blood |
| differences of neurogenic vs. hypovolemic shock and intracranial hypertension | • **neurogenic shock**—hypotension + sinus bradycardia, • **hypovolemic shock**—hypotension + sinus tachycardia, • **intracranial hypertension**—diastolic hypertension + sinus bradycardia |

*Table continued on following page*

### Table 13–1. SELECTED NEUROSURGICAL DISORDERS
*Continued*

| Most Common... | Answer and Explanation |
|---|---|
| findings in complete spinal cord injury | • **sine qua non of complete injury is the lack of anal sphincter tone and sensations in perianal area after 24 hrs,** • *flaccid motor paralysis below level of damage,* • *total anesthesia in same distribution as motor paralysis,* • *bladder dysfunction,* • *immediate onset of priapism*—delayed onset of priapism is due to an incomplete spinal cord injury that has eventually progressed to a complete spinal cord injury [**Note:** superficial reflexes and DTRs are absent below the level of the lesion, as well as sweating and skin vasomotor tone.] |
| findings in anterior cord syndrome | • **cause**—hyperflexion injury in the cervical region—e.g., * trauma, * acute central intervertebral disc disease, * anterior spinal artery occlusion, • **anterior half of the cord damaged**—includes central gray matter and fibers of lateral spinothalamic tract that cross the center, * absence of posterior column dysfunction, • **tetraparesis/-plegia,** • **bilateral pain and temperature impairment below the lesion,** • **urinary retention** |
| findings in central cord syndrome | • **cause**—hyperextension of cervical region, • **sites of damage**— * central gray matter, * fibers of lateral spinothalamic tracts that cross the center, • **quadriplegia,** • **upper extremities more involved than lower** |
| findings in Brown-Séquard syndrome | • **causes**— * **penetrating injury,** * radiation myelopathy, • **hemisection of spinal cord,** • **ipsilateral**— * loss of position and vibration sense, * spastic hemiparesis, * vasomotor paralysis below the level of the lesion, • **contralateral**— * loss of pain and temperature below the $T_{12}$ level, * loss of sensation in perineum and genitals |
| findings in posterolateral cord syndrome | • **causes**— * MS, * AIDS vacuolar myelopathy, * $B_{12}$ deficiency, • **loss of position and vibratory sensation**—posterior column dysfunction, • **preservation of pain and temperature sensation**—crossed spinothalamic tracts, • **spastic paraparesis**—lateral corticospinal tract dysfunction |

## Table 13–1. SELECTED NEUROSURGICAL DISORDERS
*Continued*

| Most Common... | Answer and Explanation |
|---|---|
| findings in the anterior commissure syndrome | • **cause**—syringomyelia, • **bilateral loss of pain and temperature sensation**, • **weakness of intrinsic muscles of hand**, • **bladder/bowel incontinence** |
| Rx of spinal cord injury | • **immobilization**—e.g., rigid cervical collar, • **correct hypotension with crystalloids or pneumatic antishock garment**, • **corticosteroids**—reduce cord edema, • **prophylactic antibiotics for penetrating injuries**, • **NG tube**—paralytic ileus occurs, • **neurosurgical consult**, • **avoid lumbar puncture**, • **prevent complications**—e.g., pressure ulcers, pneumonia, etc. |
| cause of spinal cord concussion | **high-velocity missile wounds that pass close to the spinal canal**—S/S resolve rapidly in hours to a few days |
| clinical findings of spinal cord compression | • **back pain at the level of compression**, • **difficulty with walking**, • **sensory impairment**, • **urinary retention with overflow incontinence** |
| noncompressive spinal cord lesion associated with weakness | **acute transverse myelitis** |
| cause of paraplegia following hypotension in surgery | **ischemic infarction of cord in the watershed area between the descending anterior spinal artery and aberrant ascending spinal artery of Adamkiewicz** |
| intradural spinal tumors | • **meningioma**— * **thoracic region**/foramen magnum, * increased CSF protein, • *neurofibroma*— * arise from dorsal root, * radicular pain, * association with NF, * increased CSF protein |
| intramedullary spinal tumors | • **ependymoma**, • *astrocytoma* [**Note:** intramedullary tumors are commonly associated with syringomyelia at a distant site from the tumor.] |
| sign following a cerebral concussion | **transient loss of consciousness with memory loss of events prior to or shortly after traumatic episode**— * most often caused by a nonpenetrating blunt impact, * temporary functional paralysis of neurons in reticular-activating system |

*Table continued on following page*

**Table 13–1. SELECTED NEUROSURGICAL DISORDERS**
*Continued*

| Most Common... | Answer and Explanation |
|---|---|
| cause of a cerebral contusion | **acceleration-deceleration injuries**—superficial damage to brain |
| cause of coup/ contrecoup injury | **acceleration-deceleration injury causing contusion at impact site (coup injury) and at distant site from point of injury (contrecoup injury)**—contrecoup worse than coup injury |
| sites for contrecoup injuries | **tips of frontal/temporal lobes** |
| cause of diffuse axonal injuries | **acceleration/deceleration injuries**— * shearing of axons located in white matter tracts and/or brain stem |
| secondary brain injuries in diffuse axonal injury | • **cerebral edema,** • *hypoxic brain injury,* • *meningeal tears,* • *bleeding* [**Note:** these findings occur several hours to a day or more later after trauma.] |
| fractures producing rhinorrhea | • **orbital blow-out fracture,** • **basilar skull fractures in anterior cranial fossa** |
| clinical features of basilar skull fracture in anterior cranial fossa | • **fracture through cribriform plate of ethmoid bone**—not usually seen with an x-ray, • **anosmia**— olfactory nerve rootlet transection, • **CSF leaks mixed with blood from one/ both nostrils**—blood forms a ring with a clear center called "halo sign," • **subconjunctival hemorrhage,** • **periorbital hematoma**—"raccoon sign" |
| clinical features of basilar skull fracture of middle cranial fossa | • **fracture through tegmen tympani of petrous portion of temporal bone**— * not seen by x-ray, * CT test of choice, • **hematotympanum (blood in middle ear) or ruptured membrane with otorrhea,** • **eardrum intact**—CSF moves through eustachian tube and out the nose (rhinorrhea), • **Battle's sign**— * bluish discoloration over mastoid bone, * rupture of mastoid emissary vein, • **peripheral CN VII paralysis**— * CN VII traverses temporal bone, * decreased flow of tears means injury is proximal to middle ear portion of CN VII |
| types of traumatic CNS bleeds | • **subdural hematoma,** • *epidural hematoma* |

## Table 13–1. SELECTED NEUROSURGICAL DISORDERS
*Continued*

| Most Common... | Answer and Explanation |
|---|---|
| imaging technique used to initially identify subdural/ epidural hematomas | **CT scan** |
| cause of a subdural hematoma | • **blunt trauma to skull,** • *anticoagulation* [**Note:** blunt trauma causes fracture in 50% and tearing of bridging veins between dura and arachnoid membranes → venous clot over one/both convexities of brain. Elderly patients and alcoholics are most at risk.] |
| CT finding in subdural hematoma | **high-density crescent-shaped collection of blood** |
| S/S of acute subdural hematoma | • **headache,** • *mydriasis,* • *fluctuating levels of consciousness,* • *mass effects*— * visual disturbances, * hemiparesis |
| S/S of chronic subdural hematoma | • **sustained, new headache,** • *confusion,* • *inattention,* • *dementia,* • hypersomnia, • *seizures,* • *coma* [**Note:** subdural hematomas are best diagnosed with MRI.] |
| Rx of subdural hematoma | **clot evacuation** |
| cause of epidural hematoma | **fracture of temporoparietal bone**— * fracture severs the middle meningeal artery, which courses through the bone, * the dura is separated from the periosteum by arterial blood, * ~30–50 mL accumulates over 4–8 hrs, leading to increase in intracranial pressure |
| CT finding of epidural hematoma | **high-density "lens-shaped" collection of blood with shift of brain contents** |
| S/S of epidural hematoma | • **immediate loss of consciousness, followed by a lucid interval,** • **death by herniation in 5–6 hrs** |
| Rx of epidural hematoma | **surgical evacuation of blood clot** |

*Table continued on following page*

### Table 13–1. SELECTED NEUROSURGICAL DISORDERS
*Continued*

| Most Common... | Answer and Explanation |
|---|---|
| acute post-traumatic problem of head injury | **delayed post-traumatic encephalopathy**— * occurs 15 min to 2 hrs after head injury, * patient develops N/V and becomes stuporous/obtunded, * cortical blindness (posterior cerebral artery compression) may occur from temporary uncal herniation, * most recover |
| subacute/chronic complications of head injury | • **chronic subdural hematoma**—see above, • *post-traumatic epilepsy*— * 50% chance with penetrating injuries, * 5% chance with closed injuries, * penetrating injuries are prophylactically treated with phenytoin or carbamazepine, • *delayed dementia*— * 10 × greater chance if patient has apo E ∊4 on chromosome 14, * former boxers: dementia pugilistica, • *postconcussion syndrome*— * headache, * concentration difficulties, * irritable, * dizzy |
| neurologic symptoms in patients with cancer | • **headache**—e.g., * metastasis, * hemorrhage, * drug effects, • *back pain*— * vertebral metastasis, * epidural metastasis, • *altered mental status*—metabolic encephalopathy MCC |
| neurologic complication of systemic cancer | **cerebral metastasis** |
| cancer metastatic to brain | • **lung**, • *breast*, • *colon*, • *malignant melanoma*, • *leukemia*—particularly ALL |
| CNS sites of metastasis | • **cerebral cortex**, • *cerebellum*, • *brain stem* [**Note:** most metastases are multiple and target the junction of gray/white matter or leptomeninges (particularly leukemia/lymphomas).] |
| cancers metastatic to the vertebrae/ epidural space | • **breast**, • *lung*, • *prostate* |
| cancer involving nerve plexuses | **metastatic colorectal cancer** |
| cancers metastatic to the base of the skull | **head/neck cancers** |

## Table 13–1. SELECTED NEUROSURGICAL DISORDERS
*Continued*

| Most Common... | Answer and Explanation |
|---|---|
| overall cancer with most neurologic complications | **metastatic malignant melanoma** |
| primary cancers of the brain in adults | • **glioblastoma multiforme**— * GBM, * grade IV astrocytoma, • *anaplastic astrocytoma*—grade III astrocytoma, • *astrocytoma*—grades I/II are benign, • *CNS lymphoma in AIDS patients* [**Note:** ~70% of adult primary CNS tumors are supratentorial, while ~70% of primary CNS tumors in children are infratentorial, the MC location being cerebellum (cystic astrocytoma, medulloblastoma).] |
| primary benign brain tumors in adults | • **meningioma**, • *acoustic neuroma* |
| tumors in cerebral cortex | • **metastasis**, • *GBM*, • *low-grade astrocytoma*, • *meningioma*, • *oligodendroglioma* |
| tumors in cerebellum | • **astrocytoma**, • *medulloblastoma*, • *cerebellar hemangioblastoma*—part of von Hippel–Lindau disease |
| intraspinal tumor in adults | **ependymoma** |
| location for ependymomas in adults | **lumbosacral portion of spinal cord**— * involve the filum terminale/conus medullaris, * aggressive tumors that invade nerve roots |
| primary CNS tumors seeding neuraxis | • **GBM**, • *medulloblastoma*, • *ependymoma* |
| risk factors of CNS tumors | • **AIDS**, • *neurofibromatosis*, • *Turcot's polyposis syndrome* |
| CNS tumors that calcify | • **meningioma**, • *oligodendroglioma*— * benign tumor, * frontal lobe, * often mixed in with astrocytoma |

*Table continued on following page*

**Table 13–1. SELECTED NEUROSURGICAL DISORDERS**
*Continued*

| Most Common... | Answer and Explanation |
|---|---|
| clinical findings associated with meningiomas | • **women > men,** • **neurofibromatosis association,** • **parasagittal area MC location,** • **they push surface of brain,** • **may invade overlying skull—** * increased bone density, * not a sign of malignancy, • **enlarge during pregnancy**—contain progesterone receptors, • **intraspinal location**—25%, • **MC tumor associated with new-onset focal epileptic seizures in adults,** • **contain psammoma bodies** |
| clinical findings in GBM | • *may evolve from low-grade astrocytoma or arise de novo,* • *peak in 40- to 70-yr-old age bracket,* • *target frontal lobes*—often cross the corpus callosum, • *necrotic/hemorrhagic tumors,* • *rarely metastasize out of neuraxis,* • *25–40% 5-yr survival* |
| S/S of brain tumors | • **morning headache—** * presenting symptom in 50%, * may awaken the patient at night, • *papilledema*—10%, • *vomiting—* * more common in children than adults, * projectile and not usually associated with nausea, * usually occurs in the AM before breakfast, • *altered mental status,* • *visual loss/ weakness/altered consciousness*—due to plateaus of increased intracranial pressure that come and go, • *nuchal rigidity—* * leptomeningeal spread, * CSF glucose may be decreased, • *CN palsies,* • *sensorimotor deficits depending on site* |
| diagnostic tests used in work-up of brain tumors | • **MRI,** • *lumbar puncture*—order a cytology study to look for tumor cells |
| Rx of malignant brain tumors | • **chemotherapy,** • **radiation,** • **surgery—** * meningiomas, * acoustic neuromas |
| cause of increased incidence of primary CNS lymphomas | **AIDS** [**Note:** most malignant CNS lymphomas are metastatic and involve the leptomeninges. Primary CNS lymphomas are a complication of advanced AIDS when the $CD_4$ T helper count is < 50 cells/$\mu$L. HIV/EBV viruses (100% of cases) are implicated. They are high-grade lymphomas, multifocal, and involve the CNS parenchyma (space-occupying lesion).] |

## Table 13–1. SELECTED NEUROSURGICAL DISORDERS
*Continued*

**Question:** Which of the following differentiate neurogenic shock from hypovolemic shock? **SELECT 2**
- (A) Hypotension
- (B) Sinus bradycardia
- (C) Heart and blood vessels do not respond to sympathetic response
- (D) Venoconstriction
- (E) Positive Babinski's sign

**Answers: (B), (C).** In neurogenic shock, there is hypotension and sinus tachycardia, the latter due to a lack of response to sympathetic nervous system responses **(choices B and C are correct)**. In hypovolemic shock, there is hypotension and sinus tachycardia. Activation of the sympathetic nervous system leads to venoconstriction **(choice D is incorrect)**. Both neurogenic and hypovolemic shock have hypotension **(choice A is incorrect)**. Neither neurogenic nor hypovolemic shock has a positive Babinski's sign, which is more often seen in spinal shock and damage to upper motor neurons **(choice E is incorrect)**.

AIDS = acquired immune deficiency syndrome, ALL = acute lymphoblastic leukemia, BV = blood vessels, CN = cranial nerve, CNS = central nervous system, CSF = cerebrospinal fluid, CVA = cerebrovascular accident, DTRs = deep tendon reflexes, EBV = Epstein-Barr virus, EEG = electroencephalogram, GBM = glioblastoma multiforme, GCS = Glasgow Coma Scale, HIV = human immunodeficiency, MC = most common, MCC = most common cause, MS = multiple sclerosis, NF = neurofibromatosis, NG = nasogastric, NSAIDs = nonsteroidal anti-inflammatory drugs, N/V = nausea/vomiting, R/O = rule out, S/S = signs/symptoms, UMN = upper motor neuron, VMD = ventromedial diencephalon.

## Table 13–2. SELECTED OPHTHALMOLOGIC DISORDERS

| Most Common... | Answer and Explanation |
| --- | --- |
| cause of xanthelasmas | **CH deposition in the eyelid**— * yellow plaques on the upper/lower eyelids, * may or may not indicate an underlying hypercholesterolemia |
| cause of a stye on the eyelid | ***Staphylococcus aureus***—Rx with hot packs only |
| granulomatous infection involving the eyelid | **chalazion**—involves the meibomian gland |

*Table continued on following page*

**Table 13–2. SELECTED OPHTHALMOLOGIC DISORDERS**
*Continued*

| Most Common... | Answer and Explanation |
|---|---|
| causes of acute bacterial conjunctivitis | • *Staphylococcus aureus,* • *group A Streptococcus,* • *Streptococcus pneumoniae,* • *Haemophilus influenzae*—pink eye |
| causes of viral conjunctivitis | • **adenovirus**— * viral cause of pink eye, * preauricular lymphadenopathy, • *HSV-1*— * keratoconjunctivitis with dendritic ulcers noted with fluorescein staining, * Rx with trifluridine eye drops |
| cause of conjunctivitis in neonates within 24–48 hrs | **chemical conjunctivitis from erythromycin (protects against *Neisseria gonorrhoeae* and *Chlamydia trachomatis*) or silver nitrate (protects against *Neisseria gonorrhoeae*) drops** |
| cause of bilateral conjunctivitis in neonates within 3–5 days | *Neisseria gonorrhoeae*— * symptoms of this infection usually occur in the first week after exposure, * Rx with aqueous penicillin G or ceftriaxone |
| cause of bilateral conjunctivitis in neonates after 7 days | *Chlamydia trachomatis*— * symptoms of this infection usually occur during the second week after exposure, * Rx with erythromycin |
| cause of severe keratoconjunctivitis in patients who do not clean their lenses properly | *Acanthamoeba*—Rx with propamidine 0.1% + neomycin/gramicidin/polymyxin |
| disease associated with autoimmune destruction of the lacrimal glands | **Sjögren's syndrome** |
| seasonal cause of pruritic conjunctivitis | **allergic conjunctivitis** |
| cause of arcus senilis | **CH deposition in the outer margin of the cornea** |
| cause of a pterygium | **excessive exposure to wind, sun, and sand** [**Note:** a pterygium is a raised, triangular encroachment of the conjunctiva on the nasal side of the cornea.] |

## Table 13–2. SELECTED OPHTHALMOLOGIC DISORDERS
*Continued*

| Most Common... | Answer and Explanation |
| --- | --- |
| disorders affecting visual acuity | • **retinal disorders**—e.g., * central retinal artery embolism, * diabetic retinopathy, • **optic nerve disorders**—e.g., optic neuritis, • **chiasm disorders**—e.g., * craniopharyngioma, * lesions posterior to chiasm do not affect visual acuity |
| disorders affecting visual fields | • **defects in one eye**— * globe, * retina, * prechiasmal optic nerve disorders, • **bilateral defects**—lesions at or posterior to optic chiasm, • **bitemporal field cuts**—chiasm lesions, • **papilledema**—enlarged blind spot |
| terms applied to visual field defects | • **homonymous**— * right visual field: temporal half of right eye/nasal half of left eye, * left visual field: temporal half of left eye/nasal half of right eye, • **hemianopia**—impairment of nearly half of visual field, • **quadrantanopia**—smaller impairment involving only a quarter of visual field |
| cause of a unilateral loss of vision | **damage to retina or optic nerve proximal to the chiasm**—schematic: loss of vision in left eye<br><br>Left    Right |
| cause of left/right inferior quadrantanopia | • **left**—right parietal lobe lesion, • **right**— * left parietal lobe lesion, * schematic: right inferior quadrantanopia<br><br>Left    Right |
| cause of superior bitemporal quadrantanopia | **inferior chiasmal lesion**—e.g., pituitary adenoma<br><br>Left    Right |

*Table continued on following page*

## Table 13–2. SELECTED OPHTHALMOLOGIC DISORDERS
*Continued*

| Most Common... | Answer and Explanation |
|---|---|
| cause of a visual field defect with macular sparing | **posterior cerebral artery infarct with sparing of tips of occipital lobes** Left    Right |
| cause of an enlarged blind spot (scotoma) | **increased intracranial pressure** Left    Right |
| cause of cortical blindness | **bilateral damage to the visual radiation or occipital lobe**—e.g., * basilar artery insufficiency, * hypertensive encephalopathy |
| S/S of cortical blindness | • **normal funduscopic exam,** • **normal pupillary light reflexes,** • **patient often unaware of blindness** |
| causes of sudden unilateral loss of vision | • **optic neuritis,** • *amaurosis fugax,* • *central retinal artery occlusion,* • *central retinal vein occlusion* |
| causes of optic neuritis | • **demyelinating disease**—e.g., MS: 75%, • *infection*—e.g., * measles, * mumps, * VZ, * syphilis, * TB, • *SLE,* • *methyl alcohol poisoning*—converted into formic acid |
| S/S in optic neuritis | • **retro-orbital pain when moving eyes,** • **globe tenderness to palpation,** • **flame hemorrhages around disc vessels/swollen optic disc**—if neuritis is located at nerve head, not retrobulbar location |
| Rx of optic neuritis in MS | **intravenous methylprednisolone** |
| cause of amaurosis fugax | • **retinal embolus of atheromatous plaque material**— * Hollenhorst's plaque, * often visible on retinal exam, * originates from the ipsilateral carotid artery, • **type of TIA** |
| S/S in amaurosis fugax | **described as curtain passing vertically across visual field, followed in few minutes by curtain moving up and restoring vision**—less correlation with impending stroke than other types of TIAs |

## Table 13–2. SELECTED OPHTHALMOLOGIC DISORDERS
*Continued*

| Most Common... | Answer and Explanation |
|---|---|
| causes of central retinal artery occlusion | • **embolization of plaque material from ipsilateral carotid or ophthalmic artery,** • *giant cell temporal arteritis,* • APL syndrome |
| S/S in central retinal artery occlusion | • **sudden, painless, complete loss of vision in one eye,** • **most commonly elderly patients with carotid artery stenosis,** • **pallor of optic disc,** • **"boxcar" segmentation of blood in retinal veins**—sign of stasis, • **cherry red fovea,** • **retinal edema,** • **bloodless,** • **constricted arterioles** |
| causes of central retinal vein occlusion | • **hypercoagulable state**—e.g., * PRV, * APL syndrome, * protein C or S deficiency, • *essential HTN,* • *DM,* • *glaucoma,* • *hyperlipidemia*—serum TG > 1000 mg/dL |
| S/S of central retinal vein occlusion | • **sudden, painless, unilateral loss of vision,** • **swelling of optic disc,** • **"blood and thunder" appearance of retina from hemorrhages,** • **cotton wool exudates**—microinfarctions, • **engorged retinal veins** |
| types of glaucoma | • **chronic open-angle glaucoma**— * 90% of all cases, * decreased rate of aqueous outflow into canal of Schlemm, • *acute* (angle-closure) *glaucoma*—narrow anterior chamber angle |
| S/S of a chronic open-angle glaucoma | • **increased intraocular pressure,** • *usually asymptomatic in early phases,* • *bilateral aching eyes,* • *common in African-Americans,* • *pathologic cupping of optic discs,* • *optic atrophy,* • *nyctalopia,* • *gradual loss of peripheral vision leading to tunnel vision and blindness* |
| Rx of chronic open-angle glaucoma | • **β-adrenergic blocking agents**—e.g., timolol, • **cholinergic agonist**—e.g., pilocarpine, • **adrenergic agonist**—e.g., epinephrine, • **oral/topical carbonic anhydrase inhibitor** |
| S/S of acute-angle glaucoma | • **rapid increase in intraocular pressure,** • **severe pain,** • **photophobia,** • **blurry vision**—blue or red halos around lights, • **red eye,** • **steamy cornea,** • **pupil fixed in mid-dilated position,** • **pupil nonreactive to light,** • **precipitated by**— * mydriatic agent, * uveitis, * lens dislocation |

*Table continued on following page*

**Table 13–2. SELECTED OPHTHALMOLOGIC DISORDERS**
*Continued*

| Most Common... | Answer and Explanation |
|---|---|
| Rx of acute-angle glaucoma | • **laser iridectomy,** • *carbonic anhydrase inhibitor,* • *pilocarpine* |
| causes of optic atrophy | • **optic neuritis,** • *glaucoma,* • *methyl alcohol poisoning* |
| S/S of optic nerve atrophy | • **visual field/color vision defects,** • **night blindness,** • **sluggish pupillary reactions,** • **decreased visual acuity,** • **extreme pallor of disc with sharply defined borders,** • **vessels normal**—not visible if due to increased intracranial pressure, • **visible physiologic cup**—not visible if due to increased intracranial pressure |
| causes of uveitis | • **sarcoidosis**—usually bilateral, • *AIDS*—CMV, • *ankylosing spondylitis,* • *juvenile RA,* • *ulcerative colitis,* • *TB,* • *trauma* [**Note:** uveitis is inflammation of uveal tract—iris, ciliary body, choroid.] |
| S/S of uveitis | • **pain,** • **blurry vision,** • **photophobia,** • **miotic pupil,** • **poor light reflex,** • **circumcorneal ciliary body vascular congestion,** • **normal to low intraocular pressure,** • **cornea usually clear,** • **synechiae (adhesions) between iris and anterior lens capsule** |
| Rx of uveitis | • **topical corticosteroids (anterior uveitis)/ systemic corticosteroids (posterior uveitis),** • *Rx infection if present* |
| causes of retinal detachment | • **cataract extraction,** • *myopia,* • *trauma* [**Note:** the retina usually detaches in the superior temporal area.] |
| S/S of retinal detachment | • **blurred vision in eye progressively becomes worse**—"curtain came over my eye," • **retina hanging in vitreous,** • **no conjunctival redness,** • **no pain** |
| Rx of retinal detachment | **laser photocoagulation** |
| causes of vitreous hemorrhage | • **DM retinopathy,** • *retinal tears,* • *macular degeneration,* • *trauma,* • *blood dyscrasias*—e.g., * sickle cell disease, * Hgb SC disease, • *retinal vein thrombosis* |

## Table 13–2. SELECTED OPHTHALMOLOGIC DISORDERS
*Continued*

| Most Common... | Answer and Explanation |
|---|---|
| cause of permanent visual loss in elderly patients | **macular degeneration—** * age-related, * ? relationship with cigarette smoking, * family Hx [**Note:** the macula is located lateral to the optic disc. It is normally a light red color. The central darker spot that reflects light is the fovea centralis.] |
| S/S of macular degeneration | **gradual (atrophic type) or abrupt (exudative type), progressive bilateral (atrophic type) or sequential (exudative type) visual loss (central visual loss)**—disruption of Bruch's membrane in the retina is responsible for permanent visual loss |
| Rx of macular degeneration | • **no specific Rx,** • **zinc supplements may be useful** |
| cause of blindness in AIDS | **CMV retinitis**—usually occurs when $CD_4$ T helper cell count <50 cells/$\mu$L |
| S/S of CMV retinitis | • **cotton wool exudates,** • **retinal hemorrhages,** • **visual disturbances when optic nerve involved or retinal detachment** |
| Rx of CMV retinitis | • **ganciclovir,** • *foscarnet if ganciclovir is not improving the condition* |
| causes of miotic (small, constricted) pupils | • **old age,** • *Horner's syndrome,* • *Argyll Robertson pupil,* • *barbiturates,* • *pontine hemorrhage,* • *opiate*—e.g., * heroin, * morphine, • *alcohol,* • *glutethimide,* • *pilocarpine drops,* • *sympathetic paralysis* |
| causes of mydriatic (dilated) pupils | • **anxiety,** • *parasympathetic paralysis*—e.g., uncal herniation, • *Adie's pupil,* • *amphetamines,* • *cocaine,* • *psychedelics*—e.g., * LSD, * phencyclidine, * scopolamine, • *cerebral death,* • *mydriatic drops*—e.g., atropine, • *childhood* |
| causes of anisocoria | • **normal finding in 15% of population,** • *CN III palsy,* • *Horner's syndrome* [**Note:** anisocoria refers to unequal pupil diameters.] |
| causes of Argyll-Robertson pupil | • **syphilis,** • *DM* |

*Table continued on following page*

## Table 13–2. SELECTED OPHTHALMOLOGIC DISORDERS
*Continued*

| Most Common... | Answer and Explanation |
|---|---|
| signs of Argyll-Robertson pupil | • **absence of a miotic reaction to direct or consensual light,** • **pupils constrict to near-stimulus**—accommodate, • **miotic, irregular pupil,** • **pupil does not dilate with atropine or painful stimulation in other parts of body** |
| cause of Marcus-Gunn pupil | **retrobulbar optic neuritis**—due to a lesion in the afferent limb of the pupillary light reflex |
| signs of Marcus-Gunn pupil | **using the swinging flashlight test (move light quickly from eye to eye)**— * light in normal eye causes pupillary constriction in both normal and abnormal eye, * light quickly moved to abnormal eye produces mydriasis |
| cause of Adie's tonic pupil | • **young patients with normally mydriatic pupils,** • *iris dysfunction from trauma,* • *topical mydriatics,* • *benztropine* |
| signs of Adie's tonic pupil | • **sluggish response to both direct/consensual light and accommodation,** • **unilateral or bilateral,** • **tonic pupil dilates with atropine** [**Note:** Adie's syndrome has the above signs and the absence of DTRs.] |
| cause of Horner's syndrome | **primary SCC of lung involving superior sulcus**—destruction of the superior cervical sympathetic ganglion |
| signs of Horner's syndrome | **triad of**— * ipsilateral miosis, * anhidrosis, * ptosis |
| pupil signs in subtentorial lesions | • **pinpoint**—lesion in pons, • **fixed**—lesion in tectum of midbrain, • **irregular and/or unequal**—lesion in midbrain-pontine |
| pupil signs in metabolic encephalopathy/ diencephalic damage | **small, reactive pupils** |
| symptoms of ocular muscle weakness | • **blurry vision,** • *diplopia*—double vision |
| causes of horizontal diplopia | • **lateral rectus palsy**—CN VI, • *medial rectus palsy*—CN III |
| causes of vertical diplopia | • **CN III-related palsies**— * superior/inferior rectus, * inferior oblique, • *CN IV-related palsy*—superior oblique |

## Table 13–2. SELECTED OPHTHALMOLOGIC DISORDERS
*Continued*

| Most Common... | Answer and Explanation |
|---|---|
| cause of progressive diplopia | **compressive lesion**—e.g., tumor |
| cause of sudden diplopia | **vascular lesion**—e.g., infarction |
| cause of intermittent diplopia that occurs later in the day | **myasthenia gravis** |
| causes of acute (<48 hrs) bilateral ophthalmoplegia | • brain stem stroke, • *Wernicke's syndrome*, • *botulism*, • *MG*— • *Guillain-Barré* |
| causes of acute (<48 hrs) unilateral ophthalmoplegia | • **uncal herniation**—due to CN III compression, • *DM*— * CN III: pupil spared, * CN VI palsy, • *myasthenia gravis* |
| sites responsible for voluntary/tracking conjugate eye movement | **supranuclear pathways** [**Note:** the pathway descends from the forebrain to the MLF in the brain stem. The MLF connects the CN III nucleus (MR [adducts]) with the CN VI nucleus (LR [abducts]) in the brain stem. The CN VI nucleus has a pathway connecting with the PPRF, lateral gaze center, on the same side of the brain stem. The MLF crosses in the midbrain and connects the CN III nucleus on one side with the pathway connecting the CN VI nucleus with the PPRF on the contralateral side.<br><br><br><br>LR = lateral rectus, MR = medial rectus, PPRF = pontine paramedian reticular formation |

*Table continued on following page*

**Table 13–2. SELECTED OPHTHALMOLOGIC DISORDERS**
*Continued*

| Most Common... | Answer and Explanation |
| --- | --- |
| | When the patient is asked to look right, the signal to the left CN III nucleus causes the left eye to adduct right and the signal to CN VI on the right causes abduction of the right eye. When the patient is asked to look left, the signal to the CN III nucleus on the right causes adduction of the right eye to the left and the signal to CN VI on the left to abduct the left eye. Therefore, with lesions involving the MLF, the MR is paralyzed (remains stationary) on attempted lateral gaze, whereas the LR is intact. Furthermore, the abducting eye exhibits horizontal nystagmus. Hence, with a lesion in the left MLF (lesion A, unilateral INO), conjugate gaze to the left is intact; however, conjugate gaze to the right is paralyzed (right eye abducts and has horizontal nystagmus but left eye remains stationary). A lesion in the right MLF (lesion B) allows conjugate gaze to the right, but conjugate gaze to the left is paralyzed (left eye can abduct, but the right eye remains stationary). A lesion involving both A and B is called bilateral INO. As expected, both left and right conjugate gaze are paralyzed. If one of the CN VI nuclei is destroyed and bilateral INO is present, it is called the 1 1/2 syndrome. For example, if CN VI on the left is destroyed and a bilateral INO is also present, the left eye cannot abduct when the patient looks to the left, but the right can abduct, since the nucleus is intact. Since the ability to converge both eyes (both eyes adduct) comes from a different pathway originating from the superior colliculus, in all the above lesions the ability to converge the eyes is left intact. |
| cause of unilateral INO | **ischemic damage in the brain stem affecting the MLF**—see above discussion |
| cause of bilateral internuclear ophthalmoplegia | **MS** |

## Table 13–2. SELECTED OPHTHALMOLOGIC DISORDERS
*Continued*

| Most Common... | Answer and Explanation |
|---|---|
| causes of strabismus | • **nonparalytic**—e.g., * intrinsic imbalance of muscle tone, * usually congenital, • *paralytic*—e.g., * CN III/IV/VI palsies, * MG [**Note:** strabismus is an involuntary deviation of the eyes from their normal physiologic position.] |
| complications associated with strabismus | • **headache,** • *diplopia,* • *amblyopia*— * suppression of vision in one eye in order to prevent diplopia leads to permanent reduction of vision, * more likely to occur in children with strabismus |
| causes of "floaters" in the eye | • **hemorrhages**—due to: ♦ neovascularization in diabetes mellitus, ♦ subhyaloid retinal hemorrhage secondary to a subarachnoid hemorrhage, • *tear film debris,* • *material in the vitreous*—remnants of embryonic hyaloid vascular system, • *degenerative vitreous changes*—related to aging or trauma |
| cause of cataracts | • **old age**— * age-dependent disorder, * Rx with: ♦ extracapsular extraction (MC method), ♦ intracapsular extraction, ♦ phacoemulsification, • *congenital*— * MCC of leukocoria: white eye reflex, * causes include: ♦ congenital rubella, ♦ intrauterine factors that interfere with lens development, • *miscellaneous*— * diabetes mellitus: related to osmotic damage of the lens, * hypoparathyroidism, * galactosemia: related to osmotic damage, * electrical burns, * corticosteroid eye drops, * myotonic dystrophy [**Note:** a cataract refers to any opacity in the lens.] |
| intraocular tumor in adults | **malignant melanoma**— * most frequently arises from the choroid, * other sites include: ♦ ciliary body, ♦ iris, * may cause visual disturbance, * eye must be enucleated |
| intraocular tumor in children | **retinoblastoma**— * sporadic and genetic: AD disorder, * white eye reflex on physical exam, * associated with inactivation of the Rb suppressor gene on chromosome 13: sporadic type requires mutations on both chromosomes, genetic type already has one chromosome mutated at birth, * Rx with enucleation |

*Table continued on following page*

## Table 13–2. SELECTED OPHTHALMOLOGIC DISORDERS
*Continued*

| Most Common... | Answer and Explanation |
|---|---|
| ADA recommendation for ophthalmologic exam in type I and II DM | **annual dilated eye and visual exams (ophthalmologist or optometrist) in**— * all patients 10 yrs and older with type I DM for 3–5 yrs, * all type II DM patients at time of Dx, * all DM patients who present with visual findings |
| types of eye disease in DM | • **retinopathy,** • *impaired pupillary reaction,* • *cataracts*—osmotic damage, • *glaucoma*— * 6%, * open-angle type |
| types of retinopathy in DM | • **background diabetic retinopathy**— * microaneurysms: osmotic damage of pericytes weakens vessel, * hard exudates: due to increased vessel permeability, * retinal edema, * focal macular abnormalities, • **preproliferative**— * soft exudates: due to infarction, * more diffuse retinal edema/macular disease, • **proliferative**— * capillary proliferation, * retinal detachment, * vitreous hemorrhage [**Note:** if retinopathy is present, nephropathy is present.] |
| Rx of diabetic retinopathy | • **strict glycemic control,** • *HTN control,* • *laser photocoagulation* |
| Rx of pupillary reaction abnormalities in DM | **panretinal photocoagulation** |
| findings in grade I hypertensive retinopathy | • **focal narrowing of the arterioles**— * 1:2 ratio, * normal ratio of the arteriole to the venule is 3:4, • **mild AV nicking**—depression in the wall of the venule due to sclerosis of the overlying arteriole |
| findings in grade II hypertensive retinopathy | • **more diffuse narrowing of the arterioles**—1:3 ratio, • **copper wiring of the arterioles**—sclerotic changes in the arteriole, but blood is still visible, • **more accentuation of AV nicking** |

## Table 13–2. SELECTED OPHTHALMOLOGIC DISORDERS
*Continued*

| Most Common... | Answer and Explanation |
|---|---|
| findings in grade III hypertensive retinopathy | • **more advanced arteriole narrowing**—1:4, • **silver wiring of the arterioles**—no blood is visible in the lumen, • **flame hemorrhages**—due to ruptured microaneurysms, • **soft exudates**— * microinfarctions, * look like "cotton balls" with blurry borders, • **hard exudates**— * leakage of protein from the vessels, * sharp borders, • **advanced AV nicking**—vein under the arteriole disappears, • **normal disc** |
| findings in grade IV hypertensive retinopathy | **all the above for grade III plus papilledema of the optic disc** |

**Question:** Which of the following eye disorders are associated with visual loss? **SELECT 8**
- (A) Optic neuritis
- (B) Viral conjunctivitis
- (C) Glaucoma
- (D) Methyl alcohol poisoning
- (E) Cataracts
- (F) Bacterial conjunctivitis
- (G) Argyll-Robertson pupil
- (H) Horner's syndrome
- (I) Macular degeneration
- (J) Amaurosis fugax
- (K) CN III palsy
- (L) Uveitis
- (M) Arcus senilis
- (N) Central retinal artery/vein thrombosis
- (O) Allergic conjunctivitis

**Answers:** **(A)**, **(C)**, **(D)**, **(E)**, **(I)**, **(J)**, **(L)**, **(N)**. Viral, bacterial, and allergic conjunctivitis do not affect vision **(choices B, F, O are incorrect)**. An Argyll-Robertson pupil, Horner's syndrome, CN III palsy, and arcus senilis are not associated with visual disturbances **(choices G, H, K, M are incorrect)**. Optic neuritis, glaucoma, methyl alcohol poisoning (optic neuritis), cataracts, macular degeneration, amaurosis fugax, uveitis, and central retinal artery/vein thrombosis are all associated with visual loss **(choices A, C, D, E, I, J, L, N are correct)**.

AD = autosomal dominant, ADA = American Diabetes Association, AIDS = acquired immunodeficiency syndrome, APL = antiphospholipid syndrome, AV = arteriovenous, CH = cholesterol, CMV = cytomegalovirus, CN = cranial nerve, DM = diabetes mellitus, DTRs = deep tendon reflex, Hgb = hemoglobin, HSV = Herpes simplex virus, HTN = hypertension, INO = internuclear ophthalmoplegia, LR = lateral rectus, LSD = lysergic acid diethylamide, MC = most common, MCC = most common cause, MG = myasthenia gravis, MLF = medial longitudinal fasciculus, MR = medial rectus, MS = multiple sclerosis, PPRF = pontine paramedian reticular formation, PRV = polycythemia rubra vera, RA = rheumatoid arthritis, SCC = squamous cell carcinoma, SLE = systemic lupus erythematosus, S/S = signs and symptoms, TG = triglyceride, TIAs = transient ischemic attacks, VZ = varicella/zoster.

## Table 13–3. SELECTED AUDITORY DISORDERS

| Most Common... | Answer and Explanation |
|---|---|
| causes of external otitis ("swimmer's ear") | • *Pseudomonas aeruginosa,* • *Staphylococcus aureus,* • *Aspergillus* species [**Note:** the Rx of external otitis is ear drops containing polymyxin B + neomycin + hydrocortisone.] |
| cause of malignant external otitis | *Pseudomonas aeruginosa* in elderly diabetics—Rx is imipenem or other types of antipseudomonal antibiotics |
| cause of otitis media in children | • *Streptococcus pneumoniae,* • *Haemophilus influenzae,* • *Moraxella catarrhalis* [**Note:** the Rx of choice is amoxicillin.] |
| complication of otitis media | conduction hearing loss |
| symptoms of auditory dysfunction | • **hearing loss**— * **conductive,** * sensorineural, • *tinnitus*—ringing in ears |
| sites involved in conductive hearing loss | • **external ear canal,** • *middle ear* |
| causes of conductive hearing loss | • **impacted cerumen in outer ear canal,** • *fluid in middle ear,* • *otosclerosis*—MCC in elderly people |

## Table 13–3. SELECTED AUDITORY DISORDERS *Continued*

| Most Common... | Answer and Explanation |
|---|---|
| cause of conductive hearing loss in elderly patients | **otosclerosis—** * fixation of the middle ear ossicles, * strong autosomal dominant history |
| clinical findings in conductive hearing loss | • **Weber test lateralizes to affected ear and bone conduction > air conduction (Rinne's test),** • **affected ear feels full,** • equal loss of all hearing frequencies, • **well-preserved speech discrimination** |
| sites involved in sensorineural hearing loss | • **cochlea,** • *auditory nerve—CN VIII* |
| causes of sensorineural hearing loss | • **presbycusis**—degeneration of hairs in the cochlea, • *noise trauma,* • *infection—* * viral, * bacterial, • *drugs*—e.g., * aminoglycosides: destroy cochlear hair cells, * salicylates, * diuretics, * cisplatin, • *Ménière's disease*—see below, • *acoustic neuroma* |
| clinical findings in sensorineural hearing loss | • **Weber test lateralizes to normal ear (contra-lateral ear is affected) and air conduction > bone conduction in both normal and affected ear,** • **low tones are heard better than high tones,** • **cannot hear consonants owing to high frequency loss**—loss of speech discrimination, • **cannot hear well in noisy environments,** • **recruitment**—small increases in intensity of sound cause discomfort |
| cause of Ménière's disease | • **endolymphatic HTN**—hydrops, • *loss of cochlear hairs* |
| S/S of Ménière's disease | • **fluctuating unilateral disease**—75%, • **low-frequency sensorineural hearing loss,** • **recurrent episodes of vertigo,** • **tinnitus**—low-pitched roaring, • **sense of fullness in the affected ear** |
| Rx of Ménière's disease | • **diuretics,** • *carbonic anhydrase inhibitors,* • *low-salt diet,* • *surgical decompression of excess endolymph* |

*Table continued on following page*

**Table 13–3. SELECTED AUDITORY DISORDERS** *Continued*

| Most Common... | Answer and Explanation |
|---|---|
| clinical findings of an acoustic neuroma | • **unilateral progressive sensorineural hearing loss,** • *tinnitus,* • *sensory changes in face*—trigeminal nerve irritation from large cerebellopontine angle tumor, • *abnormal corneal reflex*—loss of CN V afferent component, • *ataxia,* • *increased association with neurofibromatosis*—unilateral or bilateral acoustic neuromas, • *MRI locates lesion,* • *auditory evoked potential is useful in equivocal cases* [**Note:** acoustic neuromas are benign tumors derived from Schwann cells. They involve the VIIIth nerve. Surgery is the Rx of choice.] |
| types of tinnitus | • **subjective**—abnormal discharge in auditory system not heard by examiner, • *objective*—patient hears real sound also heard by examiner with a stethoscope |
| causes of tinnitus | • **impacted cerumen,** • *otosclerosis*—roaring sound, • *severe HTN,* • *severe anemia*—increased blood flow, • *patent eustachian tube*— * normally closed, * tinnitus corresponds with breathing, • *Ménière's disease*—loud roars or clangings, • *acoustic neuroma of CN VIII,* • *vascular disorders*— * glomus jugulare: ♦ reddish-blue mass behind tympanic membrane, ♦ pulsatile sound, * carotid artery stenosis, * compression of the vertebral artery from osteophytes in cervical osteoarthritis, • *post-traumatic*—e.g., gunshot, • *drugs*—e.g., * salicylates, * quinidine, * quinine, * indomethacin, • *raised intracranial pressure*—compression of jugular vein obliterates the sound |
| causes of dizziness | • **anxiety/hyperventilation,** • *eyes*— * eye muscle imbalance, * refractive error, • *vestibular disease,* • *carotid sinus syndrome,* • *hypotension*— * orthostatic, * arrhythmias, * aortic stenosis, • *viral labyrinthitis,* • *impaired proprioception*—e.g., pernicious anemia, • *basilar artery insufficiency* |
| S/S of dizziness | • **lightheadedness,** • **dysequilibrium when standing,** • **unsteadiness when walking** |

## Table 13–3. SELECTED AUDITORY DISORDERS *Continued*

| Most Common... | Answer and Explanation |
|---|---|
| symptom and sign of vestibular disease | • **symptom**— * vertigo, in which the patient or surroundings are whirling in a continuous direction, * symptoms related to vertigo include: ♦ N/V (not seen in dizziness), ♦ imbalance/ataxia, ♦ past pointing, • **sign**— nystagmus: ♦ rhythmic to-and-fro involuntary oscillations of eyes, ♦ horizontal/vertical/rotary types |
| mechanisms causing vertigo | • **physiologic**—e.g., * motion sickness, * heights, * visual (roller coaster ride), * neck hyperextension, • *peripheral causes involving vestibular system*— * semicircular canals, * otolithic apparatus, • *central causes*— * brain stem, * cerebellum, * CN VIII |
| pathologic causes of vertigo | • **benign positional vertigo,** • *Ménière's disease,* • *viral labyrinthitis,* • *labyrinthine concussion post-head trauma,* • *acoustic neuroma,* • *multiple sclerosis,* • *brain stem ischemia*—e.g., lateral medullary syndrome involving PICA, • *temporal lobe epilepsy,* • *cerebellar disorders*—e.g., * degenerative diseases, * tumors |
| tests to evaluate dizziness/vertigo | • **audiology,** • *ECG*—R/O arrhythmias, • *CBC*—R/O: ♦ anemia, ♦ polycythemia, • *RPR,* • *glucose/electrolytes,* • *serum ANA*— if SLE is suspected, • *MRI*—if acoustic neuroma or multiple sclerosis is suspected, • *caloric testing:* * evaluate unconscious patients, * test vestibular function, * cold water irrigation causes nystagmus away from side of stimulation, * warm water causes nystagmus to side of stimulation, • *auditory evoked potential*—R/O: * demyelinating disease, * acoustic neuroma |
| S/S of benign positional vertigo | • **precipitated by head movements**—e.g., * first lying down in bed at night or arising in AM, * turning suddenly, • *not associated with tinnitus or sensorineural hearing loss*—this is a key differentiating point from Ménière's disease, • *vertigo is accompanied by nystagmus,* • *mechanism*—dislocation of utricular macular otoliths |

*Table continued on following page*

**Table 13–3. SELECTED AUDITORY DISORDERS** *Continued*

| Most Common... | Answer and Explanation |
|---|---|
| Rx of BPV | • **positional maneuvers**—repositions displaced otoliths: e.g., move from the sitting position to lying down on the side may correct the vertigo, • *antiemetics*—e.g., meclizine, • *vestibular suppressants*—e.g., diazepam |
| mechanisms of nystagmus | *dysfunction in*— * visual perceptual area, * vestibular system, * cerebellum, * labyrinthine proprioceptive influences from neck muscles, * reticular formation in pontine brain stem [nystagmus is a type of supranuclear ocular palsy that is unrelated to problems in ocular muscles or cranial nerves III, IV, or VI.] |
| types of nystagmus | • **jerk nystagmus**—slow phase is away from visual object followed by a quick saccade (series of short jerks) back toward the target, • *pendular nystagmus*—slow, coarse, and equal in both directions: like the pendulum of a clock |
| types of jerk nystagmus | • **vestibular nystagmus**— * horizontal or rotary movement of the eyes, * sign of vestibular disease, • *convergence-retraction nystagmus*— * upward gaze causes irregular jerking of the eyes up into the orbit, * indicates midbrain tegmental damage, • *downbeat nystagmus*— * downward gaze causes irregular downward jerking of the eyes, * associated with lower medullary damage |
| types of pendular nystagmus | • **horizontal/pendular nystagmus**— * slow, steady oscillations of equal velocity around a center point, * causes: ♦ congenital, ♦ related to severe visual impairment (e.g., optic atrophy, albinism), ♦ sign of multiple sclerosis, • *vertical/seesaw nystagmus*— * rapid seesaw movement of both eyes: one rises, other is falling, * sign of optic chiasm disease |

## Table 13–3. SELECTED AUDITORY DISORDERS *Continued*

**Question:** Which of the following disorders are associated with tinnitus? **SELECT 3**
   (A) Ménière's disease
   (B) Benign positional vertigo
   (C) Acoustic neuroma
   (D) External otitis
   (E) Presbycusis
   (F) Glioblastoma multiforme
   (G) Salicylate intoxication
   (H) Otitis media

**Answers: (A), (C), (G).** A key distinction between Ménière's disease and benign positional vertigo is the absence of tinnitus in the latter condition (**choice A is correct, choice B is incorrect**). External otitis, glioblastoma multiforme, presbycusis, and otitis media are not associated with tinnitus (**choices D, E, F, H are incorrect**). Acoustic neuromas and salicylate intoxication are associated with tinnitus (**choices C, G are correct**).

ANA = anti-nuclear antibody, BPV = benign positional vertigo, CBC = complete blood count, CN = cranial nerve, ECG = electrocardiogram, HTN = hypertension, MCC = most common cause, N/V = nausea/vomiting, PICA = posterior inferior cerebellar artery, R/O = rule out, RPR = rapid plasma reagin, SLE = systemic lupus erythematosus, S/S = signs/symptoms.

# CHAPTER

# 14

# SELECTED UROLOGIC DISORDERS

## CONTENTS

### Table 14-1. SELECTED UROLOGIC DISORDERS I

| Most Common... | Answer and Explanation |
|---|---|
| cause of costovertebral angle pain | **renal disease**—e.g., * APN, * adenocarcinoma [**Note:** renal pain may radiate to the umbilicus, testicle, labium. Pain is related to swelling of the capsule and is usually constant. Pain related to obstruction (e.g., stone) is colicky (pain comes and goes). N/V commonly occur.] |
| systemic diseases associated with renal disease | • **essential HTN**— * BNS, * malignant HTN, • *DM*— * CRF, * APN, * renal papillary necrosis, • *shock*—ATN, • *peripheral vascular disease*—renal artery stenosis, • *collagen vascular disease*— * SLE, * PSS, * PAN |
| UUT (kidneys, ureter) causes of hematuria | • **renal stone**—~40%, • *GN/medullary sponge kidney/renal papillary necrosis*—~20%, • *renal adenocarcinoma*— * 10%, * MC initial finding, • *renal pelvis transitional cell carcinoma* (TCC)—7% |
| LUT (bladder, urethra, prostate) causes of hematuria | • **infection,** • *TCC*—MCC of gross hematuria in absence of infection, • *BPH* |
| cause of microscopic hematuria in adult males | **BPH** |
| drugs associated with hematuria | • **anticoagulants**—e.g., * warfarin, * heparin, • *cyclophosphamide*— * hemorrhagic cystitis, * TCC, • *drugs causing interstitial nephritis*—e.g., * methicillin, * analgesic nephropathy |

*Table continued on following page*

## Table 14–1. SELECTED UROLOGIC DISORDERS I
*Continued*

| Most Common... | Answer and Explanation |
|---|---|
| initial steps in evaluating hematuria | • **complete UA,** • *urine culture,* • *others pending results of UA/culture—* * IVP: evaluates upper urinary tract, * cystoscopy: gross hematuria, * urine cytology: R/O bladder cancer |
| lab abnormalities indicating renal disease | • **proteinuria,** • *hematuria,* • *pyuria,* • *elevated serum creatinine* |
| uses of US in renal disease | • **solid versus cystic renal mass,** • *R/O hydronephrosis/APKD,* • *assess kidney size,* • *stone work-up* |
| uses of an IVP in renal disease | • **evaluate anatomic features of urinary excretory system**—e.g., * stones, * cysts, * calyceal deformities, * ureteral obstruction, • *work-up of hematuria* |
| causes of radiocontrast-induced nephropathy | • **DM,** • *CRF,* • *multiple myeloma* |
| use of retrograde pyelography | **evaluate urinary collecting system if IVP not helpful** |
| uses of renal arteriography | • **evaluate cause of renovascular hypertension**—examples include: ♦ atherosclerosis, ♦ fibromuscular hyperplasia, • *identify—* * embolization, * thrombosis, • *evaluate vascularity of tumors* |
| use of CT scan in renal disease | **evaluate renal masses** |
| use of MRI in renal disease | • **evaluate renal masses,** • *staging of renal adenocarcinoma* |
| use of radionuclide scan | • **measure function of one kidney versus the other**—useful in the work-up of renovascular HTN, • *follow renal function in transplant kidneys* |
| uses of renal biopsy | • **work-up of GN,** • *evaluate post-transplant kidney for rejection* |
| tests used to evaluate renal function | • **urinalysis (UA),** • *serum BUN,* • *serum creatinine,* • *BUN/creatinine ratio,* • *CCr,* • *UOsm,* • *FENa$^+$* |

## Table 14–1. SELECTED UROLOGIC DISORDERS I
*Continued*

| Most Common... | Answer and Explanation |
|---|---|
| source of urea | **end-product of amino acid/pyrimidine metabolism** |
| causes of an increased serum BUN | • **decreased GFR**—e.g., * CHF, * shock, * hypovolemia, • *renal failure,* • *postrenal obstruction,* • *increased intake of protein*— * bacterial ureases convert urea into ammonia, which is reabsorbed and converted into urea in liver urea cycle, * examples include: ♦ TPN, ♦ GI bleed (blood is protein), • *glucocorticoids*—break down muscle protein, • *tetracycline*— * inhibit protein synthesis, * more amino acids are shunted into the urea cycle, * serum creatinine is normal |
| causes of a low serum BUN | • **chronic liver disease**—dysfunctional urea cycle, • *pregnancy*— * dilutional effect, * increased renal clearance, • *SiADH*— * dilutional effect, * increased renal clearance, • *malnutrition*—decreased protein intake |
| source of creatinine | *metabolism of creatine in muscle*— * underscores why creatinine is used as a measure of muscle mass, * creatinine is excreted in the kidneys at a constant rate and is neither reabsorbed nor secreted |
| pathologic causes of an elevated creatinine | • **prerenal azotemia**—decreased GFR, • *renal failure,* • *postrenal obstruction* [**Note:** creatinine is a poor screen for renal disease, since >50–70% of renal mass must be destroyed before it increases. Serum creatinine increases when GFR is <40% of normal. Creatinine increases 0.5–1.0 mg/dL/day in patients with acute renal failure.] |
| causes of a falsely high serum creatinine | • **ketoacids,** • *increased meat intake*—organic acid interference with the test, • *vitamin C,* • *drugs*— * cefoxitin, * aspirin, * cimetidine, • *rhabdomyolysis* |
| causes of a low serum creatinine | • **advancing age**—loss in muscle mass, • *cachexia*—loss in muscle mass, • *chronic liver disease*—decreased synthesis of creatinine |

*Table continued on following page*

## Table 14–1. SELECTED UROLOGIC DISORDERS I
*Continued*

| Most Common... | Answer and Explanation |
|---|---|
| clearance substance used in clinical medicine | **creatinine**— * creatinine clearance formula is: CCr = UCr × V/PCr, where V = volume of a 24-hr urine collection in mL/min, * creatinine is not a perfect clearance substance: ♦ some is secreted, ♦ some is excreted in the GI tract |
| causes of a decreased CCr | • **increasing age**— * age-dependent finding, * CCr declines by 1 mL/min/yr over the age of 40 yrs, • *inadequate 24-hr urine collection*—decreases urine volume in numerator, • *renal failure* |
| causes of an increased CCr | • **pregnancy**—increase in plasma volume increases GFR and CCr, • *early diabetic nephropathy*— * hyperfiltration is an early feature of DM, * efferent arteriole is hyalinized, which decreases blood flow out of the glomerular capillaries and increases GFR |
| effect of a decreased GFR on BUN:/ creatinine ratio | **increases normal 10:1 ratio to > 15:1** [Note: a decrease in GFR increases proximal reabsorption of urea. Urea reabsorption is flow dependent (up to 80% reabsorbed when GFR is decreased). Creatinine is not reabsorbed; however, a drop in the GFR reduces its clearance by the kidneys, so it is mildly increased. There is a disproportionate increase in urea over creatinine, leading to an increased ratio.] |
| effect of renal failure on serum BUN:/ creatinine ratio | **maintenance of 10:1 ratio** [Note: the serum BUN and creatinine are equally affected by intrinsic renal disease. Both increase at the same rate and maintain the normal 10:1 ratio (e.g., serum BUN 80 mg/dL, creatinine 8 mg/dL). This is called *renal azotemia* (uremia).] |
| effect of postrenal obstruction on serum BUN:/ creatinine ratio | **>15–20:1 ratio** [Note: in postrenal obstruction (e.g., ureters, bladder, urethra), there is a back diffusion of urea from urine into the blood and a decrease in the GFR (see below). This is called postrenal azotemia.] |
| indicator of tubular dysfunction | **inability to concentrate urine** |

## Table 14–1. SELECTED UROLOGIC DISORDERS I
*Continued*

| Most Common... | Answer and Explanation |
|---|---|
| use of UOsm | • **evaluate concentrating**—usually >800 mOsm/kg, • **evaluate diluting capacity of the kidneys**—<100 mOsm/kg, • **clinical use in oliguria (urine flow <400 mL/day, <20 mL/hr)**— * UOsm <350 mOsm/kg indicates tubular dysfunction, * UOsm >500 mOsm/kg indicates intact tubular function |
| use of FENa$^+$ (fractional excretion of sodium) | **work-up of oliguria**— * FENa$^+$ = (UNa$^+$ × PCr)/(PNa$^+$ × UCr) × 100, * values <1 indicate intact tubular function, * values >1 (usually >2) indicate tubular dysfunction |
| use of urine Na$^+$ | • **evaluation of hypo-/hypernatremia**— * UNa$^+$ <10 mEq/L indicates a nonrenal cause of hypo-/hypernatremia, * UNa$^+$ >20 mEq/L indicates a renal cause of hypo-/hypernatremia, • **work-up of oliguria**— * UNa$^+$ <20 mEq/L indicates good tubular function, * UNa$^+$ >40 mEq/L indicates poor tubular function |
| changes in UNa$^+$ in metabolic alkalosis | • **early phase**—UNa$^+$ >20 mEq/L, since excess HCO$_3^-$ anions filtered by kidney are excreted as NaHCO$_3$: alkaline urine pH, • **late phase**—when volume depletion occurs, proximal tubule HCO$_3^-$ reclamation and reabsorption of Na$^+$ increases: ♦ UNa$^+$ <10 mEq/L, ♦ acid urine pH |
| use of urine Cl$^-$ | • **identify Cl$^-$-responsive metabolic alkalosis**— * UCl$^-$ < 10 mEq/L, * e.g., vomiting, * Cl$^-$-responsive means the metabolic alkalosis is corrected by giving isotonic saline, • **identify Cl$^-$-resistant metabolic alkalosis**— * UCl$^-$ >20 mEq/L, * e.g., primary aldosteronism, * Cl$^-$-resistant means that isotonic saline will not correct the metabolic alkalosis |
| use of urine K$^+$ | **identify causes of hypokalemia**— * UK$^+$ < 20 mEq/L indicates a nonrenal cause: e.g., diarrhea, * UK$^+$ >20 mEq/L indicates a renal cause: e.g., ♦ diuretics, ♦ primary aldosteronism |

*Table continued on following page*

**Table 14–1. SELECTED UROLOGIC DISORDERS I**
*Continued*

| Most Common... | Answer and Explanation |
|---|---|
| causes of a dark-yellow urine | • **concentrated urine,** • *coloring from vitamins,* • *conjugated bilirubin (CB)*—e.g., obstructive jaundice, • *increased urobilinogen (UBG)*—e.g., extravascular hemolytic anemia |
| causes of a red urine | • **hematuria**—e.g., urinary stone, • *myoglobin*—e.g., rhabdomyolysis, • *drugs*—e.g., phenazopyridine, • *porphyrias*—e.g., AIP, • *beets* |
| causes of a black urine | • **alkaptonuria**— * AR disorder, * homogentisic acid must be oxidized on exposure to air before urine turns black, • **blackwater fever**— * *Plasmodium falciparum* infection, * Hgb changed into hematin (black pigment) in an acid pH urine |
| urine dipstick components | • **specific gravity,** • **pH,** • **protein,** • **glucose,** • **ketones,** • **bilirubin,** • **UBG,** • **leukocyte esterase,** • **nitrites** |
| use of urine specific gravity | **crude indicator of UOsm**— * hypotonic urine has a specific gravity of <1.015 (~UOsm 220 mOsm/kg), * concentrated urine has a specific gravity >1.023 (~UOsm 900 mOsm/kg), * UOsm is the best indicator of urine concentration/dilution |
| causes of a falsely high urine specific gravity | • **glucosuria,** • *proteinuria* |
| causes of isosthenuria (fixed specific gravity) | • **chronic renal failure**— * complete loss of concentration/dilution, * plasma is isosmotic with the urine at all times, • *sickle cell trait/disease*—microinfarcts in the renal medulla destroy tubular function, • *chronic interstitial nephritis*—e.g., analgesic abuse |
| dipstick urine pH findings in meat eaters and vegans | • **meat eater**—acid pH due to inorganic/organic acids from meat, • **vegan**—alkaline pH due to citrate conversion into bicarbonate |
| uses of urine pH | • **alter pH to prevent renal stones**—e.g., alkalinize urine in uric acid stones, • **alter pH to excrete drugs**—e.g., alkalinize urine to excrete salicylates, • **diagnose RTA**—urine pH > 5.5 in type I distal RTA |

## Table 14–1. SELECTED UROLOGIC DISORDERS I
*Continued*

| Most Common... | Answer and Explanation |
|---|---|
| cause of an alkaline urine that smells like ammonia | **urease producing bacterial infection**— * examples include: ♦ *Proteus* species, ♦ *Pseudomonas* species, * urease breaks urea down into ammonia, which alkalinizes the urine |
| dipstick finding indicating primary renal disease | **proteinuria**— * dipstick protein detects albumin: it does not detect globulins, * unreliable in detecting albumin <10–30 mg/dL, * +1 reading is equivalent to 30 mg/dL, which ~equals 150 mg/day, the cutoff point for normal protein excretion per day |
| confirmatory test for a positive dipstick for protein | **sulfosalicylic acid (SSA)**— * detects albumin and globulins, * detects Bence Jones protein: light chains |
| pathologic cause of a negative dipstick protein and strongly positive SSA | **Bence Jones proteinuria in multiple myeloma**— * dipstick and SSA reading for protein should be the same if only albumin is present, * a disproportionate increase in SSA over the dipstick protein (e.g., +1 dipstick, +4 SSA) indicates globulin in the urine: possibility of BJ protein |
| tests to detect microalbuminuria (30–300 mg albumin/day) | • **quantitative immunoassays,** • *microalbumin dipsticks* [**Note:** dipsticks are used as screens and are sensitive to 1.5–8 mg/dL, unlike the standard urine dipsticks, which detect only as low as 30 mg/dL. Microalbuminuria is the first sign of diabetic nephropathy.] |
| causes of a positive dipstick for glucose | • **DM,** • *normal pregnancy*— * low renal threshold for glucose, * <u>normal</u> serum glucose, • *benign glucosuria*— * low threshold, * serum glucose is normal, • *proximal RTA* [**Note:** normal threshold for glucose is 165–200 mg/dL. The test is specific for glucose, since it uses glucose oxidase.] |
| causes of a false-negative dipstick reaction | • **elevated urinary ascorbic acid**—excessive dose of vitamin C, • *increased ketones,* • *increased specific gravity* |

*Table continued on following page*

## Table 14–1. SELECTED UROLOGIC DISORDERS I
*Continued*

| Most Common... | Answer and Explanation |
|---|---|
| use of Clinitest | **detect urine-reducing substances**— * examples include: ♦ glucose, ♦ galactose, ♦ lactose, ♦ ascorbic acid, ♦ fructose, * sucrose is not a reducing sugar [**Note:** the test is too nonspecific for detection of glucose. It is commonly used in pediatrics as a screen for some inborn errors of metabolism.] |
| causes of a positive dipstick for ketones | • **volume depletion,** • *DKA,* • *normal pregnancy,* • *ketogenic diets,* • *isopropyl alcohol poisoning,* • *von Gierke's disease* [**Note:** nitroprusside in the test system reacts only with AcAc acid and acetone, not β-OHB.] |
| causes of a positive dipstick for bilirubin | • **viral hepatitis,** • *obstructive jaundice* [**Note:** only CB is detected. UCB is lipid soluble and does not enter the urine.] |
| cause of a false-negative test for CB in the urine | **high urine ascorbate levels** |
| causes of an increased dipstick reaction for UBG | • **viral hepatitis,** • *extravascular hemolytic anemia* [**Note:** in viral hepatitis, the sick liver cannot receive the recycled UBG from the large bowel. In EHA, the increase in UCB from macrophage destruction of RBCs leads to increased production of UBG in the colon. The stool is darker, and more UBG is recycled into the urine.] |
| cause of an increase in urine UBG and bilirubin | **viral hepatitis**— * liver cell necrosis causes a release of previously conjugated bilirubin into the blood stream, * see above explanation for the increase in UBG |
| cause of an increase in urine bilirubin, no change in UBG | **viral hepatitis**—this pattern occurs in the early cholestatic phase of hepatitis |
| causes of a positive dipstick for blood | • **hematuria**—, e.g., * **cystitis,** * renal stone, * renal adenocarcinoma, * bladder cancer, • *hemoglobinuria,* • *myoglobinuria*— * dipstick reagents are positive for myoglobin or Hgb, * an elevated serum CK is expected in myoglobinuria but not hemoglobinuria |

## Table 14–1. SELECTED UROLOGIC DISORDERS I
*Continued*

| Most Common... | Answer and Explanation |
|---|---|
| cause of a positive dipstick for leukocyte esterase | **cystitis**—neutrophils contain esterase |
| cause of a positive dipstick for leukocyte esterase and a negative standard urine culture | **sterile pyuria** [**Note:** pyuria refers to $\geq$ 10 WBCs/HPF in a centrifuged specimen or $\geq$ 5 WBCs/HPF in an uncentrifuged specimen. If a standard urine culture for uropathogens is negative, the term *sterile pyuria* is applied. Infectious causes include *Chlamydia trachomatis, Mycoplasma hominis, Ureaplasma urealyticum,* and renal TB. None of these organisms would grow out with the standard urine culture. Acute or chronic interstitial nephritis due to drugs or other noninfectious causes may also cause sterile pyuria.] |
| cause of a false-negative leukocyte esterase | **high urinary tetracycline levels** |
| cause of a positive dipstick for nitrites | **cystitis**— * most urinary pathogens reduce nitrates to nitrites, * the test has greater specificity than sensitivity, * *Escherichia coli* is the MC nitrate reducer and uropathogen |
| cause of a false-negative dipstick for nitrites | • **collection of urine < 4 hrs after last void**— * requires at least 4 hrs for a nitrate reducer to convert nitrates into nitrites, * most patients have increased frequency of urination, • *high urine ascorbate levels* |
| cause of dysmorphic (abnormal shapes) RBCs in the urine | **glomerulonephritis (GN)**— * dysmorphic RBCs are best seen with a phase contrast microscope, * they indicate a glomerular origin for the RBCs, * hematuria is > 2–3 RBCs/HPF |
| causes of WBCs in the urine | • **infection**— * **cystitis,** * pyelonephritis, * urethritis, • *drug-induced interstitial nephritis* [**Note:** >10 WBCs/HPF in a spun sediment is abnormal in women and >1–3 WBCs/HPF is abnormal in men.] |
| cause of eosinophiluria | **drug-induced interstitial nephritis** |

*Table continued on following page*

### Table 14–1. SELECTED UROLOGIC DISORDERS I
*Continued*

| Most Common... | Answer and Explanation |
|---|---|
| cause of oval fat bodies and free lipid in the urine | **nephrotic syndrome (proteinuria > 3.5 g/24 hrs)** [**Note:** epithelial cells or macrophages with lipid are designated oval fat bodies. If urine polarization reveals Maltese crosses in oval fat bodies, casts, or free, CH rather than TG is present in the urine. TG is identified with Sudan stains.] |
| cause of hemosiderinuria | **chronic intravascular hemolytic anemia—** * e.g., microangiopathic hemolytic anemia in a patient with aortic stenosis, * iron deficiency may occur: due to loss of iron in Hgb |
| location of urine cast formation | **diseases originating in the kidneys—**e.g., * GN, * pyelonephritis [**Note:** casts are formed in tubular lumens in the kidneys. They are composed of a protein matrix (Tamm-Horsfall protein) within which is entrapped cells, debris, or protein leaking through the glomeruli. Their presence proves a renal origin of the disease.] |
| cast in the urine | **hyaline casts—** * acellular, * clear casts, * composed of Tamm-Horsfall protein [**Note:** they usually have no clinical significance, unless present in great numbers.] |
| casts associated with the nephritic syndrome | • **RBC casts,** • *WBC casts* [**Note:** the nephritic syndrome is characterized by mild to moderate proteinuria, RBC casts, oliguria, and usually hypertension. Examples of primary nephritic GN include poststreptococcal GN, type IV SLE, IgA GN, and rapidly progressive crescentic GN.] |
| casts associated with the nephrotic syndrome | **fatty casts with or without Maltese crosses** [**Note:** the nephrotic syndrome is characterized by fatty casts and a urine protein that is ≥ 3.5 g/day. Examples include minimal change disease in children, diffuse membranous GN, membranoproliferative GN, amyloid kidney, focal segmental glomerulosclerosis (AIDS, IVDU), and diabetic nephropathy.] |
| cast associated with acute pyelonephritis | **WBC cast** |
| cast associated with ATN | **pigmented (Hgb) renal tubular cast** |

## Table 14–1. SELECTED UROLOGIC DISORDERS I
*Continued*

| Most Common... | Answer and Explanation |
|---|---|
| casts in chronic renal disease | • **broad casts**—also called renal failure casts, • **waxy casts** |
| progression of degeneration of a cellular cast in a renal tubule | • **cellular cast**—e.g., WBC cast → • **coarsely granular cast** → • **finely granular cast** → • **waxy cast**—usually after 3 months, which is why it is an indicator of chronic renal disease |
| clinically important crystals in an acid urine | • **uric acid**—e.g., * gout, * excess synthesis of purines in Rx of disseminated cancers, • **calcium oxalate**— * look like an × in a square, * examples include: ♦ Crohn's disease, ♦ ethylene glycol poisoning |
| clinically important crystal in an alkaline urine | **triple phosphate**— * looks like a coffin lid, * present in urine containing urease-producing organisms: e.g., *Proteus* species |
| inborn error of metabolism with a pathognomonic urine crystal | **cystinuria**—hexagonal crystal |
| types of proteinuria | • **hemodynamic**— * exercise, * fever, * CHF, • *glomerular*— * selective: only albumin, * nonselective: albumin + globulins, • *overflow*— * normal glomerular and tubular function, * excess amount of LMW proteins in plasma: e.g., amino acids, • *tubular*— * normal glomerular function, * tubules are damaged and cannot reabsorb normally filtered proteins |
| causes of proteinuria | • **loss of negative charge of GBM**— * the negative charge is due to heparan sulfate, * repels albumin, * e.g., nephrotic syndrome, • **alteration in size barrier of GBM**— nonselective loss of albumin + globulins: e.g., glomerular disease, • *proximal tubule abnormality*— * tubular proteinuria, * loss of amino acids, transferrin, β₂-microglobulins: e.g., ♦ proximal RTA, ♦ heavy metal poisoning, • *protein overload*— * overflow type, * e.g., loss of BJ proteins in multiple myeloma, * aminoacidurias, * liver disease: lose tyrosine and leucine |
| benign cause of proteinuria | **postural (orthostatic) proteinuria**— * proteinuria with standing, * disappears after lying down, * first AM void is free of protein |

*Table continued on following page*

## Table 14–1. SELECTED UROLOGIC DISORDERS I
*Continued*

**Question:** Which of the following test abnormalities would you expect in a patient with ischemic acute tubular necrosis? **SELECT 3**
- (A) $FENa^+ < 1$
- (B) $UNa^+ > 40$ mEq/L
- (C) UOsm > 500 mOsm/kg
- (D) Renal tubular casts
- (E) BUN/creatinine ratio < 15/1
- (F) 24-hr urine protein > 3.5 g

**Answers: (B), (D), (E).** Laboratory tests should show signs of tubular dysfunction, including an $FENa^+ > 1$, UOsm < 350 mOsm/kg, $UNa^+$ > 40 mEq/L, and renal tubular casts (choices B and D are correct, choices A and C are incorrect). The BUN/creatinine ratio should be < 15/1 owing to a proportionate increase in both the BUN and creatinine (choice E is correct). Proteinuria should be present; however, it should not be in nephrotic ranges (choice F is incorrect).

AcAc = acetoacetic, AIDS = acquired immunodeficiency syndrome, AIP = acute intermittent porphyria, APKD = adult polycystic kidney disease, APN = acute pyelonephritis, AR = autosomal recessive, ATN = acute tubular necrosis, BJ = Bence Jones, BNS = benign nephrosclerosis, BPH = benign prostatic hyperplasia, BUN = blood urea nitrogen, CB = conjugated bilirubin, CCr = creatinine clearance, CH = cholesterol, CHF = congestive heart failure, CK = creatine kinase, CRF = chronic renal failure, DKA = diabetic ketoacidosis, DM = diabetes mellitus, EHA = extravascular hemolytic anemia, $FENa^+$ = fractional excretion of sodium, GBM = glomerular basement membrane, GFR = glomerular filtration rate, GN = glomerulonephritis, Hgb = hemoglobin, HPF = high-powered field, HTN = hypertension, Ig = immunoglobulin, IVDU = intravenous drug use, IVP = intravenous pyelogram, LMW = low molecular weight, LUT = lower urinary tract, MC = most common, MCC = most common cause, N/V = nausea/vomiting, β-OHB = beta-hydroxybutyric, PAN = polyarteritis nodosa, PCr = plasma creatinine, PSS = progressive systemic sclerosis, R/O = rule out, RTA = renal tubular acidosis, SiADH = syndrome of inappropriate antidiuretic hormone, SLE = systemic lupus erythematosus, SSA = sulfosalicylic acid, TCC = transitional cell carcinoma, TG = triglyceride, TPN = total parenteral nutrition, UA = urinalysis, UBG = urobilinogen, UCB = unconjugated bilirubin, $UCl^-$ = urine chloride, UCr = urine creatinine, $UK^+$ = urine potassium, $UNa^+$ = urine sodium, UOsm = urine osmolality, UUT = upper urinary tract, V = volume.

## Table 14–2. SELECTED UROLOGIC DISORDERS II

| Most Common... | Answer and Explanation |
|---|---|
| congenital kidney disorder associated with Turner's syndrome | **horseshoe kidney**— * fused at the lower pole, * danger of infection owing to VUR, * kidney is trapped behind the inferior mesenteric artery |
| cause of urine draining from the umbilicus of a neonate | **persistent urachal sinus** |
| cause of feces draining from the umbilicus of a neonate | **persistent umbilical (vitelline) sinus** |
| cause of epispadias | **defect in genital tubercle**—associated with exstrophy of bladder |
| cause of hypospadias | **faulty closure of urethral folds** |
| nonhereditary cystic disease in adults that shows up as an IVP abnormality | **medullary sponge kidney**—striations in the papillary portion of the medulla are noted in an IVP |
| S/S of medullary sponge kidney | • **recurrent UTIs,** • *microscopic hematuria,* • *recurrent renal stones,* • *abnormal urinary concentrating ability,* • *nephrocalcinosis* |
| cause of acquired polycystic kidney disease | **renal dialysis**— * occurs in ~50% of patients on hemodialysis/peritoneal dialysis >3 yrs, * small risk for renal carcinoma |
| type of cyst in adults | **simple retention cysts**— * derived from tubular obstruction, * located in cortex/medulla, * confused with cystic renal adenocarcinoma |
| clinical findings in medullary cystic disease in adults | • **AD disease**—first manifests in adults, • **gross**— * small kidneys, * cysts at corticomedullary junction, • **clinical**— * **polyuria,** * HTN uncommon, * salt wasting, * renal failure |
| hereditary adult kidney disease | **adult polycystic kidney disease (APKD)**— * AD disease, * high penetrance, * abnormal gene on chromosome 16, * cysts noted by 20–25 yrs of age |

*Table continued on following page*

**Table 14–2. SELECTED UROLOGIC DISORDERS II**
*Continued*

| Most Common... | Answer and Explanation |
|---|---|
| S/S of APKD | • **HTN**—>80%, • *abdominal/flank pain*— * 60%, * pain from bleeding into cysts, • *bilaterally palpable kidneys*—cysts in cortex/medulla, • *hematuria*—50%, • *renal defects in concentration,* • *hepatic cysts*— * 40–60%, * cysts in spleen/pancreas, • *intracranial berry aneurysms*— * 10–30%, * subarachnoid hemorrhage, • *diverticulosis*—80%, • *risk for renal adenocarcinoma,* • *MVP*—30%, • *recurrent UTIs,* • *renal stones*—uric acid and calcium oxalate stones, • *secondary polycythemia*—increased EPO, • *CRF by 70 yrs old*—accounts for 10% of all dialysis patients |
| imaging study to diagnose APKD | • **US,** • *CT* |
| Rx of APKD | • **dialysis,** • *renal transplantation* |
| COD in APKD | • **renal failure**—50%, • *HTN complications*— * ~30%, * AMI, * stroke: ♦ intracerebral bleed, ♦ ruptured berry aneurysm |
| types of dialysis | • **hemodialysis,** • *peritoneal dialysis* |
| complications associated with both types of dialysis | • **hepatitis**—HCV most common, • **infection,** • **osteodystrophy**— * decreased 1,25-$(OH)_2$D, * increased PTH, * aluminum toxicity, • **heart disease**— * AMI, * HTN, * LVH |
| complication associated with peritoneal dialysis | **peritonitis** |
| complications associated with hemodialysis | • **N/V and headache,** • *hypotension,* • *air embolism,* • *aluminum intoxication* |
| complications associated with long-term dialysis | • **AMI/CVA**— * 50% of deaths, * risk factors: ♦ HTN, ♦ accelerated atherosclerosis, ♦ LVH, • *dialysis dementia*—relation to aluminum, • *acquired cystic disease*—see above, • *hemodialysis-related amyloidosis*— * $\beta_2$-microglobulin deposition, * spondylitis, * carpal tunnel syndrome |

## Table 14–2. SELECTED UROLOGIC DISORDERS II
*Continued*

| Most Common... | Answer and Explanation |
|---|---|
| causes of ARF | • **hypovolemia**—leads to ischemic ATN, • *AMI/CHF,* • *ureteral obstruction*— * least common cause of ARF, * most treatable, • *vascular disease*—e.g., * HTN, * vasculitis, • *rhabdomyolysis with myoglobinuria,* • *GN,* • *tubular injury*—e.g., drugs, • *tubulointerstitial disease*—e.g., drugs |
| patterns of ATN | • **ischemic ATN**— * nonoliguric: ♦ 60%, ♦ <400 mL/day or <20 mL/hr, * polyuric most common type: >800 mL/day, • *nephrotoxic ATN* [**Note:** most cases of ATN are multifactorial.] |
| cause of ischemic ATN | **prenal azotemia**— * reversible disease associated with a reduced GFR, * greatest potential for ischemic tubular damage |
| causes of nephrotoxic ATN | • **drugs**—e.g., * **aminoglycosides,** * cisplatin, * cyclosporine, • *radiocontrast agents*—patients at risk include: ♦ **DM,** ♦ multiple myeloma, ♦ old age, ♦ volume-depleted |
| mechanisms of oliguria in ATN | • **vasoconstriction of afferent arterioles,** • **tubular cells blocking lumen,** • **increased interstitial pressure from fluid leaking out through damaged BMs,** • **decreased permeability of glomerulus** |
| tests used in work-up of oliguria | • FENa⁺, • *UOsm,* • *random UNa⁺,* • *serum BUN/serum Cr ratio,* • *UA* |
| profile for good tubular function (ability to concentrate urine) | • **FENa⁺** < **1,** • *UOsm > 500 mOsm/kg,* • *random UNa⁺ < 20 mEq/L,* • *BUN:serum creatinine ratio > 15:1,* • *normal* |
| profile for poor tubular function (inability to concentrate urine) | • **FENa⁺ > 1**—usually > 2, • *UOsm <350 mOsm/kg,* • *random UNa⁺ >40 mEq/L,* • *BUN:serum creatine ratio <15:1,* • *UA with renal tubular casts* |
| causes of oliguria | • **prenal azotemia,** • *ATN,* • *postrenal azotemia,* • *acute GN* |
| causes of prenal azotemia | • **decreased EABV**—e.g., * CHF, * hypovolemia, * hypotension, • *drugs*—e.g., * NSAIDs: block intrarenal production of $PGE_2$, which vasodilates the afferent arteriole, * ACE inhibitors: block AT II and aldosterone production |

*Table continued on following page*

### Table 14–2. SELECTED UROLOGIC DISORDERS II
*Continued*

| Most Common... | Answer and Explanation |
|---|---|
| cause of postrenal azotemia in kidneys | **intratubular obstruction by crystals**—e.g., * **uric acid,** * oxalate, * drug crystals |
| causes of postrenal azotemia in ureters | • **kidney stone,** • *blood clot,* • *retroperitoneal fibrosis,* • *TCC,* • *cervical cancer*—openings of the ureters into the bladder are in close proximity to the cervix and can be blocked by invasive cancer |
| causes of postrenal azotemia in bladder | • **trauma,** • *stones,* • *TCC* |
| causes of postrenal azotemia in the urethra | • **benign prostatic hyperplasia,** • *cervical cancer* |
| causes of oliguria with preserved tubular function | • **prerenal azotemia**—normal UA, • *acute GN*— * RBC casts, * hematuria |
| causes of oliguria with tubular dysfunction | • **ATN**—pigmented renal tubular casts: "dirty urine," • *postrenal azotemia*— * normal UA, * only prolonged postrenal obstruction leads to tubular damage: initially, the tubular function is intact |
| clinical problems associated with ARF | • **excess sodium/water retention**—cause weight gain/hyponatremia, respectively, • *hyponatremia*—excess water intake in tubules that are unable to generate free water, • *increased AG metabolic acidosis*—decreased excretion of $H^+$ ions: ~1 mEq/kg/day, • *hyperkalemia*— * transcellular shift secondary to metabolic acidosis, * decreased renal excretion in the aldosterone-controlled $Na^+/K^+$ pumps in the late distal and collecting ducts, • *GI bleeding*—hemorrhagic gastritis, • *hyperphosphatemia*—decreased excretion, • *hypocalcemia*— * decreased synthesis of 1,25-$(OH)_2D$, * metastatic calcification from increased phosphate driving calcium into bone/soft tissue, • *hyperuricemia*—decreased excretion in the proximal tubules, • *anemia*—decreased production of EPO, • *uremic pericarditis*— * usually hemorrhagic, * may produce cardiac tamponade, • *uremic syndrome*—accumulation of toxic products with multiorgan dysfunction |

## Table 14–2. SELECTED UROLOGIC DISORDERS II
*Continued*

| Most Common... | Answer and Explanation |
|---|---|
| phases of ARF | • **oliguric phase**— * 1–2 weeks, * azotemia, * hyperkalemia, * increased AG metabolic acidosis, • **diuretic phase**— * usually 3rd week, * hypokalemia may occur, * severe hypercalcemia may occur if renal failure was secondary to rhabdomyolysis, • **recovery phase**—GFR improves over subsequent 3–12 mos |
| Rx of ARF | • **fluid challenge**—useful in nonvolume-overloaded oliguric patients, • **loop diuretic**— * attempts to convert an oliguric into a polyuric ARF, which has a slightly better prognosis, * flushes tubular cells out of the obstructed lumens, • **keep the patient hemodynamically stable**— * Rx volume depletion with 0.45 saline, * Rx volume excess with loop diuretics, • **low-dose dopamine**—renal vasodilator, • **daily weight**—restrict sodium if the weight increases, • **limit dietary protein**— * 0.5 g/kg/day, * reduces the urea load to the kidneys, • **Rx hyperphosphatemia**— * calcium carbonate with meals, * low-phosphate diet, • **Rx hyperkalemia**— * see Table 1–3, * Rx when serum $K^+$ is >6.5 mEq/L or if there is an abnormal ECG, • **Rx metabolic acidosis if $HCO_3^-$ is <15–16 mEq/L,** • **avoid nephrotoxic drugs,** • **dialyze when necessary**— * keep serum BUN <100 mg/dL, * best Rx for hemorrhagic pericarditis, * best Rx for peripheral neuropathy, * best Rx for volume overload resistant to diuretics, * best Rx for hyperkalemia/hyperphosphatemia when medical management is inadequate, * best Rx to reverse platelet aggregation dysfunction |
| COD in ARF | • **infection**—sepsis, • *cardiopulmonary disease* |
| time-frame for aminoglycoside-induced ATN | **5–10 days**— * some degree of ARF occurs in 10–15%, * gentamicin/amikacin most toxic, * streptomycin least toxic, * polyuric ATN, * $K^+$ and magnesium wasting commonly occur |

*Table continued on following page*

## Table 14–2. SELECTED UROLOGIC DISORDERS II
*Continued*

| Most Common... | Answer and Explanation |
|---|---|
| types of nephrotoxic ATN in which alkalinization of urine is helpful | • **amphotericin B**— * distal tubule dysfunction, * volume depletion is a major risk factor, • **methotrexate**—precipitates in the renal tubules: similar to acyclovir and some sulfa drugs, • **rhabdomyolysis**— * heme pigments produce intrarenal vasoconstriction/tubular obstruction |
| clinical findings in myoglobin-induced ATN | • **clinical settings**— * **crush injuries,** * alcoholism, * prolonged unconsciousness: particularly ♦ CO poisoning, ♦ postseizures, * heat stroke, * brown recluse spider bite, * cocaine, • **usually polyuric,** • **lab findings**— * hypocalcemia, * hyperuricemia, * hyperphosphatemia, * hyperkalemia in acute phase, * hypercalcemia in diuretic phase |
| Rx of myoglobin-induced ATN | • **forced diuresis (mannitol) to remove heme pigments,** • **alkalinize urine** |
| mechanisms of ARF due to radiocontrast dyes | • **intrarenal vasoconstriction,** • **tubular obstruction,** • **direct tubular toxicity** [Note: patients become oliguric 1–2 days after dye injection. FENa$^+$ is usually <1. It is usually reversible within a week.] |
| preventive methods to avoid radiocontrast dye-induced ARF | • **decrease dose of the dye,** • **forced diuresis with normal saline,** • **adequate hydration** |
| clinical findings of atheroembolic-induced ARF | • **most common in the elderly population,** • **spontaneous or postinvasive procedure**—e.g., angiogram, • **cardiac source of emboli is common**—particularly with chronic atrial fibrillation (AF), • **livedo reticularis,** • **CH emboli on retinal exam,** • **lab findings**— * increased ESR, * low complement levels, * eosinophilia/eosinophiluria, * thrombocytopenia, • **renal Bx demonstrates CH emboli in vessels,** • **minimal reversibility** |
| causes of ARF in pregnancy | • **severe preeclampsia,** • *abruptio placentae*—due to hypotension, • *sepsis,* • *DIC,* • *retained placenta* |

## Table 14–2. SELECTED UROLOGIC DISORDERS II
*Continued*

| Most Common... | Answer and Explanation |
|---|---|
| renal manifestation of ARF in pregnancy | **diffuse cortical necrosis—** * infarction of renal cortex, * anuria, * poor prognosis |
| causes of anuria (<50 mL/day) | • **complete obstruction,** • *RPGN,* • *renal cortical necrosis,* • *bilateral renal artery occlusion* |
| known causes of CRF in descending order | • **DM nephropathy,** • *HTN,* • *GN*—e.g., * **RPGN,** * FSG, * MPGN, • *cystic renal disease,* • *interstitial nephritis* |
| presentation of CRF | **reduction in GFR >3–6 mos—** * patients are symptomatic when the GFR is <10–15 mL/min, * constellation of findings is called the uremic syndrome, * kidneys are shrunken |
| hematologic findings in CRF | • **anemia—** * **decreased EPO,** * iron deficiency: ♦ inadequate intake of iron, ♦ loss of iron in dialysis, ♦ GI bleeds, • *qualitative platelet defects—* * ecchymoses/epistaxis/bleeding after trauma, * guanidinosuccinic acid inhibits platelet aggregation, * reversible with: ♦ dialysis, ♦ desmopressin, ♦ estrogen |
| manifestations of renal osteodystrophy in CRF | • **osteitis fibrosa cystica—** * secondary HPTH from hypocalcemia, * increased PTH resorption of bone, • *osteomalacia—* * hypocalcemia from hypovitaminosis D, * hyperphosphatemia: drives calcium into tissue, • *osteoporosis*—bone buffers excess H$^+$ ions in metabolic acidosis |
| clinical findings in renal osteodystrophy in CRF | • **spontaneous fractures/bone pain**—present in above disorders, • **skeletal deformities**—bowed legs: primarily in osteomalacia, • **pseudofractures**—primarily in osteomalacia: enlarged blood vessels in soft bone look like fractures, • **x-ray findings—** * subperiosteal resorption, * cysts, * patchy osteosclerosis: primarily in osteitis fibrosa cystica |

*Table continued on following page*

**Table 14–2. SELECTED UROLOGIC DISORDERS II**
*Continued*

| Most Common... | Answer and Explanation |
|---|---|
| cardiac findings in CRF | • **HTN**— * due to sodium retention with volume expansion, * RAA activation, • *uremic pericarditis*— * chest pain, * friction rub, * Rx with dialysis, • *CHF*— * due to volume expansion, * may be due to hypertensive heart disease, * metabolic acidosis: ♦ decreases cardiac contractility, ♦ may lead to warm shock, * butterfly fluid distribution around the hilum, • *accelerated atherosclerosis*—due to high TG levels |
| GI findings in CRF | • **anorexia**, • *N/V*, • *chronic hiccups*, • *hemorrhagic gastritis*, • *PUD* |
| neurologic findings in CRF | • **irritability**, • **inability to concentrate**, • **decreased libido**, • **asterixis**, • **peripheral neuropathy**— * less common with the advent of dialysis, * restless leg syndrome, * sensory type of neuropathy, • **myoclonus** |
| muscle findings in CRF | • **proximal myopathy**— * weakness/atrophy, * Rx with dialysis, • **cramps/twitching** |
| dermatologic findings in CRF | • **pruritus**— * due to metastatic calcification in the dermal adnexal structures, * related to the high calcium/phosphate solubility product, • *uremic frost*—urea crystals deposit on the skin, • *sallow, yellow skin*—increased urobilin deposition in the skin, • *soft tissue metastatic calcification* |
| endocrine findings in CRF | • **insulin resistance**—hyperglycemia, • *hypothermia*— * often 35.5°C, * problem in recognizing infection, since a "normal" temperature may be abnormal, • *impotence* |
| causes of normal to large kidneys in CRF | • **APKD**, • *DM*, • *amyloidosis* |
| causes of acute deterioration in CRF | • **volume depletion**, • *infection*, • *HTN*, • *urinary tract obstruction*, • *nephrotoxic drugs*, • *CH embolization*—see above |

## Table 14–2. SELECTED UROLOGIC DISORDERS II
*Continued*

| Most Common... | Answer and Explanation |
| --- | --- |
| lab findings in CRF | • **hyponatremia**— * excess water intake, * salt wasting in some CRF cases, • **hyperkalemia**—ECG is the best monitor, • **increased AG metabolic acidosis**—AG 20–24 mEq/L: normal is 8–16 mEq/L, • **hypocalcemia**—hypovitaminosis D: ♦ no 1-α-hydroxylation of vitamin D, ♦ hyperphosphatemia inhibits synthesis of 1-α-hydroxylase enzyme in proximal tubule, • **hyperphosphatemia**— * major cause of secondary HPTH: induces hypocalcemia, which stimulates the release of PTH, * increases calcium × phosphorus solubility product: metastatic calcification, • **increased intact PTH**—PTH cannot be excreted by the diseased kidneys, • **prolonged BT**— * decreased platelet aggregation, * corrected with: ♦ dialysis, ♦ estrogen, ♦ desmopressin, • **normocytic anemia**—decreased EPO synthesis by endothelial cells in the peritubular capillaries, • **isosthenuria**—see previous discussion, • **broad/waxy casts**—see previous discussion, • **increased TG**—leads to accelerated atherosclerosis, • **hyperuricemia**— * decreased excretion, * may precipitate gout, • **hypermagnesemia**— * decreased excretion, * avoid magnesium-containing antacids |
| salt-losing types of CRF | • **chronic PN**, • **medullary cystic disease**, • **hydronephrosis**, • **chronic interstitial nephritis**, • **milk-alkali syndrome**—absorbable calcium antacid + increased ingestion of milk |
| Rx of CRF | • **R/O postrenal obstruction**—e.g., * prostate hyperplasia, * order renal US, • **correct volume depletion**—due to: ♦ diuretics, ♦ decreased intake, ♦ N/V, • **limit protein intake**— * 0.6–0.7 g/kg/day: reduces urea load to the kidneys, * supplement diet with: ♦ water-soluble B vitamins (not fat-soluble), ♦ vitamin C, ♦ calcitriol (dihydrotachysterol, an analogue of calcitriol), ♦ folate, ♦ iron, ♦ calcium, • **restrict sodium**—only if pitting edema is present, • **restrict potassium, phosphorus, magnesium**, • **control HTN**— * ACE inhibitors are best unless hyperkalemia is present, * loop diuretics: best diuretic for CRF, • **Rx anemia with EPO**—keep Hct between 30 and 33%, • **Rx metabolic acidosis if bicarbonate is < 18 mEq/L**, • **dialysis** |

*Table continued on following page*

## Table 14–2. SELECTED UROLOGIC DISORDERS II
*Continued*

| Most Common... | Answer and Explanation |
|---|---|
| causes of acute interstitial nephritis | • **APN**, • *drug-induced,* • *systemic infections* —e.g., * legionnaires' disease,* CMV, * leptospirosis, • *immune disease*—e.g., * Sjögren's syndrome, * SLE, * acute transplant rejection, • *heavy metals*—e.g., * lead, * arsenic, * cadmium, * mercury |
| clinical findings of acute interstitial nephritis | • **sterile pyuria**— * 100%, * WBCs/WBC casts, • *hematuria*— * 95%, * RBC casts are rare, • *fever*—90%, • *tubular proteinuria*— * 75%, * <2 g/day, * LMW proteins, • *renal insufficiency*—60%, * oliguria, * azotemia, * $FENa^+$ >1, • *eosinophilia*— * 50%, * eosinophiluria, • *skin rash*— * 25%, * mainly drug-induced type, • *renal osteodystrophy*— see above, • *proximal tubule dysfunction*— type II proximal RTA, • *distal tubule dysfunction*— * type I RTA, * type IV RTA, * nephrogenic DI, • *hematologic abnormalities*—anemia: decreased EPO synthesis |
| causes of APN | • **ascending infection**— * urethra is initial entry site, * *Escherichia coli* derived from enteric organisms, * low $O_2$ tension in the renal medulla predisposes to infection, • *hematogenous*— * *Staphylococcus aureus,* * cortical location |
| predisposing causes of APN | • **VUR**—incompetent ureterovesical junction, • *urinary tract obstruction,* • *DM,* • *cystic kidney disease,* • *pregnancy,* • *previous LUT instrumentation* |
| test used to identify VUR | **cystourethrogram** |
| clinical and lab findings in APN | • **young woman with sudden onset of spiking fever,** • *flank pain,* • *LUT signs of infection*— * increased frequency, * dysuria, * urgency, • *UA findings*— * pyuria, * bacteria, * WBC casts, * hematuria, * positive dipstick for esterase/nitrite, • *absolute neutrophilic leukocytosis/left shift* |

## Table 14–2. SELECTED UROLOGIC DISORDERS II
*Continued*

| Most Common... | Answer and Explanation |
|---|---|
| complications of APN | • **septicemia**— * blood cultures are positive in 20%, * potential for endotoxic shock, • *chronic PN,* • *renal papillary necrosis,* • *perinephric abscess,* • *pyonephrosis*—pus in renal pelvis, • *stone formation*—urease-producing organisms produce struvite stones |
| Rx of APN | • **uncomplicated APN**— * oral FQ × 7 days, • **complicated APN**— * IV AMP + GENT for 2–3 wks |
| causes of CPN | • **reflux**— * due to VUR, * initially targets children, * more common in boys in the first year of life: usually a congenital abnormality, • *obstruction*— * causes include: ♦ tumors, ♦ prostatic hyperplasia, ♦ stones, * leads to: ♦ hydronephrosis, ♦ calyceal blunting, ♦ cortical scars |
| clinical and lab findings in CPN | • **HTN,** • *renal insufficiency,* • *tubular dysfunction*—see above |
| pathogenesis of acute drug-induced interstitial nephritis | • **type IV cellular immune reaction**—delayed type: cytotoxic T cells damage the tissue, • *antibodies directed against basement membranes*—e.g., methicillin |
| causes of acute drug-induced IN | • **methicillin,** • *rifampin,* • *sulfonamides,* • *NSAIDs*—interstitial nephritis is accompanied by the nephrotic syndrome, • *allopurinol,* • *diuretics*— * thiazides, * loop diuretics, • *cimetidine,* • *cyclosporine*—see above |
| Rx of acute drug-induced IN | • **withdraw the drug**—never use drug again, • *corticosteroids may be useful* |
| cause of chronic drug-induced interstitial nephritis | **analgesic nephropathy** |
| mechanisms of analgesic nephropathy | • **acetaminophen**—FR injury of tubules and interstitium, • **aspirin**—decreases synthesis of intrarenal $PGE_2$ (normally a vasodilator of the afferent arteriole), leading to ischemia in the renal medulla, • **cumulative ingestion ≥ 3 kg or ≥ 1 g/day for 3 years produces renal damage** |

*Table continued on following page*

## Table 14-2. SELECTED UROLOGIC DISORDERS II
*Continued*

| Most Common... | Answer and Explanation |
|---|---|
| clinical findings of analgesic nephropathy | • **woman (85%) with a long history of pain**— * chronic headaches (80%), * arthritis, * myalgia, • *anemia—85%*, • *HTN—40%*, • *renal papillary necrosis—30%*, • *PUD—40%*, • *UTI with dysuria—25%*, • *history of urinary tract obstruction—10%*, • *lab findings*— * sterile pyuria, * proteinuria: <2 g/day, * normal AG metabolic acidosis: distal tubule RTA, * small kidneys: 50% |
| complications of analgesic nephropathy | • **renal papillary necrosis**, • *HTN*, • *accelerated atherosclerosis*—due to increased TG, • *renal pelvic, ureter, bladder TCC*—bladder cancer is less common than in the other sites |
| causes of renal papillary necrosis | • **analgesic nephropathy**, • *DM*, • *APN*, • *sickle cell trait/disease*, • *chronic alcoholism with cirrhosis*, • *urinary tract obstruction*, • *TB* |
| clinical and lab findings of renal papillary necrosis | • **sudden onset of colicky flank pain**, • **gross hematuria**, • **IVP**— * calyceal clubbing, * ring sign: filling defect left behind from sloughed papilla |
| tubular abnormalities associated with aminoglycosides | **potassium/magnesium wasting** |
| tubular abnormalities associated with tetracyclines | • **nephrogenic DI**—particularly with the use of demeclocycline, • *Fanconi's syndrome*— * type II proximal tubule RTA, * outdated tetracycline |
| tubular abnormalities associated with amphotericin B | • **distal tubule dysfunction**— * type I distal tubule RTA, * nephrogenic DI, * renal potassium wasting, • *nephrotoxic ATN* |
| tubular abnormalities associated with cisplatin | • **magnesium wasting**, • *nephrotoxic ATN*, • *potassium wasting*, • *mild proteinuria* |

## Table 14–2. SELECTED UROLOGIC DISORDERS II
*Continued*

| Most Common... | Answer and Explanation |
|---|---|
| causes of urate nephropathy | **tumor lysis syndrome after Rx of disseminated cancers**— * increased production of purines, * e.g., Rx of ALL and malignant lymphomas, • *lead poisoning*— * Pb decreases uric acid secretion, * Pb produces an interstitial nephritis, • *MPD*—e.g., PRV |
| pathogenesis of urate nephropathy | **tubular obstruction by crystals**— * serum uric acid usually > 15 mg/dL, * urine uric acid > 1000 mg/day, * urine uric acid:plasma creatinine ratio > 1 on random urine |
| Rx of urate nephropathy | • **allopurinol**—inhibits xanthine oxidase–involved uric acid synthesis, • **establish urinary output > 3 liters/day**, • **alkalinize urine**—uric acid is soluble in an alkaline pH |
| clinical signs of Pb nephropathy | • **gout**— * Pb decreases uric acid secretion, * produces a chronic interstitial nephritis, • *HTN,* • *chronic renal insufficiency* |
| method of evaluating Pb stores | **IV ethylenediaminetetra-acetic acid (EDTA)**— * chelates Pb, * collect urine and measure Pb |
| heavy metals other than Pb producing interstitial nephritis | • **arsenic**, • **mercury**—organic salt of mercury, • **cadmium**—alkaline battery workers, • **gold** |
| clinical signs of lithium nephropathy | • **polyuria**— * nephrogenic DI, * usually clinically insignificant, • *incomplete distal RTA*—see below, • *renal sodium wasting,* • *chronic interstitial nephritis*—microcystic changes in renal tubules |
| causes of oxalate nephropathy | • **ethylene glycol poisoning,** • *high doses of ascorbic acid,* • *methoxyflurane*— * metabolized to fluoride and oxalate, * produces nephrogenic DI, • *pyridoxine deficiency,* • *increased GI absorption*—Crohn's disease |
| causes of nephrocalcinosis | • **primary HPTH,** • *multiple myeloma*—hypercalcemia, • *distal tubule RTA*—see below, • *hyperphosphatemia*—renal failure [**Note:** calcium deposits in the mitochondria within the tubules and within the tubular lumens.] |

*Table continued on following page*

**Table 14–2.  SELECTED UROLOGIC DISORDERS II**
*Continued*

| Most Common... | Answer and Explanation |
|---|---|
| renal effects of hypercalcemia | • **nephrocalcinosis**, • *nephrogenic DI*, • *produces intrarenal vasoconstriction* |
| clinical findings of nephrocalcinosis | • **polyuria**— * loss of urine concentration, * nephrogenic DI, • *HTN*, • *renal failure* |
| renal findings in multiple myeloma | • **hypersensitivity reaction to BJ protein**, • *nephrocalcinosis*—hypercalcemia-induced, • *amyloid nephropathy*—light chains are nephrotoxic, • *metastasis* |
| types of renal tubular acidosis | • **distal RTA**—type I, • *proximal RTA*—type II, • *hyporeninemic hypoaldosteronism*—type IV |
| causes of distal RTA (type I) | • **multiple myeloma**, • *cystinosis*, • *amphotericin B*, • *Pb poisoning*, • *outdated tetracycline*, • *lithium*, • *Sjögren's syndrome*, • *sickle cell disease* |
| pathogenesis of distal RTA (type I) | • **defect in aldosterone-enhanced H⁺/K⁺ ATPase pump in the collecting tubule**—major site for excreting excess H⁺ ions and regeneration of bicarbonate, • *inability to maintain a steep urine-to-blood H⁺ gradient*— * H⁺ ions recycle back into the blood, * mechanism of amphotericin B |
| clinical findings in distal RTA | • **muscle weakness**—hypokalemia from kaliuresis, • *polyuria*— * nephrogenic DI from hypokalemic nephropathy, * nephrocalcinosis, • *nephrolithiasis*— * due to calcium loss in urine, * usually occurs with incomplete type of distal RTA (calcium phosphate stones) |

## Table 14–2. SELECTED UROLOGIC DISORDERS II
### Continued

| Most Common... | Answer and Explanation |
|---|---|
| lab findings in distal RTA | • **hyperchloremic normal AG metabolic acidosis**—H$^+$ ions are retained and combine with Cl$^-$ anions to form HCl, • *severe hypokalemia*—H$^+$/K$^+$ pump is blocked: K$^+$ is lost in the urine, • *urine pH > 5.5*—H$^+$ ions are not excreted into the urine: decrease in formation of NH$_4$Cl and titratable acid, • *no urine acidification after infusion of NH$_4$Cl*—H$^+$ pump is defective, • *kidneys can reclaim infused bicarbonate*—predominantly a proximal, not a distal, tubule function, • *urine anion gap 0 or positive*— * urine AG = (random urine Na$^+$ + random urine K$^+$) − random urine Cl$^-$, * urine Cl$^-$ is an indirect measure of NH$_4$Cl excretion, * inability to excrete H$^+$ in urine leads to less NH$_4$Cl in the urine and a 0 to positive value for the urine AG, * urine AG is negative value in normal AG metabolic acidosis due to diarrhea, because urine acidification is normal |
| Rx of distal RTA | • **sodium bicarbonate tablets,** • *bicarbonate alternative*—Shohl's solution, which contains citrate: citrate is converted into bicarbonate |
| causes of proximal RTA (type II) | • **carbonic anhydrase inhibitors,** • *acute/chronic interstitial nephritis,* • *primary HPTH*—excess PTH inhibits reclamation of bicarbonate in the proximal tubule, • *toluene sniffing,* • *heavy metal poisoning* |
| pathogenesis of proximal RTA | **lower proximal tubule renal threshold for reclaiming bicarbonate**— * renal threshold for reclaiming bicarbonate drops to 15–18 mEq/L, * excess filtered HCO$_3$$^-$ is lost in urine in combination with Na$^+$/K$^+$: urine pH is initially >5.5 from bicarbonaturia, * plasma HCO$_3$$^-$ eventually drops to the same level as the renal threshold: HCO$_3$$^-$ is now reclaimed up to the new threshold and is not lost in the urine (urine pH < 5.5) |

*Table continued on following page*

**Table 14–2. SELECTED UROLOGIC DISORDERS II**
*Continued*

| Most Common... | Answer and Explanation |
|---|---|
| clinical findings in proximal RTA | • **related to normal AG metabolic acidosis**— * growth failure, * renal osteodystrophy, • *hypokalemia*— * muscle weakness, * polyuria: severe hypokalemia produces vacuolar nephropathy and a nephrogenic DI, * nocturia, * nephrogenic DI, * *osteomalacia*— * skeletal deformities, * fractures |
| lab findings in proximal RTA | • **hyperchloremic normal AG metabolic acidosis**, • *hypokalemia*, • *fractional excretion of infused bicarbonate >15%*—bicarbonate is lost in the urine owing to a lower renal threshold for $HCO_3^-$, • *urine pH >5.5 in early stages and <5.5 when serum and renal threshold values equilibrate*, • *urine AG is 0 to positive*—see above, • *generalized Fanconi's syndrome*— * proximal RTA, * uricosuria: hypouricemia, * phosphaturia: hypophosphatemia, * aminoaciduria, * glucosuria: hypoglycemia |
| Rx of proximal RTA | • **volume contraction with thiazides**—raises the renal threshold for reclaiming $HCO_3^-$, • *oral administration of potassium $HCO_3^-$*, • **most cases are not severe enough to warrant $HCO_3^-$ Rx** |
| causes of type IV RTA | • **DM**, • *chronic interstitial nephritis*, • *obstructive uropathy*, • *drugs*—spironolactone, • *AIDS*, • *legionnaires' disease* |
| pathogenesis of type IV RTA | **destruction of JG apparatus**— * low PRA and aldosterone, * hypoaldosteronemia: ♦ $Na^+$ loss, ♦ retention $H^+$ ions (metabolic acidosis), ♦ retention $K^+$ (hyperkalemia) |
| clinical finding in type IV RTA | **increased susceptibility to potassium intake leading to hyperkalemia**—hyperkalemia develops quickly when patients take: ♦ $K^+$ supplements, ♦ NSAIDs, ♦ ACE inhibitors |
| lab findings in type IV RTA | • **hyperkalemia**, • *hyperchloremic normal AG metabolic acidosis*, • *urine AG 0 to positive* [**Note:** it is the only normal AG metabolic acidosis with hyperkalemia.] |

## Table 14–2. SELECTED UROLOGIC DISORDERS II
*Continued*

| Most Common... | Answer and Explanation |
|---|---|
| Rx of type IV RTA | • **fludrocortisone**—mineralocorticoid replacement, • *loop diuretic,* • *restriction of K+ or drugs predisposing to K+ sparing,* • *oral administration of NaHCO₃* |
| causes of visible renal calcifications on radiographs | • **stones,** • *nephrocalcinosis,* • *calcified tumors/cysts,* • *infections*—e.g., histoplasmosis, • *medullary sponge kidney* |
| renal disease in essential HTN | **benign nephrosclerosis**—due to ischemic changes associated with hyaline arteriolosclerosis: ♦ tubular atrophy, ♦ glomerular sclerosis, ♦ small kidneys |
| lab findings in BNS | • **proteinuria,** • *hematuria,* • *renal azotemia,* • *hyaline casts* |
| causes of malignant HTN | • **preexisting BNS,** • *PSS,* • *HUS,* • *TTP* |
| cause of diffuse cortical necrosis | **pregnancy complicated by DIC** |
| causes of obstructive uropathy in UUT (above UV junction) | • **nephrolithiasis,** • *pregnancy,* • *TCC,* • *renal papillary necrosis,* • *intratubular obstruction* —e.g., uric acid, • *retroperitoneal fibrosis* |
| causes of LUT obstruction | • **prostatic hyperplasia,** • *cervical cancer*— * ureterovesical junction obstruction, • *TCC,* • *phimosis*—cannot retract prepuce over glans, • *urethral strictures* |
| kidney finding in UUT obstruction | **hydronephrosis**— * renal pelvis dilatation, * compression atrophy of cortex/medulla |
| sequence of events in renal function in postrenal obstruction | **increased tubular hydrostatic pressure → increased intraglomerular hydrostatic pressure → drop in GFR → ischemia secondary to vasoconstriction of mesangial cells and efferent arterioles by AT II/TXA₂ → tubular necrosis/atrophy** |
| clinical finding in complete obstruction | **anuria leading to ARF** |
| causes of complete urinary tract obstruction | • **urethral obstruction**—prostate hyperplasia, • *bilateral UUT obstruction*—see above |

*Table continued on following page*

## Table 14–2.  SELECTED UROLOGIC DISORDERS II
### Continued

| Most Common... | Answer and Explanation |
|---|---|
| clinical/lab findings in partial obstruction | • **polyuria**, • *flank pain*, • *tubular dysfunction*—see above, • *UTI*, • *HTN*, • *palpable mass*—hydronephrosis, • *lab findings*— * BUN/creatinine ratio >15:1, * FENa$^+$ <1, * UOsm >500 mOsm/kg, * hypernatremia: ♦ hypotonic fluid loss, ♦ urea osmotically active, * type IV RTA—see above |
| tests to confirm urinary tract obstruction | • **renal ultrasound**— * sensitivity ~98%, * specificity ~75%, • *abdominal CT with contrast + renal US*— * 100% sensitivity, * specificity confirming cause of obstruction ~85%, • *KUB*—initial step for stone evaluation, • *IVP*—good test if KUB is normal [**Note:** spiral CT is gaining popularity in large medical centers.] |
| Rx of urinary tract obstruction | **depends on the cause** |
| clinical findings in postobstructive diuresis | **osmotic diuresis leading to volume depletion and loss of electrolytes**—electrolytes include: ♦ Na$^+$, ♦ K$^+$, ♦ Mg$^{++}$ |
| metabolic cause of renal calculi | **hypercalciuria** |
| causes of hypercalciuria | • **increased GI absorption,** • *increased renal absorption*, • *increased bone resorption* |
| risk factors for renal calculi | • **low urine volume,** • *hypercalciuria*, • *male sex*, • *reduced urine citrate*—normally chelates calcium, • *primary HPTH*— * increased bone resorption, * increased vitamin D synthesis: PTH increases the synthesis of 1-α-hydroxylase in the proximal tubule, • *diet high in dairy products*—calcium phosphate stones, • *diet high in oxalates*—calcium oxalate stones, • *diet high in sodium*— * increases urine calcium excretion, * lowers urine citrate, • *diet high in protein*— * increases calcium, oxalate, uric acid excretion, * lowers urine citrate, • *Crohn's disease*—increased oxalate reabsorption, • *tumor lysis syndrome*—urate stones, • *distal RTA*—calcium phosphate stones, • *UTIs secondary to urease producers*—struvite stones, • *cystic disease*, • *genetic diseases*— * cystinuria, * gout: 25% have stones, * xanthinuria, * primary hyperoxaluria |

## Table 14–2. SELECTED UROLOGIC DISORDERS II
### *Continued*

| Most Common... | Answer and Explanation |
|---|---|
| renal stones | • **calcium oxalate,** • *calcium phosphate,* • *magnesium ammonium phosphate*— * struvite stone, * "staghorn calculus," • *uric acid,* • *cystine,* • *xanthine* |
| S/S of renal calculus | • **sudden onset of colicky pain in the flank with radiation into groin,** • *patient is constantly moving around owing to pain,* • *N/V,* • *gross/microscopic hematuria* |
| initial tests to identify stones | • **UA**— * confirms hematuria, * identify crystals, * urine pH, • *KUB*—85% of stones contain calcium, • *renal ultrasound/IVP*—if KUB is normal [**Note:** spiral CT is gaining popularity in large medical centers.] |
| confirmatory test for a stone | **stone analysis by x-ray diffraction**—patients must strain their urine |
| stones that are radiolucent | • **uric acid,** • *xanthine,* • *cystine*— occasionally radiodense |
| lab tests for recurrent stone formers | • **24-hr urine collections**— * $Ca^{++}$, * phosphate, * uric acid, * $Na^+$, * $Mg^{++}$, * citrate, • **calcium load test**—see below, • **serum PTH**—R/O primary HPTH, • **serum calcium/phosphorus**—R/O primary HPTH, • **serum electrolytes**—R/O distal RTA, • **serum BUN/creatinine**—R/O renal disease |
| method of distinguishing cause of hypercalciuria | **calcium load test**—distinguishes 3 main causes of hypercalciuria: ♦ absorptive hypercalciuria (MC overall type), ♦ resorptive hypercalciuria, ♦ primary renal disease causing hypercalciuria |
| mechanism/Rx of type I absorptive hypercalciuria | • **mechanism**— * increased jejunal reabsorption of calcium,* independent of calcium intake, * normal values for: ♦ serum calcium, ♦ phosphorus, ♦ PTH, ♦ vitamin D, • **Rx**— * cellulose phosphate: binds GI calcium, * hydrochlorothiazide: increases renal calcium reabsorption, * potassium citrate |

*Table continued on following page*

**Table 14–2. SELECTED UROLOGIC DISORDERS II**
*Continued*

| Most Common... | Answer and Explanation |
|---|---|
| mechanism/Rx of type II absorptive hypercalciuria | • **mechanism**— * increased jejunal reabsorption of calcium,* dependent on calcium intake, * normal values for: ♦ serum calcium, ♦ phosphorus, ♦ PTH, ♦ vitamin D, • **Rx**— * dietary restriction of calcium, * potassium citrate |
| mechanism/Rx of type III absorptive hypercalciuria | • **mechanism**— * increased renal loss of phosphate, * hypophosphatemia stimulates synthesis of 1-α-hydroxylase enzyme and vitamin D, * vitamin D increases GI calcium reabsorption, * serum calcium/PTH normal, * serum phosphorus low, * serum vitamin D high, • **Rx**— * oral orthophosphate: increases serum phosphate, which inhibits vitamin D synthesis, * potassium citrate |
| mechanism/Rx of resorptive hypercalciuria due to primary HPTH | • **mechanism**— * increased PTH increases bone resorption causing hypercalcemia, * calcium excreted in urine is > amount reabsorbed in urine, * serum calcium/PTH/vitamin D high, * serum phosphorus low, • **Rx**—remove parathyroid adenoma |
| mechanism/Rx of hypercalciuria due to primary renal disease | • **mechanism**— * kidney cannot reabsorb calcium, * serum calcium/phosphorus normal, * serum PTH/vitamin D high, • **Rx**— * hydrochlorothiazide, * potassium citrate |
| general Rx of stones | • **increased fluid intake**—urine output >2.5 L/day, • *analgesia*, • *stones <5 mm usually pass*, • *50% of stones 5–7 mm pass*, • *stones >7 mm usually do not pass and require surgical intervention*— * percutaneous extraction for struvite stones, * extracorporeal shock wave lithotripsy for large stones or stones in upper one-third of ureter, * extraction of stones located in lower pole of ureter |
| Rx of uric acid stones | **overproduction of uric acid (24-hr urine uric acid >1000 mg/day)**— * allopurinol: blocks xanthine oxidase, * alkalinize urine |
| Rx of hyperoxaluria | • **avoid foods high in oxalates,** • *potassium citrate*, • *magnesium gluconate* |
| Rx of hypocitraturia | **potassium citrate** |
| Rx of struvite stones | • **eradicate infection,** • **extracorporeal shock wave lithotripsy,** • **surgical removal** |

## Table 14–2. SELECTED UROLOGIC DISORDERS II
*Continued*

| Most Common... | Answer and Explanation |
|---|---|
| Rx of cystine stones | • **low methionine diet,** • **potassium citrate** |
| renal finding in tuberous sclerosis | **angiomyolipoma**— * in 50% of cases, they are hamartomas |
| malignant kidney tumor in adults | **renal adenocarcinoma**— * alias: ♦ Grawitz's tumor, ♦ hypernephroma, * they arise from proximal tubules, * >3 cm in 75–80%, * men > women, * occur during 6th–7th decade |
| causes of a renal adenocarcinoma | • **smoking,** • *von Hippel–Lindau disease*— * bilateral renal cancer develops in 50–60%, • *APKD,* • *obesity,* • *acquired renal cystic disease,* • *phenacetin abuse* |
| S/S of a renal adenocarcinoma | • **hematuria**—90%, • *pain—45%,* • *flank mass—30%,* • *fever,* • *leukemoid reaction*—benign neutrophil elevation >35,000 to 50,000 cells/μL, • *amyloidosis,* • *Staufer's syndrome*— * hepatic cell necrosis unrelated to metastasis, * hepatic lesions after nephrectomy, • *HTN*—increased renin secretion |
| ectopic hormone relationships in renal adenocarcinoma | • **erythropoietin**—polycythemia, • *PTH-like peptide*—hypercalcemia, • *renin*—HTN, • *gonadotropins*—feminization/masculinization, • *cortisol*—ectopic Cushing's syndrome |
| metastatic sites | • **lungs**— * classic "cannon ball" metastases, * hemoptysis is common, • *bone*—always lytic, • *skin*—one of a few cancers that metastasize to skin, • *liver,* • *brain,* • *general comments*— * metastasis is present in one-third when initially discovered, * renal vein invasion occurs in 50%, * regional lymph node involvement occurs in 20%, * metastases commonly occur after 10–20 yrs |
| primary organ sites that metastasize to the kidney | • **lung,** • *breast,* • *stomach,* • *malignant lymphoma* [**Note:** kidney metastasis is uncommon.] |
| method for diagnosing renal adenocarcinoma | • **CT scan,** • *US* [**Note:** most solid masses in the kidneys are renal adenocarcinoma. US is most useful in distinguishing cystic from solid masses. Percutaneous FNA is commonly performed to obtain tissue for diagnosis.] |

*Table continued on following page*

## Table 14–2. SELECTED UROLOGIC DISORDERS II
*Continued*

| Most Common... | Answer and Explanation |
|---|---|
| Rx of renal adenocarcinoma | • **radical nephrectomy,** • *metastatic disease—* * progestational agents, * α-interferon, * IL-2, * vinblastine, • *renal vein invasion does not adversely affect prognosis,* • *average 5-yr survival is 45%* |
| cancers of renal pelvis | • **TCC**—~50% have TCC in other areas of GU tract, • SCC |
| risk factors for TCC of renal pelvis | • **smoking,** • *phenacetin abuse*—high risk, • *aromatic amines—* * benzidine, * naphthylamine, • *cyclophosphamide* |
| risk factors for SCC of renal pelvis | • **stones,** • *chronic infection* |

**Question:** Which of the following conditions are associated with a FENa$^+$ < 1, UOsm > 500 mOsm/kg, and serum BUN:/creatinine ratio > 15:1? **SELECT 3**

(A) Acute interstitial nephritis
(B) CHF
(C) Nephrotoxic ATN
(D) Acute proliferative glomerulonephritis
(E) Acute pyelonephritis
(F) Volume depletion secondary to GI bleed
(G) Partial lower urinary tract obstruction
(H) Chronic renal failure

**Answers: (B), (D), (F).** Acute interstitial nephritis produces ARF with tubular dysfunction (FENa$^+$ >1, UOsm <350 mOsm/kg, BUN:creatinine ratio <15:1, **choice A is incorrect**). CHF is associated with a decreased EABV and a low GFR with preservation of tubular function (prerenal azotemia, **choice B is correct**). Nephrotoxic ATN is associated with tubular azotemia. It is most commonly caused by drugs like the aminoglycosides (**choice C is incorrect**). Acute proliferative GN is associated with oliguria, but tubular function is intact (**choice D is correct**). Acute PN has preservation of renal function, but the serum BUN:/creatinine ratio is normal (<15:1, **choice E is incorrect**). Volume depletion in general is associated with prerenal azotemia with preservation of tubular function. If left untreated, it will progress into ischemic ATN (**choice F is correct**). Partial lower urinary tract obstruction has preservation of tubular function, but the BUN:creatinine ratio is >1 (**choice G is incorrect**). Chronic renal failure is associated with tubular dysfunction (**choice H is incorrect**).

ACE = angiotensin-converting enzyme, AD = autosomal dominant, AG = anion gap, ALL = acute lymphoblastic leukemia, AMI = acute myocardial infarction, AMP = ampicillin, APKD = adult polycystic kidney disease, APN = acute pyelonephritis, ARF = acute renal failure, AT II = angiotensin II, ATN = acute tubular necrosis, BJ = Bence Jones (protein), BM = basement membrane, BNS = benign nephrosclerosis, BPH = benign prostatic hyperplasia, BT = bleeding time, BUN = blood urea nitrogen, Bx = biopsy, CH = cholesterol, CHF = congestive heart failure, CMV = cytomegalovirus, COD = cause of death, CPN = chronic pyelonephritis, Cr = creatinine, CRF = chronic renal failure, CVA = cerebrovascular accident, DI = diabetes insipidus, DIC = disseminated intravascular coagulation, DM = diabetes mellitus, EABV = effective arterial blood volume, EPO = erythropoietin, ESR = erythrocyte sedimentation rate, $FENa^+$ = fractional excretion of sodium, FNA = fine needle aspiration, FQ = fluoroquinolones, FR = free radical, FSG = focal segmental glomerulosclerosis, GENT = gentamicin, GFR = glomerular filtration rate, GN = glomerulonephritis, Hct = hematocrit, HPTH = hyperparathyroidism, HTN = hypertension, HUS = hemolytic uremic syndrome, IL-2 = interleukin 2, IN = interstitial nephritis, IVP = intravenous pyelogram, JG = juxtaglomerular, KUB = kidney/ureter/bladder (radiographs), LMW = low molecular weight, LUT = lower urinary tract, LVH = left ventricular hypertrophy, MPD = myeloproliferative disease, MPGN = membranoproliferative glomerulonephritis, MVP = mitral valve prolapse, NSAIDs = nonsteroidal anti-inflammatory drugs, N/V = nausea/vomiting, Pb = lead, $PGE_2$ = prostaglandin $E_2$, PN = pyelonephritis, PRA = plasma renin activity, PRV = polycythemia rubra vera, PSS = progressive systemic sclerosis, PTH = parathyroid hormone, PUD = peptic ulcer disease, RAA = renin angiotensin aldosterone, R/O = rule out, RPGN = rapidly progressive glomerulonephritis, RTA = renal tubular acidosis, SCC = squamous cell carcinoma, SLE = systemic lupus erythematosus, S/S = signs and symptoms, TCC = transitional cell carcinoma, TG = triglyceride, TTP = thrombotic thrombocytopenic purpura, $TXA_2$ = thromboxane $A_2$, UA = urinalysis, $UNa^+$ = urine sodium, UOsm = urine osmolality, UTI = urinary tract infection, UUT = upper urinary tract, UV = ureterovesical, VUR = vesicoureteral reflux.

## Table 14–3. SELECTED UROLOGIC DISORDERS III

| Most Common... | Answer and Explanation |
|---|---|
| cause of acute cystitis | **ascending infection secondary to *Escherichia* coli (80–90%)**—acute cystitis is more common in women (short urethra) than men |
| viral cause of hemorrhagic cystitis | **adenovirus** |

*Table continued on following page*

### Table 14–3. SELECTED UROLOGIC DISORDERS III
*Continued*

| Most Common... | Answer and Explanation |
|---|---|
| cause of acute cystitis in sexually active women | ***Staphylococcus saprophyticus***— * coagulase-negative, * accounts for ~10–20% of UTIs |
| causes of acute urethral syndrome in women (pyuria, <10⁵ CFU/mL) | • *Chlamydia trachomatis*—PCR of voided urine is currently recommended to detect the organism, • *Mycoplasma hominis*, • *Ureaplasma urealyticum*, • *Neisseria gonorrhoeae* |
| bacterial infection in elderly people | **lower UTIs** |
| general risk factors for a LUT infection | • **female sex**, • *indwelling urinary catheter*, • *sexual intercourse*—"honeymoon cystitis," • *DM*, • *pregnancy*, • *neurogenic bladder*, • *cystic renal disease*, • *instrumentation* |
| risks of indwelling urinary catheters | • **sepsis**— * indwelling catheters are the MCC of sepsis in hospitalized patients, * account for 50% of all nosocomial UTIs, * >90% have infection by 3–4 days, * prophylactic antimicrobial Rx is ineffective, * Rx if symptomatic infection |
| risk factors for LUT infections in men | • **lack of circumcision**, • *anal intercourse*, • *intercourse with a woman whose vagina is colonized with uropathogens* |
| S/S of LUT infection | • **dysuria**—painful urination, • *increased frequency*, • *urgency*, • *nocturia*, • *suprapubic discomfort*, • *gross hematuria* [**Note:** Fever is not a feature of LUT infection.] |
| lab findings in a LUT infection | • **pyuria**— * WBCs in urine, * definition —≥10 WBCs/HPF in a centrifuged specimen or ≥5 WBCs in uncentrifuged specimen, • *bacteriuria*, • *hematuria*, • *positive dipstick leukocyte esterase*, • *positive dipstick nitrite*, • *≥10⁵ colony-forming units/mL*— * gold standard criterion of infection, * midstream clean catch urine, * low colony counts with symptoms are significant, * ≥10⁵ CFU/mL correlates with 1 or more organisms/OPF on a Gram stain of unspun urine |
| urine contaminants | • *Lactobacillus*, • **α-hemolytic streptococci** |

## Table 14–3. SELECTED UROLOGIC DISORDERS III
*Continued*

| Most Common... | Answer and Explanation |
|---|---|
| causes of asymptomatic bacteriuria in women | • **pregnancy,** • *elderly women in nursing homes,* • *DM,* • *sickle cell trait,* • *cystic renal disease* [**Note:** asymptomatic bacteriuria is defined as 2 successive cultures with $\geq 10^5$ CFU/mL in an asymptomatic patient.] |
| cause of recurrent UTIs within 1–2 weeks of Rx in women | **usually exogenous reinfection in > 90%** |
| preventive measures recommended in recurrent UTIs | • **void immediately after coitus,** • *1 dose of TMP/SMX after coitus*—40 mg/400 mg after coitus, • *avoid intercourse while on Rx* |
| Rx of uncomplicated, symptomatic UTI in women and men | • **women**— * empiric Rx with TMP/SMX for 3 days, * symptoms plus microscopic examination of urine compatible with a UTI are all that is necessary to Rx the patient, • **men**— * pretreatment urine culture is necessary: UTIs are uncommon in men, * Rx with TMP/SMX for 14 days |
| Rx of asymptomatic bacteriuria | • **Rx in pregnant women**— * ampicillin or cephalosporin, * avoid sulfa drugs or tetracycline, * Rx for 10–14 days, * APN may occur in 1–2%, • **Rx in patients undergoing urologic surgery,** • **Rx in DM** [Note: Rx is not necessary in elderly, otherwise healthy women.] |
| Rx of acute urethral syndrome | • **azithromycin**— * single dose, * patient more likely to take drug with a single-dose regimen, • *doxycycline*—100 mg, PO, bid, for 7 days |
| types of bladder cancer | • **TCC**— * men > women, * majority are papillary: low-grade, * multifocality is the rule: common malignant stem cell abnormality or reimplantation of the tumor from another site, • *SCC*—association with *Schistosoma hematobium* bladder infections, • *adenocarcinoma* |
| causes of TCC involving bladder | • **smoking,** • *aniline dyes,* • *aromatic amines,* • *cyclophosphamide*—also causes hemorrhagic cystitis: prevented with mesna, • *phenacetin abuse*—less common cause in bladder than in renal pelvis TCC |

*Table continued on following page*

## Table 14–3. SELECTED UROLOGIC DISORDERS III
*Continued*

| Most Common... | Answer and Explanation |
|---|---|
| S/S of bladder cancer | • **painless gross/microscopic hematuria** —70–90%, • *irritative bladder complaints—* * dysuria, * increased frequency of urination |
| metastatic sites | • **regional lymph nodes,** • *liver,* • *lung,* • *bones* |
| methods to diagnose bladder cancer | • **cystoscopy with Bx,** • *urine cytology* |
| Rx of bladder cancer | • **unifocal disease**—cystoscopy with fulguration, • **multifocal disease**—intravesical therapy with: ♦ bacille Calmette-Guérin, ♦ mitomycin C, ♦ thiotepa, • **invasive disease**— * total cystectomy, * adjuvant chemotherapy if nodal involvement is present, • **prognosis**—5-yr survival with superficial disease 85–90% |
| causes of acute/ chronic prostatitis | • **acute prostatitis**— * *Escherichia coli,* * *Pseudomonas aeruginosa,* * *Klebsiella pneumoniae,* • **chronic prostatitis**—most cases are abacterial, • **prostate infections linked to infections of urethra and/or bladder,** • **lack of sexual intercourse,** • **prolonged sitting/bicycle riding** |
| S/S of prostatitis | • **pain**— * low back, * perineal, * suprapubic, • *painful/swollen gland on rectal exam,* • *dysuria,* • *hematuria* |
| lab findings in prostatitis | • **collect 4 specimens for culture**— * first 10 mL of urine is the urethral component, * second specimen is midstream, which is the bladder component, * third specimen is at the end of voiding, which represents the prostatic secretions, * fourth specimen represents prostatic secretions milked out of the penis after prostate massage, • **>20 WBCs/ HPF in the third specimen suggests acute prostatitis,** • **the confirmatory test is the bacterial count**—bacterial count 1 or more logarithms higher in the 3rd and 4th specimens than in specimens 1 and 2 indicates prostatitis |

## Table 14–3. SELECTED UROLOGIC DISORDERS III
*Continued*

| Most Common... | Answer and Explanation |
|---|---|
| Rx of acute prostatitis | • **≤35 yrs old**—OFLOX, 400 mg PO × 1, then 300 mg PO q12hrs × 7 days, • **≥35 yrs old**— * FQ, 500 mg bid PO × 10–14 days, * TMP/SMX, 1 double-strength bid × 10–14 days |
| Rx of chronic prostatitis | • **if bacterial**—FQ, 500 mg bid PO × 6 wks, • **if abacterial**— * doxycycline 100 mg bid × 14 days, * α-adrenergic blocking agents |
| benign disorder of the prostate | **BPH** |
| cause of BPH | **slight excess of DHT enhanced by estrogen**— * DHT causes gland/stromal/smooth muscle hyperplasia, * estrogen sensitizes prostatic tissue to androgens, * age-dependent |
| location of BPH | **transitional zone**—zone closest to the prostatic urethra |
| clinical/lab findings in BPH | • **signs of obstruction**— * trouble initiating stream, * dribbling, * incomplete emptying, * nocturia, • *hematuria,* • *PSA*— * increased in 25% of men, * rarely > 10 ng/mL: normal is 0–4 ng/mL [**Note:** the PSA is not falsely increased by a rectal exam.] |
| complications of BPH | • **obstructive uropathy**— * postrenal azotemia, * bilateral hydronephrosis, • *bladder infections,* • *prostatic infarcts*— * pain, * indurated gland, * high PSA values, • *bladder wall hypertrophy,* • *bladder diverticula,* • *no risk for progression into carcinoma* |
| Rx of symptomatic BPH | • **α₁-adrenergic blockers**— * e.g., terazosin, * reduce smooth muscle tone in bladder neck, • *5α-reductase inhibitors*— * e.g., finasteride, * blocks conversion of testosterone to DHT, * libido maintained, * increases hair growth, • *gonadotropin agonists*—e.g., leuprolide: ♦ sustained release of LH decreases androgen synthesis, ♦ impotence, • *block androgen receptor*—e.g., flutamide: ♦ libido maintained, ♦ gynecomastia, • *saw palmetto—anti-androgen effect:* ♦ blocks androgen uptake and availability without altering serum levels, ♦ shrinks the transitional zone of the prostate, • *TUR*—retrograde ejaculation common |

*Table continued on following page*

## Table 14–3. SELECTED UROLOGIC DISORDERS III
*Continued*

| Most Common... | Answer and Explanation |
|---|---|
| cancer in males | **prostate adenocarcinoma**— * age-dependent, * African-Americans > whites, * uncommon < 40 yrs old, * asymptomatic until advanced |
| risk factors for prostate cancer | • **age**, • *family history*—first-degree relatives, • *African-American*, • *smoking*, • *high-saturated-fat diet*, • *occupational exposures*— * pesticides, * rubber, * cadmium |
| location of prostate cancer | **peripheral zone**— * palpable by DRE, * obstructive uropathy is not an early finding |
| S/S of symptomatic prostate cancer | • **obstructive uropathy**, • *low back/pelvic pain*—metastases, • *compression of spinal cord*—vertebral metastasis |
| screening program for prostate cancer | **DRE/PSA annually beginning at 50 years of age**— * DRE does not falsely increase PSA but does increase PAP: PAP is no longer used, * rate of PSA change/yr is important: e.g., >0.75 ng/mL change/yr is highly predictive of cancer, * ~70% with PSA >10 ng/mL have cancer |
| confirmatory test for prostate cancer | **transrectal US with needle biopsies of suspicious sites if screening tests are abnormal** |
| spread of prostate cancer | • **perineural invasion**—method of extension of tumor to: ♦ capsule, ♦ seminal vesicles, ♦ bladder neck, • *lymphatic spread to regional lymph nodes*—obturator and iliac nodes first, • *hematogenous*— * bone: ♦ increases serum ALP, ♦ radiodense metastasis, ♦ radionuclide scans more sensitive than plain films, * lungs, * liver |
| extranodal metastatic site of prostate cancer | **vertebral column**— * 40% to lumbar spine, * osteoblastic in most cases |
| grading system for prostate cancer | **Gleason's system**—the higher the score, the more undifferentiated the cancer |

**Table 14–3. SELECTED UROLOGIC DISORDERS III**
*Continued*

| Most Common... | Answer and Explanation |
|---|---|
| staging system for prostate cancer | • **stage A**— * cannot palpate, * organ-confined, * A1 ≤ 5% of specimen involved, * A2 ≥ 5% specimen involved, • **stage B**— * organ-confined: most common stage, * palpable, • **stage C**—local extension: ♦ periprostatic tissue, ♦ seminal vesicles, • **stage D**— * pelvic nodal involvement (D1), * distant metastasis (D2) |
| Rx of stage A1 | **observed without Rx** |
| Rx of organ-confined prostate cancer (stage A2 or B) | • **radical prostatectomy**—some clinicians prefer watchful waiting if patient has < 10 yr of life expectancy, • **prognosis**—15-yr tumor-free survival rate for organ-confined cancer is ~85–90% |
| Rx of locally advanced disease (stage C) | **irradiation** |
| Rx of stage D1 prostate cancer (positive pelvic nodes) | **irradiation plus androgen deprivation**—some clinicians use only androgen deprivation: ♦ bilateral orchiectomy, ♦ antiandrogen drugs, ♦ DES |
| Rx of stage D2 prostate cancer (distant metastasis) | • **androgen deprivation**— * radiation for bone metastasis, * ketoconazole for spinal cord compression, • **prognosis**—10–40% 10-yr survival rate |
| methods for follow-up of prostate cancer | • **PSA**, • *radionuclide bone scan* |
| cause of left scrotal enlargement in an adult | **varicocele**— * always left-sided: testicular vein drains into left renal vein, not the inferior vena cava, * very common cause of male infertility: heat inhibits sperm maturation |
| cause of scrotal enlargement | **hydrocele**— * persistence of tunica vaginalis, * transillumination distinguishes a scrotal from a testicular mass, * US more accurate |
| cause of abrupt testicular pain | **testicular torsion**— * loss of cremasteric reflex, * testicle higher on the involved side |

*Table continued on following page*

## Table 14–3. SELECTED UROLOGIC DISORDERS III
*Continued*

| Most Common... | Answer and Explanation |
|---|---|
| causes of acute epididymitis | • **<35 yrs old**— * *Neisseria gonorrhoeae*, • *Chlamydia trachomatis*, • **>35 yrs old**— * *Escherichia coli*, * *Pseudomonas aeruginosa* |
| S/S of acute epididymitis | • **variable onset of scrotal pain with radiation into spermatic cord or flank**, • *scrotal swelling*, • *epididymal tenderness*, • *urethral discharge*—if STD, • *Prehn's sign*—elevation of scrotum decreases pain |
| Rx for acute epididymitis | • **STD**—ceftriaxone, 250 mg IM × 1 + doxycycline 100 mg PO bid × 10 days, • **STD ruled out**—FQ, 500 mg bid PO × 10–14 days |
| location for cryptorchid testis | **inguinal canal** |
| complication of cryptorchid testis | **potential for infertility and seminoma**—risk for seminoma applies to both the affected testicle and normal testicle |
| cause of orchitis | • **extension of acute epididymitis**, • *syphilis*, • *mumps*, • *HIV* |
| location for the urogenital diaphragm in a cystourethrogram | • **male**—located just distal to prostate, • **female**—beginning of urethra when it exits the bladder [**Note:** muscles of the urogenital diaphragm are the deep transverse perineal and sphincter muscles of urethra.] |
| functions of the detrusor muscle | • *relaxed*—storage of urine in bladder, • *contracted*—emptying of bladder |
| functions of sympathetic nervous system in bladder control | • **relaxes detrusor muscle**, • **contracts internal sphincter**—increases urine storage |
| function of parasympathetic nervous system in bladder control | **contracts detrusor muscle**—internal sphincter muscle relaxes owing to sympathetic inhibition: allows emptying of bladder |
| bladder changes that occur with aging | • **smaller bladder**, • **early contractions of detrusor muscle**—increased voiding, • **increased nocturnal urination**, • **decreased ability to suppress detrusor muscle contraction** [**Note:** urinary incontinence is not a normal age-related finding.] |

## Table 14–3.  SELECTED UROLOGIC DISORDERS III
*Continued*

| Most Common... | Answer and Explanation |
|---|---|
| factors that affect urination and urinary continence | • **diuretics**—bladder fills quickly, • **anticholinergics/narcotics impair detrusor contraction**—retain urine, • **α-adrenergics increase internal sphincter tone**—retain urine, • **α-adrenergic antagonists impair internal sphincter tone**—leak urine |
| types of urinary incontinence | • **urge incontinence**—40–70%, • *overflow incontinence,* • *stress incontinence,* • *functional incontinence* |
| mechanism of urge incontinence | **overactivity of detrusor muscle**—early detrusor contractions with low volumes of urine |
| S/S of urge incontinence | • **increased urinary frequency/urgency,** • **small volume voids,** • **nocturia** |
| causes of urge incontinence | • **bladder irritation**— * *BPH,* * atrophic urethritis, * infection, • *CNS disease*— * Parkinson's disease, * mass lesions, * stroke |
| Rx of urge incontinence | • **anticholinergics**—inhibit parasympathetic stimulation of detrusor contraction, • *behavioral training,* • *topical estrogen in urethral atrophy in women* |
| mechanism of overflow incontinence | • **outflow obstruction**—e.g., * BPH, * pelvic tumor, • *detrusor underactivity/hypotonic bladder*—e.g., autonomic neuropathy |
| S/S of overflow incontinence | • **dribbling,** • **low urine flow** |
| Rx of overflow incontinence | • **cholinergic drugs to enhance muscle tone**—increase detrusor contraction, • **Rx obstruction**—e.g., * α-adrenergic antagonist: decrease internal sphincter tone, * TUR of prostate tissue, • *indwelling urinary catheter*—try to avoid this |
| mechanism of stress incontinence | • **laxity of pelvic floor muscles with lack of bladder support**—posterior urethrovesical angle of 90–100° is not maintained, • *lack of estrogen* [**Note:** this type of urinary incontinence is primarily a disease of women.] |
| S/S of stress incontinence | **loss of urine with increases in intra-abdominal pressure**—e.g., laughing, coughing, sneezing |

*Table continued on following page*

## Table 14–3. SELECTED UROLOGIC DISORDERS III
### Continued

| Most Common... | Answer and Explanation |
|---|---|
| Rx of stress incontinence | • **increase internal sphincter tone with α-adrenergic agonists,** • **topical estrogen therapy,** • **Kegel's pelvic floor muscle exercises,** • **surgery** |
| mechanism of functional incontinence | **inability to reach toilet facilities in time**— * patients are normally continent, * commonly occurs when patients are on diuretics or drink too many caffeinated beverages |
| cause of a painless mass in the testicle | **malignancy**— * MC malignancy between 15 and 35 years of age, * majority are of germ cell origin, * seminomas MC type |
| risk factors for testicular cancer | • **cryptorchid testicle**—highest risk is an intra-abdominal cryptorchid testis, • *DES exposure of male infant* |
| clinical sign of testicular cancer | **painless enlargement of testicle** |
| tumor markers to work up testicular cancer | • **AFP**—yolk sac tumor origin, • **β-hCG**—choriocarcinoma: syncytiotrophoblast origin of β-hCG, • **LDH**—elevated in cancer |
| classification of testicular cancer | • **seminomas**— * 60%, * 30–50 yr olds, * 10% have positive β-hCG: does not alter prognosis, * spread by lymphatics, • *nonseminomas*— * 40%: mixed type MC, * spread by lymphatics/hematogenous routes, * embryonal: ♦ 20–30 yr olds, ♦ AFP elevated, * teratoma, * teratocarcinoma: see below, * choriocarcinoma: see below |
| bilateral testicular cancer | **metastatic malignant lymphoma**—most commonly occurs in men >50 yrs old |
| testicular cancer producing gynecomastia | **choriocarcinoma secreting β-hCG**— * most aggressive cancer, * usually mixed with other nonseminoma types, * pure choriocarcinomas do not enlarge the testicle |
| testicular cancer in adults containing derivatives from more than one germ layer | **teratocarcinoma**— * mixture of embryonal carcinoma and teratoma, * both AFP/β-hGG are elevated in 90% of cases, * teratomas more common in children and tend to be benign |

## Table 14-3. SELECTED UROLOGIC DISORDERS III
*Continued*

| Most Common... | Answer and Explanation |
|---|---|
| means of diagnosis of testicular cancer | • **US**— * screen for testicular cancer, * distinguish the mass as solid or cystic, • *orchiectomy*—establishes diagnosis |
| Rx of seminomas | • **low-stage disease**— * orchiectomy + irradiation of the para-aortic lymph nodes: first site of metastasis, * most radiosensitive of testicular cancers, * >95% cure rate, • **high-stage disease**—platinum-based chemotherapy |
| Rx of nonseminomas | • **low-stage disease and negative marker studies**—orchiectomy + ? observation, • **high-stage disease and positive markers**—platinum-based chemotherapy + bilateral retroperitoneal lymph node dissection, • **prognosis**—50–90% have long-term remissions |
| cancer of penis | **SCC**—HPV 16, 18 link in two-thirds of cases |
| risk factors for squamous cancer of the penis | • **lack of circumcision**, • *Bowen's disease*—shaft of the penis, • *erythroplasia of Queyrat*—red lesions on glans |
| definition of male hypogonadism | • **decreased testosterone production**, • **resistance to testosterone**—e.g., * androgen receptor deficiency: testicular feminization, * 5α-reductase deficiency: Reifenstein's syndrome |
| clinical presentations of male hypogonadism | • **impotence**—failure to sustain an erection during attempted vaginal intercourse, • *loss of male secondary sex characteristics*, • *decreased energy/stamina*, • *osteoporosis*—testosterone inhibits excessive release of interleukin-1 (osteoclast-activating factor) from osteoblasts, • *gynecomastia*—estrogen is unopposed, • *hypogonadal facies*— * facial pallor, * fine wrinkling around the mouth and eyes, • *infertility*— * not always synonymous with testosterone deficiency, * seminiferous tubule dysfunction (spermatogenesis) may be abnormal in presence of normal Leydig cell function (testosterone synthesis) |

*Table continued on following page*

## Table 14–3. SELECTED UROLOGIC DISORDERS III
*Continued*

| Most Common... | Answer and Explanation |
|---|---|
| classification of male hypogonadism | • **primary hypogonadism**— * problem with Leydig cell function, * hypergonadotropic (increased gonadotropins) hypogonadism, • **secondary hypogonadism**— * hypothalamic /pituitary dysfunction, * hypogonadotropic hypogonadism |
| tests to evaluate male hypogonadism/ infertility | • **semen analysis**— * gold standard test for infertility, * best collected by masturbation, * components: ♦ volume, ♦ sperm count (20–150 million sperm/mL), ♦ morphology, ♦ motility, • *hormone evaluation*— * FSH: responsible for spermatogenesis in seminiferous tubules, * LH: responsible for testosterone synthesis in Leydig cells, * prolactin: enhances testosterone synthesis, * total testosterone with fractionation: bound and free testosterone, * estradiol: useful in Klinefelter's syndrome, • *chromosome analysis:* useful in Klinefelter's syndrome, • *gonadotropin stimulation test*— * GnRH used to stimulate FSH/ LH, * distinguishes a pituitary from a hypothalamic problem, • *testicular biopsy*— primarily used for infertility work-ups |
| test to distinguish types of hypogonadism | **gonadotropins**— * increase in serum FSH/LH indicates a primary testicular disorder, * decrease in FSH/LH is a hypothalamic/pituitary disorder |
| components of semen | • **spermatozoa**—derive from the seminiferous tubules, • **coagulant**—seminal vesicles, • **enzymes to liquefy semen**—prostate gland |
| primary causes of seminiferous tubule dysfunction | • **varicocele**—increased heat reduces spermatogenesis, • *Klinefelter's syndrome,* • *orchitis* |
| lab findings in pure seminiferous tubule failure | • **high FSH**— * loss of inhibin from Sertoli cells, * inhibin normally has a negative feedback on FSH, • **normal LH**—Leydig cells are synthesizing testosterone, • **normal serum testosterone**, • **decreased sperm count** [Note: 90% of all cases of male infertility are due to seminiferous tubule dysfunction. Spermatogenesis is affected before Leydig cell dysfunction in testicular disorders.] |

## Table 14–3. SELECTED UROLOGIC DISORDERS III
*Continued*

| Most Common... | Answer and Explanation |
|---|---|
| causes of Leydig cell failure | • **chronic liver disease**, • **chronic renal failure**, • **irradiation**, • **orchitis**—postpubertal males |
| lab findings in pure Leydig cell failure | • **normal FSH**—inhibin is present in the Sertoli cells, • **high LH**— * low testosterone, * testosterone has a negative feedback on LH, • **low serum testosterone**, • **low sperm count** |
| causes of seminiferous and Leydig cell failure | • **chronic liver disease**, • **chronic renal failure**, • irradiation, • **orchitis** |
| lab findings in mixed seminiferous/ Leydig cell failure | • **high FSH**—inhibin is absent, • **high LH**—low testosterone, • **low serum testosterone**, • **low sperm count** |
| lab findings in Klinefelter's syndrome | • **high FSH**—loss of inhibin: seminiferous tubules are totally fibrosed, • **high LH**—low testosterone: increased FSH causes aromatization of all the testosterone into estrogens in the Leydig cells, which are hyperplastic, • **low serum testosterone**, • **high serum estradiol**, • **azoospermia**—no active seminiferous tubules |
| causes of hypothalamic/ pituitary male hypogonadism | • **constitutional delay in puberty**—testicular volume of usually > 4 mL indicates puberty has begun, • *Kallmann's syndrome*—see below, • *hypopituitarism*— * pituitary adenoma: adult, * craniopharyngioma: child, • *anorexia nervosa*—loss of body weight/fat causes a decrease in GnRH, leading to gonadotropin deficiency |
| cause of Kallmann's syndrome | **AD disorder with maldevelopment of olfactory bulbs and GnRH-producing cells** |
| clinical findings in Kallmann's syndrome | • **delayed puberty**, • *anosmia*—80%, • *color blindness*, • *cryptorchidism*, • *lab findings*— * decreased: ♦ FSH, ♦ LH, ♦ testosterone, * due to GnRH deficiency |
| Rx of Kallmann's syndrome | • **pulsatile GnRH**, • **androgen replacement** |

*Table continued on following page*

## Table 14–3. SELECTED UROLOGIC DISORDERS III
*Continued*

| Most Common... | Answer and Explanation |
|---|---|
| tests to evaluate hypogonadotropic hypogonadism | • **serum gonadotropins**—FSH/LH evaluate the degree of impairment, • **serum testosterone,** • **serum prolactin,** • MRI of the head— exclude mass lesions, • **pituitary stimulation tests**—e.g., ACTH stimulation test |
| types of androgen Rx used in male hypogonadism | • **GnRH**—induces spermatogenesis/restores fertility, • **17-hydroxyl esters of testosterone**— * long-acting, * danger of prematurely closing epiphyses in pubertal males, * R/O prostate cancer in older men |
| mechanisms of male infertility | • **decreased or abnormal sperm count**—* idiopathic: MCC, * primary testicular dysfunction: see above, * secondary hypogonadism: see above, • *ductal obstruction*—e.g., * previous vasectomy, * CF: atretic or absent vas deferens, • *disorders associated with accessory sex organs, ejaculation, or technique* [**Note:** regarding infertility in couples, one-third is related to female dysfunction, one-third to male dysfunction, and one-third is a combination of the two.] |
| tests performed in work-up of male infertility | • **sperm count/morphology**— * gold standard, * see above, • *gonadotropins*—increased serum FSH/normal LH defect in spermatogenesis, • *serum testosterone*—see above, • *serum prolactin*—R/O prolactinoma, • *vasographic studies*—R/O obstruction, • *testicular Bx*— evaluate seminiferous tubules/Leydig cells |
| causes of male impotence | • **psychogenic,** • *low testosterone*—see above, • *vascular disease,* • *neurologic disease*— * parasympathetic system for erection: $S_2$–$S_4$, * sympathetic system for ejaculation: $T_{12}$–$L_1$, • *drug effects,* • *endocrine disease,* • *alcohol* • *penis disorders* |
| cause of impotence in young men | **psychogenic**— * stress at work, * marital conflicts, * performance anxiety |

## Table 14–3. SELECTED UROLOGIC DISORDERS III
*Continued*

| Most Common... | Answer and Explanation |
|---|---|
| sign compatible with psychogenic-induced impotence | **presence of nocturnal penile tumescence**—organic/drug-induced reasons cause the loss of nocturnal erections |
| cause of impotence in men > 50 yr old | **vascular insufficiency** |
| causes of vascular insufficiency | • **Leriche's syndrome**—aortoiliac atherosclerosis involving hypogastric arteries and associated with: ♦ calf claudication, ♦ calf atrophy, ♦ diminished femoral pulse, ♦ impotence, • **penile vascular insufficiency,** • **venous leaks in corpus cavernosum** |
| neurogenic causes of male impotence | • **multiple sclerosis,** • **peripheral neuropathy**— * DM, * alcoholic, • **stroke,** • **spinal cord injury,** • **radical prostatectomy** |
| drugs causing male impotence | • **leuprolide,** • **methyldopa,** • **psychotropics,** • **cimetidine,** • **spironolactone,** • **ketoconazole** |
| endocrine disorders causing male impotence | • **DM,** • *hypothyroidism,* • *prolactinoma* |
| mechanism of alcohol-induced male impotence | • **directly inhibits the release of LH/FSH from the anterior pituitary,** • **inhibits binding of LH to Leydig cells**—decreases testosterone synthesis, • **increased liver synthesis of SHBG**— * related to hyperestrinism, * SHBG has greater affinity for testosterone than estrogen, hence lowering free testosterone levels |
| MOA of sildenafil | • **drug used for Rx of erectile dysfunction,** • **MOA**—inhibits breakdown of cGMP by type 5 phosphodiesterase: increases levels of cGMP, which causes vasodilatation in the corpus cavernosum and penis |
| penile disorders | • **Peyronie's disease**— * type of fibromatosis, * painful contractures of penis, • **trauma,** • **priapism**—e.g., sickle cell disease |

*Table continued on following page*

## Table 14–3. SELECTED UROLOGIC DISORDERS III
### Continued

**Question:** Low testosterone levels are noted in which of the following disorders? **SELECT 3**
- (A) Kallmann's syndrome
- (B) Seminiferous tubule dysfunction
- (C) Ketoconazole
- (D) Spironolactone
- (E) Testicular feminization
- (F) Peyronie's disease
- (G) Multiple sclerosis
- (H) Leriche's syndrome
- (I) Klinefelter's syndrome
- (J) Varicocele

**Answers:** (A), (C), (I). Kallmann's syndrome is an AD disease with a deficiency of GnRH, which decreases gonadotropins and synthesis of testosterone (choice A is correct). Seminiferous tubule failure causes infertility due to loss of spermatogenesis, but testosterone levels are normal (choice B is incorrect). Ketoconazole causes a decrease in testosterone synthesis (choice C is correct). Spironolactone blocks androgen receptors but does not decrease testosterone levels (choice D is incorrect). Testicular feminization is an SXR trait with a deficiency of androgen receptors. Testosterone levels are normal (choice E is incorrect). Peyronie's disease is a fibromatosis of the penis and has normal testosterone levels (choice F is incorrect). Multiple sclerosis causes impotence but testosterone levels are normal (choice G is incorrect). Leriche's syndrome is a peripheral vascular disease with impotence; however, testosterone levels are normal (choice H is incorrect). Klinefelter's syndrome is a chromosome disorder (XXY) with a deficiency of testosterone synthesis (choice I is correct). A varicocele causes infertility due to a reduction in spermatogenesis; however, testosterone levels are normal (choice J is incorrect).

AD = autosomal dominant, AFP = alpha-fetoprotein, ALP = alkaline phosphatase, APN = acute pyelonephritis, ARF = acute renal failure, β-hCG = beta-human chorionic gonadotropin, BPH = benign prostatic hyperplasia, Bx = biopsy, CF = cystic fibrosis, CFU = colony-forming units, CNS = central nervous system, cGMP = cyclic guanosine monophosphate, DES = diethylstilbestrol, DHT = dihydroxytestosterone, DM = diabetes mellitus, DRE = digital rectal exam, FSH = follicle-stimulating hormone, FQ = fluoroquinolones, GnRH = gonadotropin-releasing hormone, β-hCG = beta-human chorionic gonadotropin, HIV = human immunodeficiency virus, HPF = high-powered field, HPV = human papilloma virus, LDH = lactate dehydrogenase, LH = luteinizing hormone, LUT = lower urinary tract, MC = most common, MCC = most common cause, mesna = mercaptoethanesulfonate, MOA = mechanism of action, MS = multiple sclerosis, OFLOX = ofloxacin, OPF = oil-powered field, PAP = prostatic acid phosphatase, PCR = polymerase chain reaction, PSA = prostate-specific antigen, R/O = rule out, SCC = squamous cell carcinoma, SHBG = sex hormone–binding globulin, S/S = signs and symptoms, STD = sexually transmitted disease, SXR = sex-linked recessive, TCC = transitional cell carcinoma, TMP/SMX = trimethoprim/sulfamethoxazole, TUR = transurethral resection, UTI = urinary tract infection.

# CHAPTER

## 15

## ACQUIRED IMMUNODEFICIENCY SYNDROME, TRANSPLANTATION SURGERY

### CONTENTS

### Table 15–1. ACQUIRED IMMUNODEFICIENCY SYNDROME (AIDS)

| Most Common... | Answer and Explanation |
|---|---|
| acquired immunodeficiency (ID) in United States | **AIDS** |
| etiologic agent in the United States | • **human immunodeficiency virus (HIV)-1**— * RNA retrovirus, * HIV-2 is MCC of AIDS in West and Central America |
| steps in HIV infection | • **attachment of virus to CD$_4$ T helper cell**— * gp 120 is viral envelope protein that attaches to CD$_4$ molecule, * requires a coreceptor for fusion to host cell membrane, • **reverse transcriptase produces proviral DNA**—drug inhibitors for reverse transcriptase, • **proviral DNA integrated into host DNA**—requires viral integrase, • **viral mRNA produces codes for polyprotein,** • **polyprotein cleavage by viral proteases**—drug inhibitors for protease, • **small proteins assembled to virions at host cell membrane,** • **budding of virions off the host cell membrane** |
| cells other than CD$_4$ T helper cells infected by HIV | • **monocytes/macrophages,** • *dendritic cells,* • *astrocytes,* • *microglial cells*—CNS macrophage |
| protein surrounding viral genomic RNA | **p24 core protein**—increased in serum at two times: the initial infection and when the patient develops AIDS |
| cell lysed by HIV | **CD$_4$ T helper cell** |

*Table continued on following page*

### Table 15–1. ACQUIRED IMMUNODEFICIENCY
### SYNDROME (AIDS) *Continued*

| Most Common... | Answer and Explanation |
|---|---|
| reservoir cell for viral replication | **monocyte lineage cells**— * macrophage, * dendritic cells, * viruses replicate in these cells without killing them |
| body fluids containing the virus | • **blood**—most infective body fluid, • *saliva,* • *semen,* • *amniotic fluid,* • *breast milk*—breast feeding contraindicated, • *spinal fluid,* • *urine,* • *tears,* • *bronchoalveolar lavage material* |
| mode of transmission of HIV in United States | **intimate sexual contact between homosexual men**—blood is second MC mode: IVDU and sharing needles |
| mode of transmission of HIV worldwide | **heterosexual transmission** |
| modes of sexual transmission of HIV in United States in descending order | • **receptive anal intercourse between men,** • *vaginal intercourse male to female*—female mucosa has more surface area for exposure to infected semen, • *female to male* |
| mode of transmission of HIV in women | **heterosexual transmission in minority females who are IV drug abusers**— * sharing contaminated needles, * vaginal intercourse with HIV-positive males |
| mechanism of transmission by anal intercourse | **direct inoculation into blood from mucosal trauma or an open wound**—e.g., * syphilitic chancre, * proctitis |
| blood product containing virus | **whole blood/packed red blood cells**—1:676,000 risk of transmission per unit |
| mode of transmission of HIV in health care workers | **accidental needle stick**—0.3% risk |
| Rx recommended after needle stick from patient with HIV | • **AZT,** • **lamivudine**—prevents seroconversion in ~80%, • **high-risk exposures**— * deep punctures, * patients with advanced disease and high viral loads, * add protease inhibitor |
| mode of transmission in children | **vertical transmission (mother to fetus) from an infected mother (90%)**—most cases are transplacental, followed by breast feeding and blood contamination during delivery |

### Table 15–1. ACQUIRED IMMUNODEFICIENCY SYNDROME (AIDS) *Continued*

| Most Common... | Answer and Explanation |
|---|---|
| Rx of pregnant women who are HIV-positive | AZT—reduced neonatal rate of developing AIDS from ~25–30% to 7.6% |
| antibody detected by EIA | **anti-gp120 antibody**— * EIA sensitivity 99.5–99.8%, * poor specificity (low prevalence of HIV in general population), * EIA is usually positive in 4–8 wks |
| cause of a FP EIA | **autoimmune disease** |
| test performed if the EIA is indeterminate or positive | **western blot assay**— * positive test is p24 and gp41 antibodies and either gp120 or gp160 antibodies, * combined positive predictive value of positive EIA/western blot is 99.5% |
| recommendations for EIA if person is exposed to HIV-positive patient | **EIA at time of exposure → 6 wks → 3 mos → 6 mos** |
| test used to monitor current immune status of HIV-positive patient | **$CD_4$ T helper cell count**—e.g., count <200 cells/$\mu$L implies an increased risk for PCP |
| test to monitor viral burden in HIV-positive patient | **HIV RNA by PCR** |
| immunologic abnormalities in AIDS | • **lymphopenia**—low $CD_4$ T helper count, • **hypergammaglobulinemia**—due to polyclonal stimulation of B cells by EBV/CMV, • **anergy to skin testing**, • **decreased T cell mitogen blastogenesis**, • **decreased cytokine production**, • **dysfunctional NK cells**, • **increased p24 antigens**, • **$CD_4$:$CD_8$ ratio < 1**—normally >2:1 ratio |
| PPD skin test value considered positive for TB in HIV-positive patient | **>5 mm induration**—set for highest sensitivity owing to skin anergy |

*Table continued on following page*

## Table 15–1. ACQUIRED IMMUNODEFICIENCY SYNDROME (AIDS) *Continued*

| Most Common... | Answer and Explanation |
|---|---|
| S/S of acute retroviral syndrome | • **fever**—98%, • *generalized lymphadenopathy*—75%, • *pharyngitis*—70%, • *rash*—60%, • *myalgia*—60%, • *headache*—35% [Note: the above usually occur 3–6 wks after exposure.] |
| phase following acute HIV syndrome | **asymptomatic, clinically latent phase**—viral replication occurs in dendritic cells in lymph nodes |
| phase following asymptomatic latent phase | **early symptomatic phase**— * non-AIDS–defining infections: see below, * lymphadenopathy, * hematologic abnormalities |
| non-AIDS–defining infections in early symptomatic phase | • **oral thrush,** • *hairy leukoplakia*—EBV tongue infection: not a precancerous lesion, • *recurrent herpes simplex/herpes genitalis,* • *condyloma acuminata*—HPV, • *shingles*—*herpes zoster,* • *molluscum contagiosum*—poxvirus |
| hematologic abnormality in early symptomatic phase | **thrombocytopenia**—possible mechanisms include: ♦ immunocomplex destruction (type III hypersensitivity reaction), ♦ antibodies against platelet antigens (type II hypersensitivity reaction) |
| infections/ malignancy encountered with $CD_4$ T helper count of 200–500 cells/μL | • **hairy leukoplakia/oral candidiasis,** • *TB,* • *mucocutaneous Kaposi's sarcoma*—Kaposi's sarcoma is due to herpesvirus 8, • *recurrent bacterial pneumonia*— * *Streptococcus pneumoniae,* * *Haemophilus influenzae* |
| infections/ malignancy encountered with $CD_4$ T helper count of 100–200 cells/μL | • **PCP,** • *HSV,* • *disseminated histoplasmosis,* • *visceral Kaposi's sarcoma* |
| infections/ malignancy encountered with $CD_4$ T helper count of < 100 cells/μL | • **disseminated MAI**—usually <75 cells/μL, • *Candida esophagitis,* • *CMV retinitis/esophagitis,* • *Toxoplasma encephalitis,* • *cryptosporidiosis*—diarrhea, • *cryptococcal meningitis,* • *CNS lymphoma*—due to HIV and EBV |
| AIDS-defining conditions—HIV-positive plus | • **$CD_4$ T helper cell count < 200 cells/μL,** • *specific malignancies*—see below, • *specific infections*—e.g., PCP |

### Table 15–1. ACQUIRED IMMUNODEFICIENCY
### SYNDROME (AIDS) *Continued*

| Most Common... | Answer and Explanation |
|---|---|
| AIDS-defining malignancies | • **Kaposi's sarcoma,** • *Burkitt's lymphoma,* • *invasive cervical cancer,* • *primary CNS lymphoma*— * due to HIV, * primary CNS lymphoma is rapidly increasing in the United States due to the increase in HIV |
| AIDS-defining opportunistic bacterial infections | • **MAI**—disseminated/extrapulmonary, • *Mycobacterium kansasii*—disseminated/intrapulmonary, • *Mycobacterium tuberculosis* —any site, • *recurrent pneumonia*—usually *Streptococcus pneumoniae,* • *Salmonella* septicemia |
| AIDS-defining opportunistic fungal infections | • **PCP,** • *candidiasis*— * airways, * esophagus, • *coccidioidomycosis*—disseminated/extrapulmonary, • *cryptococcosis*—extrapulmonary, • *histoplasmosis*—disseminated/extrapulmonary |
| systemic fungal infection in AIDS | **candidiasis** |
| CNS systemic fungal infection | **cryptococcosis**—meningitis |
| opportunistic viral infections in AIDS | • **CMV**— * CMV retinitis with visual loss, * biliary tract disease, * diarrhea, • *herpes simplex*— * PUD, * esophagitis, * bronchitis/pneumonia, * diarrhea, * proctitis, • *HIV-related encephalopathy*—AIDS dementia, • *HIV-related wasting syndrome,* • *PML*—papovavirus |
| opportunistic parasitic viral infections in AIDS | • **CNS toxoplasmosis,** • *cryptosporidiosis* — *chronic intestinal infection > 1 mo,* • *isosporiasis*—chronic intestinal infection >1 mo |
| target organ involved in AIDS | **lungs**— * PCP, * *Streptococcus pneumoniae* pneumonia |
| cause of fever, night sweats, weight loss in AIDS | **MAI** |
| cause of lymphoid interstitial pneumonia in AIDS | **EBV** |

*Table continued on following page*

### Table 15–1. ACQUIRED IMMUNODEFICIENCY SYNDROME (AIDS) *Continued*

| Most Common... | Answer and Explanation |
|---|---|
| fungal organisms involving GI tract in AIDS | • *Candida*— * mouth, * esophagus, • *Histoplasma*—colon |
| viruses associated with GI disease in AIDS | • **CMV**— * esophagus, * colon, * biliary tract, • *HSV*— * esophagus, * colon, * anus, • *adenovirus*—colon |
| protozoans that are acid-fast positive and a cause of diarrhea in AIDS | • *Cryptosporidium*— * biliary tract, * Rx with paromycin, • *Isospora* |
| infectious cause of a Whipple's-like syndrome in AIDS | **MAI**—infect macrophages in lamina propria of small bowel, which in turn blocks off lymphatic drainage from the intestinal cell |
| cause of anal squamous cancer in AIDS | **HPV**—related to anal intercourse |
| cause of viral hepatitis in AIDS | **HBV** |
| electrolyte abnormality in AIDS | **hyponatremia**—SiADH |
| cause of Kaposi's sarcoma | **herpesvirus 8** |
| disease that simulates Kaposi's sarcoma in AIDS | **bacillary angiomatosis due to *Bartonella henselae*** |
| cutaneous lesion in AIDS | **Kaposi's sarcoma**—vascular malignancy |
| lymphoma in AIDS | **B cell immunoblastic lymphoma**—high-grade |
| lymphoma in AIDS related to EBV | **Burkitt's lymphoma** |
| cause of primary CNS lymphoma | **HIV in association with EBV** |
| extranodal site for lymphoma in AIDS | **CNS** |

### Table 15–1. ACQUIRED IMMUNODEFICIENCY
### SYNDROME (AIDS) *Continued*

| Most Common... | Answer and Explanation |
|---|---|
| drug-induced cause of marrow suppression in AIDS | **AZT** |
| nutritional cause of anemia in AIDS | **B$_{12}$ deficiency** |
| cause of neutropenia in AIDS | **marrow suppression from AZT** |
| renal disease in AIDS | **focal segmental glomerulosclerosis**—nephrotic syndrome |
| drugs producing nephrotoxic damage in AIDS | • **amphotericin**—Rx of systemic fungal infections, • **pentamidine**—Rx of PCP, • **foscarnet**—Rx of disseminated CMV |
| cause of weight loss of > 10%, fever, chronic diarrhea > 1 mo, and fatigue | **HIV-related wasting syndrome**—one of the top 3 causes of death in AIDS |
| source of entry of HIV into CNS | **monocytes** |
| reservoir cell for HIV in CNS | **microglial cell**—CNS macrophage |
| HIV-related CNS disease | **HIV-encephalopathy**—60% |
| causes of space-occupying lesions of CNS in AIDS | • **toxoplasmosis**, • *primary CNS lymphoma* |
| cause of focal epileptic seizures in AIDS | **toxoplasmosis** |
| cause of blindness in AIDS | **CMV retinitis** |
| Rx of CMV retinitis | **ganciclovir**—foscarnet is used if the patient is resistant to ganciclovir |
| initial drug regimen used in Rx of HIV | **2 nucleoside analogues (e.g., AZT, 3TC) + 1 protease inhibitor (e.g., indinavir)** |

*Table continued on following page*

## Table 15–1. ACQUIRED IMMUNODEFICIENCY SYNDROME (AIDS) *Continued*

| Most Common... | Answer and Explanation |
|---|---|
| tests to monitor Rx of HIV | • **HIV RNA by PCR**—monitors viral burden during Rx, * performed q3–6mos, • *CD$_4$ T helper count*— * immune status, * prophylaxis marker, * performed q3–6mos |
| MOA of nucleoside drugs | **block reverse transcriptase** |
| MOA of protease inhibitors | **suppress HIV replication by blocking protein processing later in the HIV cycle** |
| MOA of non-nucleoside reverse transcriptase inhibitors | **noncompetitively inhibit reverse transcriptase**—e.g., nevirapine |
| side effects of AZT | • **headache,** • **insomnia,** • **GI intolerance,** • **bone marrow suppression**— * macrocytic anemia unrelated to B$_{12}$ deficiency, * neutropenia, * anemia, • **proximal muscle disease,** • **dark blue nails** |
| side effects of didanosine | • **pancreatitis,** • **hepatitis,** • **peripheral neuropathy** |
| side effects of lamivudine (3TC) | • **rash,** • **peripheral neuropathy,** • **bone marrow toxicity** |
| protease inhibitor associated with renal stones | **indinavir** |
| side effect of non-nucleoside reverse transcriptase inhibitors | **rash** |
| CD$_4$ helper T cell count for prophylaxis against PCP | **<200 cells/µL**—Rx with TMP/SMX |
| CD$_4$ helper T cell count for prophylaxis against toxoplasmosis | **<100 cells/µL**— * also requires IgG antibody elevation, * Rx with TMP/SMX |
| CD$_4$ helper T cell count for prophylaxis against MAI | **<50–100 cells/µL**—Rx with azithromycin |

### Table 15–1. ACQUIRED IMMUNODEFICIENCY SYNDROME (AIDS) *Continued*

| Most Common... | Answer and Explanation |
|---|---|
| indication for prophylaxis against *Mycobacterium tuberculosis* | **PPD reaction > 5 mm**—Rx with INH + pyridoxine |
| recommendations to prevent AIDS | • **abstinence,** • *latex condoms with nonoxynol-9 viral spermicide* |
| immunizations recommended in HIV-positive patients | • **Salk's (killed) vaccine**—live vaccine not recommended, • **HBV,** • **influenza,** • **Hib,** • **pneumococcal vaccine** |
| live viral vaccine permitted in HIV-positive patients | **measles/mumps/rubella**—natural infection is worse than the potential infection from the vaccination |
| COD in AIDS | • **bacterial infection**— * *Streptococcus pneumoniae,* * disseminated *MAI,* • *wasting disease* |

**Question:** Which of the following are AIDS-defining disorders? **SE-LECT 6**

   (A) Hairy leukoplakia
   (B) Recurrent pneumonia due to *Streptococcus pneumoniae*
   (C) Oral thrush
   (D) Immune thrombocytopenia
   (E) CMV retinitis
   (F) *Pneumocystis carinii* pneumonia
   (G) Herpes zoster
   (H) Kaposi's sarcoma
   (I) *Candida* esophagitis
   (J) Primary CNS lymphoma
   (K) Cervical dysplasia due to HPV

**Answers: (B), (E), (F), (H), (I), (J).** Recurrent pneumonia due to *Streptococcus pneumoniae* is one of the most common causes of death in AIDS and is AIDS defining **(choice B is correct).** CMV retinitis is the MCC of blindness in AIDS and is AIDS defining **(choice E is correct).** *Pneumocystis carinii* pneumonia is the MC AIDS-defining disorder **(choice F is correct).** Kaposi's sarcoma is the MC cancer in AIDS and is AIDS defining **(choice H is correct).** *Candida* esophagitis is AIDS defining; however, thrush is a pre-AIDS defining lesion **(choice I is correct, choice C is incorrect).** Primary CNS lymphoma is rapidly increasing owing to HIV. It is an AIDS-defining lesion due to HIV and EBV **(choice J is correct).** Hairy leukoplakia due to EBV, immune thrombocytopenia, and herpes zoster (shingles) are pre-AIDS defining lesions **(choices A, D, G are incorrect).** Invasive cervical cancer, not cervical dysplasia, is AIDS defining **(choice K is incorrect).**

AZT = azidothymidine, CMV = cytomegalovirus, CNS = central nervous system, COD = cause of death, EBV = Epstein-Barr virus, EIA = enzyme immunoassay, FP = false-positive, HBV = hepatitis B virus, Hib = *Haemophilus influenzae* b vaccine, HIV = human immunodeficiency virus, HPV = human papillomavirus, HSV = herpes simplex virus, ID = immunodeficiency, INH = isoniazid, IVDU = intravenous drug use, MAI = *Mycobacterium avium-intracellulare*, MCC = most common cause, MOA = mechanism of action, NK = natural killer, PCP = *Pneumocystis carinii* pneumonia, PCR = polymerase chain reaction, PML = progressive multifocal leukoencephalopathy, PPD = purified protein derivative, PUD = peptic ulcer disease, SiADH = syndrome of inappropriate antidiuretic hormone, S/S = signs/symptoms, 3TC = lamivudine, TMP/SMX = trimethoprim/sulfamethoxazole.

## Table 15–2. TRANSPLANTATION SURGERY

| Most Common... | Answer and Explanation |
|---|---|
| chromosome site of the HLA system | **chromosome 6** |
| membrane glycoproteins synthesized | **HLA-A, -B, -C, -D (and its subdivisions)** |
| function of the HLA system | **markers of identity** [Note: HLA antigens are usually different in each person. One set of antigens comes from the mother and the other from the father. They are inherited in codominant fashion.] |
| class I antigens | **HLA-A, -B, -C** [Note: class I antigens are recognized by $CD_8$ cytotoxic T cells.] |
| class II antigens | **HLA-D loci** [Note: class II antigens are located on antigen-presenting cells (macrophages, dendritic cells, B cells, activated T cells) and interact with $CD_4$ T helper cells.] |
| transplantation test used to identify HLA antigens | **lymphocyte microcytotoxicity test** [Note: specific antibodies against HLA antigens plus complement are mixed together with patient lymphocytes. Lysis of the lymphocytes indicates a match. This test is useful in identifying HLA-A, -B, and some -D antigens.] |

## Table 15–2. TRANSPLANTATION SURGERY *Continued*

| Most Common... | Answer and Explanation |
|---|---|
| transplantation test used to detect preformed anti-HLA antibodies in patient serum | **lymphocyte cross-match** [Note: the patient's serum plus complement is mixed with donor lymphocytes. Lysis of the donor lymphocytes indicates that anti-HLA antibodies are present. The exact antibodies are then determined by reacting them with a panel of lymphocytes with known HLA antigens.] |
| transplantation test used to test for compatibility between the class II (D antigens) of patient and donor | **mixed lymphocyte reaction** [Note: the patient's lymphocytes are left functional, and donor lymphocytes are inactivated. Lymphocytes are mixed together in a test tube with tritiated thymidine. An increase in the radioactive count indicates dissimilar D antigens to which the patient's lymphocytes are reacting. No reaction indicates identity of the D loci.] |
| transplantation test used to test for the potential of a GVH reaction | **mixed lymphocyte reaction** [Note: the patient's lymphocytes are inactivated, and donor lymphocytes are left functional. Lymphocytes are mixed together in a test tube with tritiated thymidine. An increase in the radioactive count indicates dissimilar D antigens to which the donor's lymphocytes are reacting. No reaction indicates identity of the D loci and less chance of a GVH reaction.] |
| type of transplant with the best graft survival | • **autograft**—transfer of tissue from self to self, • *isograft*—a graft between identical twins, • *allograft*—a graft between two unrelated individuals of the same species, • *xenograft*—a graft between two different species: e.g., pig heart valve transplanted into a human being |
| source for finding compatible donors for transplantation | **siblings** [Note: there is a 25% chance of an identical 2-haplotype match, 50% chance of a 1-haplotype match, and 25% chance of a no haplotype match. A parent is always a 1-haplotype match.] |
| factors that improve graft survival | • **ABO compatibility,** • absence of *anti-HLA antibodies,* • *HLA compatibility between the D loci* |

*Table continued on following page*

**Table 15–2. TRANSPLANTATION SURGERY** *Continued*

| Most Common... | Answer and Explanation |
|---|---|
| drugs used to prevent graft rejection | • **cyclosporine**— * inhibits $CD_4$ T helper release of IL-2, * dose-related nephrotoxicity, • *prednisone*—suppresses the host immune response, • *azathioprine*—inhibits DNA and RNA production by inhibiting the conversion of inosine monophosphate to essential purines, • *tacrolimus*— * significantly more potent than cyclosporine, * inhibits T cell activation by preventing release of IL-2, * approved for use in liver transplantation, * nephrotoxic, • *OKT3*—monoclonal antibody directed against T cell antigen recognition site |
| types of transplant rejections | • **acute,** • *hyperacute,* • *chronic* |
| causes of a hyperacute rejection | • **ABO incompatibility,** • **presence of patient anti-HLA antibodies against donor tissue** [**Note:** this is an irreversible type II hypersensitivity reaction leading to immediate thrombosis of donor vessels and death of donor tissue.] |
| type of transplant rejection | **acute rejection**—usually occurs within 3 mos, * combination of CMI with cytotoxic $CD_8$ T cells producing parenchymal damage and humoral immunity, in which antibodies are directed against blood vessels, leading to thickening and ischemic damage, * rejection can be reversed: see below |
| cell types involved in acute rejection | • **donor macrophages,** • **host $CD_8$ cytotoxic T cells,** • **host $CD_4$ helper T cells,** • **NK cells** [**Note:** the class I antigens on donor macrophages interact with host $CD_8$ cytotoxic T cells, which, in turn, interact with class II antigens on host $CD_4$ T helper cells. Helper T cells release IL-2, which increases host $CD_4$ and $CD_8$ proliferation and B cell production of antibodies. $CD_8$ cytotoxic cells attack class I antigens in the graft, whereas antibodies attack vessel endothelium. NK cells also attack donor tissue.] |
| S/S of acute rejection | • **fever,** • **HTN,** • **progressive increase in serum creatinine,** • **graft tenderness,** • **reduction in urine output** |

## Table 15–2. TRANSPLANTATION SURGERY *Continued*

| Most Common... | Answer and Explanation |
|---|---|
| tests to distinguish acute rejection from other causes of loss of renal function | • **allograft biopsy**—distinguishes acute rejection from ATN, • *Doppler ultrasound*— * checks vessel patency, * R/O hydronephrosis, • *radionuclide scan*—checks blood flow and renal function, • *creatinine clearance*—most important lab parameter of acute rejection [**Note:** other causes of the above signs and symptoms must be ruled out, particularly nephrotoxicity from cyclosporine, ATN, renal artery stenosis.] |
| Rx of acute rejection | • **methylprednisolone**—high doses IV, • *antilymphocyte globulin*—sera directed against T lymphocytes, <u>or</u> • *OKT₃*—monoclonal antibody directed against T cell antigen recognition site |
| mechanism of chronic rejection | **combined humoral and CMI**— * recurrent antibody-mediated damage to vessels leads to intimal fibrosis and ischemic damage to the parenchyma, with subsequent atrophy and fibrosis, * CMI contributes to parenchymal damage |
| Rx of chronic rejection | **no specific therapy**—conservative management is used, since the changes are irreversible |
| COD in transplantation | **infection** |
| infections in first month post-transplant | • **nosocomial**—e.g., * pneumonia, * IV catheter, * wound infection, * urinary catheter-related, * usually bacterial, • *transplantation site–related infections*—e.g., * intra-abdominal, * pleura, * mediastinum [**Note:** immunosuppression is not the major cause of infection in this early time frame.] |
| infections between 1 and 6 months post-transplant | **opportunistic infections**— * CMV is the MC overall post-transplant infection: Rx with ganciclovir, * other infections include: ♦ HSV (Rx with acyclovir), ♦ HBV/HCV (predominates in liver and renal transplantation), ♦ *Pneumocystis carini* pneumonia (Rx with TMP/SMX), ♦ *Listeria monocytogenes* (Rx with ampicillin), ♦ Herpes zoster (Rx with acyclovir and immune globulin), ♦ EBV (lymphoproliferative disease, reduce immunosuppression doses) |

*Table continued on following page*

Table 15–2. **TRANSPLANTATION SURGERY** *Continued*

| Most Common... | Answer and Explanation |
|---|---|
| infections > 6 months post-transplant | • ***Cryptococcus neoformans***—meningitis: Rx with amphotericin B, • *Legionella pneumophila* |
| transplants associated with GVH reaction | • **bone marrow**—60–80%, • *liver* |
| target tissues involved in the acute GVH reaction | • **skin**— * maculopapular rash, * involves: ♦ trunk, ♦ palms, ♦ soles, • *bile duct epithelium*—epithelial cell necrosis of small bile ducts, leading to jaundice, • *GI tract*—mucosal ulceration with bloody diarrhea [**Note:** the acute GVH reaction usually occurs between 1 and 3 weeks post-transplant.] |
| cell types involved in acute GVH reaction | • **donor T lymphocytes**, • **donor NK cells** [**Note:** cytokines released by donor T cells damage host tissue and stimulate proliferation of $CD_8$ cytotoxic T cells, which also attack host tissue. IL-2 released from donor $CD_4$ T cells activates host NK cells, which become lymphokine-activated killer cells that lyse normal host cells. Mortality is > 80%.] |
| Rx of acute GVH reaction | • **donor tissue treated with OKT3 to remove donor T lymphocytes**, • **cyclosporine**—prevent release of IL-2 |
| cause of chronic GVH reaction | **immunocompetent lymphocytes develop in the recipient and attack skin and liver** |
| tissue transplant with the best overall survival | **corneal transplant**— * the cornea is avascular, * there is a danger of transmitting Creutzfeldt-Jakob disease |
| source for a living donor | **siblings**— * 25% chance for 2-haplotype match, * 50% chance for 1-haplotype match, * 25% chance for 0-haplotype match, * parents are 1-haplotype matches |
| types of renal transplant | • **cadaver**—1-yr graft survival rate is 80%, • *living donor*—1-yr graft survival rate is 90%, • *transplantation is Rx of choice for end-stage renal disease* |
| types of compatibility necessary for renal transplantation | • **ABO compatible**, • **class I, class II compatible**—should be at least 6 antigen matches in both class I and II HLA antigens for cadaveric kidney transplantation |

## Table 15–2. TRANSPLANTATION SURGERY *Continued*

| Most Common... | Answer and Explanation |
|---|---|
| tests employed for renal transplantation | • **cross-match test**—patient serum against donor leukocytes to R/O anti-HLA antibodies against donor leukocytes, • **HLA typing** |
| types of renal disease requiring transplantation in descending order | • **DM with renal failure**, • *hypertensive renal disease*, • *GN* |
| type of GN with highest rate of recurrence in graft | • **FSG**—20–30%, • *MPGN*, • *membranous GN*, • *DM*, • *HUS*, • *IgA GN*—mild and not usually significant |
| absolute contraindications for renal transplantation | • **malignancy**, • **severe atherosclerosis**, • **pulmonary disease**, • **active hepatitis** |
| immunosuppressants used in renal transplant patients | • **cyclosporine**—inhibits IL-2 release from $CD_4$ T helper cells, • **azathioprine**—inhibits proliferation of activated T cells, • **prednisone**—blocks IL-1 and cytokine production from T cells, • **OKT₃**—monoclonal antibody against T cell antigen receptor |
| side effects of cyclosporine | • **dose-related nephrotoxicity**—interstitial fibrosis, • *gum hyperplasia*, • *hypertrichosis*, • *HUS*, • *TTP*, • *hepatotoxicity*, • *HTN*, • *lymphoproliferative malignancy*, • *hyperkalemia* |
| tests to evaluate renal transplant rejection | • **renal biopsy**, • *renal scans* |
| COD in renal transplant patients | • **opportunistic infections**— * **CMV**, *Aspergillus*, • *AMI* |
| type of renal transplant with the best survival | **transplant between living donors with a 2-haplotype match**— * 90–95% 1-yr survival rate, * e.g.: ◆ sibling, ◆ identical twin [**Note:** cadaver transplants have an ~80% 1-yr survival.] |
| effect of multiple blood transfusions to recipients prior to renal transplant surgery | **improves graft survival** |
| indications for liver transplantation | • **chronic liver disease**, • *fulminant hepatic failure*, • *Rx of severe hemophilia A*—liver synthesizes most of the VIII components |

*Table continued on following page*

## Table 15–2. TRANSPLANTATION SURGERY *Continued*

| Most Common... | Answer and Explanation |
|---|---|
| 1-yr survival rate for liver transplantation | ~**80%** |
| indications for heart transplantation | • **ischemic cardiomyopathy,** • *congestive cardiomyopathy* |
| test used to document heart transplant rejection | **endomyocardial biopsy** |
| 1-yr survival rate for heart transplantation | **80–90%** |
| indications for lung transplantation | • **emphysema,** • *CF,* • *primary PH* |
| test used to document lung transplant rejection | **IV methylprednisolone to see whether pulmonary function improves** |
| 1-yr survival rate for heart-lung transplant | **60–75%** |
| malignancies associated with immunosuppressive Rx in transplant patients | • **squamous cell carcinoma of the skin,** • *cervical cancer,* • *malignant lymphomas,* • *BCC* |

**Question:** A 25-yr-old-woman with postpartum congestive cardiomyopathy develops immediate rejection of a heart transplantation. The possible mechanisms for the rejection of the heart most likely involve . . . **SELECT 2**

  (A) Donor NK cells
  (B) Donor macrophages
  (C) Recipient $CD_4$ T helper cells
  (D) Recipient anti-HLA antibodies against donor HLA antigens
  (E) ABO mismatch

**Answers: (D), (E).** The patient has a hyperacute rejection of the donor heart, which, though uncommon, is most often due to the recipient having anti-HLA antibodies against donor HLA antigens (e.g., a mistake involving an ABO mismatch (e.g.), patient is blood group A and the donor heart is blood group B, **choices D and E are correct**). Donor NK cells are involved in GVH reactions **(choice A is incorrect)**. Donor macrophages are involved in acute transplant rejection **(choice B is incorrect)**. Recipient $CD_4$ T helper cells are primarily involved in acute transplant rejection **(choice C is incorrect)**.

AD = autosomal dominant, AMI = acute myocardial infarction, ATN = acute tubular necrosis, BCC = basal cell carcinoma, CD = cluster designation, CF = cystic fibrosis, CMI = cell-mediated immunity, CMV = cytomegalovirus, COD = cause of death, DM = diabetes mellitus, EBV = Epstein-Barr virus, FSG = focal segmental glomerulosclerosis, GN = glomerulonephritis, GVH = graft versus host (reaction), HBV = hepatitis B virus, HCV = hepatitis C virus, HLA = human leukocyte antigen, HSV = herpes simplex virus, HTN = hypertension, HUS = hemolytic uremic syndrome, IL = interleukin, MOA = mechanism of action, MPGN = membranoproliferative glomerulonephritis, NK = natural killer, PH = pulmonary hypertension, R/O = rule out, SLE = systemic lupus erythematosus, S/S = signs/symptoms, TMP/SMX = trimethoprim/sulfamethoxazole, TTP = thrombotic thrombocytopenic purpura.

# ■ INDEX